Psychiatric Nursing

Psychiatric Nursing:
A Comprehensive Reference

SECOND EDITION

Suzanne Lego, RN, PhD, CS, FAAN
Editor

Private Practice, Pittsburgh, Pennsylvania,
and Kent, Ohio

with
42 Contributors

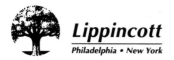
Lippincott
Philadelphia • New York

Acquisitions Editor: Margaret Zuccarini
Editorial Assistant: Emily Cotlier
Production Editor: Molly E. Dickmeyer
Production: Berliner, Inc.
Cover Designer: Thomas M. Jackson
Printer/Binder: Courier/Westford

Second Edition

Library of Congress Cataloging in Publications Data
Psychiatric nursing : a comprehensive reference / [edited by] Suzanne Lego. — 2nd ed.
    p.   cm.
    Rev. ed. of: The American handbook of psychiatric nursing / Suzanne Lego, editor, c1984.
    Includes bibliographical references and index.
    ISBN 0-397-55266-1
    1. Psychiatric nursing—Handbooks, manuals, etc.   I. American handbook of
psychiatric nursing.
    [DNLM: 1. Psychiatric Nursing—handbooks.   WY 49 P974 1996]
    RC440.A55   1996
    610.73'68—dc20
    DNLM/DLC
    for Library of Congress   95-26303
                                                            CIP

The material contained in this volume was submitted as previously unpublished material, except in the instances in which credit has been given to the source from which some of the illustrative material was derived.

Any procedure or practice described in this book should be applied by the health-care practitioner under appropriate supervision in accordance with professional standards of care used with regard to the unique circumstances that apply in each practice situation. Care has been taken to confirm the accuracy of information presented and to describe generally accepted practices. However, the authors, editors, and publisher cannot accept any responsibility for errors or omissions or for any consequences from application of the information in this book and make no warranty, express or implied, with respect to the contents of the book.

The authors and publisher have exerted every effort to ensure that drug selection and dosage set forth in this text are in accordance with current recommendations and practice at the time of publication. However, in view of ongoing research, changes in government regulations, and the constant flow of information relating to drug therapy and drug reactions, the reader is urged to check the package insert for each drug for any change in indications and dosage and for added warnings and precautions. This is particularly important when the recommended agent is a new or infrequently employed drug.

Materials appearing in this book prepared by individuals as part of their official duties as U.S. Government employees are not covered by the above-mentioned copyright.

9   8   7   6   5   4   3   2   1

To

Hildegard E. Peplau,
The Mother of Psychiatric Nursing

and to

S. Lee Spray,
My husband, colleague, and friend

Contributors

CATHERINE ADAMS, RN, EdD
   Professor of Nursing, Russell Sage College, Troy, New York

LINDA S. BEEBER, RN, PhD, CS
   Professor, College of Nursing, Syracuse University, Syracuse, New York

CAROLYN V. BILLINGS, RN, MSN, CS
   Private Practice, Raleigh, North Carolina

MARGERY M. CHISOLM, RN, EdD
   Associate Professor and Graduate Coordinator, Psychiatric Mental Health Nursing Program,
      Northeastern University, Boston, Massachusetts

MICHELLE CONANT, RN, MSN, CS
   Clinical Specialist, West Essex Community Health Services, Verona, New Jersey

ROSE EVA BANA CONSTANTINO, RN, PhD, JD, FAAN
   Associate Professor, University of Pittsburgh, School of Nursing, Pittsburgh, Pennsylvania

CLAIRE BURKE DRAUCKER, RN, PhD
   Associate Professor, School of Nursing, Kent State University, Kent, Ohio

ANNE BARKER DUNN, RN, MSN, CS, CARN
   Clinical Nurse Specialist, VA Medical Center, Brecksville, Ohio

KAREN EVANCZUK, RN, PhD, CS
   Clinical Director, Critical Incident Stress Management, University of Pittsburgh Medical Center,
      Pittsburgh, Pennsylvania

MARY GRACE FITZGERALD, RN, MSN, CS
   Clinical Nurse Specialist, University of Pittsburgh Medical Center, Pittsburgh, Pennsylvania

LINDA M. FITZSIMONS, RN, BS, CS
   Research Nurse Coordinator, ECT Service, Department of Biological Psychiatry, New York
      State Psychiatric Institute, New York, New York

EDITH BROGAN DE LA FUENTE, RN, MSN, CS
   Psychiatric Clinical Nurse Specialist, Visiting Nurse Service, Akron, Ohio

LOU ANN FULMER, RN, MSN, CS
   Coordinator of Geriatric and Mental Health Services, Visiting Nurse Service, Akron, Ohio

DONNA A. GAFFNEY, RN, DNSc, CS, FAAN
   Assistant Professor, Columbia University School of Nursing, New York, New York

ANNE GALLENSTEIN, RN, MS, CS, NPP
Private Practice, New York, New York

SUSAN L. GLODSTEIN, RN, MSN, CS
Psychiatric Nurse Manager, St. Barnabas Hospital, Bronx, New York

CHRISTINE A. GRANT, RN, PhD, CS
Director, Center for Psychiatric Nursing Research, Melbourne, Australia

JUDITH HABER, RN, PhD, CS, FAAN
Private Practice in Family Therapy, Stamford, Connecticut

CHRISTINE A. HEIFNER, RN, MSN
Clinical Nurse Specialist, Partial Hospitalization Program, Akron General Medical Center, Akron, Ohio

MARY BETH HUSSEINI, RN, MSN, CS
Instructor in Psychiatric Nursing, Kent State University, Kent, Ohio

BONNIE S. JOYCE, RN, MSN
Nurse Clinical Manager, Western Psychiatric Institute and Clinic, Pittsburgh, Pennsylvania

CATHERINE KANE, RN, PhD
Associate Professor, University of Virginia, Charlottesville, Virginia

SUSAN L. W. KRUPNICK, RN, MSN, CARN, CS
Psychiatric Liaison Nurse, Bay State Medical Center, Bay State Health System, Springfield, Massachusetts

SUZANNE LEGO, RN, PhD, CS, FAAN
Private Practice, Pittsburgh, Pennsylvania, and Kent, Ohio

WENDY LEWANDOWSKI, RN, MSN, CS
Psychiatric Clinical Nurse Specialist, Visiting Nurse Service, Akron, Ohio

MAXINE E. LOOMIS, RN, PhD, CS, FAAN
Distinguished Professor Emerita, University of South Carolina College of Nursing, Columbia, South Carolina

KEM BETTY LOUIE, RN, PhD, CS, FAAN
Chair, Graduate Program, College of Mount St. Vincent School of Nursing, Riverdale, New York

DONNA FELBER NEFF, RN, MSN
Instructor in Psychiatric Nursing, Kent State University, Kent, Ohio

ANITA WERNER O'TOOLE, RN, PhD, CS, FAAN
Private Practice, Kent, Ohio

HILDEGARD E. PEPLAU, RN, EdD, FAAN
Professor Emerita, Rutgers University, New Brunswick, New Jersey

KATHRYN R. PUSKAR, RN, DrPH, CS, FAAN
Assistant Professor of Psychiatric Nursing, University of Pittsburgh School of Nursing, Pittsburgh, Pennsylvania

FATIMA RAMOS, RN, MSN, CS
Director of Psychiatric Nursing, St. Barnabas Hospital, Bronx, New York

ONA Z. RIGGIN, RN, EdD, ARNP
   Professor and Chair, Graduate Program in Psychiatric–Mental Health Nursing, University of
      South Florida, Tampa, Florida

JOSEPHINE SAPP, RN, MSN, CS
   Assistant Professor, Columbia University School of Nursing, New York, New York

PEGGY A. SAWYER, RN, MSN, MBA, CS
   Manager, Health Systems Integration Practice, KPMG Peat Marwick, White Plains, New York

JOYCE A. SELZER, RN, MSN, CARN, CS
   Clinical Nurse Specialist, VA Medical Center, Brecksville, Ohio

MARIE C. SMITH-ALNIMER, RN, MA, CS
   Assistant Professor of Nursing, Bronx Community College, Bronx, New York

CAROL TAYLOR, RN, PhD, CSFN
   Assistant Professor of Nursing, Clinical Ethicist, Holy Family College, Philadelphia, Pennsylvania

PATRICIA M. TOMCHO, RN, MSN, CS, CCJS
   Clinical Nurse Specialist, VA Medical Center, Brecksville, Ohio

KATHLEEN TUSAIE-MUMFORD, RN, MSN, CS
   Research Associate, University of Pittsburgh School of Nursing, Pittsburgh, Pennsylvania

ELIZABETH M. VARCAROLIS, RN, MA
   Professor of Nursing, Borough of Manhattan Community College, City University of
      New York, New York, New York

ROTHLYN P. ZAHOUREK, RN, MS, CS
   Private Practice and Consultation, Amherst, Massachusetts

Foreword

The last quarter of the 20th century is remarkable for far-reaching transformations in all fields of endeavor and in virtually all societies. One consequence is that great stress is experienced by individuals and families. The need for help in facing and coping with personal psychosocial problems is more apparent than ever before.

New forms of health care services are particularly evident. Most notably there are changes in the nature and scope of psychiatric–mental health nursing care. At the turn of the century, psychiatric nursing consisted mainly of companionship and basic nursing procedures adapted to the care of the mentally ill. Today, psychiatric nursing practices tend to be derived from theoretical constructs that provide nurses with an understanding of the problems clients present to them in nursing situations.

It is only since the mid-1900s that the nursing profession has been enriched and its practices guided by research and scholarly theorizing by nurses. In the last few decades this trend has enlarged considerably. Psychiatric nursing practices which are derived from theory that illuminates the client's problems and enable the person to live within the community are a primary aim of psychiatric nursing. This important trend is an evolving process that requires psychiatric nurses to keep current with new developments. Commitment to psychiatric nursing services of the highest quality requires of the nurse an intense interest in the nature of the client's difficulties. Such interest is rooted in knowledge. Commitment also requires the nurse's persistence and sustained knowledgeable support of clients' struggles to overcome their difficulties, to move toward self-understanding and self-care. Intense interest also requires the nurse to have a practical grasp of the utility of theoretical constructs in their application toward remedial outcomes in every nurse–patient relationship.

The second edition of *Psychiatric Nursing: A Comprehensive Reference* is a major resource for nurses whose commitment is toward continuous learning and self-improvement, so that nursing of the highest quality is provided for the mentally ill. It is a definitive edited work written by 42 experts in the field of psychiatric nursing.

It provides comprehensive authoritative knowledge of human difficulties and treatment modalities. This text is therefore a resource for continuous learning for students and practicing nurses, as well as a significant reference source for staff use within the workplace.

The shifting tides of change suggest that the conspicuous feature of the upcoming 21st century will be knowledge. This work puts all that is new and useful into the hands of psychiatric nurses.

Hildegard E. Peplau, RN, EdD, FAAN
Professor Emerita, Rutgers, The State University of New Jersey

Preface

When I sat down to plan the second edition of *Psychiatric Nursing: A Comprehensive Reference*, I realized just how much has changed in the decade since the first edition. The biomedicalization of psychiatry, the industrialization of health care, the emphasis on consumer-centered care, the importance of psychoeducation for the client and family, and new technology have all changed and expanded the role of the psychiatric–mental health nurse. In planning the book and writing my 11 chapters I have attempted to include all that is new but to hold on to those old values that endure. One thing that has not changed is the importance of the nurse–patient relationship. In fact, it might be argued that the emergence of new chemistry, new technology, and new financial incentives makes clients' interpersonal relations with the nurse more important than ever.

The book begins with psychiatric nursing assessment, diagnosis, and use of the DSM-IV. In Part II, 19 different modalities are described. Part III describes the psychiatric nurse's work with specific clients. Part IV is devoted to designing programs for the treatment of clients in hospitals, outpatient agencies, the community, jails and prisons, and at home. Part V describes distinct, specific nursing procedures. Part VI describes psychopharmacology for a variety of categories of disorders. Part VII concerns special broad issues of psychiatric nursing that deserve individual examination: legal, ethical, cultural, and women's issues.

Again in this volume the matter of *patient* versus *client* arose. This time I left it up to each author to decide which term to use.

Like the first edition, the book is written in simple, practical terms designed to make the material immediately usable. Information is presented in outline form and in tables and boxes.

In the past 10 years many nurses have told me they use a copy of this book in the nurses' station at work and have a copy at home. Given the changes in the past 10 years, the book will now be found in the advanced-practice nurses' private practice offices or in their cars as they make home visits.

The book is intended to help practitioners at every level: students, teachers, and administrators. I hope it will help beginners as well as seasoned clinicians.

Suzanne Lego, RN, PhD, CS, FAAN
Sewickley, Pennsylvania

Acknowledgments

I would like to thank the contributors to both editions, without whom this book would not have been possible, as well as my friends Anita O'Toole and Janet Muff, for reviewing sections. I thank Dr. Hildegard Peplau for the foreword and Stewart Brisby for his incredible computer and word-processing expertise in preparing the manuscript. At Lippincott–Raven Publishers, I owe thanks to my editor, Margaret Zuccarini, and her assistant, Emily Cotlier. My biggest thanks go to my husband and colleague, Lee, who discussed the book with me almost daily for 10 months and who made many valuable suggestions. His good-natured help and support, intelligence, and sense of humor are the wind beneath my wings.

Suzanne Lego, RN, PhD, CS, FAAN
Sewickley, Pennsylvania

Contents

PART ONE

Assessment
and
Planning

1

ONE

Psychiatric Nursing Assessment

Josephine Sapp

INTRODUCTION

Hildegard Peplau best defined the practice of psychiatric nursing in *Interpersonal Relations in Nursing* (1991) when she wrote:

> Nursing is a significant, therapeutic, interpersonal process. It functions cooperatively with other human processes that make health possible for individuals in communities. In specific situations in which a professional health team offers health services, nurses participate in the organization of conditions that facilitate natural ongoing tendencies in human organisms. Nursing is an educative instrument, a maturing force that aims to promote forward movement of personality in the direction of creative, constructive, productive, personal and community living. (Peplau, 1991, p. 16)

Psychiatric nursing practice begins with the nurse's assessment.

DEFINITION

The psychiatric nursing assessment is the phase of the nursing process in which health status information of a patient is systematically obtained, organized, recorded, and communicated. The psychiatric nursing assessment is based on the nurse's knowledge of biological, cultural, behavioral, social, pharmacological, and neurological sciences.

DESCRIPTION

The psychiatric nursing assessment process is multidimensional and multifaceted in scope. The assessment is a systematic process for gathering patient data in a fluid, ongoing process. Establishing a therapeutic relationship with the client and family or significant others is critical to the assessment process as it enhances data gathering. The advanced practice nurse uses psychotherapy principles and practices to acquire the comprehensive information needed to accurately and effectively formulate a DSM-IV diagnostic impression, conclusions, and treatment recommendations. The assessment and evaluation data become part of the multidisciplinary treatment team's assessment and an integral part of multidisciplinary treatment planning.

PURPOSE

The psychiatric nursing assessment is completed to assure the patient's problems are identified so that appropriate nursing care can be rendered.

INFLUENCING FACTORS

Factors that influence the assessment process include:
1. Source of the referral
2. The patient's level of cooperativeness
3. The family's level of cooperativeness
4. The setting of the assessment and evaluation
5. The patient's medical status
6. The patient's mental status
7. The nature of the nurse–patient interaction
8. The level of the nurse's education and expertise
9. The patient's ego functions
10. The nurse's understanding of the patient's cultural and ethnic beliefs, practices, and patterns

SETTINGS

Nurses may provide assessment in the following settings:
1. Crisis intervention programs
2. Mobile crisis units
3. Emergency room programs
4. Partial hospital programs
5. Inpatient programs
6. Brief treatment programs
7. Outpatient programs including intensive evening and day programs
8. Home care programs
9. Employee assistance programs
10. Counseling/psychotherapy centers
11. Consultation/liaison programs
12. Health promotion programs
13. High risk screening programs
14. Rehabilitation services including vocational rehabilitation services
15. School-based clinics
16. Private practices

ASSESSMENT PROCESS

The assessment and evaluation process varies according to where the patient is evaluated. The assessment may occur in a single, initial interview or may occur over several sessions. The psychiatric assessment and evaluation can also be woven into a physical assessment process when the patient presents with a physical illness as is frequently the case with the addictive illnesses. In most instances the nurse must complete the assessment of the patient within 8 hours of admission to an inpatient program and within 24 hours for an outpatient program. Table 1-1 shows nursing actions and rationale during the assessment process.

TABLE 1-1
Nursing Actions and Theoretical Rationale When Interviewing

NURSING ACTION	THEORETICAL RATIONALE
The nurse introduces herself* by name, title, and role. The nurse addresses the patient by name and asks how he prefers to be addressed.	Addressing the patient by name and introducing herself by name and title is a way for the nurse to convey respect for the patient.
The nurse provides an interview room that is private and quiet, and does not contain distracting objects. When a room is unavailable, as in the CCU, some measure of privacy is provided by using curtains and screens. Interruptions and interference by other staff members are kept to a minimum.	Privacy encourages the reticent, embarrassed patient to disclose his personal problems and feelings. It also eliminates some of the patient's concerns about confidentiality. Distracting objects may prove disturbing to a confused, disoriented, or psychotic patient. The psychiatric interview is demanding of both the patient and the nurse and requires concentration.
The nurse provides two chairs of equal size and comfort and a choice of seating. Additional seating should be available for family interviews and consultations.	The choice of where he sits provides clues to the patient's need for personal space, fears of interpersonal closeness, and possible suspiciousness.
The nurse makes prior arrangements and establishes a protocol to provide for safety and security for the patient and herself. This is particularly important in the emergency room or other medical treatment settings.	Medical paraphernalia is potentially dangerous and may also frighten the patient. Help is sometimes needed to manage the confused, assaultive, or suicidal patient. Prior arrangement for this help will allay the nurse's anxiety. Limit setting is also reassuring to the disturbed or impulsive patient.
The nurse begins with an open-ended question (a question that indicates a general inquiry, defines an area of interest, but leaves a wide range of interpretation possible). Ex: "What brought you here today?" The nurse uses the kind of response, verbal or nonverbal, that encourages the patient to say more. The response may be anything from an expectant look to a request to "tell me more about that."	The open-ended question is broad and allows the patient to verbalize his views, thoughts, and feelings. The closed question tends to elicit facts only. Direct, more specific questions are asked (to get additional information) after the patient has told his story. This response is nonrestrictive and does not sharply define the answer for the patient, but rather elicits spontaneous and individualistic responses that describe how he sees his problem.
The nurse communicates with the patient by the use of silences. Silences, on the part of both the patient and the nurse, are accompanied by facial and bodily expression, gestures, or postures that convey meaning. If, for example, the patient transmits a feeling of anger, the nurse might state something about the anger and ask the patient to put it into words.	The nurse's silence can convey concern and interest, and can facilitate continued communication. The nurse can determine the possible meaning of the patient's silences by observing his nonverbal communication and by examining her empathic response.
The nurse uses responses that convey support, empathy, and understanding. Ex: "You seem to feel guilty about being unable to work."	This type of response affirms that the nurse accepts the feelings and information the patient has offered with concern but without criticism.
The nurse uses confrontation and interpretation to make explicit a connection between a feeling or symptom and the patient's interpersonal or intrapsychic life. Ex: "You seem to have these headaches at times when you are most angry."	This encourages the patient to make his own additional connections and to explore matters further.
The nurse pays attention to the interview content (words spoken), as well as to the process (what is happening) between the patient and the nurse. Ex: The patient states that he feels relaxed but fidgets in his chair and cannot make eye contact.	By attending to the two levels of a message, the content and the process, the nurse may more accurately assess the patient, what is occurring in the interview, and what may be occurring in his life.

*The female pronoun will be used for the nurse, and the male pronoun for the patient.

From Webster, M. (1984). Psychiatric nursing assessment. In S. Lego (ed.), *The American Handbook of Psychiatric Nursing* (pp. 3–17). Philadelphia: J. B. Lippincott.

THE PSYCHIATRIC INTERVIEW

The psychiatric interview is a therapeutic process that occurs between the nurse and the patient but may include the family as well. The interaction during this process is not casual but rather is a planned interaction based on scientific, psychotherapeutic principles. The use of these psychotherapeutic principles by the nurse becomes an art through the use of the nurse's ability to instill trust and empathy in the patient and family or significant others. The patient is always made aware of the confidential nature of the nurse–patient relationship before the initial interview. The nurse asks for the following.

CHIEF COMPLAINT

The chief complaint is often obtained by asking patients to say in their own words why they are seeking help, that is, what is the problem that brings them here today? If the patient is unable to provide the information, the chief complaint is the predominant reason why the assessment was requested. For example, "Patient was admitted following a suicide attempt by drug overdose."

DEMOGRAPHIC DATA

Demographic information about the patient is then collected. See Box 1-1.

HISTORY OF PRESENT ILLNESS

The patient is asked about the duration of present symptoms and recent stressors. The patient's perception of the problem or illness as well as other perceptions of the informant are requested, including patient and family beliefs regarding the illness. The patient is asked about:

1. The first sign of a problem
2. Symptom development
3. The course of the illness
4. Current use of prescription medication, illicit drugs, alcohol, caffeine, nicotine, over-the-counter medications, and anabolic steroids
5. A recent change or an identified trauma in the patient's life

PAST PSYCHIATRIC HISTORY

The patient describes past psychiatric, psychological, or addiction treatment. See Box 1-2. The patient is also asked to describe psychiatric illness that was *not* treated, if any, as well as drug allergies, adverse drug effects, and personal preferences in psychopharmacological treatment, if appropriate.

MEDICAL HISTORY

The nurse obtains a detailed medical history, including review of past systems problems. Especially noted are high-risk benchmarkers that may indicate a medical illness that can present as a psychiatric problem. These areas include history of high fevers, convulsions, seizures, head injuries, thyroid dysfunction, and other neurological concerns. See Box 1-3 for a medical history form.

FAMILY MEDICAL AND PSYCHIATRIC HISTORY

Especially helpful is the use of a genogram (see Chapter 6) to document addictions, medical and psychiatric illnesses, as well as family and marital history. Special concerns are given to family history of suicide and homicide. The securing of therapeutic pharmacological treatment responses of first-degree (biological) family members for related problems is important information for treatment considerations.

BOX 1-1: Demographic Data Form: Psychiatric Nursing Assessment

THE FOLLOWING INFORMATION WAS GATHERED FROM: _____

PATIENT'S NAME: _____ AGE: _____ DATE OF BIRTH: _____

ADMISSION: Voluntary: _____   Commitment: _____

NUMBER OF PRIOR PSYCHIATRIC HOSPITALIZATIONS: _____

RESIDENCE: _____

RELIGIOUS AFFILIATIONS: _____

ETHNIC IDENTIFICATION: _____

HIGHEST EDUCATIONAL LEVEL: _____

NAME OF SCHOOL/LOCATION: _____

CURRENT OCCUPATION: _____

NAME OF EMPLOYER/LOCATION: _____

MARITAL STATUS: Single: _____   Married, how long: _____   Number of marriages: _____

Widowed, how long: _____   Separated, how long: _____   Divorced, how long: _____

CURRENT FAMILY COMPOSITION:

NAME	RELATIONSHIP	AGE	OCCUPATION OR GRADE IN SCHOOL	WHERE LIVING

SIGNIFICANT OTHERS LIVING OUTSIDE THE HOME:

NAME	RELATIONSHIP	AGE	OCCUPATION OR GRADE IN SCHOOL	WHERE LIVING

PSYCHOSOCIAL AND DEVELOPMENTAL HISTORY

See Box 1-4 for a form used to gather psychosocial and development history.

MENTAL STATUS EXAMINATION

The mental status examination is designed to assess the patient's mental functioning level and estimate the effectiveness of the patient's mental capacities. Because the mental status can change quickly, the nurse does a mental status exam in the initial assessment to collect baseline data. See Box 1-5 for a formal mental status exam form.

BOX 1-2: History of Past Psychiatric Treatment Form

INPATIENT TREATMENT AND/OR RESIDENTIAL TREATMENT:

NAME & LOCATION OF FACILITY	DIAGNOSIS	DATES	TREATMENT	RESPONSE

OUTPATIENT TREATMENT:

THERAPIST	LOCATION	DATES	TREATMENT	RESPONSE

PSYCHIATRTIC MEDICATIONS:

DRUG	DOSAGE	DATES	LENGTH OF TRIAL	RESPONSE	SERUM LEVELS

MINI–MENTAL STATUS EXAM

The Mini–Mental State Examination (MMSE) is the most widely used screening evaluation for cognitive impairment. The MMSE used to screen for dementia and delirium grossly quantifies the degree of cognitive impairment, and serially measures cognitive changes over time. It should be emphasized that the MMSE is only a screening measure, and it should not be used as the sole criterion for diagnosing dementia. The MMSE is reprinted in Box 1-6. Scores range from 0–30, and values of 23 or less suggest the presence of cognitive impairment. Some authorities recommend three levels of cognitive impairment be delineated: 24–30 = no cognitive impairment; 18–23 = mild cognitive impairment; and 0–17 = severe cognitive impairment. MMSE scores are correlated with years of education, and the established cutoff points are probably not valid if the patient has less than a ninth-grade education.

PHYSICAL ASSESSMENT

The physical assessment is essential to the psychiatric nursing assessment. Some physical disorders can present with psychiatric symptoms and some psychiatric disorders can result in physiological complications (Kaplan, Sadock, & Grebb, 1994). In addition, chronically mentally ill patients often do not receive primary health care services. If they are homeless they may not have had a physical exam for a long time, and will probably have physical problems. At the basic nursing level the following physical assessment skills include:

❍ Performing a physical assessment with ability to perform general techniques of inspections, observations, measurement of vital signs

BOX 1-3: Medical History Form

MEDICAL HISTORY   (Include dates and treatment of identified problems)

CHILDHOOD ILLNESSES: _____

_____

_____

HIGH, PROLONGED FEVER: _____

ACCIDENTS OR TRAUMA: _____

HEADACHES: _____

FRACTURES: _____

_____

HEAD INJURIES: _____

SEIZURES: _____

MEDICAL HOSPITALIZATIONS: _____

_____

SURGERY: _____

VENEREAL DISEASE: _____

THYROID DISEASE: _____

HEPATITIS: _____

SPEECH DIFFICULTIES: _____

HEARING DIFFICULTIES: _____

VISION DIFFICULTIES: _____

COLOR BLINDNESS: _____

OTHER SIGNIFICANT MEDICAL PROBLEMS: _____

_____

NUTRITIONAL STATE: _____

_____

MENOPAUSE: _____

MENSES: _____

BIRTH CONTROL: _____

PREGNANCIES: _____

ABORTIONS: _____

TOBACCO USE: _____

ALCOHOL USE (I): _____

SUBSTANCE ABUSE (I): _____

ALLERGIES (FOOD, DRUG OR CONTACT): _____

OTHER: _____

○ Review of laboratory data and tests
○ Survey of health history/systems

Advanced practice nurses who have these skills may perform a physical exam and according to state regulations may order further diagnostic procedures.

BOX 1-4: Psychological and Developmental History Form

COMPOSITION OF FAMILY OF ORIGIN

    MOTHER: LIVING? IF NOT, PATIENT'S
AGE WHEN SHE DIED: _____

    FATHER: LIVING? IF NOT, PATIENT'S AGE
WHEN HE DIED: _____

    SIBLINGS IN ORDER OF BIRTH (include
patient in chronological list): _____

    _____

    _____

    _____

CULTURE/ETHNICITY: _____

RELIGION: _____

DESCRIPTION OF FAMILY LIFE: _____

_____

DESCRIPTION OF MOTHER'S
PREGNANCY WITH PATIENT: _____

DESCRIPTION OF BIRTH: _____

DEVELOPMENTAL MILESTONES: _____

    AGE PATIENT   AGE PATIENT
    WALKED: _____   TALKED: _____

SCHOOL PERFORMANCE
(retentions, average grades, etc.): _____

DIFFICULTIES IN:

    FINE OR GROSS MOTOR SKILLS: _____

    LEFT-RIGHT DISCRIMINATION: _____

    ATTENTION/CONCENTRATION: _____

    LETTER REVERSAL: _____

HISTORY OF:

    HEADBANGING/ROCKING: _____

    FIRE SETTING: _____

    ENURESIS: _____

    ENCOPRESIS: _____

    CRUELTY TO ANIMALS: _____

    SCHOOL TRUANCY: _____

JOB HISTORY: _____

_____

FINANCIAL STATUS: _____

SOCIAL RELATIONSHIPS: _____

COMMUNITY INVOLVEMENT: _____

MARITAL HISTORY: _____

_____

SEXUAL HISTORY
(including sexual preference): _____

MILITARY HISTORY: _____

LEGAL PROBLEMS/PENDING
COURT DATES: _____

SIGNIFICANT LOSSES/SEPARATIONS: _____

SPORTS/HOBBIES: _____

_____

_____

VOCATIONAL/CAREER INTERESTS OR PLANS: _____

_____

PATIENT'S PERCEPTION OF FAMILY
RELATIONSHIPS/ISSUES: _____

_____

_____

_____

_____

PATIENT'S PERCEPTION OF RELATIONSHIPS WITH
SIGNIFICANT OTHERS: _____

_____

_____

_____

PHYSICAL OR SEXUAL CHILD ABUSE: _____

_____

SIGNIFICANT LOSSES IN LIFE: _____

_____

_____

_____

ADDITIONAL COMMENTS: _____

_____

_____

_____

STANDARDIZED PSYCHIATRIC RATING SCALES

Once a tentative diagnosis has been made, rating scales may be used to determine the severity of the illness. Besides determining severity of the illness, rating scales are used to:

1. Provide a baseline rating
2. Compare and evaluate changes in symptoms
3. Measure clinical responses to treatment interventions, especially psychopharmacological response scales
4. Validate a tentative diagnosis
5. Provide quantitative data

BOX 1-5: Formal Mental Status Examination

1. Orientation to   time: _____
                    place: _____
                    person: _____

2. Fund of knowledge: Level I

   A. Who were the last three presidents of the
      United States? _____

   B. What is a telephone for? _____

   C. Name three countries in the Middle East. _____

   _____

   D. How many miles is it from Los Angeles to
      New York City? _____

3. Recent Memory

   A. Name three objects to the patient: rose, paper clip,
      bulletin board.

      Tell patient you will ask him to recall these three objects
      5 minutes from now.

   B. Have patient count from 1 to 23 out loud.

4. Calculations:

   Serial 7s $100 - 7 = 93$, etc.   _____

   Serial 3s $100 - 3 = 97$, etc.   _____

5. Digital span—Forward

   Ask patient to repeat series of numbers after you. Give
   numbers in a series in 1-second intervals.

   6–1–2   7–9–6–4–8–3
   6–1–5–8   9–8–5–2–1–6–3
   5–2–1–8–6

6. Digital Span—Backward

   Interviewer lists numbers forward; ask patient to list
   numbers backward.

   2–5–9   3–6–7–1–9–4
   8–4–9–3   4–5–7–9–2–3–1
   9–7–8–5–2

7. Fund of Knowledge

   A. Thoreau was a famous man;
      what was he famous for? _____

   B. Where is Belgium? _____

   C. What do we celebrate on
      the Fourth of July? _____

   D. What is a barometer? _____

   E. What causes iron to rust? _____

   F. Who wrote *The Adventures of
      Tom Sawyer*? _____

      or: Who wrote *Paradise Lost*? _____

8. Recent Memory

   A. Ask patient to recall 3 objects:

      Rose: _____
      Paper Clip: _____
      Bulletin Board: _____

   B. What number did patient
      count up to by ones? _____ (23)

9. Ability to Abstract

   A. Similarities:

      1. Plum and Peach   _____
      2. Piano and Violin   _____
      3. Paper and Coal   _____
      4. Ankle and Wrist   _____
      5. Laughter and Tears   _____
      6. Mountain and Lake   _____
      7. First and Last   _____

   B. Proverbs:

      What does it mean when I say:

      1. People in glass houses shouldn't
         throw stones._____

      _____

      2. A rolling stone gathers no moss. _____

      _____

      3. Every cloud has a silver lining. _____

      _____

10. Social and Personal Judgment

    A. What should you do if you lose a book belonging to the
       library? _____

       _____

    B. What should you do if you see a train approaching a
       broken track? _____

       _____

    C. Why are criminals locked up? _____

       _____

11. Intelligence: Below Average _____, Average _____,
                   Above Average _____

12. Judgment: Appropriate _____, Impaired _____

13. Insight: Absent _____, Poorly Developed _____,
              Adequate _____, Well Developed _____

14. Three Wishes:

    1. _____
    2. _____
    3. _____

15. Where do you see yourself in five years? _____

    _____

16. If you could change one thing about yourself, what would
    it be? _____

    _____

17. Additional Comments: _____

    _____
    _____
    _____
    _____
    _____
    _____

BOX 1-6: Instructions for Administering Mini–Mental State Examination

Orientation

1. Ask for the date. Then ask specifically for parts omitted (e.g., "Can you also tell me what season it is?"). One point for each correct.
2. Ask in turn, "Can you tell me the name of this hospital (town, county, etc)?" One point for each correct answer.

Registration

Ask the patient if you may test his memory. Then say the names of three unrelated objects (e.g., car, house, book), clearly and slowly, about 1 second for each. After you have said all three, ask him to repeat them. This first repetition determines his score (0–3), but keep saying them until he can repeat all three, up to six trials. If he does not eventually learn all three, recall cannot be meaningfully tested.

Attention and Calculation

Ask the patient to begin with 100 and count backward by 7s. Stop after five subtractions (93, 86, 79, 72, 65). Score the total number of correct answers.

If the patient cannot or will not perform this task, ask him to spell "world" backward. The score is the number of letters in correct order (e.g., dlrow = 5, dlorw = 3).

Recall

Ask the patient if he can recall the three words you previously asked him to remember. Score 0–3.

Language

Naming—Show the patient a wristwatch and ask him what it is. Repeat for pencil. Score 0–2.

Repetition—Ask the patient to repeat the sentence after you. Allow only one trial. Score 0–1.

Three-stage command—Give the patient a piece of plain, blank paper and repeat the command. Score 1 point for each part correctly executed.

Reading—On a blank piece of paper print the sentence "Close your eyes" in letters large enough for the patient to see clearly. Ask him to read it and do what it says. Score 1 point only if he actually closes his eyes.

Writing—Give the patient a blank piece of paper and ask him to write a sentence for you. Do not dictate a sentence; it is to be written spontaneously. It must contain a subject and verb and be sensible. Correct grammar and punctuation are not necessary.

Copying—On a clean piece of paper, draw intersecting pentagons, each side about 1 inch, and ask the patient to copy it exactly as it is. All 10 angles must be present and 2 must intersect to score 1 point. Tremor and rotation are ignored. Estimate the patient's level of sensorium along a continuum, from alert on the left to coma on the right.

Adapted from Folstein, M., et al. (1975). Mini–mental state: A method for grading the cognitive state of patients for clinicians. *Journal of Psychiatric Research, 12,* 189. Copyright Pergamon Press, Ltd. Reprinted with permission.

See Kaplan, Sadock, and Grebb (1994, p. 333) for a list of psychiatric rating scales and their sources.

SUICIDE ASSESSMENT

If the patient is depressed or the nurse has some reason to believe the patient is suicidal, a suicide assessment is paramount. Box 1-7 shows a scale used to rate the patient's potential for suicide. (See also Chapter 24.)

OTHER SOURCES OF DATA

With the patient's permission, data may also be gathered by:
1. Interviews with the family and significant others
2. Contacts with the referring person
3. Contacts with a former therapist
4. Contacts with school guidance counselors
5. Contacts with crisis counselors
6. School records

BOX 1-7: Sad Children—A Suicide Potential Scale

S	Support system	Who is at home? How does the client get along with them? Are there others in the environment who can be called upon?
A	Alcohol	Is alcohol abuse involved in the attempt? Is the client a known alcoholic? Is the client sober enough for a final assessment?
D	Depression	How clinically depressed is the client?
C	Communication	Is the client communicating with you? With the family?
H	Hostility	How hostile or angry is the client? Is the anger so strong that the client might commit suicide in order to "punish" significant others?
I	Impulsivity	How impulsive was the suicidal act? Is the client generally impulsive?
L	Lethality	Is the client aware of the lethality of the method? Was the plan well thought out to avoid rescue?
D	Demography	Do demographic variables such as age, sex, and socioeconomic status place the client in a high-risk category?
R	Reaction of evaluator	Is your empathic response to the client a feeling of hopelessness or depression? Is there something about the client that makes you feel angry?
E	Events	What events led to the attempt? Has the client had any significant life changes, particularly the loss of a spouse?
N	No hope	Does the client believe there is no hope of things improving? Do you feel hopeless upon hearing about the client's life?

From DiVasto, P., et al. (1979). A framework for the emergency evaluation of the suicidal patient. *Journal of Psychosocial Nursing, 17*, 15–19. Reprinted by permission of Journal of Psychosocial Nursing and Mental Health Services, Slack, Incorporated, Medical Publisher.

7. Prior and current medical records
8. Legal records

Once all the data has been collected, the nurse formulates a clinical picture of the patients' problems in the context of their lives.

FORMULATION

The nurse's formulation of the patient depends largely on the nurse's theoretical orientation, practice paradigm, and epistemology (Sperry, Gudeman, Blackwell, & Faulkner, 1992). There are four major psychiatric orientations to psychiatric formulations. These four psychiatric formulation models are as follows:

1. Biological Orientation
2. Psychodynamic Orientation

3. Behavioral Orientation
4. Biopsychosocial Orientation

The formulation is the culmination of the psychiatric nurse's assessment. The formulation must support the nurse's diagnostic impressions. No matter what the orientation of the formulation, it is recommended that the formulation follow the DSM-IV Multiaxial Evaluation format. (See Chapter 2.)

REFERENCES

DiVasto, P., et al. (1979). A framework for the emergency evaluation of the suicidal patient. *Journal of Psychosocial Nursing. 17,* 15–19.

Folstein, M., Folstein, S., & McHugh, P. (1975). Mini–mental state: A method for grading the cognitive state of patients for clinicians. *Journal of Psychiatric Research, 12,* 189–200.

Kaplan, H. I., Sadock, B. J., & Grebb, J. A. (1994). *Kaplan and Sadock's Synopsis of Psychiatry* (7th Ed.). Baltimore: Williams & Wilkins.

Peplau, H. E. (1991). *Interpersonal Relations in Nursing.* New York: Springer.

Sperry, L., Gudeman, J. E., Blackwell, B., & Faulkner, L. R. (1992). *Psychiatric Case Formulations.* Washington, DC: American Psychiatric Press, Inc.

Webster, M. (1984). Psychiatric nursing assessment. In S. Lego (ed.). *The American Handbook of Psychiatric Nursing* (pp. 3–17). Philadelphia: J. B. Lippincott.

TWO

Diagnosis and the DSM-IV

Josephine Sapp

OVERVIEW:

INTRODUCTION

The psychiatric–mental health field has made great leaps since the early 1970s in the area of psychiatric diagnosis. Perhaps the most significant has been the publishing in 1980 of the *Diagnostic and Statistical Manual of Mental Disorders,* 3rd edition. This manual, better known as the DSM-III, introduced several new concepts in the area of psychiatric diagnosis including explicit diagnostic criteria, a multiaxial assessment system, and a descriptive diagnostic approach that attempted to present a "common" behavioral language while being unbiased toward theories of psychiatric etiologies. Since its publication the DSM-III and its successors—the DSM-III-R published in 1988 and the DSM-IV published in 1994—have become the cornerstone of psychiatric diagnosis for both clinicians and researchers in the United States.

    The main function of psychiatric diagnosis is to provide a succinct means of communicating information about the patient's illness. The accuracy of a psychiatric diagnosis is based on a comprehensive collection of data including physical, neuropsychiatric, psychopharmacological, and psychosocial assessment as well as data about cultural, spiritual, and ethnic dimensions of the patient. The psychiatric–mental health nurse must have the knowledge, skill, and ability to conduct and interpret the patient's assessment to plan and provide the appropriate treatment plan for patients and their families.

    To achieve this goal the psychiatric–mental health nurse is educated in the biopsychosocial approach, advocated as the best paradigm for psychiatric assessment (Fink, 1988). In this approach equal emphasis is placed on the assessment and evaluation of the psychological, social, and biological factors influencing the patient's presentation (Yates, Kuthol, & Carter, 1994). To perform a psychiatric assessment within the biopsychosocial assessment framework, the advanced practice psychiatric nurse needs strong clinical training at the master's level. Assessment results in an accurate multiaxial diagnosis leading to a comprehensive treatment plan, including the possible need for specific patient referral. The psychiatric mental health nursing assessment and evaluation is a sophisticated process that mirrors all the diagnostic advances achieved over the last 25 years in the psychiatric–mental health field.

HISTORIC OVERVIEW

Until the publication of the first *Diagnostic and Statistical Manual of Mental Disorders* in 1952, psychiatric disorders were diagnosed unsystematically. For example, factors such as the patient's geographical location or the practitioner's own etiological thinking influenced the diagnosis and treatment. As behavioral, biological, psychosocial, and genetic theories evolved along with the increased ability to perform specific laboratory testing, a clear need was indicated to categorize psychiatric diagnosis into a common, useful language among practitioners, researchers, and providers. Although the American Psychiatric Association began addressing this need in 1952, it did not begin to look at diagnosis based on behavioral criteria and a theoretical framework until the publication of the DSM-II in 1968. With the subsequent publication of the DSM-III, DSM-III-R, and DSM-IV, the focus, scope, and significance of psychiatric diagnosis changed through the development of diagnostic classifications for all mental disorders.

The DSM-IV

The fourth edition of the *Diagnostic and Statistical Manual of Mental Disorders* (DSM-IV) published in 1994 presents the most current classification of mental disorders. This edition correlates with the 10th revision of the World Health Organization's International Classification of Disease and Related Health Problems (ICD-10), developed in 1992. Diagnostic systems used in the United States must correlate with the ICD to ensure uniform reporting of national and international health statistics (Kaplan, Sadock, & Grebb, 1994).

Each diagnostic classification is grounded in research using diagnostic field trials with a multiaxial evaluation system. The DSM-IV diagnostic classification system consists of a set of clinically significant behaviors or psychological syndromes. The mental disorder represents a behavioral, psychological, or biological dysfunction in the individual. The clinician is always reminded that what is being classified is a disorder, and not the patient (American Psychiatric Association, 1994). The DSM-IV manual allows both clinicians and researchers with vastly varied frameworks to speak a universal language in the diagnostic arena, to transmit key information through the use of multiaxial diagnosis in a succinct format, and to comprehend the vital patient information.

BASIC FEATURES OF THE DSM-IV

DESCRIPTIVE APPROACH

The DSM-IV manual presents an atheoretical approach with regard to the psychiatric disorder's etiology or pathophysiological process. The manual does not focus on case management or suggest treatment protocols, but rather attempts to describe the manifestations of mental disorders. Although there are instances in the DSM-IV when etiological factors are listed, as with dementia, for the most part the disorders consist of descriptions of clinical features.

DIAGNOSTIC CRITERIA

Each mental disorder is described by a list of clinical features called diagnostic criteria. These criteria are based on extensive research including data reanalysis, review of relevant literature, and field trials.

SYSTEMATIC DESCRIPTION

The DSM-IV systematically describes each disorder and includes the following:
- Associative descriptive features and mental disorders
- Associative laboratory findings
- Associative physical examination findings and general medical conditions
- Specific culture and age features
- Prevalence
- Course
- Differential diagnosis

DIAGNOSTIC UNCERTAINTIES

Diagnosis in the DSM-IV is deferred or provisional when the information is insufficient. This also occurs when the patient's history or clinical presentation does not meet the full criteria of a prototypical category such as Not Otherwise Specified (NOS) within a diagnostic classification.

MULTIAXIAL ASSESSMENT

The multiaxial assessment system was the second area of contribution to the DSM-III, and its successors, the DSM-III-R and DSM-IV, added to the refinement of psychiatric diagnosis. This multiaxial assessment system evaluates the patient on each of five axes representing different classes of information. The five axes provide clinically useful information that helps the practitioner determine the patient's treatment plan and possible treatment outcomes. This function expands the psychiatric diagnosis beyond diagnosing and treating the patient's present problem. The multiaxial assessment enhances the treatment planning process while succinctly listing the most urgent areas affecting the patient's treatment outcomes.

The multiaxial assessment system is comprised of:

Axis I	Clinical disorders
	Other conditions that may be a focus of clinical attention (See Box 2-1)
Axis II	Personality disorders
	Mental retardation (See Box 2-2)
Axis III	General medical conditions (See Box 2-3)
Axis IV	Psychosocial and environmental problems (See Box 2-4)
Axis V	Global assessment of functioning (See Box 2-5)

USING THE DSM-IV

MULTIAXIAL EVALUATION REPORT FORM

The DSM-IV includes a DSM-IV multiaxial evaluation form. This form is helpful in recording the data collected during the multiaxial assessment. The form and examples of how to record the results of a DSM-IV multiaxial evaluation are given in Boxes 2-6 and 2-7.

PRINCIPAL DIAGNOSIS

When the patient presents with more than one diagnosis, the principal diagnosis is the diagnosis established after the patient assessment and evaluation. The principal or primary diagnosis is the diagnosis that will be the primary focus of the individual's treatment. (See Appendix for Axis I and Axis II disorders with code numbers.)

(Text continues on page 21)

BOX 2-1: Classes or Groups of Conditions in DSM-IV, Axis I

Disorders usually first diagnosed in infancy, childhood, or adolescence
(excluding Mental Retardation, which is diagnosed on Axis II)
Delirium, dementia, and amnestic and other cognitive disorders
Mental disorders due to a general medical condition
Substance-related disorders
Schizophrenia and other psychotic disorders
Mood disorders
Anxiety disorders
Somatoform disorders
Factitious disorders
Dissociative disorders
Sexual and gender identity disorders
Eating disorders
Sleep disorders
Impulse-control disorders not elsewhere classified
Adjustment disorders
Other conditions that may be a focus of clinical attention

From DSM-IV, *Diagnostic and Statistical Manual of Mental Disorders* (4th ed.). Copyright
American Psychiatric Association, Washington, DC, 1994. Used with permission.

BOX 2-2: Classes of Groups of Conditions in DSM-IV, Axis II

Mental Retardation

Personality Disorders
Paranoid personality disorder
Schizoid personality disorder
Schizotypal personality disorder
Antisocial personality disorder
Borderline personality disorder
Histrionic personality disorder
Narcissistic personality disorder
Avoidant personality disorder
Dependent personality disorder
Obsessive-compulsive personality disorder
Personality disorder not otherwise specified

From DSM-IV, *Diagnostic and Statistical Manual of Mental Disorders* (4th ed.). Copyright
American Psychiatric Association, Washington, DC, 1994. Used with permission.

BOX 2-3: Axis III: General Medical Conditions (with ICD-9-CM codes) in DSM-IV

Infectious and parasitic diseases (001–139)

Neoplasms (140–239)

Endocrine, nutritional, and metabolic diseases and immunity disorders (240–279)

Diseases of the blood and blood-forming organs (280–289)

Diseases of the nervous system and sense organs (320–389)

Diseases of the circulatory system (390–459)

Diseases of the respiratory system (460–519)

Diseases of the digestive system (520–579)

Diseases of the genitourinary system (580–629)

Complications of pregnancy, childbirth, and the puerperium (630–676)

Diseases of the skin and subcutaneous tissue (680–709)

Diseases of the musculoskeletal system and connective tissue (710–739)

Congenital anomalies (740–759)

Certain conditions originating in the perinatal period (760–779)

Symptoms, signs, and ill-defined conditions (780–799)

Injury and poisoning (800–999)

From DSM-IV, *Diagnostic and Statistical Manual of Mental Disorders* (4th ed.). Copyright American Psychiatric Association, Washington, DC, 1994. Used with permission.

BOX 2-4: Axis IV: Psychosocial and Environmental Problems in DSM-IV

Problems with primary support group

Problems related to the social environment

Educational problems

Occupational problems

Housing problems

Economic problems

Problems with access to health care services

Problems related to interaction with the legal system/crime

Other psychosocial and environmental problems

From DSM-IV, *Diagnostic and Statistical Manual of Mental Disorders* (4th ed.). Copyright American Psychiatric Association, Washington, DC, 1994. Used with permission.

BOX 2-5: Global Assessment of Functioning (GAF) Scale

Consider psychological, social, and occupational functioning on a hypothetical continuum of mental health–illness. Do not include impairment in functioning due to physical (or environmental) limitations.

Code   (Note: Use intermediate codes when appropriate, e.g., 45, 68, 72.)

100
91   Superior functioning. In a wide range of activities, life's problems never seem to get out of hand; is sought out by others because of his or her many positive qualities. No symptoms.

90
81   Absent or minimal symptoms (e.g., mild anxiety before an exam), good functioning in all areas, interested and involved in a wide range of activities, socially effective, generally satisfied with life, no more than everyday problems or concerns (e.g., an occasional argument with family members).

80
71   If symptoms are present, they are transient and expectable reactions to psychosocial stressors (e.g., difficulty concentrating after family argument); no more than slight impairment in social, occupational, or school functioning (e.g., temporarily falling behind in schoolwork).

70
61   Some mild symptoms (e.g., depressed mood and mild insomnia) OR some difficulty in social, occupational, or school functioning (e.g., occasional truancy, or theft within the household), but generally functioning pretty well, has some meaningful interpersonal relationships.

60
51   Moderate symptoms (e.g., flat affect and circumstantial speech, occasional panic attacks) OR moderate difficulty in social, occupational, or school functioning (e.g., few friends, conflicts with peers or co-workers).

50
41   Serious symptoms (e.g., suicidal ideation, severe obsessional rituals, frequent shoplifting) OR any serious impairment in social, occupational, or school functioning (e.g., no friends, unable to keep a job).

40

31   Some impairment in reality testing or communication (e.g., speech is at times illogical, obscure, or irrelevant) OR major impairment in several areas such as work or school, family relations, judgment, thinking, or mood (e.g., depressed man avoids friends, neglects family, and is unable to work; child frequently beats up younger children, is defiant at home, and is failing at school).

30

21   Behavior is considerably influenced by delusions or hallucinations OR serious impairment in communication or judgment (e.g., sometimes incoherent, acts grossly inappropriately, suicidal preoccupation) OR inability to function in almost all areas (e.g., stays in bed all day; no job, home, or friends).

20

11   Some danger of hurting self or others (e.g., suicide attempts without clear expectation of death: frequently violent; manic excitement) OR occasionally fails to maintain minimal personal hygiene (e.g., smears feces) OR gross impairment in communication (e.g., largely incoherent or mute).

10
1   Persistent danger of severely hurting self or others (e.g., recurrent violence) OR persistent inability to maintain minimal personal hygiene OR serious suicidal act with clear expectation of death.

0   Inadequate information.

The GAF Scale is a revision of the GAS (J. Endicott, R. L. Spitzer, J. L. Fleiss, J. Cohen (1976). The Global Assessment Scale: A procedure for measuring overall severity of psychiatric disturbance. *Arch Gen Psychiatry. 33*, 766), and CGAS (D. Shaffer, M. S. Gould, J. Brasic, P. Ambrosini, P. Fisher, H. Bird, S. Aluwahlia (1983). Children's Global Assessment Scale (CGAS). *Arch Gen Psychiatry. 40*, 1228S). They are revisions of the Global Scale of the Health-Sickness Rating Scale (L. Luborsky (1962). Clinicians' judgments of mental health. *Arch Gen Psychiatry. 7*, 407).

From DSM-IV, *Diagnostic and Statistical Manual of Mental Disorders* (4th ed.). Copyright American Psychiatric Association, Washington, DC, 1994. Used with permission.

BOX 2-6: Multiaxial Evaluation Report Form

AXIS I: Clinical Disorders
          Other Conditions that May Be a Focus to Clinical Attention

Diagnostic code   DSM-IV name

---- ---- ---- ---- ----   _____
---- ---- ---- ---- ----   _____
---- ---- ---- ---- ----   _____

AXIS II: Personality Disorders
          Mental Retardation

Diagnostic code   DSM-IV name

---- ---- ---- ---- ----   _____
---- ---- ---- ---- ----   _____

AXIS III: General Medical Conditions

ICD-9-CM code   ICD-9-CM name

---- ---- ---- ----   _____
---- ---- ---- ----   _____
---- ---- ---- ----   _____

AXIS IV: Psychosocial and Environmental Problems

Check:

_____ Problems with primary support group—Specify: _____

_____ Problems related to the social environment—Specify: _____

_____ Educational problems—Specify: _____

_____ Occupational problems—Specify: _____

_____ Housing problems—Specify: _____

_____ Economic problems—Specify: _____

_____ Problems with access to health care services—Specify: _____

_____ Problems related to interaction with the
      legal system/crime—Specify: _____

_____ Other psychosocial and environmental problems—Specify: _____

AXIS V: Global Assessment of Functioning Scale

Score: ____ ____ ____

Time frame: _____

From DSM-IV, *Diagnostic and Statistical Manual of Mental Disorders* (4th ed.). Copyright
American Psychiatric Association, Washington, DC, 1994. Used with permission.

SEVERITY AND COURSE SPECIFIERS

"A DSM-IV diagnosis is usually applied to the individual's current presentation and is not typically used to denote previous diagnosis from which the individual has recovered. The following specifics indicating severity and course may be listed after the diagnosis: Mild, Moderate, Severe, In Partial Remission, In Full Remission, and Prior History." (American Psychiatric Association, 1994, p. 2)

"*Mild.* Few, if any, symptoms in excess of those required to make the diagnosis are present, and symptoms result in no more than minor impairment in social or occupational functioning.

"*Moderate.* Symptoms or functional impairment between mild and severe are present.

"*Severe.* Many symptoms in excess of those required to make the diagnosis, or several symptoms that are particularly severe, are present, or the symptoms result in marked impairment in social or occupational functioning.

"*In Partial Remission.* The full criteria for the disorder were previously met, but currently only some of the symptoms or signs of the disorder remain.

"*In Full Remission.* There are no longer any symptoms or signs of the disorder but it is still clinically relevant to note the disorder. The differentiation of in full remission from recovered requires consideration of many factors, including the characteristic course of

---

BOX 2-7: Examples of How to Record the Results of a DSM-IV Multiaxial Evaluation

Example 1:

Axis I	296.23	Major depressive disorder, single episode, severe without psychotic features
	305.00	Alcohol abuse
Axis II	301.6	Dependent personality disorder, frequent use of denial
Axis III		None
Axis IV		Threat of job loss
Axis V	GAF = 35	(current)

Example 2:

Axis I	300.4	Dysthymic disorder
	315.00	Reading disorder
Axis II	V71.09	No diagnosis
Axis III	382.9	Otitis media, recurrent
Axis IV		Victim of child neglect
Axis V	GAF = 53	(current)

Example 3:

Axis I	293.83	Mood disorder due to hypothyroidism, with depressive features
Axis II	V71.09	No diagnosis, histrionic
Axis III	244.9	Hypothyroidism
	365.23	Chronic angle-closure glaucoma
Axis IV		None
Axis V	GAF = 45	(on admission)
	GAF = 65	(at discharge)

Example 4:

Axis I	V61.1	Partner relational problem
Axis II	V71.09	No diagnosis
Axis III		None
Axis IV		Unemployment
Axis V	GAF = 83	(highest level past year)

From DSM-IV, *Diagnostic and Statistical Manual of Mental Disorders* (4th ed.). Copyright American Psychiatric Association, Washington, DC, 1994. Used with permission.

the disorder, the length of time since the last period of disturbance, the total duration of the disturbance, and the need for continued evaluation or prophylactic treatment.

"*Prior History.* For some purposes, it may be useful to note a history of the criteria having been met for a disorder even when the individual is considered to be recovered from it. Such past diagnosis of mental disorder would be indicated by using the specifier Prior History (e.g., Separation Anxiety Disorder, Prior History, for an individual with a history of Separation Anxiety Disorder who has no current disorder or who currently meets criteria for Panic Disorder)." (American Psychiatric Association, 1994, p. 2)

"*Nonaxial Format.* Clinicians who do not use the multiaxial format to list the diagnosis serially may simply list the appropriate diagnosis. The *Principal Diagnosis* or the *Reason for Visit* should always be listed first." (American Psychiatric Association, 1994, p. 35)

Examples are listed in Box 2-8.

PROVISIONAL DIAGNOSIS

"The specifier *provisional* can be used when there is a strong presumption that the full criteria will ultimately be met for a disorder, but not enough information is available to make a firm diagnosis. The clinician can indicate the diagnostic uncertainty by recording 'Provisional' following the diagnosis. For example, the individual appears to have a Major Depressive Disorder, but is unable to give an adequate history to establish that the full criteria are met. Another use of the term *provisional* is for those situations in which differential diagnosis depends exclusively on the duration of illness. For example, a diagnosis of Schizophreniform Disorder requires a duration of less than 6 months and can only be given provisionally if assigned before remission has occurred." (American Psychiatric Association, 1994, pp. 3–4)

BOX 2-8: Reporting Diagnosis Without Using the Multiaxial System

Example 1:

296.23	Major depressive disorder, single episode, severe, without psychotic features
305.00	Alcohol abuse
301.6	Dependent personality disorder, frequent use of denial

Example 2:

300.4	Dysthymic disorder
315.00	Reading disorder
382.9	Otitis media, recurrent

Example 3:

293.83	Mood disorder due to hypothyroidism, with depressive features
244.9	Hypothyroidism
365.23	Chronic angle-closure glaucoma, histrionic personality features

Example 4:

V61.1	Partner relational problem

From DSM-IV, *Diagnostic and Statistical Manual of Mental Disorders* (4th ed.). Copyright American Psychiatric Association, Washington, DC, 1994. Used with permission.

NOT OTHERWISE SPECIFIED CATEGORIES

"Because of the diversity of clinical presentation, it is impossible for the diagnostic nomenclature to cover every possible situation. For this reason, each diagnostic class has at least one Not Otherwise Specified (NOS) category and some classes have several NOS categories. Four situations in which an NOS diagnosis may be appropriate are:

"1) The symptom picture is atypical.

2) The symptoms lead to a symptom pattern not included in the DSM-IV. [See Box 2-9.]

3) There is uncertainty about etiology (i.e., whether the disorder is caused by a medical condition, a substance, or is primary). [See Table 2-1.]

4) There is insufficient opportunity for complete data collection." (American Psychiatric Association, 1994, p. 4)

BOX 2-9: Criteria Sets and Axes Provided for Further Study

Postconcussional disorder
Mild neurocognitive disorder
Caffeine withdrawal
Alterative dimensional descriptors for schizophrenia
Postpsychotic depressive disorder of schizophrenia
Simple deteriorative disorder (simple schizophrenia)
Premenstrual dysphoric disorder
Alternative criterion B for dysthymic disorder
Minor depressive disorder
Recurrent brief depressive disorder
Mixed anxiety-depressive disorder
Factitious disorder by proxy
Dissociative trance disorder
Binge-eating disorder
Depressive personality disorder
Passive-aggressive personality disorder (negativistic personality disorder)
Medication-induced movement disorders
    Neuroleptic-induced parkinsonism
    Neuroleptic malignant syndrome
    Neuroleptic-induced acute dystonia
    Neuroleptic-induced acute akathisia
    Neuroleptic-induced tardive dyskinesia
    Medication-induced postural tremor
    Medication-induced movement disorder not otherwise specified
(Note: These categories are included in the "Other Conditions That May Be a Focus of Clinical Attention" section. Text and research criteria sets for the conditions are included here.)

Defensive Functioning Scale
Global Assessment of Relational Functioning (GAF) Scale
Social and Occupational Functioning Assessment Scale (SOFAS)

TABLE 2-1
Ways of Indicating Diagnostic Uncertainty

TERM	EXAMPLES OF CLINICAL SITUATIONS
V Codes (for Other Conditions That May Be a Focus of Clinical Attention)	Insufficient information to know whether or not a presenting problem is attributable to a mental disorder, e.g., Academic Problem; Adult Antisocial Behavior
799.9 Diagnosis or Condition Deferred on Axis I	Information inadequate to make any diagnostic judgment about an Axis I diagnosis or condition
799.9 Diagnosis Deferred on Axis II	Information inadequate to make any diagnostic judgment about an Axis II diagnosis or condition
300.9 Unspecified Mental Disorder (nonpsychotic)	Enough information available to rule out a Psychotic Disorder, but further specification is not possible
298.9 Psychotic Disorder Not Otherwise Specified	Enough information available to determine the presence of a Psychotic Disorder, but further specification is not possible
[Class of disorder] Not Otherwise Specified, e.g., Depressive Disorder Not Otherwise Specified	Enough information available to indicate the class of disorder that is present, but further specification is not possible, either because there is not sufficient information to make a more specific diagnosis or because the clinical features of the disorder do not meet the criteria for any of the specific categories in that class
[Specific diagnosis] (Provisional), e.g., Schizophreniform Disorder (Provisional)	Enough information available to make a "working" diagnosis, but the clinician wishes to indicate a significant degree of diagnostic uncertainty

From DSM-IV, *Diagnostic and Statistical Manual of Mental Disorders* (4th ed.). Copyright American Psychiatric Association, Washington, DC, 1994. Used with permission.

CRITICISMS OF THE DSM-IV

As critical thinkers it is important that nurses be aware of some of the criticisms of the DSM-IV. Ross and Pam (1995) write the following:

> The DSM-IV diagnostic system arises from the reductionistic philosophy of late twentieth-century North American psychiatry . . . psychiatric disorders are largely treated as separate entities, consistent with the hypothesis that there is one gene for schizophrenia, a gene for depression, and another separate gene for alcoholism. Although there are groupings of disorders, and various exclusion rules based on the pressure of other disorders, the main purpose of the system is to sort patients out into discrete categories. The way in which diagnoses are placed in categories, rather than being phenomenologically based, is highly determined by historical artifacts, the residual effects of Freudian theory, and political turf disputes among different subcommittees. (pp. 122–123)

Political disputes have arisen between the APA and special-interest groups over the years who wanted categories either deleted or included in the DSM. Examples of these categories are homosexuality, rape perpetration, and premenstrual syndrome (PMS). In this way the DSM has bowed to a departure from science.

NURSING DIAGNOSIS

Advanced practice psychiatric nurses use the DSM-IV categories to assess clients and plan treatment. Nurses also use nursing diagnoses to categorize phenomena for which nursing interventions are appropriate. Appendix A shows the list of psychiatric nursing diagnoses developed by a task force of the American Nurses Association Council on Psychiatric Mental Health Nursing in cooperation with the North American Nursing Diagnosis Association (NANDA) (O'Toole & Loomis, 1989).

As the DSM-IV provides a common diagnostic language for all mental health clinicians, so does the nursing diagnosis provide a common diagnostic language for the nursing professional. The development of the DSM-IV diagnoses and nursing diagnoses parallel each other in goal, purpose, and intent. (See Box 2-10.) The accuracy of diagnoses in both is dependent on the accuracy and comprehensiveness of the assessment data. It is essential that the nurse as a member of the multidisciplinary team command an understanding of the DSM-IV and multiaxial diagnoses. The nurse will then be able to translate the DSM-IV diagnoses into the appropriate nursing diagnoses. These nursing diagnoses based on comprehensive nursing assessment will be assimilated into the patient's multidisciplinary treatment plan.

BOX 2-10: Common Elements of the DSM-IV Diagnoses and Nursing Diagnoses

- Based on comprehensive assessment findings
- Behaviorally oriented in definition
- Atheoretical in etiological causes
- Focus on the patient's needs and problems
- Improve interdisciplinary communications
- Diagnostic criteria validated through research

REFERENCES

American Psychiatric Association (1994). *Diagnostic and Statistical Manual of Mental Disorders* (4th ed.). Washington, DC: American Psychiatric Association.

Fink, P. J. (1988). Response to the presidential address: Is "biopsychosocial" the psychiatric shibboleth? *Archives of General Psychiatry, 145,* 1061–1067.

Kaplan, H. I., Sadock, B. J., & Grebb, J. A. (1994). *Kaplan and Sadock's Synopsis of Psychiatry* (7th ed.). Baltimore: Williams & Wilkins.

O'Toole, W. W., & Loomis, M. E. (1989). Revision of the phenomena of concern for psychiatric mental health nursing. *Archives of Psychiatric Nursing, 3* (5), 288–299.

Ross, C. A., & Pam, A. (1995). *Pseudoscience in Biological Psychiatry: Blaming the Body.* New York: John Wiley & Sons.

Yates, W. R., Kuthol, R. G., & Carter, J. (1994). Psychiatric assessment, DSM-IV, and differential diagnosis. In A. Stoudemire (ed.), *Clinical Psychiatry for Medical Students* (2nd ed.) (pp. 1–77). Philadelphia: J. B. Lippincott Co.

BIBLIOGRAPHY

Morrison, J. (1995). *DSM-IV Made Easy: The Clinician's Guide to Diagnosis.* New York: Guilford Press.

II
PART TWO

Therapeutic Modes

Psychodynamic Individual Psychotherapy

Suzanne Lego

OVERVIEW:

INTRODUCTION

The advent of managed care as a method of reducing health care costs has had a profound effect on the practice of psychodynamic individual psychotherapy. Clients who must rely on their health insurance are usually limited to brief therapy (see Chapters 12–15) or to group therapy (see Chapter 4). Table 3-1 shows a number of myths that account for a reduction in interest in psychodynamic individual psychotherapy, and corresponding facts.

DEFINITION

Psychodynamic individual psychotherapy refers to a confidential relationship between a therapist and client aimed at the alleviation of symptoms and distress through the exploration and investigation of the client's interpersonal life.

QUALIFICATIONS

The nurse who practices individual psychotherapy:
1. Is certified by the American Nurses Association as a clinical specialist in psychiatric and mental health nursing or is in the process of becoming certified
2. Is undergoing personal psychotherapy or has done so
3. Is participating in peer review or other supervision

TABLE 3-1
Myths and Facts about Individual Psychotherapy

MYTH	FACT
1. Individual psychotherapy is not cost-effective.	1. Research shows that the provision of mental health services reduces overall health care expenses (Jones & Vischi, 1979; Mumford, Schlesinger & Glass, 1982). Mumford, Schlesinger, Glass, Patrick & Cuerdon (1984) performed a meta-analysis on 58 studies of medical utilization following psychotherapy. Decreases in medical use following psychological intervention were reported in 85% of these studies (Giles, 1993).
2. If mental disorders are caused by a chemical imbalance, psychotherapy is not needed, just medication.	2. Even when a chemical imbalance occurs, e.g., as sometimes happens with depression, the imbalance can be triggered by an interpersonal event or ongoing situation. While medications can control the symptoms of the imbalance, they do not change the situation or its meaning to the client. Psychotherapy empowers individuals to take control of their lives and to maximize their potential. An NIMH study showed a combination of medications and psychotherapy works best with depression.
3. If mental disorders are caused by genetics, individual therapy is not going to be effective.	3. There is much speculation about the role of genetics in mental disorder, especially by geneticists (Horgan, 1993; Hubbard & Wald, 1993; Lewontin, 1992; Lewontin, Rose, & Kamin, 1984; Mender, 1994; Ross & Pam, 1995). Even if genetics play a part, the disease causes interpersonal sequelae that can be helped through psychotherapy.
4. Psychotherapy itself can be iatrogenic, for example, in cases of "false memory," where therapists convince clients they have been victims of incest when they have not.	4. Therapists who create false memories make up a very small percentage of caregivers. On the other hand, recent research shows the act of talking to another person produces physiological changes in the brain that are experienced as pleasurable (Hammond, 1990) and may cause permanent differences in brain functioning (Gabbard, 1992).
5. People get worse when they go into therapy, because they now have an explanation or "excuse" for their deviant behavior.	5. Often clients do get "worse" before they get better. This is because as they slowly give up defenses they become more anxious. As they begin to feel empowered and in control of their lives, they begin to feel and act better. In addition those who judge the client to be "worse," may have a stake in keeping the client the same for their own reasons, or may disapprove of the new behavior.

SETTINGS

Even with the restrictions of managed care, there are some settings where psychodynamic individual psychotherapy still takes place:
   1. Private practice with clients using their insurance as allotted, usually 20 sessions or $1000, and then paying out of pocket for the rest of the year
   2. Public mental hospitals and outpatient departments
   3. Outpatient clinics

GOALS

The goals of psychodynamic individual psychotherapy are:
1. Alleviation of symptoms
2. Alteration of character structure
3. Ego strengthening
4. Emotional and interpersonal maturation
5. The creation of new enabling potentials

ROLE OF THE THERAPIST

The role of the therapist is to help the client experience consciously those aspects of life that are unconscious or dissociated, but that appear in the form of symptoms or unsatisfactory life patterns. This is done through the establishment of an intimate professional relationship between the client and nurse over time.

PHASES

INTRODUCTORY PHASE (Lego, 1984)

In the introductory phase, which may last several months, the client and therapist examine each other closely to assess the "boundaries" of the relationship. The therapist is alert to the problems of the client and the characteristic ways of handling them. At the same time the client's strengths and attributes are being measured. The client, in turn, is closely watching the nurse's ability to hear and understand what is being said. Both are aware of their different ways of relating and are making the slight adjustments necessary to be understood. Once this method of communicating openly is established, the working phase of the relationship begins.

WORKING PHASE (Lego, 1984)

In the working phase, the client comes to the session prepared to talk about what is bothersome that day. This may include something that is currently happening, a memory of a past event or relationship, a recent dream, a recent fantasy, or thoughts or feelings about the therapist. Anything the client brings up is considered "grist for the therapeutic mill." That is, all thoughts, feelings, dreams, and fantasies offer an entrance into the client's unconscious or dissociated experience. By talking about them, clients become aware of wishes, feelings conflicts, and desires of which they were not wholly aware. Over time, this material fits into a general pattern that becomes clear to the nurse long before it is clear to the client, by virtue of the fact that the nurse is an objective, though participating, observer. As the pattern becomes clear, the nurse helps the client see how the pattern manifests itself.

TERMINATION PHASE (Lego, 1984)

1. The client and therapist agree that the client has reached maximum benefit (mutual termination).
2. The nurse must cease treating the client owing to geographical move, job change, and so forth (forced termination).
3. The client decides to stop treatment prematurely owing to resistance (premature termination).

During this period, if the first or second reasons are responsible, the sessions may be concerned with separation and the reawakening of early painful separations. If the client is stopping therapy prematurely, the nurse attempts to explore the reasons for the resistance.

Tables 3-2, 3-3, and 3-4 show client behaviors, interventions, and theoretical rationale in the introductory, working, and termination phases of individual therapy.

TABLE 3-2
Possible Client Behaviors, Interventions, and Theoretical Rationale in the
Introductory Phase of Individual Therapy

CLIENT BEHAVIOR	INTERVENTION	THEORETICAL RATIONALE
1. The client enters the room and sits down, looking expectantly at the therapist.	1. The therapist may ask "Why don't you tell me what brings you here today?" or "Tell me what has happened to bring you into the hospital."	1. Clients are very anxious at this time and need structure and a task to help them begin and to relax.
2. The client tells about the symptoms or problems that have led to the need for treatment. (This may continue for weeks or months.)	2. The therapist mostly listens but may ask clarifying questions from time to time, carefully observing the client's demeanor, attitude, level of anxiety, and ways of relating, carefully assessing the situation (see Chapters 1 and 2).	2. Observations in the first session are very important, because they are "fresh" or "pure," that is, uncontaminated by the client's unconscious conformity to what is "expected."
3. The client asks explicitly or implicitly if there is any hope for change in the situation.	3. The therapist states that individual therapy is indicated and can be helpful. "I believe that by talking over what you are going through, things can change for the better. I suggest you come once a week."	3. The client's anxiety is reduced somewhat on learning that the situation is not terribly unusual and can be improved with therapy.
4. The client needs to know the practical details of therapy.	4. The therapist tells the client the time, place, and fee for therapy as well as how the therapist can be contacted. The client is told that it is important to attend sessions every time and to inform the therapist 24 hours in advance of any cancellation.	4. A professional contract conveys to the client the importance of the endeavor upon which they are about to embark, and clarifies mutual responsibilities.

KEY CONCEPTS

The following are definitions of key concepts in individual therapy.

CONTENT AND PROCESS

The content of a therapy session includes all that is *said,* and the process includes all that is *done.* Elements of process include the sequence of topics, body language, voice level and tone, and so forth.

TRANSFERENCE

Transference is the attribution to the therapist of feelings, wishes, and attitudes originally felt *toward* or *by* the client's parents or significant others.

COUNTERTRANSFERENCE

Countertransference occurs when the therapist experiences irrational, exaggerated, or unrealistic feelings toward the client, based on the therapist's own past life or current situation with the client, as in projective identification.

RESISTANCE

Resistance occurs when powerful, often unconscious factors prevent clients from giving up defenses and distortions, often when the client is on the brink of insight (Lego, 1984). Examples include silence, missed sessions, lateness, excessive intellectualization, and abrupt change of subject.

TABLE 3-3
Possible Client Behaviors, Interventions, and Theoretical Rationale in the
Working Phase of Individual Therapy

CLIENT BEHAVIOR	INTERVENTION	THEORETICAL RATIONALE
1. The client begins the session by discussing • Symptoms • Problems • Dreams • Fantasies • Recent occurrences • Thoughts or feelings about the therapist	1. The therapist listens carefully, eliciting information as needed, for example: • The client's notion of the meaning of the dream, symptom, and so forth • The client's associations to the dream, symptom, and so forth • What happened right before or on the day of the dream, symptom, and so forth	1. The therapist is vigilant not to take over the session or make premature interpretations. The less active the therapist, the more active the client. The therapist does offer associations and connections that are not readily available to the client by virtue of the client's resistance.
2. The client falls silent.	2. The therapist gently encourages the client to verbalize thoughts and feelings.	2. The therapist demonstrates that the time is used to discuss any thoughts or feelings, even uncomfortable ones.
3. The client demonstrates in relating to the therapist the interpersonal problems that have brought the client into therapy (for example, manipulation or intimidation).	3. The therapist is careful not to fall into the client's pattern, but rather points out what is happening, even though this may cause the client to become angry, for example, "Are you trying to manipulate me now into doing what you want?"	3. The therapist is often the only person in the client's life who can be honest, straight, and direct with the client, since the therapist has no vested interest, that is, nothing to gain or lose by being honest.
4. The client demonstrates transference, resistance, acting out, and insight and may elicit countertransference responses.	4. See Table 3-5.	4. See Table 3-5.

ACTING OUT

Acting out occurs when the client relives or reproduces through actions, rather than words, the feelings, wishes, or conflicts operating unconsciously (Lego, 1984).

INSIGHT

Insight occurs when the client connects unconscious feelings, wishes, and conflicts to conscious behavior. This connection is emotional and experiential, not merely intellectual (Lego, 1984).

Table 3-5 shows an example of each of the key concepts, the intervention, and theoretical rationale.

THE VALUE OF SELF-DISCLOSURE

Individual psychotherapy was originally called "the talking cure." For an explanation of how talking about the self with a therapist over time brings about a "cure," see Table 3-6. In addition to these 15 steps, built on Peplau's steps of the learning process (Peplau, 1989a), there are three concepts that run through the process and have not been mentioned earlier. These are:
1. *The Whorfian hypothesis* that "language influences thought." Peplau (1989b) extended this idea, writing that:
   o Language influences thought.

TABLE 3-4
Possible Client Behaviors, Interventions, and Theoretical Rationale in the
Termination Phase of Individual Therapy

CLIENT BEHAVIOR	INTERVENTION	THEORETICAL RATIONALE
Mutual Termination The client's symptoms have disappeared, interpersonal relationships are satisfying, work is rewarding, and the client is able to change things that need to be changed and let alone those that cannot be changed. The client looks forward to the future with pleasure.	The therapist reinforces the client's accomplishments, pointing out that "ups and downs" may occur as a natural part of life, but that the client will be able to handle these.	No one is ever totally free of all irrationality, and to expect this will lead to disappointment and frustration.
Forced Termination The client may experience strong positive feelings along with negative feelings toward the therapist for leaving.	The therapist encourages the expression and exploration of both, connecting these to earlier feelings. "You must feel abandoned by me and very angry," and then, "Does this remind you of an earlier time?"	The therapist's leaving is bound to arouse earlier feelings of actual separation or emotional abandonment. The client profits from expressing these feelings and "surviving" them and from seeing that separation can also be survived.
Premature Termination The client states that therapy is not working or that another therapist or another kind of therapy would be better. Often the client states, "I need a vacation from therapy."	The therapist helps the client to explore the client's feelings in great detail, alert to the signs of unconscious resistance. Attention is paid to what has been discussed recently and to what has been happening in *process* between the client and therapist.	Premature termination is usually caused by resistance. Resistance occurs when the client is on the brink of change or insight. If this prospective change can be examined and allowed to happen, the client may not need to terminate. Sometimes clients are reluctant to change and grow in front of one therapist and must move on to the next. This is because the client fears the withdrawal of parental love if separation and growth occur.

    ○ Thought then evokes action.

    ○ Thought and action taken together evoke feelings in relation to a situation or context.

Individual therapy provides an opportunity for clients to examine their true thoughts and feelings and take action.

2. *Catharsis and taking the role of the other.* People often report that the simple act of talking about their troubles makes them feel better. Bohart (1977) found that catharsis works best when combined with some attempt to understand what happened, why it was upsetting, and how it must have seemed to the others involved.

3. *Validation and empathy* regarding inner experience as well as actions. Clients often feel understood for the first time in therapy. One of the reasons this phenomenon can take place is that the therapist has no personal stake in the client's life, and no axe to grind.

TABLE 3-5
Key Concept, Example Intervention, and Theoretical Rationale in Individual Therapy

EXAMPLE OF CONCEPT	INTERVENTION	THEORETICAL RATIONALE
Content and Process Interplay The client complains in her session that her husband is always mad at her for her irresponsibility and that he constantly demeans her and treats her like a child. In process, she is late for every session, often misses sessions, forgets her insurance forms, forgets to pay the therapist, and so forth.	The therapist points out that the client portrays for the therapist the very behavior she is describing that annoys her husband. An attempt is made to help the client figure out how she learned to use this childlike behavior in earlier life and how it continues to serve her unconsciously now in her adult life. The therapist is careful not to pass judgment on the behavior, or to urge the client to stop.	It is inevitable that the client exhibit in the nurse–client relationship those behaviors that have brought the client into treatment. If the therapist has a stake in getting the client to stop acting a certain way, the client will either conform simply to please the therapist or will rebel. Neither behavior is growth-promoting.
Transference (positive) The client tells the therapist that he was kind to the therapist in a past session because he did not want to hurt or disappoint the therapist. His mother was an erratic person who frequently used guilt to control the client.	The therapist points out that the client is treating the therapist as though she were his mother, and questions whether this occurs in other situations.	Because the therapist is seen as an authority figure by the client, the situation is reminiscent of the parent–child relationship. The inevitable distortions, when analyzed in therapy, help the client to recognize the distortions that occur in all aspects of the client's life.
Transference (negative) The client accuses the therapist of disliking her and treating her meanly because she holds a different opinion from the therapist. The client has an overbearing mother.	1. The therapist points out that this behavior would be in keeping with the mother's usual behavior, and that the therapist is not aware of any such feelings. There is an examination of how this might occur in other situations. 2. The therapist is always careful to entertain the possibility that there may be some truth to the client's assertion. If there is, and countertransference does occur, this is explored in the manner described below.	1. It is both inevitable and useful when the client distorts the therapist's behavior in line with the past behavior of parents or significant others. It is through this distortion and its exploration that the client begins to see a pattern of distortions in all relationships. Early longings, fears, and other strong feelings are brought to light in the process. 2. Clients who are schizophrenic or borderline are actually attuned to the therapist's unconscious.
Countertransference (positive) The therapist finds herself being overly protective and "helpful" to the client, and feels happy when the client appears to appreciate her.	1. The therapist examines why it is important to her that the client appreciate and love her. 2. She is alert to the behaviors in the client that elicit this kind of helping behavior. For example, does the client seem helpless in situations when he is not? She does not hide her reaction if it has been observed by the client.	1. Positive feelings from the client often supply narcissistic gratification for the therapist, and provide needs that the therapist missed early in life. 2. However, it is useful for the client to see how his behavior affects others in a situation in which the therapist is open and direct.

(continued)

TABLE 3-5 (continued)

EXAMPLE OF CONCEPT	INTERVENTION	THEORETICAL RATIONALE

Countertransference (negative)
 	
The therapist becomes exasperated and angry when the client acts narcissistic, provocative, and controlling. These are all behaviors the therapist has struggled to give up himself with some but not total success.
	1. The therapist examines internally, with a therapist, supervisor, or colleague, the meaning of his overreaction to the client's behavior. He realizes that he is resentful that the client is still able to "get away" with this behavior that he is working so hard to overcome. He is mad at the "unfairness" of the situation and at being reached by the client, and reminded of his *own* humanness.
	
	2. He examines with the client the meaning of the client's behavior vis-à-vis their relationship. For example, what does it mean to the client? He does not attempt to deny his reaction when it has been observed by the client.
		1. Therapists become irrationally angry at clients when clients
		  a. Display behavior they are displeased with in themselves
		  b. Display the therapist's own defenses or unconscious behavior in a clumsy, transparent way
		  c. Display behavior toward the therapist reminiscent of behavior the therapist's parents or significant others displayed
		2. The therapist tries to represent a stable, realistic reference point uncontaminated by the therapist's distortions. However, it is useful for the client to see how his behavior affects others, in a situation in which the therapist is open and direct.

Acting Out
 	
The client, who is struggling with ambivalent feelings about her parents and strong sibling rivalry, enters an affair with her college professor.
	The therapist helps the client to recognize those feelings that are being acted upon, without attempting to stop the client's acting out.
	As the feelings are explored and openly experienced by the client, the acting out stops.
		Acting out provides excellent grist for the therapeutic mill. As it progresses, feelings are brought to the surface for exploration.
		If the therapist attempts to stop the acting out, the client
		  a. Is deprived of valuable analytic material
		  b. May conform or rebel and leave treatment
		  Neither is useful.

Insight The client tells of an incident that in the past would have intimidated him and caused much anxiety. He reports that instead he was able to handle it in an adult, direct way by simply stating his needs and how he planned to proceed. "I found I didn't need to act like a scared child. I could be an adult and no harm came to me."	The therapist reinforces this positive behavior and brings up any other aspects of the situation that could be further explored.	Insight is the anticipated end result of reconstructive therapy. True emotional insight has occurred when, by and large, the problem behavior or symptoms stop. However, regressions occur from time to time, and no one is ever perfectly "healthy" or absolutely "cured."

EVALUATION   The nurse is constantly evaluating the client's progress throughout therapy. Evaluation is tricky because the relief of symptoms does not always mean the client is better and an increase of anxiety does not always mean the client is worse. Typically the therapy runs the course as described below.

TABLE 3-6
The Curative Process of Self-Disclosure

STEPS	EXAMPLE OF PSYCHOTIC CLIENT	EXAMPLE OF ANXIOUS CLIENT	EXAMPLE OF BORDERLINE CLIENT
1. Clients* enter therapy with symptoms of mental illness or difficulties in living.	1. The client is withdrawn, hallucinating, and delusional.	1. The client exhibits anxiety, phobias, obsessive behavior.	1. The client is needy, angry, narcissistic.
2. It becomes clear to both the client and therapist that the client cannot "name" or describe the problem, or that the client sees the problem only in very concrete terms. Thoughts, feelings, and actions are elusive and unconnected.	2. The client is often bewildered, confused, frightened, lonely, the victim of unexplained terror. She stays home, can't work, has no relationships and no pleasures.	2. The client is often anxious, fearful, depressed, and generally dissatisfied with life. She manages to work and go to school but believes her chronic anxiety has held back her life.	2. The client works on and off but loses jobs because of her inability to get along with others.
3. The nurse reassures the client that others have felt as she does and that talking about her life can be helpful.	3. The nurse tells the client that anxiety often causes alterations in thoughts and perceptions and that these will change for the better as her anxiety decreases.	3. The nurse tells the client that talking about one's thoughts and feelings reduces anxiety and symptoms.	3. The nurse tells the client that understanding the nature of the inner turmoil will bring relief.
4. Clients begin to describe their lives including their thoughts, actions, and feelings.	4. The client tells of her hallucinations beginning at night when she was alone. Because she had no relationships she began to review the day in her mind every night before going to sleep. Soon this review came not in the form of her own thoughts but rather as "voices." At first they were reassuring but in time they became hostile and derogating.	4. The client tells of going to a party the previous evening. She had a glass of wine, was relaxed, laughing and talking. The next day was spent obsessing over all that had happened, fearing she'd made a fool of herself. She was afraid to leave the house, fearing she'd see someone she knew from the party.	4. The client tells of a big fight with a friend. She says she wants to call her up again and give her a piece of her mind. She used to be her best friend but now she hates her.
5. This attention paid to description starts a pattern of increased self-observation, as well as observation of significant others in the client's life.	5. The client begins to notice she is very angry when her parents tell her what to do, what to eat, how to dress, how to act in public.	5. The client notices she becomes especially anxious if she is given special attention or praise in her work.	5. The client notices she becomes particularly anxious when people are nice to her or show an interest in getting to know her better.
6. This observation widens to include both actual conversations and interchanges as well as wishes, fantasies, dreams, and accompanying thoughts and feelings. As clients observe and describe their lives, they "hear" themselves saying things they have never said before, also evidence of increased self-observation.	6. The client describes in detail an interchange with her sister who told her not to talk to people on the street anymore, as she is embarrassing her family.	6. The client describes a meeting at work, where a speaker invites her to move closer so she can hear. All eyes in the room are on her but she does not move. Her face is on fire with embarrassment.	6. The client tells of a date she was supposed to have had the evening before. Instead she got into a power struggle with the date over whether they would go to his place, her place, or a cafe.

*The female pronoun is used, as clients are more often females.   *(continued)*

TABLE 3-6 (continued)

STEPS	EXAMPLE OF PSYCHOTIC CLIENT	EXAMPLE OF ANXIOUS CLIENT	EXAMPLE OF BORDERLINE CLIENT
7. The relationship between client and therapist becomes more trusting, laying the groundwork for the client to become more open and honest.	7. The client says, "I don't hear those voices anymore now that I have you to talk to."	7. The client says "I'm waiting for you to criticize me or make me feel bad, but so far you haven't."	7. The client says, "I *hate* you when you say my behavior is unusual, but I know you're right."
8. The client and therapist begin to connect the pieces that in the beginning seemed random and unconnected.	8. The client says, "I have always felt different from others, and afraid they could tell what I was thinking. When my sisters tell me not to talk to people I think it's because I'm a freak."	8. The client says, "I've always feared that if people saw the real me they'd be very disappointed. I'm careful to cover up what I think and feel."	8. The client says, "If I get close to a man, I can't let go. I get too clingy and attached. If he leaves I'm devastated!"
9. Patterns emerge that are seen to be self-destructive or that lead to dissatisfaction.	9. The client says, "I stay in my room so people can't boss me around or torture me. I'm pretty lonely."	9. The client says, "I don't ever speak up in class or ask questions so people won't see how dumb I am. I guess I miss out on some things."	9. The client says, "If a man acts interested in me I run!"
10. The client and therapist formulate hypotheses about these patterns and the phenomena that underlie them, such as anger, loneliness, envy, jealousy, dependency, self-loathing, and so forth.	10. The client says, "They always said I was weird and now I dress and talk funny to prove they're right."	10. The client says, "My sister was retarded, and I always had to be careful not to outshine her. I'm still being careful not to draw attention to myself."	10. The client says, "I'm so needy and angry that I cling to people so hard I drive them away."
11. The therapist seeks validation from the client by asking, "Are you saying that . . .?" Also the client seeks validation from the therapist.	11. The client asks, "I wonder if I refused to go to the wedding just to make my family mad. What do you think?"	11. The client asks, "I was invited to a party but I don't want to go. Do you think I'm just afraid I'll have too much fun and show too much of myself?"	11. The client says, "I'm thinking of calling the guy who asked me out last week, but I'm afraid it's still that I want to *win*, not that I really want to see him. Do you agree?"
12. The client tests new, less self-destructive, more satisfying patterns of behavior.	12. The client applies for a job, taking care to wear appropriate clothing.	12. The client receives a grade she thinks is unfair, and makes an appointment to see the teacher.	12. The client calls her friend and asks if he'd like to get together, agreeing to go wherever he wants to go.
13. The client's life improves.	13. The client gets the job.	13. The client gets her grade raised.	13. The client goes on the date and enjoys it.
14. The client integrates these new behaviors into everyday life.	14. The client does well in her job, makes some friends, and moves into her own apartment. She begins a life apart from her family but still sees them without the anxiety she used to have around them.	14. The client begins to relate to her classmates and talk a bit in class. She develops new friends and takes a vacation with them.	14. The client begins to date more often and goes out more with friends, adjusting to their idiosyncrasies without fighting with them.
15. The client uses this process to manage hard times, foresee future problems, and to forestall them.	15. The client says, 'A party is coming up at work. I want to go but my sister's invited. She's never seen me with these friends. I hope she won't boss me around. I think I can handle this. I'm going."	15. The client says, "I have to give a class presentation. I'm prepared but I'm nervous. But, my friends are all there. They'll back me up."	15. The patient says, I'm invited away for the weekend. I've never spent a whole weekend with anyone. I'm sure I'll get anxious but I'll be okay."

HONEYMOON STAGE

A honeymoon stage occurs, during which the client feels amazingly better. This is caused by the feeling of relief at being heard and understood and the richness of honest, open communication.

AGGRESSIVE STAGE

During an aggressive stage, the client experiences long-buried anger and resentment, which may be expressed toward the therapist or significant others.

REGRESSIVE STAGE

During a regressive stage, the client begins to give up defenses that have warded off anxiety and begins to feel very anxious and almost "raw."

ADAPTIVE STAGE

During an adaptive stage, the client has begun to resolve major problems and is trying out new kinds of behavior.

Evaluation at any of these stages could be misleading. Freud once said that therapy is successful if the client is able to love and to work. This remains a good general criterion for positive outcome in individual psychotherapy.

REFERENCES

Bohart, A. (1977). Role playing and interpersonal conflict reduction. *Journal of Counseling Psychology, 24,* 15–24.

Gabbard, G. O. (1992). Psychodynamic psychiatry in the "Decade of the Brain." *American Journal of Psychiatry, 149* (8), 991–998.

Giles, T. R. (1993). *Managed Mental Health Care: A Guide for Practitioners, Employers, and Hospital Administrators.* Needham Heights, MA: Allyn and Bacon.

Hammond, M. (1990). Affective maximization: A new macro-theory in the sociology of emotions. In T. D. Kemper (ed.), *Research Agendas in the Sociology of Emotions* (pp. 58–81). Albany, NY: State University of New York Press.

Horgan, J. (1993). Eugenics revisited. *Scientific American,* June, 123–131.

Hubbard, R., & Wald, E. (1993). *Exploding the Gene Myth.* Boston: Beacon Press.

Jones, K., & Vischi, T. (1979). Impact of alcohol, drug abuse and mental health treatment on medical care utilization. *Medical Care, 17* (December supplement).

Lego, S. (1984). Psychoanalytically oriented indivdual and group therapy with adults. In D. L. Critchley & J. T. Maurin (eds.), *The Clinical Specialist in Psychiatric Mental Health Nursing: Theory, Research, and Practice.* New York: John Wiley & Sons.

Lewontin, R. C. (1992). *Biology as Ideology: The Doctrine of DNA.* New York: Harper-Perennial.

Lewontin, R. C., Rose, S., & Kamin, L. J. (1984). *Not in Our Genes: Biology, Ideology, and Human Nature.* New York: Pantheon Books.

Mender, D. (1994). *The Myth of Neuropsychiatry: A Look at Paradoxes, Physics, and the Human Brain.* New York: Plenum Press.

Mumford, E., Schlesinger, H., & Glass, G. (1982). The effects of psychological intervention on recovery from surgery and heart attacks: An analysis of the literature. *American Journal of Public Health, 72,* 141–151.

Mumford, E., Schlesinger, H., Glass, G., Patrick, C., & Cuerdon, T. (1984). A new look at evidence about reduced cost of medical utilization following mental health treatment. *American Journal of Psychiatry, 141,* 1145–1158.

Peplau, H. E. (1989a). Process and concept of learning. In A. O'Toole & S. R. Welt (eds.), *Interpersonal Theory in Nursing Practice* (pp. 348–352). New York: Springer.

Peplau, H. E. (1989b). Theory: The professional dimension. In A. O'Toole & S. R. Welt (eds.), *Interpersonal Theory in Nursing Practice* (pp. 21–41). New York: Springer.

Ross, C. A., & Pam, A. (1995). *Pseudoscience in Biological Psychiatry: Blaming the Body.* New York: John Wiley & Sons.

BIBLIOGRAPHY

Greenberg, L. S., & SaFran, J. D. (1987). *Emotion in Psychotherapy. Affect, Cognition, and the Process of Change.* New York: Guilford Press.

Havens, L. (1993). *Coming to Life: Reflections on the Art of Psychotherapy.* Cambridge, MA: Harvard University Press.

Levenson, E. (1995). *The Ambiguity of Change.* Northvale, NJ: Jason Aronson.

Mendelsohn, R. (1992). *How Can Talking Help?* Northvale, NJ: Jason Aronson.

Weiss, J. (1993). *How Psychotherapy Works: Process and Technique.* New York: Guilford Press.

FOUR

Psychodynamic Group Psychotherapy

Suzanne Lego

OVERVIEW:

INTRODUCTION

Psychodynamic group psychotherapy was not meant to stand on its own, but was originally thought of as an adjunct to individual therapy. While that still remains its best use, managed care organizations promote group therapy as a single treatment, as it is cost-effective.

DESCRIPTION

Psychodynamic group psychotherapy is a method of therapeutic intervention based on the exploration and analysis of both individual and intrapsychic structures and the group process. As individuals interact in a group over time, they are able to observe their own and each other's secret wishes, conflicts, and motivations. An understanding of these unconscious processes and the way they are acted upon with others can help clients to adopt more satisfying modes of interaction. In psychodynamic group psychotherapy, members' behavior is continually examined, keeping in mind that the group is a microcosm of the larger world.

| **OTHER TYPES OF GROUP PSYCHOTHERAPY** | **EDUCATIVE THERAPY** |

Leader presents fixed content in lectures or written material, which is then discussed by clients, for example, medication education groups. See Chapters 49 and 62.

SUPPORTIVE THERAPY

Supportive therapy uses clients' present ego strength and further strengthens it through support and encouragement to help clients cope with a crisis. Emphasis is placed on mobilizing clients' own inner resources and on helping one another. Examples are bereavement groups and groups for HIV-infected clients or their caregivers (Lego, 1993, 1994a, 1994b).

SELECTION OF MEMBERS

NUMBER

Seven has been found to be the ideal number for maximum interaction in a therapy group. It is helpful to select 10 clients, because some attrition will occur. If there are more than 10 members, the group tends to subdivide.

HETEROGENEITY

The more heterogeneous the group, the better. Members should vary in age, gender, and psychodynamics. Exceptions to this rule are psychotic, alcoholic, and drug-addicted clients, who do best in homogeneous groups.

1. *Age*—Members should be 20 and over. When clients come from different "generations," there is a greater likelihood of transference of feelings about their own parents or children.
2. *Gender*—Interaction with both genders helps clients to recognize and work through feelings about both men and women.
3. *Psychodynamics*—A variety of styles helps members to view their own lives from different vantage points and to help one another do so.
4. *Difficult clients*—In the past, schizophrenics and borderline clients have been considered inappropriate for group psychotherapy. This is not necessarily so (Geller, 1963; Lego, 1979; Nehls, 1991, 1992). However, it is recommended that beginning therapists refrain from treating borderline clients in group, since they present many challenging problems. Clients with antisocial personality disorder are not appropriate for group psychotherapy because they are often disruptive to the group and are unable to relate in a way helpful to themselves.

CREATION OF THE GROUP

Table 4-1 lists nursing actions in organizing a psychotherapy group and gives a theoretical rationale for each action.

GROUP LEADERSHIP

ROLE

The role of the group leader is to stimulate group interaction and the group's analysis of the interaction. This is done by making observations of individual dynamics and group dynamics. The leader never does anything for the group that members can do for themselves. For example, members are not called upon by the leader to speak and are not introduced to one another. Instead of asking, "John, why don't you tell us about yourself?" the leader would wait several sessions for John to speak. If he failed to do so, the leader would comment, "John, I notice you seem to have trouble talking here. Do you have any idea why?" The principle here is that, rather than being a boss or guide,

TABLE 4-1
Nursing Actions and Rationale When Organizing Psychotherapy Groups

NURSING ACTION	THEORETICAL RATIONALE
All prospective members are seen at least once individually before admission to the group. (The more times they are seen, the better.)	A libidinal tie will develop between the client and nurse. This tie helps clients to remain in the group later, when they become anxious. This also provides a time for assessment.
Clients are not seen in group only, without individual sessions as well, unless combined therapy is impossible.	Group psychotherapy produces anxiety, which spills over at times outside the group. This anxiety can motivate clients to explore their reactions in individual sessions, and later in the group.
Before entering the group, the client is not prepared for what happens in the group or who will be there. Only a general statement is made such as, "The group is a place to discuss feelings, problems, or reactions."	If the client knows a great deal about the group in advance, spontaneous reactions are lost to exploration. These spontaneous reactions are "grist for the therapeutic mill."
Group members are not told about new members before they appear.	Their spontaneous or irrational response to the new member is useful to explore, for example, this may be reminiscent of the birth of a sibling.
Group members sit in chairs in a circle. No table is used, nor does anyone sit on the floor.	All members should be visible to one another. This increases anxiety slightly, which leads to more irrational behavior and its subsequent observation. It also aids in the observation of nonverbal communication, which can then be explored.
The leader changes seats each session, causing other members to shift seats.	Members should not be able to find a comfortable "niche" in which to hide.
Weekly sessions last 1½ hours, and daily sessions last 1 hour.	When groups meet only once a week, resistance builds between sessions, and it may take 45 minutes for work to begin. When groups meet daily, the resistance is less.
Sessions begin and end on time.	Clients pace their reactions according to this time frame. This pacing in itself is interesting to note, for example, when a client reports in the last 5 minutes that he has quit his job.
The same leader leads the group.	Group process is based on a balance of forces that takes the leader into account. Changing leaders seriously changes this balance and makes interaction more superficial.
Observers do not sit in the group.	This disturbs the ongoing balance and process, causing more superficiality.
Open-ended groups are more effective than time-limited groups. The group continues indefinitely, with replacements made as members leave.	When members know there are only a certain number of sessions left, they remain more controlled and superficial.

the leader is a stimulator. Table 4-2 shows the relationship between the leader's behavior and the group's development.

From this table it can be seen that the leader must remain somewhat behind the scene in regard to what happens in the group. The first session sets the stage for this. The leader lets the group begin on its own, instead of suggesting introductions or describing the purpose of group therapy. In this way, members will catch on from the beginning that the group is their responsibility. The leader avoids an "I am the expert" attitude and comments only with observations that no one else has made or seems ready to make. Table 4-3 shows behaviors of the leader that inhibit growth and those that promote growth.

TABLE 4-2
Relationship Between Leadership of Group and Group's Development

TYPE OF LEADER	GROUP INTERACTION PHENOMENA	PRODUCTION RANGE OF THE GROUP
Boss: Plans, controls, directs, and decides autocratically.	Group submits, conforms when told what to do, has little influence on things except in a passive way.	From nothing useful to support of leader's irrational needs.
Guide: Plans, controls, and steers, usually subtly and indirectly.	Group can register differences, initiate complaints, and make requests. Group participates in thinking and forming opinions, makes minor decisions. Group has some active influence, but little responsibility.	Limited to leader's capacity.
Stimulator: Educates, facilitates production and communication, balances group forces, and shares leadership.	Group generates ideas, sets limits. and establishes methods. Group sets no limits on productivity and development of members. Group has primary responsibilities, uses self-evaluation, has healthy group spirit, is creative and productive.	Can be expected to go beyond leader's capacity to members' maximum potential.

From Lego, S. Group psychotherapy. In Haber, J., et al. (eds.), *Comprehensive Psychiatric Nursing*, 2nd ed. New York: McGraw-Hill, 1982. Reproduced with permission.

TABLE 4-3
Growth-Inhibiting Behaviors and Growth-Promoting Alternatives

GROWTH-INHIBITING BEHAVIORS	GROWTH-PROMOTING BEHAVIORS
Starting sessions by introducing members or explaining the purpose of group therapy.	Waiting for members to begin on their own. Avoiding lengthy explanations of anything.
Bringing food or drink for group members.	Exploring dependency needs in the context of the group and the members' lives outside the group.
Calling on specific members to talk.	Allowing silences to continue until a group member breaks them, or after a few minutes, commenting on the silence. Allowing other members to deal with consistently silent members.
"Going around" the group, requiring that each member talk in turn.	Allowing members to talk at random as they please.
Pushing for closure on a topic or summing up sessions at the end.	Realizing that there is no "final solution." Allowing issues to be discussed, explored, examined by anyone in the group, with interest and respect shown to all. Allowing sessions to end "up in the air," with some members feeling anxious.

From Lego, S. Group psychotherapy. In J. Haber, et al. (eds.), *Comprehensive Psychiatric Nursing,* 2nd ed. New York: McGraw-Hill, 1982. Reproduced with permission.

QUALIFICATIONS

1. The American Nurses Association suggests that nurses who practice group psychotherapy should hold a master's degree in psychiatric nursing.
2. Nurses who are group psychotherapists should be certified as clinical nurse specialists, or should be in the process of becoming certified.

TABLE 4-4
Leader's Expectations of Clients, Possible Client Behavior, and Leader Intervention

EXPECTATION	POSSIBLE CLIENT BEHAVIOR	APPROPRIATE LEADER INTERVENTION
Members will attend every session or tell leader beforehand if they must miss one. (Voiced by leader)	Leave message with another client, secretary, or answering service.	Tells members they must speak to leader directly. Explores need to avoid leader in this case.
	Miss sessions without notice.	Asks members about absence. Explores meaning if appropriate.
	Call to cancel with vague excuse ("I'm not feeling up to it.").	Strongly encourages members to come anyway, pointing out that not feeling well may be related to feelings about the group.
Members will be as open as possible. (Not voiced by leader)	Conscious deception. Members feel one way (for example, angry) but act another (for example, sweet).	Points out inconsistency: "You look angry, but you're acting sweet."
	Unconscious deception. Member seems to feel one way but does not seem aware of it and acts another.	Points out inconsistency or questions in a gentle way: "Are you sure you're not angry?"
No physical violence will occur. (Not voiced by leader)	Members threaten violence.	States that physical violence is not allowed, but encourages verbal exploration of reason for violent feelings.
Members will not discuss group matters outside the group with those who are concerned in these matters. (Not voiced by leader)	Members break group confidentiality.	Explores this in the group.
Members will not meet outside the group, or if they do, they will discuss their meetings in the group. (Not voiced by leader)	Two members form a sexual relationship.	Explores in the group the meaning of the relationship vis-à-vis the group itself, the leader, and past relationships with significant others.
	Two members of the group appear to be attracted to one another.	Explores in the group the relationship with a view to "nipping it in the bud" and dealing with the motivation rather than having it acted out.

From Lego, S. Group psychotherapy. In J. Haber, et al. (eds.), *Comprehensive Psychiatric Nursing*, 2nd ed. New York: McGraw-Hill, 1982. Reproduced with permission.

3. As a part of graduate study, certification, and professional development in general, nurses will find these activities helpful in their preparation:
   a. Didactic preparation—courses in group theory and group psychotherapy theory
   b. Ongoing intensive supervision over time
   c. A personal group experience over time

LEADER'S EXPECTATIONS OF CLIENTS

The leader has certain expectations of clients, some of which are voiced by the leader at the outset and others that are discussed as the event occurs. This is because giving a list of rules at the beginning creates an authority-subordinate atmosphere and because the expectations might cause undue anxiety in the clients. Table 4-4 shows a leader's expectations of clients, possible client behavior, and appropriate leader interventions.

PROBLEMS OF BEGINNING LEADERS

Beginning leaders often feel anxious. This anxiety is reflected in a need to maintain a good self-image and the need to maintain control of the group. Box 4-1 lists ways in which each of these irrational needs may be expressed in the leader's behavior. Supervision is helpful in working through these problems (Lego, 1982).

BOX 4-1: Common Irrational and Nonproductive Needs of Beginning Group Psychotherapists

Need to Maintain a "Good" Self-Image
   Need to be liked
   Need to avoid exposing self as "human"
   Need to impress group with knowledge and authority

Need to Maintain Control of the Group
   Need to prevent group disintegration
   Need to prevent regressive behavior
   Need to prevent resistance
   Need to prevent expression of hostility
   Need to prevent acting out
   Need to avoid "taboo" topics
   Need to prevent intensive, multiple transference reactions
   Need to prevent the examination of individual or subgroup problems
   Need to restrict process that does not "go through" the therapist

From Lego, S. Group psychotherapy. In J. Haber, et al. (eds.), *Comprehensive Psychiatric Nursing*, 2nd ed. New York: McGraw-Hill, 1982. Reproduced with permission.

PHASES OF DEVELOPMENT

The growth of a group follows four stages of development. There is sometimes overlap, but in general the group moves through phases of uncertainty, overaggressiveness, regression, and adaptation. When new members join an ongoing group, they move through these phases as individuals.

Uncertainty (1–20 sessions)

In this phase, group members are anxious and attempt to carve out a place for themselves in the group. Many demands are made on the leader to provide structure. When the leader does not give in to these demands, members become angry. Table 4-5 shows typical client behaviors and leader interventions with each (Lego, 1982).

Overaggression

In this phase, members have begun to understand how the group operates. As a defense against the regression and adaptation soon to follow, the members become aggressive toward one another and toward the leader. Often the aggression expressed toward one another is actually meant for the leader. In this phase, members also begin to feel attracted to one another. This, in turn, leads to aggression, for members uncon-

TABLE 4-5
Behavior, Examples, and Leader Intervention in the Uncertainty Phase

BEHAVIOR	EXAMPLE	LEADER INTERVENTION
Initial anxiety	Pacing the floor. Leaving and returning. Hallucinations and delusions. Excessive intellectualization. Organization of a "group plan."	Comment about the anxiety. Question what members fear happening in the group.
Demands on leader to explain purpose or provide structure	"Do we begin now?" "What is supposed to happen here?" "How does this work?"	Communicate to members that it is their group. ("Let's see how things go.")
Competition	Comparison among members of past group experience, past number of years of psychotherapy, knowledge of the leader, and so forth.	Point out that competition is taking place, being careful to communicate that it is not wrong and should not necessarily stop just because it is noted.
Excessive politeness	Members feel anxious and angry about the lack of structure from the leader, but they are afraid to show this. Instead, they react with inappropriate kindness. To a monopolizer: "You certainly are talkative today."	Note the covert feeling and ask if it is present. ("Are you a little irritated by all that talking?") Encourage openness rather than politeness.
Silence	All members sit for 5 minutes staring at the floor or occasionally glancing at each other.	Comment on the silence. ("I guess everyone is afraid to start.") Comment on some nonverbal behavior. ("Mary, I notice you're staring at John. Do you wish he'd speak?")
Questions about the leader's personal life, qualifications, and competence	Member asks: "Are you a mother?" Member asks: "Are you an MD?"	Comment, "No. Are you afraid I won't know how to care for you because I'm not?" Comment, "No, I'm a psychiatric nurse. Are you afraid I won't know enough to do things right?"
Avoidance of involvement in the group	Schizophrenic member talks to voices instead of other group members. Members intellectualize about their problems. Members adopt roles that were used in their families to reduce anxiety but that are not appropriate in the current group (for example, the buffoon, the boss, the incompetent person, the ingenue).	Comment that these are methods to avoid reacting emotionally to the current group. Explore why this is feared and avoided.
Strong, irrational reactions to the leader	The leader is seen as a "savior" with all the answers. The leader is seen as using power to manipulate or humiliate members and as having a secret reason for every comment or move.	Explore why a "savior" is necessary. Explore the meaning of these ideas in the context of the members' lives.

From Lego, S. Group psychotherapy. In J. Haber, et al. (eds.), *Comprehensive Psychiatric Nursing,* 2nd ed. New York: McGraw-Hill, 1982. Reproduced with permission.

TABLE 4-6
Behavior, Examples, and Leader Intervention in the Overaggressive Phase

BEHAVIOR	EXAMPLE	LEADER INTERVENTION
Criticism of one another	One member who is very lonely but who leads the life of the happy, sophisticated swinger is critical of another member whose isolation and loneliness are all too stark and evident.	Ask whether the "swinger" is reminded of herself by the isolated member. Explore their similarities and the resultant anxiety.
	One member becomes enraged when another acts stubborn and impenetrable.	Ask whether there was someone else in the member's life he could not "get through" to.
Anger at one another for using their own defenses in a clumsy way	One obsessional member begins sentences with "Please don't think I'm trying to be controlling but . . . ." Another obsessional says, "Don't warn us so obviously. It only calls our attention to the fact that you are!"	Point out the dynamic that people feel their own defenses should be used only in their own unique way and are spoiled or "exposed" if used "incorrectly."
Ganging up	One member who is secretly anxious about almost everything arrives late to group each week, giving various weak excuses. He refuses to acknowledge that he might have wanted to miss part of a session or that he may have wanted to stir everyone up.	Examine and explore both sides of the process, why the member is so provocative as well as why members cannot resist being provoked.
Hostility toward the leader	Clients distort the leader's behavior. ("You do nothing to help us.") Clients point out real eccentricities of the leader. ("You are too compulsive!")	Accept their hostility in a nondefensive way. Avoid a win–lose approach. Weaknesses and eccentricities may be acknowledged freely. It is often a great relief to members to see that the leader is human and does not mind if this shows.

From Lego, S. Group psychotherapy. In J. Haber, et al. (eds.), *Comprehensive Psychiatric Nursing*, 2nd ed. New York: McGraw-Hill, 1982. Reproduced with permission.

sciously fear the closeness that may result from the attraction. See Table 4-6 for behaviors and leader interventions in the overaggressive phase (Lego, 1982).

Regression

At this point in group development, earlier defenses are put aside and members experience pure anxiety, anger at more primitive sources, dependency, fear, longing, envy, jealousy, and other forms of pain. Members no longer feel the need to be in control, although there may still be unconscious resistance. Regression is no longer used as manipulation, but rather occurs spontaneously. Members are often surprised at the emotional reactions they experience when others regress. Members who regress are often surprised at the support they receive, because they have previously believed that to lose control would be disastrous. In this phase, the leader comes to be seen as a resource person and as a human being (Lego, 1982).

TABLE 4-7
Signs of Group Cohesiveness

SIGN	EXAMPLE
Meetings outside the group	Members want to go for coffee after meetings.
Resentment of new members	Old members act closer than usual and discuss, without an explanation, matters that are unknown to new member or that are sexually or highly emotionally charged.
Rescuing the leader when under attack	When one member is critical of the leader for giving "bad advice," other members point out that it was not advice but rather exploration.
Control of monopolizers	When one member monopolizes, the others point this out and do not permit it to continue.
Looking down on those outside the group	Members state how lucky they are to be in this particular group.
Acceptance of other members even though they are disliked	One member is domineering. The others work around her bossiness and, without strong hostility, cheerfully tease her about it.

From Lego, S. Group psychotherapy. In J. Haber, et al. (eds.), *Comprehensive Psychiatric Nursing,* 2nd ed. New York: McGraw-Hill, 1982. Reproduced with permission.

Adaptation

Members in this phase accept one another in spite of their weaknesses and faults. As a result, defenses are lowered, and in this atmosphere of acceptance, members are able to explore their conflicts more openly. This mutual acceptance can be a disadvantage because members may become *immune* to one another's neuroses. This is why the leader must continue to "stir up the dust" and poke at members' defenses. Open-ended groups are advantageous in that new members are occasionally admitted and bring a fresh perspective to old patterns (Lego, 1982).

GROUP COHESIVENESS

Group cohesiveness is a feeling of "belonging" that is very important in group life. Cohesiveness is the phenomenon that occurs when group members feel a strong attachment to the group. Forces to remain in the group may come from the following:

1. The group members tend to encourage one another to remain in the group. All want to believe the group is right for them and must validate this by convincing one another.
2. The tie to the leader acts upon members to keep them in the group. This tie may have both healthy and neurotic aspects.
3. Significant others outside the group may urge the members to continue, observing that the group is having a positive effect on the member.
4. The client may experience internal pulls based on the satisfactions felt in the group.

When group cohesiveness has occurred, there are observable signs. These appear in Table 4-7 (Lego, 1982).

TABLE 4-8
Ways to Promote Cohesiveness, with Examples

WAYS TO PROMOTE COHESIVENESS	EXAMPLES
Make group personally rewarding.	Clarifying observations about group or individual behavior that help members understand themselves better. Pointing out to members that they seem healthier or different.
Promote usefulness of other members whether they are liked or not.	Pointing out that an unpopular member is only a symbol of significant other or oneself and therefore useful in helping work out one's own conflicts. Pointing out the "good" qualities of an unpopular member.
Make activities attractive.	Subtly rewarding clients for helping others to recognize distortions or clarifying issues by saying, "Marv has a good point," and so on.

From Lego, S. Group psychotherapy. In J. Haber, et al. (eds.), *Comprehensive Psychiatric Nursing*, 2nd ed. New York: McGraw-Hill, 1982. Reproduced with permission.

Group cohesiveness cannot be artificially produced through exercises that are designed to move members quickly through the phases of development. Positive and negative emotions must be experienced in their own good time as they emerge naturally. There are, however, ways to promote cohesiveness within the natural group process. These are listed in Table 4-8 (Lego, 1982).

CONTENT AND PROCESS

The *content* in group psychotherapy consists of all that is *said* in a session, and the *process* is all that *occurs*. Examples of process include:
1. All nonverbal communication, such as body posture, who speaks to whom, and so forth
2. The order in which topics are brought up

Clients often act out in process what they have described in content. For example, a client may present herself as a "victim" in her relations with her family. However, as she talks and interacts in the group it becomes clear through process that she unconsciously sets up situations in which she plays the victim role, although actually she powerfully controls events. The group therapist is alert to this interweaving of content and process and carefully points this out when it is appropriate.

CENTRAL CONCEPTS OF GROUP PSYCHOTHERAPY

There are five central concepts that are crucial to the practice of psychodynamic group psychotherapy. They are transference, countertransference, resistance, acting out, and insight. In Table 4-9 each concept is defined, an example is given, and guidelines for intervention are presented.

TERMINATION

Termination ideally occurs when both the client and the therapist believe the client has reached maximum benefit. Freud believed this is when the client is able to "love and work." Prior to termination, clients usually relate to others in a nondefensive way and show other signs of healthy self-esteem. There is satisfaction with life on the whole and

TABLE 4-9
Concept, Example, and Intervention in Group Psychotherapy

EXAMPLE OF CONCEPT	EXAMPLE OF INTERVENTION
Transference The client says that the therapist prefers all the other members over her. In reality, this has never entered the therapist's mind, and on reflection, she does not believe this to be true.	The leader asks the client what this is all about. As other members explore this with the client, it is learned that she had a "Cinderella" role in her large family. When the client's distortion is questioned by a group of people who do not believe the distortion, the client is able to view the situation more realistically.
Countertransference The therapist experiences the client as hostile, or very special, or inadequate, and feels strongly about these attributes.	The leader explores silently, or with a therapist, supervisor, colleague, or so forth, what this is about. It is likely that the client does show some of these attributes and that these serve some neurotic purpose for the client. This should be explored openly in the group, for example: "Mary, you seem to be trying to control what happens here today." The strong emotional reaction of the leader to the client must be worked through by the leader, apart from the client.
Resistance The client begins to miss sessions or to come late just after the birth of her first child. She tells the group that she is so happy at home with her husband and new baby that she hates to come to group and get all "stirred up" again.	The leader encourages a discussion of the resistance in the group. Most members enter into discussion because this is a familiar feeling. It is revealed that the client identifies with the new infant's own narcissism and omnipotence and is especially sensitive to the disruptions of this fantasy world that occur in group sessions. This discussion continues for a few sessions, and the resistance passes.
Acting Out A client secretly desires a close, special relationship with the therapist. Instead, she enters an affair with a group member.	The leader brings this matter up in the group or encourages the members who are involved to do so. The meaning of the behavior is explored and analyzed by the group. As this is discussed, members become aware consciously of the real feelings, wishes, and conflicts that were previously only acted on without an understanding of their meaning. The acting out loses its "kick" as understanding occurs, and the acting out stops.
Insight A client has been very angry at her husband, whom she loves and admires. She is puzzled by the anger because she experiences him as loving and kind. She finds herself picking on him for no reason.	The client describes the situation in group, saying, "I thought that marriage to a wonderful person would make my life complete. But it hasn't. He hasn't! He has let me down by not giving me total fulfillment!" As she tells this, she is very moved, as are all the group members. This insight into her irrational anger is further enhanced by continuing discussion of her experience.

a realization of those unsatisfying areas that cannot be changed. There is contentment in self-directed pleasures as well as happiness in relationships with others. Group members can be helpful to clients who want to terminate by pointing out resolved as well as unresolved areas (Lego, 1982).

REFERENCES

Geller, J. J. (1963). Group psychotherapy in the treatment of schizophrenic syndromes. *Psychiatric Quarterly, 63* (1).

Lego, S. (1979). Treatment of the acting out borderline patient in private practice. In *American Nurses Association, Clinical and Scientific Sessions. Nashville, 1979* (pp. 333–344). Washington, DC: American Nurses Association.

Lego, S. (1982). Group psychotherapy. In J. Haber, et al. (eds.), *Comprehensive Psychiatric Nursing* (2nd ed.) (pp. 142–160). New York: McGraw-Hill.

Lego, S. (1993). Group psychotherapy with HIV-infected persons and their caregivers. In H. Kaplan & B. Sadock (eds.), *Comprehensive Group Psychotherapy* (pp. 470–476). Baltimore: Williams & Wilkins.

Lego, S. (1994a). Group therapy with HIV-infected persons. In *Fear and AIDS/HIV: Empathy and Communication* (pp. 45–54). Albany, NY: Delmar Publications.

Lego, S. (1994b). AIDS-related anxiety and coping methods in a support group for caregivers. *Archives of Psychiatric Nursing, 8* (3), 200–207.

Nehls, N. (1991). Borderline personality disorder and group therapy. *Archives of Psychiatric Nursing, 5* (3), 137–146.

Nehls, N. (1992). Group therapy with borderline personality disorder: Interventions associated with positive outcomes. *Issues in Mental Health Nursing, 13* (3), 255–269.

BIBLIOGRAPHY

Bonnivier, J. F. (1992). A peer supervision: Let's put countertransference to work. *Journal of Psychosocial Nursing, 30* (5), 5–8.

Byers, P. H., Mullis, M. A., & Lipe, D. M. (1990). Psychiatric nurses' and patients' perceptions of discussion topics in therapeutic groups. *Issues in Mental Health Nursing, 11* (2), 185–191.

Clark, C. C. (1994). *The Nurse as Group Leader* (3rd ed.). New York: Springer.

Drew, N. (1991). Combating the social isolation of chronic mental illness. *Journal of Psychosocial Nursing, 24* (6), 14–17.

Ganzarain, R. (1989). *Object Relations Group Psychotherapy: The Group as an Object, a Tool, and a Training Base.* Madison, CT: International Universities Press.

Kaplan, H. I., & Sadock, B. J. (eds.) (1993). *Comprehensive Group Psychotherapy* (3rd ed.). Baltimore: Williams & Wilkins.

Lego, S. (1984). Psychoanalytically-oriented individual and group therapy with adults. In D. Critchley & J. Maurin (eds.), *The Clinical Specialist in Psychiatric Mental Health Nursing.* New York: John Wiley.

Lego, S. (1987). Therapeutic groups. In J. Haber, et al. (eds.), *Comprehensive Psychiatric Nursing* (3rd ed.). New York: McGraw-Hill.

Lego, S. (1995). Group therapy in nursing practice. In *Psychiatric Nursing: 1946–1994. A Report on the State of the Art.* Columbus, OH: Ohio State University.

MacKenzie, K. R. (ed.) (1992). *Classics in Group Psychotherapy.* New York: The Guilford Press.

Ormont, L. R. (1992). *The Group Therapy Experience.* New York: St. Martins Press.

Shields, J. D., & Lanza, M. L. (1993). The parallel process of resistance by clients and therapist to starting groups: A guide for nurses. *Archives of Psychiatric Nursing, 7* (5), 300–307.

Couple Therapy

Margery M. Chisholm

OVERVIEW:

Description
Criteria for Couples
Formats
Indications

Assessment
Theoretical Frameworks
Outcomes

DESCRIPTION

Couple therapy is a way of resolving tension or conflict in a dyadic relationship. The phenomena of emotional bonding, role enactment, communication, sexuality, and the broader system that provides the context for the relationship become the focus of therapy. With the goal of changing troublesome behavior and dysfunctional interaction patterns in the couple, the nurse creates a climate that allows for discussion and acceptance of differences, increases empathic understanding of each individual's specific vulnerabilities, and fosters communication and engagement that is direct and facilitative to the relationship while allowing individual growth and fulfillment.

CRITERIA FOR COUPLES

The nurse considers the following criteria of couples before assessing them for couple therapy:

1. Both individuals define themselves as a couple (e.g., married, nonmarried, or a homosexual or heterosexual pair).
2. The couple sees the source of tension/conflict as residing in their relationship.
3. The relationship is embedded in a sociocultural context that has affected the behavior of the individuals (e.g., issues of gender, race, age, ethnicity, religious, cultural, or economic differences).
4. The behavior is enacted in a cyclical pattern in which action by one person evokes a reaction in the other person and vice versa. The pattern may or may not be known by the persons in the relationship.
5. Individual behavior has been influenced by prior learning from the family of origin and cultural context of each member of the couple, and is now influencing their current perceptions and actions.
6. Life cycle and developmental events have precipitated changes in emotional, interactive, and functional aspects of the relationship.

FORMATS

Formats used in therapy include:
1. One therapist works with both members of the couple in the same session.
2. One therapist alternates sessions between the members with periodic conjoint meetings.
3. Two therapists collaborate on the couple's problem, one working with one member and one working with the other. Periodic conjoint sessions are held with the couple and therapists together.
4. One or two therapists facilitate a couples' group.

Decision about the appropriate format is based on the following:
1. Focus of therapy—communication/interaction, sexual problems, or family of origin influences
2. Intensity—crisis or noncrisis approach
3. Frequency—one or twice a week or month
4. Duration—short term or long term
5. Current treatment system—other therapists working with the couple in individual or group sessions
6. Extended family network—inclusion of children or parents of either partner

INDICATIONS

Couple therapy is indicated when (Glick & Kessler, 1980):
1. The presenting problem is a breakdown in communication and trust with a predominance of dysfunctional interaction.
2. The presenting problem is a sexual dissatisfaction or difficulty.
3. The emotional tension in the couple's conflict is serious enough to jeopardize the relationship, health, job stability, or parenting of either member of the couple (e.g., child abuse/neglect, extramarital affairs, spouse battering).
4. There is a clear recent crisis (e.g., illness, death, or job loss) or a family developmental shift (e.g., graduation, marriage, retirement) that causes emotional disruption and role change for one or both partners.
5. A child or adolescent is the presenting patient.
6. Individual or group treatment is not effective in addressing the identified problems.
7. Improvement in an individual patient results in symptom formation in the partner or deterioration in the relationship.

ASSESSMENT

Before beginning the actual assessment, several critical questions are asked. These are shown in Table 5-1 along with the rationale for each question. Table 5-2 shows the dimensions of couple assessment with examples and rationales.

THEORETICAL FRAMEWORKS

Three major theoretical frameworks underpin couple therapy, providing a lens to view interactional phenomena and to generate hypotheses from which to base interventions. These frameworks have spawned contextual therapy, object-relations therapy, and marital behavioral therapy. Boxes 5-1, 5-2, and 5-3 show each theoretical orientation, basic concepts with examples, responsivity, and typical interventions with examples.

OUTCOMES

Couple therapy is considered successful when:
1. Original goals have been met.
2. Couples are satisfied with the outcome, even if it means termination of the relationship.
3. Partners are able to generalize growth to other relationships.

TABLE 5-1
Critical Questions in Preassessment of Couple and Rationale

QUESTION	RATIONALE
1. What does each partner see as the current problem?	1. Often partners blame each other for the problem and may expect only the partner to change.
2. Why is treatment sought now?	2. Whether the current problem is a reactive situation or a chronic problem can influence the format for the treatment.
3. Who referred the couple?	3. The referral source (i.e., doctor, minister, self-referral) indicates the couple's initial view of the problem and approach to problem-solving.
4. Is there violence in the relationship?	4. An extremely explosive relationship requires individual contracts for safety. An assessment of the capacity for delay in action, self-control measures, and the provocative stimulus for each partner is critical.
5. Is either partner addicted to drugs or alcohol?	5. The degree to which the interactions, conflicts, and problems are influenced by substance abuse will determine the focus of the treatment and the format (i.e., conjoint or two therapists). Sexual dissatisfaction may also be a problem.
6. Has either partner been sexually or physically abused?	6. When a partner has been sexually or physically abused there often is an associated problem with intimacy and sexual expression in the couple's relationship.
7. Is hospitalization or individual therapy indicated for either partner?	7. If a partner has a psychiatric illness (DSM-IV, Axis I diagnosis) or a personality disorder (DSM-IV, Axis II diagnosis) the focus of the treatment may require a psychoeducational, supportive approach initially until acute symptoms subside and the partner has stabilized in individual functioning.

TABLE 5-2
Dimensions of Comprehensive Couple Assessment, Examples, and Rationale

DIMENSION	EXAMPLE	RATIONALE
Demographic 1. Composition of nuclear and extended family 2. Ethnic, cultural, sexual, religious orientation of both partners 3. Age and current health status of partners 4. Occupations and financial status 5. Individuals occupying current household 6. Neighborhood/environmental impact on lifestyle	1. Ages, gender, and health status of children and grandparents. 2. Mixed race, ethnic (Italian/Russian), religious (Jewish/Catholic), or heterosexual/ bisexual couple. 3. Older female/younger male attachment or vice versa. 4. Dual-career marriage or husband or wife unemployed. 5. Cohabiting friends, parents, children, stepchildren. 6. Crowded living space, unsafe neighborhood.	These elements are often external to the couple's relationship, yet influence their interaction as do expectations embedded in cultural stereotypes and prohibitions. Pressure for conformity by either creates conflict. Living conditions can contribute to stress of partners.
Historical 1. History of the relationship, including sexual 2. Prior difficulties in the relationship and sources of help 3. Physical or mental illness of both partners 4. Family of origin experiences for both partners	1. How and where partners met, initial attraction, development of shared interests, sexuality, relationships with family and friends. 2. Recency or chronicity of difficulties, resources available to couple (i.e., minister, friends, lawyer, therapist for individual/partner). 3. Occurrences of illness during relationship, impact on both partners, duration of illness, residual adjustments in relationship. 4. Belief system, emotional cues, learned behavioral responses drawn from earlier relationships with significant others.	These elements help determine the phase of development of the coupleship, expectations for therapy, and the impact of prior individual and couple experiences on the current interactions and stated problems.

(Continued)

TABLE 5-2 *(continued)*

DIMENSION	EXAMPLE	RATIONALE

Developmental
 1. Couple development phase
 	
 2. Adult development issues of both partners.
 	
 3. Family life cycle phases
 	
 4. Developmental phases of any children
	1. Newlyweds enthralled with each other or disillusioned midlife couples.
	 2. Young adult issues of career goals and developing intimacy; midlife reordering of priorities; late-life issues of aging, illness, retirement, death.
	 3. Engagement, marriage, birth of children, school-age children, teens, children leaving, couple alone, illness of parent, death.
	 4. Infant schedules, toddler negativity, school-age competence, teen rebelliousness.
		Relationships change over time in terms of emotional closeness, shared goals, and need for individuality. Individual development can affect the stability of a relationship as the desire for change in life course affects the partner.
		    Couples with children are influenced by family life cycle changes, requiring changes in typical patterns of adjustment.
		    Developmental demands of differing age children strain the typical roles of partners and the time for mutual interests. The interaction of these elements in treating problems is important to assess.

Relationship Interaction Patterns 1. Communication 2. Role assumption 3. Boundaries 4. Problem-solving 5. Power structure	1. Directness, clarity, tolerances for differences of opinion, responsiveness, capacity for disagreement. 2. Spousal, parental, partner, occupational, and congruence between partners' perceptions. 3. Diffuse with partners speaking for each other or rigid with little togetherness; difficulty with "I" positions, bringing others into conflicts. 4. Ability to bring relevant information to issue, weigh alternatives, and reach a decision that considers wishes and ideas of both. 5. Symmetrical with shared power, minimizing of differences, and role similarity or asymmetrical with authoritarian, domineering, and nonequal relationships; partner assumes parental role.	Relationship dimensions are derived from verbal and nonverbal observations and include intuitive hunches and the affective experience of the nurse and are a measure of how the relationship works more than what problems are about.
Emotional Expression 1. Affect/mood/tone 2. Intimacy/affiliation 3. Anger/conflict	1. Quick paced—anger, hostility, excitement; or slow paced—depression, withdrawal, despair. 2. Signs of affection, i.e., hand-holding, or sitting near each other; degree to which feelings can be shared. 3. Ability to modulate emotional exchanges or the tendency for escalation that can end in abusive exchanges.	The emotional climate established by the couple and the degree to which it is satisfying to both is a key element in marital satisfaction/dissatisfaction. The absence of positive emotional exchanges can lead to dissolution of the relationship.
Meaning Structure 1. Values 2. Relational ethics	1. Honoring loyalty expectations, adherence to contractual assumptions, congruence between personally held values and those of partner (decision to have/not have children, how to spend money). 2. Perceptions of fairness/unfairness in the relationship; balance between giving and taking, contributions to welfare of partnership.	Meanings are attached to events in the couple's life together and reflect personally held beliefs or are based on accommodation to a spouse's value choices. Trust develops as values are mutually determined, adhered to, and demonstrated in the relationship.
Treatment 1. Couple's goals and expectations 2. Couple's motivation and resistance	1. Couple wants to enhance the sexual relationship/communication or decision-making or to dissolve the relationship. 2. One partner wants to improve the relationship and the other shows no interest or desire to try new behaviors, or both identify problems but do not carry out suggestions for change.	Designing an approach for helping a couple must take into account their desires for change and ability to enter into the work. The nurse considers the information in the other dimensions to determine the best approach and to set the treatment contract.

TABLE 5-2 *(continued)*

DIMENSION	EXAMPLE	RATIONALE
3. Formulation of problem areas	3. Based on demographic, historical, developmental, and relationship concerns.	
4. Therapeutic approach	4. In a couple with previous sexual abuse of one of the partners, a therapy group focusing on the impact of abuse is offered in addition to couple therapy.	
5. Treatment contract	5. The place, frequency, time, length of session, cost, and inclusion of other family members are explained to the couple, eliciting their agreement.	

BOX 5-1: Contextual Therapy: Goals, Concepts, Responsivity, and Interventions

Goals

Establish trust and trustworthiness

Balance issues of fairness and unfairness

Resolve loyalty conflicts

Identify resources in couple relationship

Couple Problems Responsive

Power imbalances or abuses

Spouse abuse

Child abuse

Extramarital affairs

Unresolved parental involvement in couple relationship

All phases of couple development

Basic Concepts and Examples

Loyalty—a bond of relationship and responsibility between partners

Filial loyalty—a bond of relationship and responsibility toward one's own parents by each partner

Split loyalty—a conflict between competing bonds and responsibilities to others

Parentification—an expectation by parents that their offspring provide excessive support or concern for them

Justice—the balance of fairness, giving and getting in relationships over time

Legacy—the effort to correct past injustices in current relationships

Ledger—the family story of a partner that includes what is "owed" to family members and who is obligated

Destructive entitlement—seeking of retribution or reparation for past injuries in current relationships

Exoneration—understanding past experiences of personal injustice through acknowledgment of patterns from generation to generation

Interventions

Multidirected partiality—directing concern toward both partners for actual injuries and sense of injustice and acknowledging contributions made to the relationship

Reviewing sources of entitlement—focusing on the experiences of care and consideration or lack thereof in a spouse's family and current relationships; children may be included to address their roles in the family

Redefining loyalty obligations—helping an overresponsible partner sort out competing interests and giving to parents, spouse, children, and work

Fostering mutuality—challenging partners to engage in negotiating standards of fairness

Crediting—identifying and recognizing ways the partners contribute to the relationship

Siding—backing up each partner to facilitate the discussion of fairness

Confronting legacies—encouraging a partner to face conflicts and establish a new relationship with family of origin; invite own parents for interview with partner excluded

Unlocking past ledgers—helping each partner understand how the past relationship burdens are reflected in the current relationship; shifting focus back and forth between past and present sense of injustice

Seeking resources—fostering couple's recognition and pursuit of activities, relationships, and personal dialogue that validates the relationship

Grunebaum, J., 1990.

BOX 5-2: Object Relations Therapy: Goals, Concepts, Responsivity, Interventions, and Examples

Goals

Establish empathic relatedness.

Identify roots of self-vulnerability.

Contain rageful exchanges.

Refocus misperceptions of partner.

Basic Concepts and Examples

Projection—placing one's own feelings, moral transgressions, self-expectations on partner— e.g., husband who is angry says to his wife, "You're angry."

Introjection—taking in the partner's projections and making it a part of one's self-image—e.g., wife says, "I'm an angry person" and feels angry.

Projective identification—infusing one's partner with one's own unwanted feelings—e.g., the husband feels angry, acts upon the wife until *she* feels and acts angry, and then walks away feeling much better.

Collusion—partners reenact the cycle of disowning feelings by one person and acting out the feelings by the other: "I'm not angry— you're angry." "How dare you?" "See, you're angry."

Vicarious identification—the projector enjoys and condemns the partner's display of the disowned feeling. "She's angry—this is not right—she probably won't stop."

Couple Problems Responsive

Chronic marital dissatisfaction.

Child or adolescent complaint.

Escalating interactions and emotional patterns.

Symptoms in partners owing to poor self-esteem.

Interventions and Examples

Modeling empathic listening—listening attentively to partners and reflecting their position.

Containing projections—helping projector reflect on the meaning of the projection and the recipient to delay in responding, "I wonder what's behind the concern with anger." "Do you really feel angry?"

Empathy training—recognizing what was said that aroused hurt feelings in the partner; partners identifying what they wish the partner had said instead. "What did (your partner) say that made you feel bad?" "What could she have said instead?"

Teaching anger control—calming self-statements, deep breathing, leaving scene. "Can you try to calm yourself on your own or leave the room for a while?"

Fostering internalization of conflicts—asking partners to pay attention to what was frustrating from their partners and its relation to their current feelings. "What happened to cause such low feelings?"

Relating current interaction to family of origin experiences—identifying specific vulnerabilities each person has experienced in the past and their relationship to current fears, interactions, and feelings. "Has this ever happened before? With whom?"

Teaching defocusing on self—helping one partner to observe the other partner and use own feelings as a signal for what partner is feeling. "What do you think she must be feeling?"

Fostering personal contracts for change—identifying the disowned self-image one needs to work on. "Have you thought about how you might address your own tendency to criticize? What will you practice?"

Mallouk, 1982.

REFERENCES

Follette, V., & Jacobson, N. S. (1990). Treating communication problems from a behavioral perspective. In D. Chasin, H. Grunebaum, & M. Herzig (eds.), *One Couple, Four Realities: Multiple Perspectives on Couple Therapy.* New York: Guilford Press.

Glick, I. D., & Kessler, D. R. (1980). *Marital and Family Therapy* (2nd ed). New York: Grune & Stratton.

Grunebaum, J. (1990). From discourse to dialogue: The power of fairness in therapy with couples. In D. Chasin, H. Grunebaum, & M. Herzig (eds.), *One Couple, Four Realities: Multiple Perspectives on Couple Therapy.* New York: Guilford Press.

Mallouk, T. (1982). The interpersonal context of object relations: Implications for family therapy, *Journal of Marital and Family Therapy*, October, 429–441.

BOX 5-3: Behavioral Marital Therapy: Goals, Concepts, Responsivity, and Interventions

Goals

Increase positive behaviors.

Consolidate a collaborative set between the pair.

Foster better listening and expressive skills.

Enhance sexual intimacy.

Basic Concepts and Examples

Behavior exchange—partners engage in behaviors that are pleasing to each other on a daily basis.

Directives—nurse tells partners specific behaviors in which to engage to enhance positive exchanges.

Response generation—partners are told to identify behaviors in own repertoire that please partner, and increase positive responses: "What do you do that makes him pay attention?" "Keep a list."

Reinforcement—partners are encouraged to increase their pleasing behaviors toward spouse to receive more positive responses: "Can you increase what you are doing in order for her to treat you nicely more often?"

Feedback—nurse elicits comments about how it feels when new behaviors are tried and experienced in the relationship.

Generalization—partners are encouraged to engage in positive interactions in natural environment—home, shopping, problematic settings.

Maintenance—periodic relationship meetings are held posttermination to remind each other of new skills; periodic booster sessions with therapist are held regarding skills.

Couple Problems Responsive

Negative day-to-day interactions.

Communication problems.

Problem-solving conflicts.

Sexual dissatisfaction.

Interventions

Self-report measures—identifying own behaviors that are positive and negative for spouse.

Pinpointing skills—focusing on what each can do to enhance the relationship for partner; generation of lists, menus of behaviors.

Homework assignments—deciding during the week which behaviors each will enact, being careful to avoid behaviors that increase own resentment.

Communication training—teaching receptive and expressive skills to foster closeness and intimacy, i.e., paraphrasing, validation of partner's position, making "I" statements.

Modeling—nurse demonstrating both poor attention skills and ways of showing that one has attended to partner's ideas.

Problem-solving training—teaching partners to focus on problem definition and problem resolution, emphasizing affective issues and pros and cons of options.

Journals—asking couples to keep a written account of sexual exchanges and engage in expressions of affection mentioned by partner.

Imaging and fantasy exercises—generating new ideas about pleasurable behaviors from perspective of each spouse.

Change agreements—identifying behavior each will modify on a temporary basis, assuring how and when with provisions for reevaluating.

Follette & Jacobson, 1990.

BIBLIOGRAPHY

Freeman, D. S. (1992). *Family Therapy with Couples: The Family-of-Origin Approach.* Northvale, NJ: Jason Aronson, Inc.

Givelber, F. (1990). Object relations and the couple: Separation-individuation, intimacy and marriage. In D. Chasin, H. Grunebaum, & M. Herzig (eds.), *One Couple, Four Realities: Multiple Perspectives on Couple Therapy.* New York: Guilford Press.

Goldner V., Penn, P., Sheinberg, M., & Walker, G. (1990). Love and violence: Gender paradoxes in volatile attachments. *Family Process, 29* (4), 343–364.

Gurman, A. S. (1985). *Casebook of Marital Therapy.* New York: Guilford Press.

Gurman A. (1992). Integrative Marital Therapy: A time sensitive model for working with couples. In S. H. Budman, M. F. Hoyt, & S. Friedman (eds.), *The First Session in Brief Therapy.* New York: Guilford Press.

Heusden, A. van, & Eerenbeemt, E. van den (1987). *Balance in Motion: Ivan Boszormenyi-Nagy and His Vision of Individual and Family Therapy.* New York: Brunner/Mazel.

Jacobson, N. S., & Holtzworth-Munroe, A. (1986). Marital therapy: A social learning–cognitive perspective. In N. S. Jacobson & A. S. Gurman (eds.), *Clinical Handbook of Marital Therapy.* New York: Guilford Press.

Kantor, D., & Okun, B. (eds.) (1993). *Intimate Environments: Sex, Intimacy, and Gender in Families.* New York: Guilford Press.

Lerner, H. G. (1989). *The Dance of Intimacy.* New York: Harper and Row.

Schnarch D. M. (1992). *Constructing the Sexual Crucible: An Integration of Sexual and Marital Therapy.* New York: W. W. Norton & Company.

6
SIX

Family Therapy

Judith Haber

OVERVIEW:

Introduction
Family Therapy Models
Family Assessment
   Description
   Purpose
   The Genogram
   Family Assessment Guide

Indications
Contraindications
Attendance
Setting
Techniques
Evaluation

INTRODUCTION

All family therapy models are systemic in nature in that they recognize the interconnectedness of individual, family, and social phenomena. The family is viewed as a system instead of a group of separate individuals. Family functioning cannot be understood fully by simply understanding each of the parts because the whole is greater than the sum of its parts. Symptoms emerge from dysfunctional interaction, behavior, relationship, and structural patterns within the family system. Family dysfunction is also reflected in relationships and interactions that family members have in larger social contexts such as school, work, friendship, and community networks. All family therapists agree that the first purpose of family therapy is improvement in family functioning (Bowen, 1976a; Madanes, 1991; Minuchin, 1974; Wheeler, Avis, Miller, & Chaney, 1991).

Generally, the therapeutic goal is to expand the family members' repertoire of responses to the complexities of life. Interventions are therefore geared toward understanding behavior patterns that arise from, and feed back into, the family system.

FAMILY THERAPY MODELS

While all models of family therapy are systemic in nature, they differ in their emphasis on certain dimensions of family functioning, definition of therapeutic goals, preferred type of intervention, and underlying beliefs about the nature of the family system (Guttman, 1991). Table 6-1 compares the models.

FAMILY ASSESSMENT

DESCRIPTION

Family assessment is a holistic, comprehensive process that involves evaluation of the structural, functional, and developmental aspects of a family system as illustrated in Figure 6-1. Family assessment is a map of the family system over at least two generations,

TABLE 6-1
A Comparison of Family Therapy Models

MODEL	DESCRIPTION	GOALS
Psychodynamic	Regards family pathology as resulting from internal intrapsychic forces manifested in intimate interactions. Symptoms result from family projection processes stemming from unresolved conflicts and losses in the family of origin (Boszormenyi-Nagy & Spark, 1973).	To bring about reconstructive personality change achieved by a working through of unconscious transference distortions among family members and with the therapist. Over an extended period, clients explore the connection between past relationships and current problems (Bentovin & Kinston, 1991).
Bowen	Regards family pathology as resulting from lack of differentiation and high anxiety. Those who lack differentiation are emotionally reactive, anxious, and dysfunctional (Bowen, 1976a).	To promote differentiation and less reactivity. Therapy focuses on the family of origin within a multigenerational context. The therapist coaches family members to resolve undifferentiated relationships with the family of origin (Kerr & Bowen, 1988).
Structural	Regards family pathology as resulting from stresses on a family that cannot nurture its members owing to faulty social organization and structure as well as dysfunctional interactions among members (Minuchin, 1974).	To transform family structural patterns by challenging the family's idea of where the problem lies and how it should be solved. The therapist joins the family to challenge the system from within, transforming the structure, patterns, and behavior (Colapinto, 1991).
Strategic	Focuses on the social context of human dilemmas and idiosyncrasies, avoiding the use of psychiatric labels. Instead problems are seen as solvable by the use of directives to change how family members relate to one another (Lankton & Lankton, 1983).	To organize family members to take charge of problems, to facilitate the ability of family members to love and be loved, to promote the family's ability to reframe the distribution of power and responsibility, to promote shifts between hierarchy and equality, and to address personal gain and altruism that contribute to maintaining or resolving family problems (Madanes, 1991).
Behavioral	Problems are defined as overt behavioral acts rather than emotional states or cognitions. Combines training strategies with individuals and conjoint problem-solving among members (Falloon, 1991).	To change reinforcements so family members are rewarded for desired behavior instead of maladaptive behavior. This is achieved through education, training, conditioning, and management strategies (Patterson, 1975).
Feminist	Problems are seen as resulting from the unique problems women face as a result of socialization. Enacts a political, institutional, gender-sensitive viewpoint aimed at gender equality in defining and changing family structure and function (Goodrich, 1991).	To equalize access to influence, control, choice, resources, opportunity, and status. Uses role modeling, education, rebalancing of relationship power and authority, reframing authority, and reinforcing of new beliefs (Avis, 1991).

together with information relevant to the identified client's presenting problem. A family assessment is completed during the initial session(s), but is "fleshed out" over time as family relationship and interaction patterns are examined. Family assessment provides a great deal of data for the therapist and is also therapeutic for family members who invariably discover information about each other that was not known before (Leach-McMahon, 1992; Pendagast & Sherman, 1977).

PURPOSE

1. To collect data about structural aspects of the family system over at least two generations
2. To observe and collect data about family relationship and interaction patterns
3. To observe and collect data about the "identified" client or clients in relation to the family system as a whole
4. To identify functional and dysfunctional aspects of the family system
5. To formulate a "working hypothesis(es)" to explain the family's dysfunction
6. To help the family understand the interactional and relationship patterns operating to generate and maintain problem behaviors by the family as a whole and by any individual family members

THE GENOGRAM

A genogram is a diagrammatic historical "map" of a family over two or more generations. The genogram illustrates internal and external family structure data, including family demographic information (see Figure 6-1). It is also a starting point for assessing

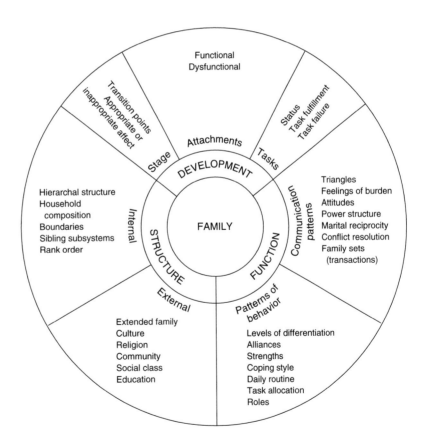

FIGURE 6-1   Components of a Family Assessment

Adapted with pemission from: A. Leach-McMahon (1992). Family therapy and intervention. In J. Haber, A. Leach-McMahon, P. Price-Hoskins, & B. F. Sideleau (eds.), *Comprehensive Psychiatric Nursing* (4th ed.) (pp. 211–242). St. Louis, MO: Mosby.

family function. The genogram data are connected to the identified client's presenting problem when the therapist says, "The information I am asking you about will help me understand how the problem you are describing developed." Preparing a genogram begins at the initial session with one or more family members. Universally recognized symbols that are used to note facts about a family are illustrated in Figure 6-2. The advantage of a genogram is that it visually organizes complex data, which then become a "living map" that is never complete. New information is uncovered and reviewed by the therapist and family as the data collection continues and the family system evolves (Leach-McMahon, 1992). Organization of the genogram is illustrated in Figure 6-3.

FAMILY ASSESSMENT GUIDE

The family assessment guide presented in Box 6-1 is a conceptual outline used to organize the data collection process to facilitate the systemic identification of internal and external family structural information (Pendagast & Sherman, 1977). The assessment questions are also designed to elicit data about multigenerational function and dysfunctional developmental, communication, behavior, and relationship patterns. Questions related to the presenting problem of the family are also included. Data about the presenting problems are often connected to family data that emerge in other areas of the family assessment.

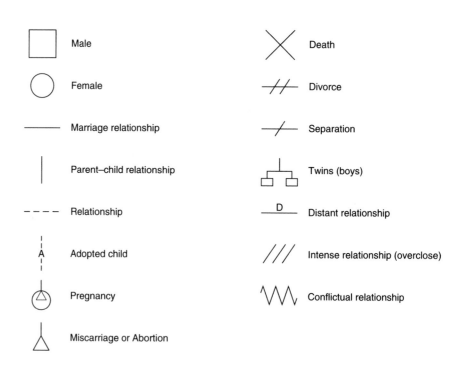

FIGURE 6-2 Genogram Symbols

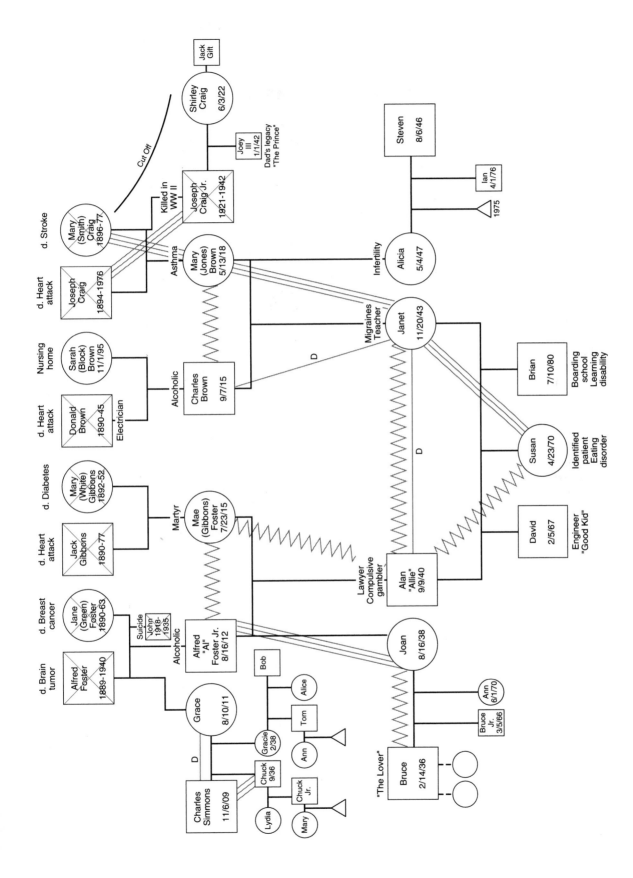

FIGURE 6-3 Four-Generational Family Genogram

BOX 6-1: Family Assessment Guide

A. Family structure (using family genogram)
 1. Parents of nuclear family members
 2. Children—ages and sibling position
 3. Personality description of each individual
 4. Extended family members (e.g., grandparents, aunts, uncles, cousins)
 5. Nonbiological significant others (e.g., special friend, boyfriend, girlfriend)

B. Family in relation to the community
 1. Level of education
 2. Ethnicity
 3. Religion
 4. Socioeconomic status
 5. Geographic location of family members

C. Presenting problem
 1. Each family member's perception of the problem
 2. Each family member's perception of their contribution to the problem
 3. Each family member's perception of how they would like to see things change
 4. Each family member's perception of the positive aspects of the family

D. Communication patterns
 1. Who speaks to whom, when, and in what manner or tone
 2. Emotional climate
 3. Family themes and values
 4. Manner in which anger and hostility are expressed
 5. Frequency (e.g., daily, weekly, monthly, holidays only, annually) and type (letter, phone, tapes, videos, visits) of contact between family members
 6. Conflict resolution style and skills
 7. Triangles

E. Family roles
 1. Which members are supportive, antagonistic, critical, blaming, rescuers, victims, codependent?
 2. Are there family coalitions, alliances, cutoffs, triangles, pairings?
 3. What is the power structure?
 4. What is the nature of the family boundaries (e.g., rigid, blurred, enmeshed, fused)?
 5. How do members feel about their relationships with each member of the family?

F. Family behavior patterns
 1. Level of differentiation
 2. Strengths
 3. Coping style
 4. Task allocation
 5. Daily routine

G. Developmental history
 1. What is the family's life-cycle stage?
 2. What is the:
   a. History of the family of origin of each parent?
   b. History of courtship of parents?
   c. History of birth and rearing of each child in nuclear family?
 3. What is the developmental history of the presenting problem?
   a. Early behavioral symptoms of the problem
   b. Persons involved in the problem
   c. Behavioral problems involved in the problem

H. Family's expectations of therapy

INDICATIONS

Table 6-2 lists indications for family therapy and examples.

CONTRAINDICATIONS

Family therapy is contraindicated:
 1. When key family members are unavailable or unwilling to attend family sessions
 2. When one family member is so dysfunctional that the family approach is unworkable because this member is disruptive in family sessions

ATTENDANCE

 1. Some family therapists contend that the entire family should attend all sessions over the course of therapy (Haley, 1976). Others contend that family therapy can take place with only one family member present (Bowen, 1976a). Most therapists use various combinations of persons attending the sessions over the course of therapy.

TABLE 6-2
Indications for Family Therapy and Examples

INDICATIONS	EXAMPLES
1. The identified problem reflects dysfunction in the family system (Bowen, 1976b).	1. Mary, a 25-year-old mother, develops agoraphobia following the death of her 2-year-old. The family does not discuss the child.
2. The family is involved in an overfunctioning/underfunctioning pattern that is no longer acceptable to one or more family members (Guerin, Fay, Burden, & Kautto, 1987).	2. Jane has been an alcoholic for 10 years and is increasingly unable to care for her children. Her husband becomes unwilling to work, take care of the house, and parent the children alone.
3. A child is the symptom-bearer, masking family conflict (Barrangan, 1976).	3. A 5-year-old manifests bedwetting, nightmares, school problems, and acting out when his parents are considering divorce.
4. A family member is being treated for a serious mental disorder, requiring family crisis intervention and psycho-education (Keefler & Koritar, 1994). (See Chapter 49.)	4. Bob has suffered his first schizophrenic break and is in an inpatient unit.
5. The family experiences an acute situational crisis (Wright & Leahey, 1994).	5. Ella's husband is diagnosed with a terminal illness. She has three children in high school.
6. Individual therapy outcomes are not satisfactory (Guttman, 1991).	6. Bill has been depressed over his marriage, and has not improved in individual therapy.
7. The family must make a difficult decision (Minuchin, 1974).	7. Lynn has been disruptive throughout childhood. Her parents want her to attend college away from home. She wants to live at home.

2. The entire nuclear family is usually present for the initial assessment session(s). Exceptions might occur when a couple with marital problems initially seeks therapy for a dyadic problem. In other situations extended family members, such as grandparents, may attend assessment sessions when multigenerational issues concerning parenting boundaries are the presenting problem.
3. Children over 4 are sometimes included in most, if not all, of the family therapy sessions, especially when the presenting problem is child-focused. For example, when the "identified" client is a 10-year-old child who has a school phobia, the child will attend a number of family sessions. However, meetings with the adults alone are scheduled to focus on the marital dyad and deal with covert marital conflict, explore sensitive issues such as sex, or help parents see themselves as marital partners rather than as just parents (Minuchin, 1974).
4. Children under 4 may attend some early sessions to evaluate the nature of parent–child interactions but do not come to every session during the middle stage of therapy.

SETTING

1. Office—Some family therapists prefer to see the family in their community-based office to create a professional and formal atmosphere for the meeting.
2. Inpatient units—Some family therapists meet with the family prior to discharge from an inpatient setting. In such cases multiple family therapy may take place in a meeting room on the inpatient unit. In other cases, the family may meet with therapists in their offices or another designated location.

3. Home—Some therapists prefer to see the family in the home. The advantage is that the therapist can evaluate the families in their natural environment and observe family structure and function in a relaxed and characteristic manner.

TECHNIQUES   Table 6-3 lists typical family therapy techniques, a description, and an example.

(Text continues on page 71)

TABLE 6-3
Major Techniques, Descriptions, and Examples of Family Therapy

TECHNIQUE	DESCRIPTION	EXAMPLES
Focusing on here-and-now interactions	Family members talk about current rather than past thoughts, feelings, and behaviors with the goal of arousing more profound responses than those involving the past (Falloon, 1991).	1. *To work through a present relationship*—Mrs. Green, a single parent, and her 15-year-old son are in family therapy with the presenting problem of acting-out behavior by the adolescent. During one session, the son screams at his mother, "I hate your guts. Just get out of this room!" Mrs. Green ignores her son's behavior, smiles at the therapist, and proceeds to angrily denounce her ex-husband for being a negligent parent. The therapist interjects, "Mrs. Green, your son just told you that he hates you and told you to get out of the room, yet you smiled, ignored his statement, and then got angry about something else. What were your feelings when your son screamed at you? Talk with your son about these feelings." 2. *To work through a past relationship*—Nancy and Jack Smith are in family therapy because of marital conflict. The conflict is related to Jack's feeling of being ignored emotionally by Nancy, who seems to have time to take care of everybody's emotional needs but his. After observing an interaction during a therapy session, the therapist responds, "You say, Jack, that you feel neglected and unloved by Nancy, yet I see you choosing to sit on a chair by yourself rather than on the couch next to Nancy. Tell me, what was your relationship like with your mother?"
Restructuring family interactional patterns	This technique is based on the premise that it is more effective to enact family interaction patterns than to describe them. Therapists help family members to transact, in their presence, ways in which they naturally interact and resolve conflicts, support each other, enter into alliances and coalitions, diffuse stress, and solve problems. Reenacting interaction patterns helps family members experience their behaviors with heightened awareness. From the therapist's perspective, it also helps them see family members in action, and it is through such observation that the family structure becomes apparent, thereby providing the basis for transforming family structure and function (Minuchin, 1974).	1. "Talk with your mother about that." 2. "Discuss with your husband how the children might help with household chores." 3. "I want you and your wife to plan a budget now." 4. "I know you care about Johnny's feelings, but I want to hear from *him* now."

TABLE 6-3 *(continued)*

TECHNIQUE	DESCRIPTION	EXAMPLES
Clarifying communication	Family members often communicate one thing verbally and another nonverbally. The therapist helps family members to sort out what they mean to say and to say it accurately (Haley, 1976).	1. A couple is in therapy because of marital conflict. A central issue is the power imbalance in the relationship, reflecting a traditional male balance of power. The goal of therapy is to equalize the power structure in the marital relationship. The couple is discussing the possibility of the wife switching from part to full-time employment now that the children are older. The husband frowns and responds, "I really don't care if you work full-time, if you can still run the household. You make the decision." The verbal communication level is, "Yes, work full-time." However, based on past experiences in the marital relationship and other subtle nonverbal cues like his frowning facial expression, the nonverbal, metacommunication level indicates, "No, don't work full-time because it will disrupt the household." The therapist has the couple discuss the husband's response to allow the incongruent message to become obvious, or the therapist points out the seeming incongruence between the husband's verbal and nonverbal message. 2. The Gray family recently initiated family therapy because of their 14-year-old son Jamie's declining grades. Always a high-achieving student, Jamie received 2 Cs, 2 Ds, and one F on his mid-year report card. During a family session, Jamie speculates that his grades may be the result of parental pressure and unrealistic expectations. His father responds, "We love you whatever you do, but we know you have what it takes to be the very best." Jamie confronts his father about the contradictory nature of his message, highlighting the underlying demand to be the "best." He goes on to indicate how much pressure this creates for him and how he worries that his parents will never be satisfied if his choices are different from theirs.
Reframing	To emphasize the positive aspects of interpersonal assumptions, feelings, and behaviors, the therapist renames seemingly dysfunctional behavior as reasonable and understandable. This causes the family members to shift their thoughts, perceptions, and evaluations of a problem (Wheeler, Avis, Miller, & Chaney, 1991).	1. In a family session, a young woman tells her mother how ostracized she felt as a child because she did not dress like the other girls. The mother begins to cry. The daughter assumes she is the cause of her mother's tears and says she didn't mean to hurt her mother by being critical. The therapist reframes the "hurt" by calling it "freedom to share pain in a climate of emotional acceptance." 2. Family therapists who work with abused women may use reframing to highlight women's strengths by relabeling as strengths what women regard as deficits, deviance, or pathology. While not condoning remaining in an abusive relationship, the therapist may marvel at the incredible strength a woman must have had to survive and to help her children survive under such devastating circumstances. This may provide needed recognition about also having the strength to leave the abusive relationship.

(continued)

TABLE 6-3 *(continued)*

TECHNIQUE	DESCRIPTION	EXAMPLES
Challenging the client's internal belief system	Addresses family members' beliefs that their problems are of their own making, a result of their inadequacy, unworthiness, or ignorance. Though they may be unsure of these feelings consciously, they produce guilt and shame. Open-ended questions challenge and disassemble these irrational beliefs and explore their foundations (Avis, 1991).	1. "Where did you learn that you are responsible for making other people happy?" 2. "Who told you that you shouldn't ask directly for what you want?" 3. "It sounds as if you believe your anger is bad. Where does this belief come from? Does it still make sense?" 4. "What do you believe would happen if you said 'No'?" 5. "What do you believe a husband's responsibilities are in a marriage?"
Paradoxical techniques	The therapist asks the family to behave in a way that is seemingly contradictory, hoping the family members will resist and in so doing change their behavior. Through assignment the therapist is asking the family not to change while telling them covertly that they should change. These techniques are based on the assumption that families who come for help are also resistant to the help being offered, providing potential for a power struggle (Selvini-Palazzoli, Boscolo, Cecchin, & Prata, 1978).	
1. Prescribing the symptom	The therapist "orders" the family members to continue and perhaps increase the symptoms. The rationale is that whereas symptoms previously may have seemed out of anyone's control, after the therapist gives the directive the symptoms begin to lose their autonomy, mystery, and power. They appear to come under the therapist's control. The participants in the behavior become increasingly conscious of them, and the dysfunctional behavior may disappear (Selvini-Palazzoli, Boscolo, Cecchin, & Prata, 1980).	A marital couple that has engaged in nonproductive arguing finds that the therapist has asked them to continue fighting and to increase the fighting. The couple is told to fight about the menu before dinner so that they can enjoy the food. This injunction jars the continuing process and they may rebel against the therapist's orders.
2. Reductio ad absurdum	A symptom is reduced to absurdity by discussing it endlessly (Selvini-Palazzoli et al., 1980).	A mother and father in family therapy with their acting-out 13-year-old son, who is the identified client. The primary conflict is between the mother and the son. The therapist commiserates with the mother about the cross she bears and the scientific fact that anyone else would have been completely crushed by it. The goal is to force the mother to say, "I didn't say it was *that* bad!" highlighting the fact that the child has more redeeming features than indicated by the therapist, thereby rebelling against the perspective suggested by the outsider.

TABLE 6-3 *(continued)*

TECHNIQUE	DESCRIPTION	EXAMPLES
Family sculpting	Derived from psychodrama, the family is asked to create a tableau that is a representation of specific relationships among them. In this way, they use the physical during the session to re-create the emotional space between them. Because sculpting involves activity and body movement, it can be a means of engaging children for whom nonverbal modes of expression are natural (Papp, 1976).	The Adams family, consisting of mother, father, and three children, is in therapy because the 12-year-old wets the bed repeatedly. During one session, the therapist introduces sculpting. He first outlines the nature of the activity, then chooses the sculptor (the identified client), and then instructs all of the family members to move out of their seats so that the sculpting can begin. The sculptor physically arranges each member of the family in relation to each other member. During this time, the therapist encourages the identified client, observing and commenting on the manner in which she sculpts each person. After the physical activity is complete, the entire family talks about how they felt during the activity, the extent to which they agree with the sculptor's physical representation of the family, and how they might have sculpted the family differently. At times it is helpful to have more than one family member sequentially sculpt the family and then discuss differences in representation.

EVALUATION

Family therapy is considered successful when:

1. Family communication is open and direct.
2. Families resolve conflicts effectively.
3. Family members enact roles flexibly and effectively.
4. Problem-solving skills are evident.
5. Anxiety and stress are managed through use of effective coping skills.
6. Family power structure reflects balanced influence, authority, and control.
7. Family members demonstrate functional interaction patterns.

REFERENCES

Avis, J. M. (1991). Power politics in therapy with women. In T. J. Goodrich (ed.), *Women and Power: Perspectives for Family Therapy* (pp. 183–200). New York: Norton & Company.

Barrangan, M. (1976). The child-centered family. In P. Guerin (ed.), *Family Therapy: Theory and Practice* (pp. 232–248). New York: Gardner Press.

Bentovin, A., & Kinston, W. (1991). Focal family therapy: Joining systems theory with psychodynamic understanding. In A. S. Gurman & D. P. Kniskern (eds.), *Handbook of Family Therapy*, vol. 2. New York: Brunner/Mazel.

Boszormeyni-Nagy, I., & Spark, G. (1973). *Invisible Loyalties: Reciprocity in Intergenerational Family Therapy.* New York: Harper & Row.

Bowen, M. (1976a). Theory in the practice of psychotherapy. In P. Guerin (ed.), *Family Therapy: Theory and Practice* (pp. 42–90). New York: Gardner Press.

Bowen, M. (1976b). Family reaction to death. In P. Guerin (ed.), *Family Therapy: Theory and Practice* (pp. 335–348). New York: Gardner Press.

Colapinto, J. (1991). Structural family therapy. In A. S. Gurman & D. P. Kniskern (eds.), *Handbook of Family Therapy*, vol. 2 (pp. 417–443). New York: Brunner/Mazel.

Falloon, I. R. H. (1991). Behavioral family therapy. In A. S. Gurman & D. P. Kniskern (eds.), *Handbook of Family Therapy*, vol. 2 (pp. 65–95). New York: Brunner/Mazel.

Goodrich, T. J. (1991). Women, power, and family therapy: What's wrong with this picture? In T. J. Goodrich (ed.), *Women and Power: Perspectives for Family Therapy* (pp. 3–35). New York: W. W. Norton & Company.

Guerin, P. J., Fay, L. F., Burden, S. L., & Kautto, J. G. (1987). *The Evaluation and Treatment of Marital Conflict.* New York: Basic Books.

Guttman, H. A. (1991). Systems theory, cybernetics, and epistemology. In A. S. Gurman & D. P. Kniskern (eds.), *Handbook of Family Therapy*, vol. 2 (pp. 41–64). New York: Brunner/Mazel.

Haley, J. (1976). *Problem Solving Therapy*. San Francisco: Jossey-Bass.

Keefler, J., & Koritar, E. (1994). Essential elements of a family psychoeducation program in the aftercare of schizophrenia. *Journal of Marriage and Family, 20* (4), 368–380.

Kerr, M. E., & Bowen, M. (1988). *Family Evaluation: An Approach Based on Bowen Theory*. New York: W. W. Norton & Company.

Lankton, S. R., & Lankton, C. H. (1983). *The Answer Within: A Clinical Framework of Ericksonian Hypnotherapy*. New York: Brunner/Mazel.

Leach-McMahon, A. (1992). Family theory and intervention. In J. Haber, A. Leach-McMahon, P. Price-Hoskins, & B. F. Sideleau (eds.), *Comprehensive Psychiatric Nursing* (4th ed.) (pp. 211–242). St. Louis, MO: Mosby.

Madanes, C. (1991). Strategic family therapy. In A. S. Gurman & D. P. Kniskern (eds.), *Handbook of Family Therapy*, vol. 2 (pp. 396–416). New York: Brunner/Mazel.

Minuchin, S. (1974). *Families and Family Therapy*. Cambridge: Harvard University Press.

Papp, P. (1976). Family choreography. In P. J. Guerin (ed.), *Family Therapy: Theory and Practice* (pp. 465–477). New York: Gardner Press, Inc.

Patterson, G. (1975). *Families: Applications of Social Learning to Family Life*. Champaign, IL: Research Press.

Pendagast, E. G., & Sherman, C. O. (1977). A guide to the genogram family systems training. *The Family, 5* (1), 3–14.

Selvini-Palazzoli, M., Boscolo, L., Cecchin, G., & Prata, G. (1978). *Paradox and Counterparadox*. New York: Jason Aronson.

Selvini-Palazzoli, M., Boscolo, L., Cecchin, G., & Prata, G. (1980). Hypothesizing–circularity–neutrality: Three guidelines for the conductor of the session. *Family Process, 19* (1), 3–12.

Wheeler, D., Avis, J. M., Miller, L. A., & Chaney, S. (1991). Rethinking family therapy training and supervision: A feminist model. In M. McGoldrick, C. M. Anderson, & F. Walsh (eds.), *Women in Families: A Framework for Family Therapy*. New York: W. W. Norton & Company.

Wright, L. M., & Leahey, M. (1994). Calary family intervention model: One way to think about change. *Journal of Marital and Family Therapy, 20* (4), 381–395.

BIBLIOGRAPHY

Boszormeyni-Nagy, I., Grunebaum, J., & Ulrich, D. (1991). Contextual therapy. In A. S. Gurman & D. P. Kniskern (eds.), *Handbook of Family Therapy*, vol. 2 (pp. 200–238). New York: Brunner/Mazel.

Friedman, E. H. (1991). Bowen theory and therapy. In A. S. Gurman & D. P. Kniskern (eds.), *Handbook of Family Therapy*, vol. 2 (pp. 134–170). New York: Brunner/Mazel.

Gilbert, J. (1981). After the drinking stops: Working with the "sober" family. *The Family, 9* (1), 11–14.

Guerin, P. J. (1976). Family therapy. The first twenty-five years. In P. J. Guerin (ed.), *Family Therapy: Theory and Practice* (pp. 2–22). New York: Gardner Press.

Haber, J. (1993). A construct validity study of a differentiation of self scale. *Scholarly Inquiry for Nursing Practice: An International Journal, 7* (3), 165–178.

Madanes, C. (1981). *Strategic Family Therapy*. San Francisco: Jossey-Bass.

McFarlane, W. R. (1991). Family psychoeducational treatment. In A. S. Gurman & D. P. Kniskern (eds.), *Handbook of Family Therapy*, vol. 2 (pp. 363–395). New York: Brunner/Mazel.

Satir, V. (1964). *Conjoint Family Therapy*. Palo Alto, CA: Science & Behavior Books.

Seaburn, D., Gawinski, B., Harp, J., McDaniel, S., Waxman, D., & Shields, C. (1993). Family systems therapy in a primary care medical setting. The Rochester experience. *Journal of Marriage and Family Therapy, 19* (2), 177–190.

Walters, M., Carter, B., Papp, P., & Silverstein, O. (1988). *The Invisible Web: General Patterns in Family Relationships*. New York: The Guilford Press.

7

Crisis Intervention

Wendy Lewandowski

OVERVIEW:

Introduction
Basic Concepts
Types of Crises
Crisis Intervention—
    Individual Approach
      General Guidelines
      Specific Guidelines

Myths and Facts About Crisis
    Intervention
Other Models of Crisis Intervention
Evaluation

INTRODUCTION

Crises occur in every person's life. Often people cope by drawing upon their inner resources alone, or with family and friends. Severe crises, however, present baffling, upsetting conditions that defy usual problem-solving techniques and prior experience. Crisis theory evolved as a basis for intervention through the study of people confronted with such situations. The hope is that people in crisis will emerge from the crisis experience in a positive, healthy way.

Caplan (1964) suggests that "a crisis occurs when an individual is confronted with a problematic situation for which his typical way of operating in the world and his usual supports are not sufficient. The person's problem-solving behavior is not adequate to produce a satisfactory resolution to the difficulty at hand. A crisis produces a temporary disruption in a person's normal pattern of living and is characterized by high tension" (p. 40). Table 7-1 shows typical changes in behavior of people in crisis.

In nearly all crises, the following occurs (Swanson, 1984):
1. There is a suddenness about the event. Often there is no warning whatsoever, and there is inadequate preparation.
2. The crisis is experienced as life-threatening, even when it is not.
3. Communication with significant others is cut off or decreased.
4. There is some displacement from familiar surroundings or significant others.
5. There is actual or perceived loss of a person, object, idea, or hope.

BASIC CONCEPTS

Those who have contributed to the formulation of crisis theory describe a state of equilibrium, progressing to a state of disequilibrium, and then returning again. The total sequence of events, from equilibrium to disequilibrium and back again, is the "crisis situation." The crisis situation is characterized by five components shown in Table 7-2.

TABLE 7-1
The Crisis Response: Typical Changes in Behavior

BEHAVIOR	DESCRIPTION
Signaling	Sends a "distress signal" to significant others through verbal and nonverbal behaviors.
Attention	Is typically preoccupied with the crisis situation. Expresses disinterest in current interactions unless they pertain to the crisis.
Affectional attachments	Drops out of ordinary patterns of social interaction. At the same time, there is a desire to be close. May be perceived as "clinging" or "demanding."
Identity	Seems diffused, vague, volatile. Loses clear concept of self.
Role performance	Performance of usual roles becomes random and unpatterned; however, is very open to "putting on new roles."
Network attitude	Reports significant others discounting crisis behavior. Feels disqualified.
Memory	Becomes random.
Decision-making	Makes decisions in a random trial-and-error fashion. Cannot sort through or select from a range of choices.

Hansell, 1976.

TABLE 7-2
Components of the Crisis Situation

COMPONENT	DESCRIPTION	EXAMPLE
Hazardous event	A specific, stressful occurrence experienced by a person in a state of physical and psychological stability.	Mr. C's wife undergoes coronary artery bypass surgery and is placed in the surgical intensive care unit postoperatively.
Vulnerable state	The person's subjective response to the hazardous event.	Mr. C experiences high anxiety and feelings of helplessness as he waits for his wife's surgery to conclude, and visits her for the first time following surgery.
Precipitating factor	The link in the chain of stress-provoking events. Converts the vulnerable state into an active crisis state.	Two days following open-heart surgery, Mrs. C goes into respiratory failure and must be placed back onto a ventilator.
Active crisis state	The person's subjective experience when homeostatic mechanisms have broken down. State of disequilibrium in which emotional discomfort and psychic pain are great.	Mr. C is found crying uncontrollably in the waiting room. He calls into the unit many times each hour for a report of his wife's progress. He seems "dazed" and unable to think clearly.
Reintegration	A new form of adjustment and reintegration either above or below precrisis functioning.	After several weeks, Mr. C is able to make decisions related to his wife's care and his outside work interests. He attends the ICU family support group. He verbalizes anger related to his wife's setbacks.

These components or stages are mere abstractions; they cannot actually be isolated, and many times they overlap.

TYPES OF CRISES

Table 7-3 lists the types of crises, descriptions, and examples of each.

CRISIS INTERVENTION— INDIVIDUAL APPROACH

Table 7-4 shows the characteristics of crisis intervention, descriptions, and examples.

GENERAL GUIDELINES

Crisis intervention requires that the nurse:

1. Listen carefully to both the content and the affective quality of the client's presentation (Swanson, 1984).
2. Use a direct, straightforward approach to elicit the fullness of the situation, including what is thought, what is felt, and what has been happening. Keep the focus on the present. Help the person to begin to reorganize while assessment is still in progress (Swanson, 1984).

TABLE 7-3
Types of Crises, Descriptions, and Examples

TYPE OF CRISIS	DESCRIPTION	EXAMPLE
Developmental	Expected, natural changes as one moves from childhood to adulthood.	A child starts school, an adolescent leaves home for college, a young adult marries, a first child is born.
Situational	Unexpected, disruptive changes.	Death of a loved one, divorce, acute illness.
Adventitious	Unexpected, uncommon, accidental changes often involving loss and environmental disruption.	Airplane crashes, floods, hurricanes, mass murders.

TABLE 7-4
Characteristics of Crisis Intervention, Descriptions, and Examples

CHARACTERISTIC	DESCRIPTION	EXAMPLE
Crisis intervention is active.	Nurse listens carefully and connects client with support systems. Nurse encourages and helps client to be active in all steps of the crisis intervention process.	"It sounds like you are very upset. Is there someone who can stay with you tonight?" "Tell me again how you see your role in your daughter's illness." "Tell me your plans."
Crisis intervention is focused.	Nurse focuses on the crisis here and now, avoiding distracting data.	"What are you thinking about now?" "Let's focus on what your options are now."
Crisis intervention has a specific time structure unique to each crisis.	Nurse intervenes immediately when a client is in crisis. Nurse schedules subsequent appointments in fairly quick succession. Nurse lengthens the time between appointments as the client improves.	"I want to talk with you about what you're experiencing." "I would like to set up another appointment this week to talk with you." "I sense your anxiety has been reduced greatly over the past 4 weeks. You also see your situation more realistically. What about coming back in 2 weeks to see me?"

3. Listen without condemnation or judgment (Swanson, 1984).

4. Help to reframe or normalize life events when possible.

5. Provide an opportunity for the client to release anxiety and tension and to express feelings. Use ventilation of feelings to the client's advantage after they are expressed. For example, anger can be used to decrease a sense of helplessness. Help the client integrate these responses with experience.

6. Give clients frequent validation that you have heard them and that you understand the situation (Swanson, 1984).

7. Use language to demonstrate your active listening, or paraphrase. Allow space for clients to correct your reflected perceptions when they are not congruent with what they are trying to express (Swanson, 1984).

8. Avoid overidentification with the client's problem or need. Conversely, avoid detachment. Keep boundaries clear.

9. Connect the client with support systems, being aware of previously untapped support systems.

10. Help clients regain use of cognitive functions, identify choices, and make decisions. Provide a logical discussion of the situation.

11. Support existing patterns of coping until new patterns can be learned. Unless you can offer the client an alternative way of functioning or coping, do not tear down existing patterns.

12. Identify and use the client's strengths; for example, intellectual functions, interpersonal assets, and emotional responses.

SPECIFIC GUIDELINES

1. If the person is clearly on the verge of total collapse or self-destructiveness, institute emergency interventions, but only for as long as is necessary to sustain life (Swanson, 1984).

   a. Be authoritative; for example, "I want you to do as I say."

   b. Be directive; for example, "Tell me your plans."

   c. Involve others; for example, telephone a family member or community agency, direct the client to contact a support system.

2. If the client is clearly distressed but not in danger of death (Swanson, 1984):

   a. Have the client further clarify and focus on the major current problem.

   b. Elicit from the client experience that might successfully be applied to the current situation.

   c. Support the client's idea if it is a feasible one.

   d. Mutually decide upon a timetable for appointments and action on the problem.

   e. Elicit ideas from the client about possible action.

MYTHS AND FACTS ABOUT CRISIS INTERVENTION

Table 7-5 lists common myths about crisis intervention and corresponding facts.

OTHER MODELS OF CRISIS INTERVENTION

Crisis intervention does not always take place on a one-to-one, nurse–client basis or in a consultation room. Table 7-6 describes other accepted models of crisis intervention.

TABLE 7-5
Crisis Intervention: Myths and Facts

MYTH	FACT
Crisis intervention is only for responding to psychiatric emergencies.	Crisis intervention is practiced and used effectively in a wide variety of settings and in response to a variety of hazardous events.
Crisis intervention is a "one-shot" form of therapy.	Crisis intervention often has the continuity and follow-through of two to eight sessions during a period when the person is open to help.
Crisis intervention is a form of therapy practiced only by paraprofessionals.	Crisis intervention has become respected and practiced by extensively trained as well as lay professionals. Crisis theory has its roots in psychoanalytic and ego psychology; however, crisis theory and intervention is vastly different from long-term, analytic-oriented therapy.
Crisis intervention represents only a "holding action" until longer-term therapy can begin.	Crisis intervention may be the treatment of choice, especially for persons whose precrisis level of functioning is productive.
Crisis intervention is effective only for primary prevention programs.	Crisis intervention is applicable in primary, secondary, and tertiary programs.
Crisis intervention does not produce lasting change.	Crisis intervention has been shown effective in preventing future crises.
Crisis intervention requires no special skills for the therapist.	Crisis intervention includes responses not typical of other therapies.

Swanson, 1984.

TABLE 7-6
Other Models of Crisis Intervention

MODEL	DESCRIPTION	EXAMPLE
Environmental crisis intervention	Manipulating the client's environment to provide a chance to reorganize in an environment of less stress.	Moving a family from unsafe quarters after a flood. Providing shelter to a battered wife.
Generic crisis intervention	Teaching clients to weather a change by using material or strategies shown helpful to others in similar situations.	Teaching classes for new mothers.
Network development	Helping clients connect with others who can help prevent crisis or facilitate resolution of crisis in progress.	Leading a discussion of family members in an ICU waiting room.
Debriefing (See Chapter 42)	A psychologic and educational group discussion immediately following a critical incident that has potential to evoke a crisis response.	Debriefing a group of staff nurses following an assault of a co-worker.

Swanson, 1984.

EVALUATION

There are two ways of evaluating crisis intervention. The first is to determine whether the crisis has been resolved and the client returned to a precrisis, or perhaps a higher, level of functioning. The second is to determine whether similar hazardous events lead the client back into crisis, or whether the client handles the event using strength, skills, and coping obtained through the crisis intervention (Swanson, 1984).

REFERENCES

Caplan, G. (1964). *Principles of Preventive Psychiatry.* St. Louis: C. V. Mosby.

Hansell, N. (1976). *The Person in Distress: On the Biosocial Dynamics of Adaptation.* New York: Human Sciences Press.

Swanson, A. R. (1984). Crisis intervention. In S. Lego (ed.), *The American Handbook of Psychiatric Nursing* (pp. 235–240). Philadelphia: J. B. Lippincott.

BIBLIOGRAPHY

Coler, M. S., & Hafner, L. P. (1991). An intercultural assessment of the type, intensity and number of crisis precipitating factors in three cultures: United States, Brazil and Taiwan. *International Journal of Nursing Studies, 28,* 223–235.

Erikson, K. (1994). *A New Species of Trouble: Explorations in Disaster, Trauma, and Community.* New York: W. W. Norton.

Evans, J. V. (1993). Crisis, grief and loss. *Canadian Nurse, 89* (8), 40–43.

Hayes, G., Goodwin, T., & Miars, B. (1990). After a disaster: A crisis support team at work. *American Journal of Nursing, 90,* 61–64.

Puskar, K. R., & Obus, N. L. (1989). Management of the psychiatric emergency. *Nurse Practitioner: American Journal of Primary Health Care, 17* (7), 9–10.

Rew, L., Agor, W., Emery, M. R., & Harper, S. C. (1991). Intuitive skills in crisis management. *Nursing Connections, 4* (2), 3–12.

Rosenzweig, L. (1992). Psychiatric triage: A cost-effective approach to quality management in mental health. *Journal of Psychosocial Nursing and Mental Health Services, 30* (6), 5–8.

Shires, B., & Tappan, T. (1992). The clinical nurse specialist as brief psychotherapist. *Perspectives in Psychiatric Care, 28* (4), 15–18.

Stanley, S. R. (1990). When the disaster is over: Helping the healers to mend. *Journal of Psychosocial Nursing and Mental Health Services, 28* (5), 12–16.

Whoolley, N. (1990). Crisis theory: A paradigm of effective intervention with families of critically ill people. *Journal of Advanced Nursing, 15,* 1402–1408.

8
EIGHT

Individual Therapy with Children

Donna A. Gaffney

OVERVIEW:

Introduction
Qualifications and Preparation of the
    Therapist
Settings
Assessment
Goals

Developmental and Therapeutic
    Functions of Play
Techniques
Countertransference
Evaluation

INTRODUCTION

Children who are coping with stress or crises in their lives often require time to understand and work through these potentially traumatizing experiences. The therapeutic relationship provides children with the opportunity and the means to express thoughts and feelings, facilitating optimal psychological and emotional growth. Therapy also provides time for children to gain a sense of control as they test strategies and learn new skills.

QUALIFICATIONS AND PREPARATION OF THE THERAPIST

The nurse who provides child psychotherapy possesses:
1. Theoretical and experiential knowledge of child development: cognitive, emotional, moral, spiritual, and physical
2. Assessment and evaluation skills in child psychiatric–mental health nursing
3. Knowledge of cultural differences and family development
4. Theoretical and clinical expertise in the therapeutic use of self in establishing and maintaining a therapeutic clinician–child relationship
5. Knowledge of various therapeutic modalities: play, games, activities, art, story-telling, bibliotherapy, drama (puppets or role-play), and one-to-one interviewing
6. Awareness of the clinician's responsibility as an advocate and activist for children and families on local, regional, and national levels
7. Realization of transference and countertransference and their impact on treatment
8. Certification as a child and adolescent clinical specialist in psychiatric–mental health nursing

SETTINGS   Individual therapy with children may take place in:
1. Inpatient and outpatient psychiatric facilities
2. Schools and school-based clinics
3. Pediatric units in hospitals and children's hospitals
4. Private practice
5. Community-based programs (social and service)

ASSESSMENT   See Box 8-1 for the overall assessment and Box 8-2 for questions to ask the child. These questions need not be asked in the order in which they appear.

GOALS   The goals of individual therapy with children include:
1. Identification of interaction of developmental issues and crisis/stress issues in the child's life
2. Recognition of the child's challenges, assets, and liabilities
3. Use of various developmentally appropriate therapeutic modalities to address process, content, and themes
4. Promotion of optimal functioning and growth-promoting behaviors

DEVELOPMENTAL   Play is used (Welt, 1984, pp. 244–245):
AND THERAPEUTIC   1. To work out problematic experiences
FUNCTIONS OF PLAY   2. To learn about interpersonal relations
3. To learn to compete, cooperate, and collaborate
4. To assimilate and gain mastery over unpleasant and new experiences
5. To learn about the culture
6. To act out an uncomfortable emotion symbolically or gradually enough so ultimately it can be felt
7. To represent an absent object—people or things
8. To represent an observation of a part of the external world
9. To represent an observation of a situation in the external world
10. To represent the internal world—a thought or a feeling, a wish, an attitude
11. To accommodate to reality
12. To organize experience privately and with others
13. To develop the capacity to gratify oneself and to delay gratification
14. As an expression of cognitive status
15. As a contributor to the character of cognition
16. As a bridge between concrete experience and abstract thought
17. As a creative act

TECHNIQUES   1. *Engagement:* Connect with the child in developmentally appropriate ways while recognizing the issues bringing the child into therapy.

Toddler/Preschooler: Use physical reassurance as children explore the new environment, remain in close proximity, sitting in a chair not standing above the children's height, not approaching physical contact until children initiate first, usually regarding the mechanics of a toy or activity. Communication should be sensitive and consistent with the children's experiences.

BOX 8-1: Essentials of Child Assessment

Problem/Reason for Referral
- Who referred child?
- What was precipitating event? Chronology?
- How long prior to initial session did event occur?
- What are specific parameters of problem?
  — Intensity, frequency, precipitants, involvement of others
  — Specific behaviors, responses of others

Family/Child History—Use detailed genogram (See Chapter 6)
- Roles, relationships, communication styles
- Cultural, religious observances
- Previous mental illness, psychiatric illness, crisis, losses
- Significant illness/health events/sleep patterns
- Parental childhood experiences

Developmental History
- Cognitive stage assessment/school performance
- Emotional stage assessment
- Play patterns
- Significant prenatal, birth, physical events

Environmental Changes/Events
- Personal changes (death in the family, separation or divorce, relocation to a new area, change of schools)
- Personal violation (abuse, violence, accidents, theft)
- Community influences (violence, disaster, isolation)
- National/internal influences (war, violence, disaster)

Emotional Assessment
- Mood, affect, responses to stressful events
- Interactions with others
- Maturity
  — Responsibility for self
  — Help-seeking behaviors
  — Health-seeking behaviors

Mental Status Exam (West & Evans, 1992)
- Appearance
- Speech quality/pattern
- Defenses
- Attitude
- Perceptions
- Creativity/fantasy
- Mood lability
- Motor activity (hypoactivity, hyperactivity)
- Thought patterns (content, age appropriate)
- Coping skills
- Sensory status

Note: Comprehensive assessment of the child and family should span several sessions. Data are best obtained through semistructured, open interviews. This allows the child time to acclimate to the therapeutic process and become more comfortable with the therapist. Family data can be obtained through separate family interviews, telephone consultation, and input from other significant adults (teachers, coaches, neighbors).

BOX 8-2: Interpersonal/Emotional Life Questionnaire for Children

1. If you could have three magic wishes, what would they be?

2. What is your ambition when you grow up?

3. Do you ever think about what it would be like to leave home?

4. What would you do with $1? With $100?

5. What is the best thing that has happened to you?

6. What is the best thing that could happen to you?

7. What is the worst thing that has happened to you?

8. What is the worst thing that could happen to you?

9. What is the thing you like best about kids?

10. What is the thing you would like to change about kids?

11. What is the thing you like best about adults?

12. What is the thing you would like to change about adults?

13. What is the thing you like best about yourself?

14. What is the thing you would like to change about yourself?

15. If you could be an animal, which one would you like to be?

16. What animal would you never want to be?

17. When do you get angry? How do you show it?

18. When do you get sad? How do you show it?

19. When do you get happy? How do you show it?

20. When do you get nervous? How do you show it?

21. When do you get upset? How do yo show it?

22. What are you afraid of?

23. Who is your best friend? What do you like about him or her? What do you dislike about him or her?

24. What do you and your friends do together?

25. Are you on any teams? In any clubs?

26. What would you say are some problems you have with your sisters or brothers?

27. What would you say are some problems you have with your mother?

28. What would you say are some problems you have with your father?

29. If you could change your life, what would you have it be?

Welt, 1984, p. 243.

Latency, early: Invite children into the room and tell them to look around and touch or explore anything they wish. Offer to answer any questions while also asking how they came to see the therapist. Acknowledge that "first times" are often confusing.

Latency, later: Invite children to enter the therapist's office and to choose any place they'd like to sit. Offer any of the materials in the room to explore or the option of asking the therapist questions. Address confidentiality in a brief but reassuring manner.

Preadolescence: Be patient and sensitive to fears or preconceived ideas. Ask the child: "Tell me the reason you think you are here." Explain the structure of the therapy session. Reinforce the idea that what is said to the therapist is confidential and information will only be shared with people chosen by the child.

2. *Observation:* Study the children's actions and words and maintain active listening as they engage in their communication and play activities. These interventions do not require verbal communication with the child or proximity to the child. Supportive eye contact may be all that is necessary to convey a sense that the office is a safe and nonjudgmental environment.

3. *Guidance:* When using play materials and activities, literature or games, provide minimal directions and brief suggestions for the use of material. (See Boxes 8-3 and 8-4 for suggestions about play and activity tools.) The use of play materials is not intended to replace therapeutic communication but facilitate it. The younger the child, the more the therapist may have to interpret the meaning of play behaviors. Choice of materials should be made by the child.

> "What would you like to do today?"
> "Why don't you look around? You can chose anything you like."

The therapist keeps all materials at eye level so they are easy to remove from shelves or cabinets. Any equipment with small pieces is kept in transparent or labeled containers.

BOX 8-3: Building a Playroom

Tools for Provocative Play

Activities	Optimal Ages
Art:	**3 to 11**
paper (white, colored)	
finger paints	
tempera paints	
brushes	
sponges	
scissors	
clay, play dough	
crayons, pencils	
Imagination/Pretend:	**4 to 12**
doll house, furniture, family	
miniatures (food, birthday cake, cleaning tools, books)	
telephone	
lock box	
"Felt Faces"	
Dramatic:	**3 to 10**
stage	
puppets	
costumes/props	
stuffed animals	
Puzzles/Games:	**all ages**
checkers	
tic-tac-toe	
The Storytelling Game (Richard Gardner copyright 1988)	
The Talking, Feeling, and Doing Game (Richard Gardner copyright 1973)	
Books:	**all ages**
children's literature (featuring heros or heroines)	

BOX 8-4: Special Additions and Adaptations of Play Equipment for the Playroom

Doll House	Unlike manufactured doll houses these houses can be viewed from two sides. Any four-sided box creates a room. Wallpaper, wrapping paper, and self-stick paper add the finishing touches. Boxes can be placed vertically or horizontally (an "apartment" or a "suburban home"). The therapist has a clear view of the children's faces as they play. Boxes are available from wine sellers, unpainted furniture stores, and lumber yards. Rooms should be 12" H x 12" W x 8" D. Children can participate in the construction of the house as well.
Library	Avoid stocking your library with "advisement" books. These are brief stories that make the problem the center of the story, as opposed to children's literature, which centers on the lives of the characters who encounter various problems. Consult with children's librarians, the American Library Association, or booksellers. Use *The Horn Book* or *Book Links* to become familiar with the newest children's books. Read them first. (See Chapter 9 for a list of children's books.)
Lock Box	A wooden box with compartments and doors that latch/lock. Children may use it to keep "secrets." A wooden box with a key will also serve the same propose. A lock box is available at The Children's General Store.
Felt Faces	Use wooden paddles (similar to the type with rubber band and rubber ball) and cover with felt. Create felt facial smiles, frowns, eyes, etc. As they are removable, the young child can change the facial expressions.

Other Equipment and Suppliers

Moody Bear	A wooden puzzle (boy or girl) with changeable faces and clothes (Schylling Associates, P.O. Box 667, Ipswich, MA 01938).
Tabletop Theater	Wooden theater facade comes with hand-held stick puppets (Rhyme & Reason, 184 Kinsley Avenue, Providence, RI 02903).
Worry Dolls	Soft fabric dolls, 1½" high, multicultural.
	(All above are available from The Children's General Store, 2473 Broadway, New York, NY 10025.)
Decor	An entire room or portion of an office can be used. Use neutral warm tones, carpeting, artwork hung at eye level, a bulletin board, folders for each child to store paintings, etc.
Food	An apothecary jar filled with pretzels. A water cooler with small paper cups.

4. *Exploration:* Use probing statements and open-ended questions to further illuminate issues occurring in the child's life.

> "You are scrubbing the dollhouse floor so much, I wonder, does that happen in your home too?"

> "Tell me what is happening in your picture:
> > Who are the people?
> > What are their names?
> > What are they doing?
> > What are they saying to each other?
> > What do you think will happen next?

> "You said you really don't like your teacher. Tell me more about that."

5. *Interpretation:* Listen to the child's descriptions of feelings, thoughts, and actions and elucidate when appropriate.

"You are crying. Tell me what you are thinking about."

"It seems as if you and your friend had a really big fight. Was that the first time?"

"Tell me another time you had this same feeling."

6. *Validation:* When children connect thoughts and feelings to the situations causing them the most difficulty in their lives, the therapist confirms this information with the children.

"It sounds like you are very angry that your dad is not living with you anymore."

"I hear some sadness in your voice when you talk about your friend."

"You begin to cry when you talk about your brother."

7. *Reframing resistance:* When the therapist recognizes resistant behaviors (lateness, acting out, etc.), intervention must be accomplished in a nonthreatening manner. For older children this can be verbally addressed.

"It must be difficult to be here."

"You'd probably rather be somewhere else right now."

"Sometimes new experiences are tough to get used to."

8. *Empowerment:* Encourage the children to identify or suggest ways of approaching people or problems in their lives. The therapist lets the children know that they are not only capable of talking about feelings but can resolve the issue as well.

"What could you do if this happens again?"

"Is there any other way you could tell your mom how you feel?"

"What would you like to do in this situation?"

COUNTER-TRANSFERENCE

Countertransference may take the form of (Welt, 1984, p. 248):

1. Overidentification with the child
2. Competition with the parents
3. Competition with the child; the need to be "right"; the need to win or the need to lose
4. Hatred, anger, and disgust, and defenses against these feelings
5. Overconcern about the child's "productions"
6. Too much or too little limit setting regarding play behavior: cheating, hitting, breaking, spitting, changing game rules
7. Engaging in power struggles with children to "straighten them out"
8. Engaging in power struggles with the parents to "straighten them out" (actually or in fantasy)
9. Control of the child: fear of parental anger and disapproval or fear of the child's anger and disapproval
10. Control of the child through interpretation of behavior
11. Control of the child through control of the direction of the session: lack of therapist–child resonance

12. Control of the child through control of the child's direction or vehicle of expression: fear of the child's loss of control
13. Intrusiveness: lack of respect for the child's needs and desires
14. Emotional detachment: lack of therapist–child resonance or anxiety about the "nonintellectual" approach
15. Feeling fraudulent: anxiety about the "nonintellectual" approach

Countertransference reactions are not necessarily detrimental to treatment, especially those reactions induced by the child rather than the therapist's unconscious reactions.

EVALUATION

The child is evaluated as therapy progresses, through behavior in the play therapy and reports about school and home behavior. When it appears the child has resolved the problems and conflicts that prompted therapy, termination is planned. In a schedule decided on by the child and therapist, the therapy is tapered off until the child no longer wants the contact (Welt, 1984).

REFERENCES

Welt, S. R. (1984). Individual therapy with children. In S. Lego (ed.), *American Handbook of Psychiatric Nursing* (pp. 241–250). Philadelphia: J. B. Lippincott.

West, P., & Evans, C. (1992). *Psychiatric Mental Health Nursing with Children and Adolescents*. Gaithersburg, MD: Aspen Publications.

BIBLIOGRAPHY

Brown, D. T., & Prout H. T. (1990). *Counseling and Psychotherapy with Children and Adolescents* (2nd ed.). Brandon, VT: Clinical Psychology Publishing Co.

Chethik, M. (1990). *Techniques of Child Therapy*. New York: The Guilford Press.

Clunn, P. (1991). Child psychotherapy and play therapy. In P. Clunn (ed.), *Child Psychiatric Nursing* (pp. 396–418). St. Louis: Mosby.

9
NINE

Group Therapy with Children

Donna A. Gaffney

OVERVIEW:

Introduction
Purpose
Leadership
Types of Groups
Working with Parents and Teachers
Transference and Countertransference

Problems and Strategies
Bibliotherapy
Theme-Centered Groups
Development of a Group Therapy
    Proposal
Evaluation

INTRODUCTION

The clinician who is working with children in groups must address the key concepts of child development, group dynamics, and the various types of psychotherapy groups appropriate to children's problems and needs. The clinician's selection of group type is dependent on the mental health, development, situational, and emotional needs of children as they relate to the group experience.

PURPOSE

Group therapy provides a secure therapeutic environment for:
1. The expression and maturation of developmental turning points
2. The expansion and enhancement of growth-promoting coping skills in children who face excessive stressors in family, school, and social arenas
3. The identification of actual or potential psychopathology
4. Playing out relationship problems outside of school, family, and social settings
5. A shared experience with other children who are undergoing similar special situations and challenges

LEADERSHIP

The group therapist must be able to:
1. Identify the developmental phases of a psychotherapy group
2. Develop a contract with children regarding group behavior (see Box 9-1 for a sample contract)
3. Recognize and intervene appropriately when the following occur:
   - Transference
   - Subgrouping

BOX 9-1: A Sample "Contract" with Second-Grade Children

Our Rules

1. No hurting each other.
2. No eating or drinking in the group.
3. Don't speak when someone else is speaking.
4. Have respect for each other.
5. No fighting.
6. Treat others as you want to be treated.
7. Go to the bathroom and get a drink of water before or after group, not during.
8. Group meets from 1:30 to 2:15 P.M.

Members: (list of names)

Signatures:

- Resistance
- Acting out
4. Recognize group process and cohesion
5. Integrate developmental needs with group process
6. Establish working relationships with administrators, parents, and teachers
7. Comfortably use several leadership styles:
   - Supportive
   - Limit-setting
   - Interpretive
   - Role-modeling
8. Seek supervision and guidance with a qualified professional to discuss:
   - Countertransference
   - Technique clarification and development
   - Problematic members

Table 9-1 shows the ages of children, developmental needs, types of groups, and leader goals in therapy groups. Table 9-2 shows the phases of development in group therapy with children, behaviors in each phase, and leadership approaches.

TYPES OF GROUPS

Discussion Groups: The focus in the group is on the verbal and nonverbal exchange between the members. Older children are better suited to this situation. The leader facilitates discussion, interprets content, and helps the participants renew relationships with each other.

Play Therapy Groups: These groups are most effective for younger children who rely on play materials and tools to express their concerns. Toys that stimulate imagination, identification, and imitation are most appropriate. The therapist structures the sessions to provide a stimulating environment that will help children work through their conflicts.

TABLE 9-1
Age of Children, Developmental Behavior, Types of Groups, and Leader Goals in Group Therapy

AGE RANGE	DEVELOPMENTAL BEHAVIOR	TYPES OF GROUPS	LEADER GOALS
2–3 years— Toddler	Parallel play, limited comprehension of language.	Play and simple activity.	Facilitation of shared and singular play activities, assessment.
4–5 years— Preschooler	Developing fine motor skills. Capacity for shared imaginary play, increased attention span, and identification with others.	Play, activity, story-telling, primitive art techniques (finger painting, etc.).	Observation and assessment of behaviors, selection of stories, organization of play materials. Begins to address verbalized issues.
6–8 years— Early Latency	Competition and cooperation, need for structure and rules, group roles begin to emerge.	Activity, games, role-play, story telling, art activities (painting, sculpture), primitive discussion.	Assessment, helps group structure rules, provides appropriate games and activities.
9–12 years— Latency	Ability to learn about others and approaches to special needs and situations, social group becomes very important, group cohesion and roles evident.	Activity, art therapy, bibliotherapy, discussion, role-play (drama), psychoeducational, "natural" group of classroom.	Assessment, sets limits and helps group establish rules, role model for communication skills, points out process and relationship issues.

TABLE 9-2
Phases of Development in Group Therapy with Children

PHASE	BEHAVIORS OF CHILDREN	LEADERSHIP APPROACHES
Beginning	Some acting out or hyperactivity. Missed sessions, subgrouping or other attention-getting behaviors.	Gentle reminders of purpose of group and limit-setting, consistency, and support. Role-modeling.
Working	Increased communication in group, establishment and adherence to contract rules. Empathetic and supportive responses to each other.	Facilitates relationships in group, confronts and interprets as necessary. Points out problem-solving approaches useful to others in group.
Termination	Members begin to ask when "the last time" will occur. Request to continue or extend group. Plan a party for the last day. Content may focus on other times of separation.	Reminds group of the last day 3 weeks in advance. Interprets request for extension and facilitates discussion of their own feelings regarding termination. Allows for some "celebration" of the work the group has accomplished but not to exclude or diminish "goodbyes."

Activity Groups (Art Therapy):   Activities include art projects, dramatic play, games, and structured experiences. In some cases music, movement, or dance techniques are also used. The therapist should be skilled in the techniques being used in the group.

Social Skills Training Groups: Children who have difficulty negotiating social situations and often find themselves in conflict with significant adults or peers are most appropriate for this type of group. The therapist provides activities and a safe environment to "practice" skills used in the outside world. Conflict resolution and skills of negotiation are often the focus of social skills training groups.

WORKING WITH PARENTS AND TEACHERS

Forming an alliance with significant adults in the child's life is imperative for the long-term success of the group. Establishing a working relationship with administrators and teachers in school settings provides a foundation for their continued support of group work. Ongoing information sessions can be provided without compromising the confidentiality of the group members. Through weekly contact the therapist can demonstrate to the administrators concern and involvement in the larger system as well as provide a comfortable forum for communication. Parents also require contact from the therapist as they are eager to know the group therapy is helping their children. Reassurance that they have made wise choices by bringing their child to group is supportive for both parent and child.

TRANSFERENCE AND COUNTER-TRANSFERENCE

The primary issues of transference and countertransference with children individually and in groups center around nurturing and parenting. Parents may view the therapist as a parent substitute who in some ways is perceived as "better" than the natural parent. Children also view the therapist as a "parent" and, in fact, may even call the therapist "Mom" or "Dad." The child group member may cling to or hold hands with the therapist and in the group there is often "jockeying" for position next to the therapist. The therapist acknowledges the child's behavior in a positive way but also clearly establishes that theirs is not a parent–child relationship.

PROBLEMS AND STRATEGIES

Destructive Behavior: Occasionally the therapist will have to remove or exclude certain children from the group. For example, these children may exhibit behaviors that would be destructive to the entire group (violent behaviors, foul language, arguing with the leader, leaving the room). If the therapist must spend a great amount of the time attempting to control the behaviors of the child, then it is time to consider removing the participant from the group. The therapist should not focus on the negative activity—"Don't run around the room while we are having group"—but on the desired behaviors—"Everyone needs to be seated before we can begin." The therapist must adequately prepare the child for the consequences of destructive behaviors. The child should be told very specifically what they are: "If you cannot follow the rules of our group, you will not be able to come anymore. If you can continue to follow the rules the group has made, you can continue to be a part of it. If you do not choose to follow the rules, you will not be a member of the group anymore. We will see how things go this week." It is best to talk to the child individually since the acting-out behavior may be an effort to pull the leader away from the rest of the group. The other members will most likely be aware of the situation and will be watching to see if the leader can resolve the difficulty.

Withdrawn and Silent Members: Children often do not speak in early sessions. Rather than address any one child's nonparticipation in the group, the leader refers to nonparticipation as an occurrence with which other group members can help: "Do you think all of the members feel this way? I'm not sure we've heard everyone in the group." The therapist's nonverbal behavior is critical here. Looking around the group as a whole will not put any one child "on the spot."

Violent or Aggressive Behavior: Children who hit or in any way compromise the safety of group members must be dealt with quickly and firmly. Clear limit-setting with consequences for bad behavior is imperative. Throwing or breaking equipment, toys, or art materials is destructive to the group and threatening to the participants. Removing the materials from the child and encouraging group response and sanctions should be encouraged: "In our contract we talked about no breaking or hurting anything. What do you think about what has happened here? What can we do?"

Overactive Members: Children who are anxious may become restless, fidget in their seats, wander around the room, or become very talkative. In addition to gentle limit-setting, the leader encourages the group to respond to this member's behavior and assesses if there is a particular stressor influencing the child. The leader points out to the group that using words instead of actions helps others understand what is going on with the overactive participant. However, the leader should realize that younger children may be incapable of articulating their concerns.

Outside Objects and Clothing: Children sometimes bring books, toys, and outer clothing to the group session. The therapist can explain that there are materials that are used during the group sessions and items that are from home or school. A separate area for these objects will aid in setting boundaries for the participants. For younger children the need to "show and tell" may be very strong. Early school-age children like to "share" parts of their lives with classmates, allowing bonding with their peers. The group leader can structure a separate time focusing on "telling" more than "showing." The group leader may want to set aside time at the beginning of each session for the sharing experience.

Subgrouping: Children who are latency age and who may know each other prior to the group experience bring a natural bond to the group. There will be a tendency to form a tight unit and share words and secretive nonverbal responses with each other. Pointing this behavior out to group members in a nonthreatening way encourages others to respond as well. The therapist may address this issue early in the group work: "Some of you may know each other from (class, your neighborhood, the unit). In the beginning it's nice to have friends here but we will all get to know each other in a few weeks." Actually identifying who the friendship dyads are during group is useful for the therapist and the other children.

BIBLIOTHERAPY

Description: This approach uses the successes of fictional heroes/heroines in children's literature as a focal point for group sessions with children in the early elementary school grades (3rd, 4th, 5th). More than a book review or a reading group, this experience provides an opportunity for children to express feelings and identify the roles of the characters they learn about in stories. Selection of the literature is based on prior analysis and evaluation of stories by the therapist and experts in the field of children's books (librarians, booksellers, and specialized journals). It is important to select and thoroughly evaluate each book. Group leaders should particularly focus on the published works portraying children as effective, competent problem-solvers who are confronted with difficult circumstances such as loss, separation, illness, and family conflict. The ideal protagonist not only copes in an exemplary manner but is capable of mobilizing the actions of others.

Children Who May Benefit: These groups are often used for children undergoing loss, separation, or extreme stress, e.g., following a natural disaster, or children with parents and siblings who are HIV-positive (Lovrin, 1995), children living in abusive or otherwise dangerous settings, etc.

Appropriate Books:
1. Books drawn from the lists of the American Library Association (the Newberry Award) and *Horn Book Magazine* and the Coretta Scott King Awards. See Box 9-2.
2. Books usually quite popular with teachers, critics, librarians, and bookstore owners. Avoid the so-called "advice" books; these tend to make the problem the focal point of the story. Carefully review books that are part of a popular series. These should be saved for fun and enjoyment.

BOX 9-2: Suggested Books for Bibliotherapy

Recommended for Girls

Fenner, C. (1978). *The Skates of Uncle Richard.* New York: Random House.

Lowry, L. (1990). *Number the Stars.* New York: Houghton.

MacLachlan, P. (1986). *Sarah, Plain and Tall.* New York: Zolotow/Harper.

Mohr, N. (1989). *Felita.* New York: Scholastic Books.

Paterson, K. (1978). *Bridge to Terabithia.* New York: Crowell.

Rylant, C. (1993). *Missing May.* New York: Jackson/Orchard.

Taylor, M. (1977). *Roll of Thunder, Hear My Cry.* New York: Dial.

Voight, C. (1983). *Dicey's Song.* New York: Atheneum.

Recommended for Boys

Bauer, M. (1987). *On My Honor.* New York: Clarion.

Brooks, B. (1985). *The Moves Make the Man.* New York: Harper.

Brooks, B. (1993). *What Hearts.* New York: Harper Collins.

Cleary, B. (1984). *Dear Mr. Henshaw.* New York: Morrow.

Conly, J. (1994). *Crazy Lady.* New York: Harper Collins.

Fox, P. (1985). *One Eyed Cat.* New York: Bradbury.

Meyers, W. (1993). *Somewhere in the Darkness.* New York: Scholastic.

Naylor, P. (1992). *Shiloh.* New York: Atheneum.

Paterson, K. (1978). *Bridge to Terabithia.* New York: Crowell.

Reviewing Books: Analysis of the book being reviewed should include:
1. Identification of the conflicts and issues confronting the main character
2. Support systems
3. Coping skills
4. Relationships
5. Behaviors
6. Outcomes or resolution of the situation or problems

Goals of the Group: Through the vicarious experiences of fictional characters and group process children will:
1. Explore their own coping skills
2. Share the conflicts and problems facing their fictional counterparts
3. Learn how to successfully navigate relationships using assertiveness and honesty

4. Examine their own problem-solving skills in relationship to approaches used by characters in the stories

5. Validate their own growth-promoting behaviors when dealing with conflict in everyday life

6. Establish empathetic relationships with other group members

Setting: Groups are most appropriately situated in school settings. Forty-five- to 55-minute sessions can be planned during the school day or even in after-school programs. Other community settings such as girls' clubs, scouting groups, libraries, community centers, and mental health settings can also be used.

Implementation: The program can take place throughout the calendar year or follow the academic schedule. The therapist will:

1. Meet with the administration of the agency or school

2. Work with teachers or guidance counselors to select children who can benefit from the group

3. Send permission/consent forms to parents and guardians indicating that:
   - Weekly group meetings will be held
   - Groups will be led by a qualified mental health professional
   - A total of four to six books will be read over the course of the year
   - The children will keep the books for their own libraries
   - Children will discuss the stories and the characters in the books

4. Select the books

5. Maintain a working relationship with the school or agency administration

The Role of the Therapist in Group Sessions: The group leader must recognize that while the setting may take place in an educational institution the groups are not library or reading sessions. The group leader functions as a "story teller" during the group sessions. Reading out loud and story-telling enhance the therapeutic process by:

1. Increasing participant response and attention

2. Decreasing anxiety and competition over reading skills

3. Allowing the therapist to use provocative passages to stimulate process

The children will establish their own contract for behavior in their group sessions. Participation is not rewarded or penalized through the student's academic record. The children keep personal journals where they can write their thoughts, feelings, and words or language they do not understand in the book. While reading outside of the group is encouraged, it is not required. Group discussions address themes in the books and applicability to personal situations in the lives of each of the participants. Each group meeting can be transcribed or taped and the data discussed with the clinical supervisor.

Evaluation: Evaluation for the group is best accomplished through assessment of participant feedback, responses of teachers, and parent communication.

THEME-CENTERED GROUPS

In addition to the shared experience of accomplishing developmental milestones, children may also have special needs related to crisis situations in their own lives. The therapist can organize groups for children with similar life occurrences. However, to enhance mutual support and understanding, the age range of participants should be limited to 12–18 months. These groups can be ongoing in nature as children may need to rejoin the groups at various times. Theme-centered groups might include the following.

Loss/Bereavement: Categorization of types of loss may be necessary: parental loss versus sibling loss; sudden death versus long-term illness. These groups may be most effective if established in a time-limited framework (6–8 weeks) with follow-up groups for those in later stages of bereavement.

Chronic Illness: Children who have chronic illnesses may benefit from sharing their experiences and problem-solving strategies with each other. The hospital or clinic provides a natural setting to bring the members together.

Sibling Groups: Children who have siblings with special situations (illness, substance abuse, etc.) need a forum to talk about their feelings. These concerns are usually not verbalized to parents who may be too emotionally or physically involved with the sibling. Competition, jealousy, fear, and anxiety often arise in these groups.

Children of Substance-Abusing or Mentally Ill Family Members: Children who have mental illness, alcoholism, or substance abuse within their families need to have their own fears addressed in a shared experience. There is often a need for education and reinforcement of treatment approaches. Anger, fear, worry, and distancing from the family unit are not uncommon for these children.

Children of Divorce and Separation: Parents who are divorcing or separating need to consider the needs of their children. Talking with others who are in similar situations helps the group participants understand that their differences with other families are not insurmountable. Parental competition, custody, and geographic changes in the family are important concerns for the therapist to note.

Children Who Have a Family Member with HIV/AIDS: Perhaps the greatest support the therapist can provide to children who are confronted with HIV/AIDS in their lives is to allow them a sense of competency and connectedness to others. For this reason, long-term group work may be the most effective approach. After-school programs incorporating discussion time, recreational and other activity therapies provide support for these children.

DEVELOPMENT OF A GROUP THERAPY PROPOSAL

Table 9-3 provides a guide for developing a plan or proposal for a children's therapy group.

TABLE 9-3
Developing a Plan and Proposal for a Children's Therapy Group

PROPOSAL COMPONENT	CONTENT
Overview of Group	Describe: • Type of group • Purpose • Time, dates • Number of sessions • Place • Number of members • Population characteristics • Leadership person

TABLE 9-3 *(continued)*

PROPOSAL COMPONENT	CONTENT
Needs Assessment	Identify the reason or rationale for implementing groups for children: • Community needs • Individual needs • Shared event/situation • Systems needs • Theoretical rationale Integrate relevant literature
Goals of Group	Provide measurable, behavioral outcomes for participants, personnel, systems: • Outcomes may be translated into cost benefits • Include goals: succinct and limited to 4–5
Structure of System (Agency)	Demonstrate how the group will interface with other therapeutic modalities in system
Agency/Community Population	Describe children in the community: • Developmental characteristics • Family characteristics • School characteristics • Free lunch program participation • Pregnancy rates • Socioeconomic statistics
Developmental Needs of Participants	Describe physical, psychosocial, cognitive characteristics of participants and how those characteristics will be addressed in the group
Possible Problems/Issues	Identify and describe anticipated problems implementing the group: • Administration • Group process • Population
Supervisory/Leadership Issues	Indicate who will lead the group, who will provide supervision, and the scheduling of supervisory sessions
Documentation	Describe how the group work will be recorded—by audio, video, or written records
Evaluation	Identify the process to be used for evaluation of group effectiveness: • Written instrument • Participant report • System outcomes Identify outcomes
Appendices	Include letters to participants/families Letter to agency administrator Necessary materials: • Books • Play equipment/materials Bibliography Personnel qualifications

EVALUATION

Group therapy with children is considered successful when:
1. Symptoms subside.
2. School performance improves.
3. The child relates well to peers.

REFERENCES

Lovrin, M. (1995). Interpersonal support among 8-year-old girls who have lost parents or siblings to AIDS. *Archives of Psychiatric Nursing 9* (2), 92–98.

BIBLIOGRAPHY

Charach, R. (1983, July). Brief interpretive group psychotherapy with early latency-age children. *International Journal of Group Psychotherapy, 33* (3), 349–364.

Clifford, M. W. (1991). A model for group therapy with latency-age boys. Special Issue: Child and adolescent group psychotherapy. *Group, 15* (2), 116–124.

Corder, B. F., Haizlip, T., & DeBoer, P. (1990). A pilot study for a structured, time-limited therapy group for sexually abused preadolescent children. *Child Abuse and Neglect, 14* (2), 243–251.

Critchley, D. L. (1982, April–June). Therapeutic group work with abused preschool children. *Perspectives in Psychiatric Care, 20* (2), 79–85.

Kitchur, M., & Bell, R. (1989). Group psychotherapy with preadolescent sexual abuse victims: Literature review and description of an inner-city group. *International Journal of Group Psychotherapy, 39* (Special Issue), 285–310.

Krietemeyer, B. C., & Heiney, S. P. (1992). Storytelling as a therapeutic technique in a group for school-aged oncology patients. *Children's Health Care, 21* (1), 14–20.

Mallery, B., & Navas, M. (1983). Engagement of preadolescent boys in group therapy: Videotape as a tool. *International Journal of Group Psychotherapy, 32* (4), 453–468.

Mosholder, A., Burke, W., & Carter, W. (1988). Insight-oriented group psychotherapy of latency-age children in an acute care setting. *Group, 12* (4), 226–232.

Pfeifer, G., et al. (1985). Continued individual and group psychotherapy with children: An ego development perspective. *International Journal of Group Psychotherapy, 35* (1), 11–35.

Reister, A. (ed.) (1986). *Child Group Psychotherapy: Future Tense.* New York: American Group Psychotherapy Association.

Rose, S. D., & Edelson, J. L. (1987). *Working with Children and Adolescents in Groups.* San Francisco: Jossey-Bass.

Schacht, A. F., Kerlinsky, D., & Carlson, C. (1990). Group therapy with sexually abused boys: Leadership, projective identification, and countertransference issues. *Journal of Group Psychotherapy, 36* (3), 447–469.

Schamess, G. (1992). Reflections on a developing body of group-as-a-whole theory for children's therapy groups: An introduction. *International Journal of Group Psychotherapy, 42* (3), 351–356.

Slavson, S. R., & Schiffer, M. (1975). *Group Psychotherapies for Children.* New York: International Universities Press.

van der Kolk, B. A. (1987). The role of the group in the origin and resolution of the trauma response. In B. A. van der Kolk (ed.), *Psychological Trauma* (pp. 153–171). Washington, DC: American Psychiatric Press.

Walsh, R. T., Richardson, M. A., & Cardey, R. M. (1991). Structured fantasy approaches to children's group therapy. Special Issue: Group work with suburbia's children: Difference, acceptance and belonging. *Social Work with Groups, 14* (1), 57–73.

The Bibliotherapy section refers to the Growing Heroes/Growing Heroines Program, New York, New York, created, designed, and coordinated by Donna A. Gaffney, and supported in part by the American Association of University Women Educational Foundation, Washington, DC.

10
TEN

Individual Therapy with Adolescents

Kathryn R. Puskar

OVERVIEW:

INTRODUCTION

With the problems of depression, suicide, violence, and drug abuse in adolescents, there is a concurrent need for mental health services, including individual psychotherapy. The prevalence of mood disorders in adolescents is 5% (Kaplan & Sadock, 1991). Psychiatric mental health nurses are in unique positions to provide psychotherapy to adolescents because of the nurse's knowledge of both biological and psychological aspects of adolescent development.

DEFINITION

Psychotherapy is defined as "a formally structured, contractual relationship between the therapist and client(s) for the explicit purpose of effecting change in the client system" (American Nurses Association, 1994). This approach attempts to treat mental disorders, alleviate emotional distress, reverse or change maladaptive behavior, and facilitate personal growth and development.

THE THERAPEUTIC CONTRACT

The therapeutic contract with the client is discussed in the first session, and includes purpose of the therapy, time, place, fees, confidentiality, and access to emergency after-hours help. To assure quality, the nurse continually scrutinizes the therapy sessions in relation to the content, process, and theoretical rationales for interventions.

Proficiency in psychotherapy is an outgrowth of specialized educational experience, efforts to refine psychotherapy skills through practice, continuing education, and the use of competent consultation with other psychotherapists. Consultation minimizes personal inferences on the part of the therapist, and enhances the therapist's competence in the conduct and evaluation of therapy.

SETTINGS

Advanced practice psychiatric nurses may conduct individual psychotherapy with adolescents in a variety of settings such as:

1. Outpatient clinics
2. Private offices
3. Group practice settings
4. Inpatient units
5. The client's home
6. School-based offices

QUALIFICATIONS OF THE THERAPIST

A psychiatric–mental health advanced practice nurse who conducts individual psychotherapy with adolescents:

1. Has a master's degree in psychiatric mental health nursing
2. Is nationally certified by the American Nurses Association either as an adult clinical specialist in psychiatric and mental health nursing or as a specialist in child and adolescent psychiatric mental health nursing

MYTHS ABOUT ADOLESCENTS

Two myths that can have a negative impact on the nurse's approach to therapy with adolescents are (Lewis, 1985, p. 36):

1. *Myth:* Adolescence is a time of turmoil, rebellion, and hostility toward parents.
   Fact: A moderate degree of rebelliousness may be characteristic of some adolescents, but the majority remain close to parents.
2. *Myth:* Adolescents have an extraordinary need for privacy such that a therapist's contact with a parent is likely to jeopardize the development of a therapeutic relationship.
   Fact: Most adolescents expect their parents to be involved in their treatment to at least some extent.

DEVELOPMENTAL TASKS OF ADOLESCENTS

Nurses must be knowledgeable about the developmental tasks of the adolescent phase of development. The theoretical base underpinning individual therapy with adolescents incorporates adolescent development (Lidz, 1968; Blos, 1979; Anthony, 1983; Erikson, 1963; Miller, 1983). Lidz (1968) identifies three tasks of adolescence:

1. To gain an ego identity
2. To gain independence
3. To become capable of intimacy

In the process of completing these tasks adolescents must:

1. Struggle between dependence and independence
2. Individuate from the family
3. Adjust to bodily changes
4. Develop a sexual identity

Owing to these tasks and changes, it is helpful for adults working with adolescents to ask at least three questions:

1. What is the teen likely to be feeling right now?
2. How has this feeling been modified by interviews with me and other authority figures in the past?
3. What are the adolescent expectations of the situation? How has the adolescent been told about them? What is his or her perception of the interview role? (Miller, 1983, p. 284)

PHASES OF THERAPY AND INTERVENTIONS

1. *Beginning phase*—Lasts from one to six sessions, and is a chance for the therapist and client to get acquainted. The therapist uses this phase to assess the client's problems and establish a beginning relationship. See Table 10-1 for nursing interventions, theoretical rationales, and examples.

2. *Middle phase*—Extends from the establishment of a firm or at least workable therapeutic alliance to the serious introduction of termination. It is the main phase of exploring, analyzing, working through, and resolving the adolescent's emotional symptoms. It is the heart of treatment and is the longest period of therapeutic work. See Table 10-2 for nursing interventions, theoretical rationales, and examples.

3. *Termination phase*—In the termination phase, the therapist attempts to bring closure to the therapy. A review of progress in therapy, a discussion of plans for the future, and the formal goodbye are aspects of termination. During this phase, the therapist may expect some regressive behavior as a reaction to the termination. Finally, a sharing of the experience of loss related to the ending of the relationship is reviewed by the nurse and the adolescent.

TABLE 10-1
Nursing Interventions, Theoretical Rationale, and Examples in the Beginning Phase of Individual Therapy with Adolescents

NURSING INTERVENTION	THEORETICAL RATIONALE	EXAMPLE
1. The nurse identifies the problem.	1. It is important to understand how the adolescent sees the problem, as opposed to parents or teacher.	1. "Peter, it sounds like you've been having a tough time at school. What's happening?"
2. The nurse takes a psychiatric history, developmental history, and does a mental status exam arriving at a DSM-IV diagnosis.	2. A complete assessment helps the therapist determine treatment needs.	2. (See Chapters 1 and 2 for assessment guide.) "I'm going to ask you some questions to get to know you better."
3. The nurse explains psychotherapy to the client, describing it as a collaborative effort.	3. While adolescents long for independence, they are still dependent. They will be reassured that the therapist is "in charge" but also glad to be considered a partner in treatment. Adolescents frequently exhibit ambivalence that is manifested in the shifts in moods, and in the desires to be themselves versus desires to be like their peers.	3. "You and I will work together to figure out what this is all about and how to make things easier for you."
4. The nurse clarifies the contract, working out the time, place, and frequency. Explains confidentiality.	4. Clients will be reassured by the structure and the chance to have a part in planning the therapy. Confidentiality allows freedom to discuss all thoughts, actions, and feelings.	4. "So we will meet here every Saturday at noon for 45 minutes. Everything you say will be between us, unless you are feeling like harming yourself."
5. The nurse demonstrates understanding and empathy, taking care not to appear overly solicitous or naive.	5. Adolescents don't want to feel they are being manipulated or that the therapist is a "pushover."	5. "It sounds like you've been pretty unhappy."

TABLE 10-2
Nursing Interventions, Theoretical Rationale, and Examples in the
Middle Phase of Individual Therapy with Adolescents

NURSING INTERVENTION	THEORETICAL RATIONALE	EXAMPLE
1. The nurse waits for the client to begin the session.	1. This helps clients to see it is their time, and the nurse has no "agenda."	1. The nurse sits quietly, looking at the client in a relaxed, calm way.
2. The nurse listens to the client's stories, usually of the week's events, asking questions, clarifying, exclaiming, and at times confronting.	2. This helps clients hear themselves, clarify their thoughts and feelings, and challenges them to explore the events of their lives, particularly their own part in the troubles they may have.	2. "So you and Tim pulled a practical joke on your teacher, and he blew up at you? You thought this prank would endear him to you?"
3. The nurse identifies resistance.	3. This is an inevitable part of therapy, and exploration often leads to further insight. Resistance often comes because insight is around the corner.	3. "Let's try to figure out why you were late today. Is there something you don't want to talk about?"
4. The nurse permits regression.	4. Clients often regress when anxiety occurs over separation and individuation.	4. "You sound pretty mad at yourself for screwing up at school. Did you get scared over doing so well recently?"
5. The nurse is alert to the "all better" phenomenon.	5. Clients will report feeling "all better" in an attempt to avoid dealing with anxiety-producing material.	5. "You said you are feeling fine, but you look sad. Let's talk about it."
6. The nurse makes interpretations.	6. Clients will feel understood. Leads to insight.	6. "So you're afraid if you do well, more and more will be asked of you, and you'll turn into your dad?"
7. The nurse validates the client's insight.	7. Encourages clients to go on, rewards their work.	7. "That makes sense and explains why you've had so much trouble with Mr. Smith."
8. The nurse verbally rewards positive changes.	8. Encourages client, increases self-esteem, offers hope.	8. "You sure handled that a lot better than you would have when you came here!"

EVALUATION   Therapy with adolescents is considered successful when the client:
1. Experiences decrease or removal of symptoms
2. Relates to parents in a more mutually satisfying way
3. Relates to peers in a more mutually satisfying way
4. Improves school performance
5. Looks forward to the future

REFERENCES   American Nurses Association (1994). *A Statement on Psychiatric Mental Health Clinical Nursing Practice and Standards of Psychiatric–Mental Health Clinical Nursing Practice.* Washington, DC: American Nurses Publishing.
Anthony, J. (Speaker) (1983). *Between Yes and No: The Potentially Neutral Area Where the Adolescent and His Interviewer Can Meet* [Audiotape Short Course in Adolescent Psychiatry]. New York: Psychiatric Institute Foundation, American Audio Association.
Blos, P. (1979). *The Adolescent Passage.* New York: International Universities Press.
Erikson, E. (1963). *Childhood and Society.* New York: Norton.

Kaplan, H., & Sadock, B. (1991). *Synopsis of Psychiatry. Behavioral Sciences* (6th ed.). Baltimore: Williams & Wilkins.

Lewis, D. (1985). The neuropsychiatric assessment of the adolescent. *Psychiatric Annals, 15* (1), 36–38.

Lidz, T. (1968). *The Person.* New York: Basic Books.

Miller, D. (1983). *The Age Between Adolescence and Therapy.* New York: Jason Aronson.

BIBLIOGRAPHY

Adams, G. R., Montemayor, R., & Gullotta, T. P. (eds.) (1994). *Substance Misuse in Adolescence. Advances in Adolescent Development* (vol. 7). Newbury Park, CA: Sage.

Archer, S. L. (ed.) (1994). *Interventions for Adolescent Identity Development. Sage Focus Editions* (vol. 169). Newbury Park, CA: Sage.

Bukstein, O. G. (1995). *Adolescent Substance Abuse.* New York: John Wiley & Sons.

Eisen, A., Kearney, C., & Schaefer, C. (1994). *Clinical Handbook of Anxiety Disorders in Children and Adolescents.* New York: Jason Aronson.

Fox, K. (1980). Adolescent ambivalence: A therapeutic issue. *Journal of Psychiatric Nursing and Mental Health Services, 18* (9), 29–33.

Godenne, G. (Speaker) (1983). *Outpatient Treatment of the Adolescent* [Audiotape. Short Course in Adolescent Psychiatry]. New York: Psychiatric Institute Foundation, American Audio Association.

Ghuman, H. S., & Sarles, R. M. (eds.) (1994). *Handbook of Adolescent Inpatient Psychiatric Treatment.* New York: Brunner–Mazel.

Gonet, M. M. (1994). *Counseling the Adolescent Substance Abuser: School-Based Intervention and Prevention. Sage Source Books for the Human Services* (vol. 29). Newbury Park, CA: Sage.

Lewis, D. (1985). The neuropsychiatric assessment of the adolescent. *Psychiatric Annals, 15* (1), 36–38.

Meeks, J. E. (1971). *The Fragile Alliance.* Baltimore: Williams & Wilkins.

Semrud-Clikeman, M. (1995). *Child and Adolescent Therapy.* Boston: Allyn and Bacon.

Zimmerman, J. K., & Asnis, G. M. (eds.) (1995). *Treatment Approaches with Suicidal Adolescents.* New York: John Wiley & Sons.

11

Group Therapy with Adolescents

Kathryn R. Puskar
Kathleen Tusaie-Mumford

OVERVIEW:

Definition
Process and Content
Types of Groups
   Activity
   Psychoeducational
   Cognitive-Behavioral
   Problem-Solving Counseling
   Psychodrama
   Socialization
   Interpersonal Psychodynamic
      Psychotherapy

Therapeutic Factors
Qualifications of Group Leader
   Psychotherapy
   Counseling and Health Teaching
Designing and Starting the Group
Group Leadership
Stages of Group Development
Special Issues
Evaluation

DEFINITION

In a society recently focused on the escalating problems of violence among youth, teen pregnancy, and a high rate of teen suicide and substance abuse, mental health professionals are concerned with ways of preventing and treating adolescents with emotional distress. Group therapy is an ideal intervention for the treatment of adolescents, as teens have a natural tendency to form and communicate in groups, often experience discomfort in one-to-one situations with adults, and have a tendency to use peers as a source of emotional support. Group therapy is a method of therapeutic intervention based on the exploration and analysis of both individual intrapsychic structure and the group process (Lego, 1984).

PROCESS AND CONTENT

Recognizing the relationship between process and content is one of the major tasks of group leaders. *Content* consists of what is said and *process* looks at the ways in which the group deals with the task and maintenance, the ways members assume roles, how decisions are made, how conflicts are handled, how leadership and authority are exercised, and all nonverbal communication. In interpersonal psychotherapy groups the leader guides the group toward discussing content and processing here-and-now issues. If the group is participating in an activity, the activity is seen as the content.

TYPES OF GROUPS

ACTIVITY

The leader chooses an activity that will foster the therapeutic goals of the members, e.g., drawing to encourage self-expression and concentration, volleyball to encourage teamwork and coordination, blind trust walks to build trusting relationships, music to increase cohesiveness, feedback, and self-discovery. Group time is structured and action-oriented.

PSYCHOEDUCATIONAL

These groups are extensions of educational and vocational services and are designed to provide information and prevent developmental problems. Instructional aides, lectures, and informal exercises are used to help adolescents build social skills, coping skills, problem-solving abilities, and cognitive control. Groups may be organized to teach parenting skills, sexuality, anger control, or other specific themes. These groups may also be expanded to a multiple family format.

COGNITIVE-BEHAVIORAL

Cognitive therapy is a form of psychotherapy that is structured, directive, collaborative, and focused on the here-and-now (Beck, 1976). The role of an individual's perceptions, thoughts, and beliefs about feelings and behavior is stressed. Cognitive restructuring of real life events with adolescents can lead to a decrease in the sense of urgency for immediate gratification and a move from all-or-nothing thinking to a more graduated position. This increases accommodation and decreases reactivity. Also the Socratic dialogue helps teens to see the difference between possibility and probability. This sets the groundwork for new responses to old problems (Wilkes, Belsher, Rush, & Frank, 1994). With a group of adolescents in varying stages of intellectual development, there is an emphasis on incorporating cognitive restructuring techniques into behavioral coping skills through the use of homework assignments.

PROBLEM-SOLVING COUNSELING

These groups have a short-term secondary prevention focus. Common crises may be a pregnancy, a traumatic event such as the death of a friend or relative, or sexual or physical abuse. The goal is to return to the level of functioning preceding the crisis, or higher.

PSYCHODRAMA

This is a form of psychotherapy in which verbalization is secondary to action. Adolescents may be unmotivated or verbally unsophisticated, rendering them unable to benefit from traditional talk-oriented treatment. Psychodrama that provides an enactment of real or fantasized events that have produced emotional discomfort in a group member may facilitate the therapeutic process.

SOCIALIZATION

These groups are designed to help adolescents maintain or develop appropriate social skills through involvement in a positive peer culture. These groups may be used as primary prevention in the community, and include scout troops, campfire girls, 4-H clubs, church groups, YMCA or YWCA. Or, these groups may be at the tertiary level and be located in a residential treatment center or an inpatient facility.

INTERPERSONAL PSYCHODYNAMIC PSYCHOTHERAPY

These groups focus on the dynamics of the individual's development as well as the group process. The goal is interpersonal insight and an appreciation of the need to change behavioral patterns. A constant processing of the here-and-now behavior occurring in the group facilitates personal growth.

THERAPEUTIC FACTORS

Adolescents have reported being helped in therapy groups by experiencing universality, cohesiveness, and guidance (Puskar & Martsolf, 1995) as well as interpersonal learning, catharsis, and positive recapitulation of the primary family group (Chehler & Burns, 1987). Adolescents in an inpatient group experienced catharsis, universality, and guidance (Riddle, 1994).

QUALIFICATIONS OF GROUP LEADER

PSYCHOTHERAPY

According to the American Nurses Association (1994), psychotherapy may be performed only by nurses who are certified clinical specialists in psychiatric–mental health nursing. Furthermore, there must be a therapeutic contract with the client, knowledge of personality theory, growth and development, psychopathology, social systems, small group dynamics, stress and adaptation, and theories related to the therapeutic methods used.

COUNSELING AND HEALTH TEACHING

An ANA certified psychiatric mental health nurse (RNC) may lead groups designed to help adolescents with problem solving, the development of simple coping skills, and health teaching.

DESIGNING AND STARTING THE GROUP

The steps taken to set up a group of adolescents are shown in Table 11-1 along with rationales for each intervention. See also Chapter 9 for a proposal to lead groups in school-based programs. Table 11-2 shows interventions, rationales, and examples of interventions in an ongoing group.

GROUP LEADERSHIP

The group leader functions as both a participant and an observer. As a participant, the group leader's functions are to provide structure and support, and to process the here-and-now. Comments about group process help members to change. For example, "Sandy, I notice whenever Judy makes a comment about her boyfriend, you make a face." By focusing on both content and process, the group members learn to see themselves as others do, understand their own behavior, and become aware of their effect on others.

As an observer, the leader "steps out" of the group dynamics to observe what is happening and how to intervene. After group, the leader may discuss the session with the coleader or, if alone, use a standard form or videotape to identify member roles that facilitate or interfere with group task/maintenance, communication patterns, and underlying themes (hostility, fight–flight, togetherness–separateness).

STAGES OF GROUP DEVELOPMENT

Yalom's (1985) stages in adolescent groups include:
1. Hesitant participation and search for meaning
2. Conflict, dominance, and rebellion
3. Cohesiveness and work
4. Termination

TABLE 11-1
Leader Interventions, Theoretical Rationales, and Examples in Starting Adolescent Therapy Groups

INTERVENTION	THEORETICAL RATIONALE	EXAMPLE
Meet with adolescent individually and review records to identify range of symptoms, age, personal style, and motivation for group. Discuss rationale for group.	Cohesiveness is facilitated by similar age range, similar symptoms, a balance in personal styles, and a size of 7–9 members (Yalom, 1985). Problems for younger teens include separation, sexual anxieties, and movement out of childhood. Older teens are concerned with identity, dating, vocation, drugs, and money. Older adolescents may regress in groups with younger adolescents. Therefore, the age range of members should be approximately 2 years (13–15 years, 15–17, 17–19) (Dato, 1984).	The nurse organizes a group of teens aged 15–17 who are adjusting to high school, a blended family group, or teens who have lost a parent to AIDS.
Balance talkative teens with those who are more introspective.	The group functions more effectively when members have varied verbal attitudes, degrees of withdrawal, and developmental social skills.	The group consists of three teens who are very open and talkative, two who are depressed and quiet, and two teens who are angry and only moderately verbal.
Arrange the size of the group according to ages of the members. Younger adolescent groups would include 5–6 members and older adolescent groups would include 6–9 members.	More than 9 members in a group leads to subgrouping and disruption. Older adolescents often have poor attendance.	A 10-week group of 15–17-year-olds coping with depression has an average attendance of 7–8 members.
During the individual session have teen sign a consent that includes ground rules and rationale for group.	Adolescents vary in their ability to exercise control and the presence of external limits is presented to ensure safety. If the group's goal and expected behaviors are ambiguous, the group will be less cohesive and less productive, and members will be more anxious, defensive, and prone to terminate (Yalom, 1985).	Form includes time, place, number of sessions, and member expectations, such as no violence, no drugs, no sexual activity, no leaving the room, no interrupting others, issues of confidentiality, and the specific purposes of the group (improving coping skills, expressing feelings about parent's death, problem-solving, sharing feelings, etc.).
Administer a pregroup measurement tool that will be used before and after group intervention to measure outcome.	Effectiveness can be demonstrated through rapid assessment instruments that measure objective outcomes. Structured interviews or self-reports focusing on internal frames of reference may be used to measure process changes in members (Azima & Richmond, 1989).	Members fill out a checklist measuring self-esteem before the first session and after the last.
Arrange appropriate space and timing of 90-minute sessions for a specific number of weeks.	Adolescent groups are often scheduled to correspond to the school calendar. Ideally 10–20 sessions are needed for members to gain full value from the group, but this is often unrealistic in today's cost-conscious environment.	A 10-week group for high school seniors to improve coping skills meets every Monday 9 A.M. to 10:30 A.M. in the conference room.

TABLE 11-2
Leader Interventions, Theoretical Rationales, and Examples in the
Working Phase of Adolescent Therapy Groups

INTERVENTION	THEORETICAL RATIONALE	EXAMPLE
Mix confrontation with empathy.	Confrontation is meant to alter and heighten the awareness of the group members and adolescents are especially receptive to empathetic confrontations. Empathy decreases denial and the impact is on every member present. But therapists working with adolescents must recognize the danger of being perceived as a parent and must take a less scholarly, less controlling position than with adults (Azima & Richmond, 1989).	"John, I notice you have not spoken today. That is somewhat different from your initial behavior in the group" (scholarly and parental), versus "So, John, how come you're so quiet today?"
Use self-disclosure as appropriate.	Self-disclosures make the adolescents recognize the therapist is not omnipotent and facilitate group action. This helps work through transference–countertransference reactions and allows members to face their dissatisfaction and primitive rage.	"I really don't know the answer to that question. What do the rest of you think?"
Be aware of the feelings of members as well as your own reactions to what is happening.	By developing a trusting relationship through the use of empathy, the group therapists can engage and reengage members and provide anchoring in the transition to adulthood. For adolescents, the process of empathic confrontation is the most therapeutic form of communication (Azima & Richmond, 1989).	"That must be difficult for you." "I hear what you are saying."
Demonstrate activity and spontaneity. Provide feedback on group progression, frequent reinforcement of positive statements, and reflective statements.	Adolescents often use play and jokes when dealing with anxiety-laden topics. Clear, consistent communication is necessary to decrease proud anxiety and reinforce basic rules. Adolescents want to be understood as individuals and are narcissistic. Therefore, it is important to reflect back to them more frequently than adults.	"So, now you feel comfortable enough to share the real reason you've been feeling depressed." "What is different today from the first group session?" "You are saying that . . . ." "Is anyone else experiencing . . . ?" "That is interesting."
Encourage group members to confront and interpret acting-out behaviors in the group.	Adolescents need to learn how to conceptualize and problem-solve to enable separation from an angry, dependent relationship with authority.	One boy makes strange sounds while others are talking. Another member says, "Tom, I used to try to be a clown all the time, but it's better to talk."
Accept fluctuations in moods— yes/no, love/hate, to be like others/to be different.	Adolescents make developmentally based attempts at separation and individuation and experience rapidly shifting emotional states that cause difficulties for therapists.	Following an especially emotional discussion, one member begins to giggle and soon the whole group is laughing. The leader comments, "Isn't it interesting how we all affect each other's moods?"

TABLE 11-2 *(continued)*

INTERVENTION	THEORETICAL RATIONALE	EXAMPLE
Make interpretations to group members, to the group as a whole, and encourage member-to-member interpretations. This occurs only after there has been adequate empathetic confrontation.	Interpretation gives meaning to the underlying unconscious conflicts that have been identified in the transferences of the individual (Azima & Richmond, 1989). Interpretation is a powerful therapeutic technique to help with self-understanding and change.	"Nancy, I notice that whenever Joe speaks, you make a comment about your father."
Use role-playing, music, dance, games, art, or videos.	Active techniques can heighten interaction by providing an experience to share as opposed to talking about a feeling (Carrel, 1993). Some groups may also include an educational component, for example, a video on sexuality and discussion of thoughts and feelings after the film.	Following two extremely quiet group sessions, the leader brings in art supplies. Each member creates a painting and has the group choose a title. There is active discussion and an experience of cohesiveness.

SPECIAL ISSUES

Group leaders need to be cognizant of phenomena unique to adolescent groups. Puskar (1982) has identified six issues, coined the six "Cs," in providing therapy to teens:
1. Clear communication
2. Clarity of rules
3. Consistency in rule-keeping
4. Clear consequences
5. Liberal use of consultation
6. Examination of countertransference

EVALUATION

In today's cost-conscious health care environment, it is wise to determine ways to demonstrate clinical outcomes. The following may be used:
1. Pregroup and postgroup diagnostic scales in groups designed to decrease symptoms
2. Pregroup and postgroup quizzes in psychoeducation groups
3. Reports from home and school about school attendance, number of fights at home, number of disciplinary actions required
4. Self-report of members at the end of the group

REFERENCES

American Nurses Association (1994). *Statement on Psychiatric–Mental Health Clinical Nursing Practice and Standards of Psychiatric–Mental Health Clinical Nursing Practice.* Washington, DC: American Nurses Publishing Co.

Azima, F. J., & Richmond, L. H. (1989). *Adolescent Group Psychotherapy* (Monograph 3, American Group Psychotherapy Association Monograph Series). Madison, CT: International Universities Press.

Beck, A. T. (1976). *Cognitive Therapy and Emotional Disorders.* New York: International Universities Press.

Carrel, S. (1993). *Group Exercises for Adolescents: A Manual for Therapists.* Newbury Park, CA: Sage Publications.

Chehler, J., & Burns, M. J. (1987). Anorexia, bulimia and sexuality: Case study of an adolescent inpatient group. *Archives of Psychiatric Nursing, 1* (3), 163–170.

Dato, C. (1984). Therapy with adolescents. In S. Lego (ed.), *The American Handbook of Psychiatric Nursing.* Philadelphia: J. B. Lippincott.

Lego, S. (1984). Group therapy In S. Lego (ed.), *The American Handbook of Psychiatric Nursing* (pp. 206–217). Philadelphia: J. B. Lippincott.

Puskar, K. (1982). The client needing improved parenting skills. In J. Durham and S. Hardin (eds.), *Nurse Psychotherapist in Private Practice* (pp. 265–272). New York: Springer.

Puskar, K., & Martsolf, D. (1995). Adolescent Relocation Support Groups. Unpublished manuscript, University of Pittsburgh, Pittsburgh, PA.

Riddle, C. R. (1994). Development of an adolescent inpatient sexual abuse group: Application of Lewin's model of change. *Journal of Child and Adolescent Psychiatric Nursing, 7* (1), 17–24.

Wilkes, T. C., Belsher, G., Rush, J., & Frank, E. (1994). *Cognitive Therapy for Depressed Adolescents.* New York: The Guilford Press.

Yalom, I. (1985). *The Theory and Practice of Group Psychotherapy.* New York: Basic Books.

12
TWELVE

Behavior Therapy

Maxine E. Loomis

OVERVIEW:

INTRODUCTION

Behavior therapy focuses on removal of overt symptoms, without regard for the patient's private experience or inner conflicts.

CLINICAL APPLICATIONS

Behavior therapy is used to treat:
1. Agoraphobia through graded exposure (Martin & Pear, 1992)
2. Alcohol dependence by the use of disulfiram (Antabuse), other aversive conditioning, stimulus exposure and extinction, contingency management, and social learning (Martin & Pear, 1992)
3. Anorexia nervosa by observing eating and weight gain (Hersen & Detre, 1994)
4. Bulimia nervosa by observing eating and weight gain (Kaplan, Sadock, & Grebb, 1994)
5. Other phobias through systematic desensitization (Marks, 1987)
6. Paraphilia through aversive stimulation (Maletzky, 1990)
7. Schizophrenia through token economy (Kaplan, Sadock, & Grebb, 1994)
8. Sexual dysfunction through relaxation, desensitization, and graded exposure (Masters & Johnson, 1970)

9. Obesity through the use of hand-held computers (Agras, Taylor, Feldman, Losch, & Burnett, 1990)
10. Cocaine dependence through chemical aversion therapy (Frawley & Smith, 1990)
11. Chronic nightmares (Kellner, Neidhardt, Krakow, & Pathak, 1992)

PSYCHIATRIC NURSING FUNCTIONS

Psychiatric nursing can be viewed as a process of altering the behaviors of clients, their families, and their environments. This alteration should provide for an increasingly more rewarding living situation for the clients and their families. Nurses perform four functions in the process of altering behavior:

1. Increasing the strength of clients' adaptive behaviors
2. Decreasing the strength of clients' maladaptive behaviors
3. Teaching clients new behaviors for living with themselves, their families, and their environments
4. Teaching clients new ways of adjusting to their environments

BASIC PRINCIPLES

OPERANT BEHAVIOR

Definition

Operant behavior is behavior that operates on the environment in such a way as to produce a change in that environment. (For example, a client, Don, randomly hits clients whom he sees in the dayroom.)

Operant Responses

Operant responses are individual units of operant behavior that are objectively defined and can be measured along some dimension such as frequency, duration, or intensity. (The frequency, duration, and intensity of Don's hitting behavior can be measured.)

Response Class

Response class is a grouping of operant responses according to some common characteristic (e.g., social interaction). A response class may be broken down into many specific behavioral components. (Don's behavior could be classified as "social interaction," hitting, or making contact.)

STIMULI

Definition

Stimuli are environmental events that interact with and influence a person's behavior.

Discriminative Stimuli

Discriminative stimuli precede a response and influence it by signaling or setting the stage for the response to occur. (Don's hitting occurs when clients are laughing together.)

Reinforcers or Punishers

Reinforcers or punishers follow or provide the consequences for a response and thereby influence the future rate of occurrence of that response. (Don is either scolded or secluded when he hits clients.)

OPERANT CONDITIONING

Definition

Operant conditioning is the learning process by which discriminative stimuli, operant responses, and environmental consequences become linked together in an orderly way.

Contingency System

A contingency system is represented in the following manner:

Discriminative stimulus	$\rightarrow$	Operant response	$\rightarrow$	Environmental consequences
(Other clients laugh)		(Don hits them)		(He is scolded or secluded)

What this model indicates is that certain discriminative stimuli set the stage for the occurrence of a behavior response, which is followed by environmental consequences that either increase or decrease the future probability that the response will occur. Nurses must identify and manipulate the discriminative stimuli, the responses (or human behavior), and resulting consequences to achieve the goal of change in client behavior.

REINFORCING STIMULI

Positive Reinforcement

Positively reinforcing stimuli are those consequences that increase or maintain the behaviors that they follow. Thus, a reinforcer is any event that increases the probability of the response that immediately precedes it. Reinforcement is one of the most direct ways of increasing behavior. Positive reinforcement is the presentation of desirable consequences following a behavior.

Negative Reinforcement

Negative reinforcement is the removal of an aversive condition (such as alleviating pain) in order to strengthen behavior. This is classified as reinforcement because it increases the future probability of the response it follows.

Learning

Learning can occur whether we plan for it or let it take place accidentally. Much of the bizarre behavior demonstrated by psychiatric clients has been learned accidentally and is reinforced by attention. (Don's hitting other clients was followed by being placed in seclusion. For Don, seclusion was the reinforcer that maintained hitting behavior. That is, he hit clients in order to get into seclusion where he felt more in control.)

Specificity of Reinforcers

Reinforcers are individually specific, that is, an event that will serve as a reinforcer for one person may not do so for another person. (For some clients, seclusion is punishment; for others, like Don, it is a relief to have his behavior controlled.)

Premack Principle

The Premack principle states that a more frequently occurring behavior can be used to increase the probability of a less frequently occurring behavior. (In Don's case, being in seclusion occurred more frequently than being with the other clients, so the former could be used to reinforce the latter.) The assumption underlying this principle is that activities in which people spend most of their time have some reinforcing properties. In other words, people choose activities that they like. These activities can be used as reinforcers.

Conditions Influencing Reinforcer Effectiveness

1. Deprivation will increase the potency of a reinforcer (e.g., thirst or hunger). (Don is more likely to control the hitting if he is hungry and is promised dinner if he controls his behavior.)
2. Satiation will decrease the potency of a reinforcer, e.g., food loses its reinforcing power following a big meal. (After dinner, Don is less likely to conform.)
3. Primary reinforcers, which fulfill biological needs (e.g., food, sex, sleep, warmth), are more or less effective at predictable intervals. (Don gets hungry or sleepy at predictable times.)
4. Conditioned, or secondary, reinforcers (e.g., money, grades, praise) acquire their reinforcing value as a result of experience and are harder to satiate. (Once Don learns to accept praise for talking with other clients instead of hitting them, he can accept this secondary reinforcer at any time.)
5. Immediacy of reinforcement is required to increase the strength of behavior; therefore, a token or praise given immediately following a behavior is a potent reinforcer. (Praise of Don's control upon seeing clients laugh must be given at once.)

EXTINCTION

Definition

Extinction is the withholding of positive reinforcers following a response, which eventually decreases the response rate. (Theoretically, if Don's hitting behavior could be ignored, it would decrease and finally stop.)

Problematic Side Effects of Extinction (or Ignoring Behavior)

1. The rate or intensity of the response subject to extinction may increase before it decreases. This is especially dangerous with self-destructive behavior. (If it were ignored, Don's hitting would initially increase, endangering him and others, before it began to decrease.)
2. There may be an increased variability in clients' behavior as they randomly search to produce the desired reinforcement. Emotional (crying or yelling) escalations are not uncommon. (Don could become more and more verbally abusive.)
3. Staff may engage in a process of *differentiated reinforcement* as the client does more and more extreme behaviors to get attention. (The staff may ignore less intense behaviors, for example, asking for medication, but be forced to respond to more upsetting behaviors, for example, hysterical crying or thrashing around.)

AVERSIVE STIMULI

Definition

Aversive stimuli are stimuli that follow a response and result in a decrease of the future probability of that response. These aversive stimuli are commonly called punishers. When an aversive stimulus is used to decrease the future probability of the response that it follows, the operation is called punishment.

Primary Aversive Stimuli

Primary aversive stimuli directly threaten biological needs or existence (e.g., extremes of heat or cold, physical blows).

Conditioned or Secondary Aversive Stimuli

Conditioned aversive stimuli acquire their punishing potential as a result of experience (e.g., frowns or bad grades).

Punishment

Punishment can be delivered by the presentation of an aversive stimulus immediately following a response or by the withdrawal of an ongoing positive reinforcer immediately following a response. The use of punishment requires ongoing, accurate assessment of the consequences. When the response is not rapidly suppressed, the punishment should be stopped, or if safe, the magnitude of the aversive stimulus should be increased enough to produce rapid suppression.

Conditions Influencing Effectiveness

Effective punishment results in a suppression of the target response.
1. Punishment is less effective if the person is used to a high level of this punishment. Examples:
    a. Football players are gradually trained to tolerate increasing amounts of physical abuse. This is thought of as "conditioning."
    b. Abused children often become habituated to lower levels of punishment so that it takes increasingly severe abuse to get them to respond.
2. Punishment is less effective when positive reinforcers are mixed in with the aversive stimuli in an unplanned manner.
3. Punishment is more effective when aversive stimuli for specific responses are clearly combined with positive reinforcement for other specific responses.

Disadvantages of Punishment

1. The effects of punishment tend to be situationally specific, that is, associated with a place as the discriminative stimulus. (If Don were punished repeatedly by scolding in the dayroom, he might avoid the dayroom.)
2. Punishment tends to serve as the discriminative stimulus for escape responses. (If Don were scolded by the nurses frequently, he would avoid them.)
3. The use of punishment may sometimes result in the client's exhibiting aggressive responses. (Don could become assaultive to staff who scold him.)
4. The aversive properties of the punishment may be generalized to the person delivering the punishment. (If the same nurse scolded Don each time, he might become unable to relate to this nurse in a positive way at other times.)
5. Punishment has little holding power in relation to long-term behavior change unless the response has been totally suppressed. (As long as Don continues to hit clients even though scolding follows, the punishment has not been successful and will not be.)
6. While punishment can be an effective technique for changing behavior, few professionals are prepared to use it safely and ethically. Staff members would most likely not call the scolding "punishment" but rather refer to it euphemistically as "presenting reality through confrontation."

ISSUES OF CONTROL   Whether a person's behavior is considered appropriate or inappropriate depends on whether that behavior has a high or low probability of being well received (reinforced) by others in the environment. Thus, the ability to discriminate when reinforcement is forthcoming is a basic function in successful interpersonal behavior.

RESPONDING IN APPROPRIATE ENVIRONMENTAL CONDITIONS

Discriminative Stimuli

Discriminative stimuli are stimuli that precede the emission of responses and serve to "set the occasion" for a particular response to occur. Discriminative stimuli do not cause a response to occur; instead they indicate when a response has a high probability of being reinforced. (When the nursing staff has helped Don change, he enters the dayroom, sees clients laughing and talking, and joins them, "knowing" that this response will be reinforced by staff members.)

Stimulus Control

Stimulus control exists when a given response is more likely to occur under the desired stimulus conditions than when these conditions are not present. (Don is more likely to respond appropriately when staff who tend to reinforce this behavior are present.) When a person's behavior is controlled by the situation in which he finds himself, the person is said to be able to *discriminate*.

Stimulus Generalization

Stimulus generalization occurs when an environmental situation similar to, yet different from, the situation in which the response was originally reinforced acquires the capacity to set the stage for the occurrence of that response. (Once Don has learned that socially appropriate [nonhitting] behavior will be reinforced in the dayroom, he generalizes this response to the dining room as well.)

Response Generalization

Response generalization is a process whereby there is an increase in the reinforced response as well as in responses that are members of the same response class. (Once Don has learned that nonhitting behavior is reinforced, he generalizes to other socially appropriate behavior such as eating and dressing properly.)

RESPONDING WITHOUT IMMEDIATE REINFORCEMENT

People frequently respond without reinforcement. This is essential because the environment is not always capable of producing reinforcement every time a response occurs.

REINFORCEMENT SCHEDULES

Continuous Reinforcement

The continuous reinforcement schedule is a special case in which every occurrence of the target response is followed by reinforcement. Continuous reinforcement is used primarily in the initial phases of generating new responses.

Problems

1. The person delivering the reinforcement must be continuously present to monitor the occurrence of the target response.

2. Because of the possibility of satiation, generalized secondary reinforcers (e.g., money, points, tokens) must be selected that will maintain their reinforcing potential over time.
3. When continuous reinforcement is withdrawn, extinction occurs quickly.

Intermittent Reinforcement

Intermittent reinforcement schedules are used to combat the above problems. There are four types of intermittent reinforcement:

1. A *fixed ratio schedule* is a method of delivering reinforcement following a set number of responses. (Don is given a token every time he eats a meal in the dining room without hitting anyone.)
2. A *variable ratio schedule* is a method of delivering reinforcement in which the number of responses required varies from reinforcement to reinforcement. (Don is given a token after some meals when he has not hit anyone, but not every meal.)
3. A *fixed interval schedule* is a method of delivering reinforcement for behavior following a set period of time. (Don is given a token at the end of every hour during which he has hit no one.)
4. A *variable interval schedule* is a method of delivering reinforcement in which the time interval varies from reinforcement to reinforcement. (Don is given a token at various times during the day when he is observed talking to clients without hitting them but not every time he spends time without hitting anyone.)

Clinical Application

1. A continuous schedule of reinforcement is necessary for the initial strengthening of weak responses.
2. *Ratio schedules* are more useful when a transition step is necessary to move from a continuous reinforcement schedule to a more real-life schedule, or when the target response occurs in well-specified and infrequently occurring situations (e.g., preparing meals, washing the car, or doing the laundry). Ratio schedules are often impractical and inefficient in clinical situations because they require that the person delivering the reinforcement keep the client under constant observation in order to know when to deliver the reinforcement.
3. *Interval schedules* are practical in a clinical setting because the staff does not have to stay with the client between reinforcement intervals. Most everyday behavior is reinforced on an interval schedule. The variable interval schedule is the most resistant to extinction and can therefore be used to maintain behaviors that are not likely to be naturally reinforced every time they occur. For example, the instructor who wants her nursing students to be informed at all times about the conditions of their clients will spot check her students at randomly selected times. Students must then remain informed at all times, because they never know when they will be questioned.

RESPONSE CHAINS

Normal behavior consists of numerous *response chains* with multiple links made up of discriminative stimuli, discrete responses, and conditioned reinforcers. At the end of this series of links is a very potent reinforcer. For example, a nurse may go to work every day and enjoy the daily reinforcement of a job well done, or of at least being able to go home at the end of the shift. Occasionally she receives a compliment from a supervisor (variable interval schedule), and every other week she receives a paycheck (fixed interval schedule). After a longer chain of working responses, she may receive an annual raise (fixed interval schedule) or a promotion (variable ratio schedule).

Response chains are learned in the reverse order from that in which they are eventually performed when they become a complex behavior. That is, the last behavior is taught first and reinforced, then preceding behaviors are added to the chain. For example, in toilet training, going in the toilet is reinforced first and then all of the behaviors for getting to the toilet in time are added in stages.

MODIFICATION TECHNIQUES

In order to apply the principles of behavior modification (operant conditioning) the nurse must consider these basic questions:

1. What is the target behavior, and how will all staff members recognize it when it occurs?
2. In what setting does the target behavior occur?
3. What are potent reinforcers or punishers for this client?
4. Can staff members control the reinforcers? the punishers?
5. What schedule of reinforcement or punishment should be used?

Table 12-1 can be used as a guide for the selection of appropriate behavior modification techniques.

TABLE 12-1
Problems, Goals, Techniques, and Technical Considerations in Behavioral Modification

BEHAVIORAL PROBLEM	GOAL	TECHNIQUES	TECHNICAL CONSIDERATIONS
Response too infrequent (for example, client will not leave his room to socialize with others)	Increase frequency of ongoing response	1. Positive reinforcement 2. Negative reinforcement	1. Response definition, reinforcer identification, reinforcer control. 2. What is the aversive stimulus? Who will initiate it? What client response will result in the termination of the aversive stimulus?
Response too frequent (for example, client constantly washes her hands)	Decrease frequency of ongoing response	1. Punishment 2. Extinction 3. Reinforce incompatible responses 4. Satiation	1. Response definition, definition of consequence, presentation of an aversive or removal of a positive stimulus? Delivered by whom? Strength of the punisher? Emotional side effects and generalization—how will they be prevented or dealt with? With which other modification techniques will punishment be combined? 2. Response definition, definition of consequences, reinforcer control. What other responses will be reinforced? 3. Response definition of incompatible response, reinforcer quantity and quality. 4. By what means will the client be satiated? Is this practical?

TABLE 12-1 *(continued)*

BEHAVIORAL PROBLEM	GOAL	TECHNIQUES	TECHNICAL CONSIDERATIONS
		5. Time-out from positive reinforcement	5. Definition of responses (a) being punished, (b) being extinguished, and (c) being negatively reinforced. Definition of consequences for (a), (b), and (c) above.
		6. Response cost	6. Definition of response, determination of cost, potential for desirable responses to occur.
Response never occurs (includes never did or used to occur) (for example, client is mute except for primitive sounds)	Teach or retrain response	1. Shaping	1. Target response definition; identify prerequisite response currently in client's repertoire. Define sequential response steps of successive approximation. Reinforcer identification, differentially reinforce each successive step until target response reached.
		2. Chaining	2. Response definition, analyze response in relation to its temporal sequence, define backward or forward chain. Teach response at end of chain that results in reinforcement, and then add on the next step.
		3. Imitation	3. Does the client imitate? Response definition, reinforcer identification, generalization of imitative responding.
		4. Behavioral rehearsal	4. How, where, and by whom will the behavioral rehearsal be conducted? How closely does rehearsal situation simulate real-world situation?
Response occurs but inappropriately:			
1. Occurs when it should not occur (for example, bed-wetting)	Stimulus discrimination	1. Discrimination training	1. What is the stimulus setting in which the response is desired? What will be used to reinforce the response when it occurs in that setting? What will happen when the response occurs in an inappropriate setting?
2. Occurs in some but not all instances when it should	Generalization of response to all appropriate situations	2. Generalization training	2. Define current stimulus situation in which response is emitted. Define other situations in which response should occur and identify any aspects that are similar to situations where response already occurs. Identify reinforcers for use in new situations.

Adapted from Loomis, M., & Horsely, J. A. (1974). *Interpersonal Change: A Behavioral Approach to Nursing Practice.* New York: McGraw-Hill. Reproduced with permission.

BEHAVIORAL NURSING PROCESS

Box 12-1 shows a complete and individualized way to treat specific clients using the principles and techniques of operant conditioning and applying a problem-solving process.

▌BOX 12-1 Nursing Process Outline for Behavior Modification

1. *Statement of behavioral problem*
   a. What is the problem?
   b. Who defined the problem?
      (1) The identified patient?
      (2) An external agent? (for example, the patient's mother)
      (3) Society?

2. *Behavioral history*
   a. Responses
      (1) What are the appropriate responses present within the patient's behavioral repertoire?
      (2) What are the inappropriate responses present within the patient's behavioral repertoire?
      (3) What are the age-appropriate responses absent from the patient's behavioral repertoire?
   b. Consequences
      (1) What are reinforcers for this patient?
      (2) What are punishers for this patient?
      (3) What are potential mediators for this patient?
   c. Discriminative stimuli
      (1) Under what conditions do appropriate responses occur?
      (2) Under what conditions do "inappropriate responses" occur?
      (3) Under what conditions is it hoped that the response will occur?
   d. Control
      (1) Can the nurse control the stimulus to the patient's response?
      (2) Can the nurse control the reinforcers?

3. *Baseline*
   a. Select problem response(s) and stimulus condition(s)
      (1) Define objectively. (When Don sees patients laughing together in the dayroom, he hits a patient.)
      (2) Quantify response(s). (This happens about once an hour.)
   b. Empirically validate potential reinforcers

       (1) Apply Premack principle. (Note how Don spends most of his time.)
       (2) Manipulate reinforcers under consideration. (Reward Don with what he likes best.)

4. *Assessment*
   a. Are the empirical baseline data different from the "armchair" behavioral history information?
      (1) Are there newly identified problems?
      (2) Are the originally defined problems substantiated by the data?
   b. Can the problem be redefined and therefore eliminated?
   c. What type of learning problem is involved?
      (1) Response too frequent?
      (2) Response too infrequent?
      (3) Response never occurs?
         (a) Never did occur?
         (b) Used to occur but does not currently?
      (4) Response occurs but in inappropriate stimulus situations?
         (a) Discrimination problem—response occurs when it should not occur?
         (b) Generalization problem—response occurs only in some of the instances when it should occur?

5. *Intervention*
   a. What is the behavioral goal?
   b. What behavioral technique can be used to accomplish this goal?
   c. How can the technique be operationalized?

6. *Evaluation*
   a. Was the goal reached?
      (1) Yes
         (a) Plan for maintenance of the change.
         (b) Is there another behavior that requires modification?
      (2) No
         (a) Is more time required?
         (b) Is the plan in need of alteration? If so, return to assessment step and continue.

Adapted from Loomis, M., & Horsley, J. A. (1974). *Interpersonal Change: A Behavioral Approach to Nursing Practice.* New York: McGraw-Hill. Reproduced with permission.

EYE MOVEMENT DESENSITIZATION AND REPROCESSING

EMDR is a cognitive behavioral therapy technique that employs specific, repetitive eye movements similar to those used in rapid eye movement (REM) sleep. While executing the rapid eye movements, the client holds in mind distressing visual memories or worries, negative self-statements, and unpleasant feelings. "EMDR has been shown to promote rapid processing (working through) of traumatic memories, with subsequent relief of anxiety, depression, somatic disorders and other symptoms" (Grainger, 1992, p.18).

USES

EMDR has been used to treat:
1. Posttraumatic stress disorder (PTSD) (Lipke & Botkin, 1992; Thomas & Gafner, 1993)
2. Phobias (Doctor, 1994; Kleinknecht, 1993)
3. Panic disorder (Goldstein & Feske, 1994; O'Brien, 1993)
4. Sexual dysfunction (Levin, 1993; Wernik, 1993)
5. Chemical dependency (Shapiro, Vogelmann-Sine, & Sine, 1994)
6. Dissociative disorders (Young, 1994)

ROLE OF PSYCHOTHERAPY

EMDR is seen as "an adjunct to, not a substitute for, good solid psychotherapy" (Grainger, 1992). Though the exact mechanism is not known, EMDR appears to "thin out the amnesic barrier" that protects clients from traumatic memories (Grainger, 1992, p. 18). As clients retrieve the memories it is vital they have a trusted therapist to work through this painful material.

REFERENCES

Agras, W. S., Taylor, C. B., Feldman, D. E., Losch, M., & Burnett, K. F. (1990). Developing computer-assisted therapy for the treatment of obesity. *Behavior Therapy, 21,* 99–109.

Doctor, R. (1994, March). Eye Movement Desensitization and Reprocessing with Personality Disorders. Paper presented at the 10th annual meeting of the Anxiety Disorders Association of America, Santa Monica, CA.

Frawley, P. J., & Smith, J. W. (1990). Chemical aversion therapy in the treatment of cocaine dependence as part of a multimodal treatment program: Treatment outcome. *Journal of Substance Abuse Treatment, 7,* 21.

Goldstein, A., & Feske, V. (1994). Eye movement desensitization and reprocessing for panic disorder: A case series. *Journal of Anxiety Disorders, 8,* 351–362.

Grainger, R. D. (1992). Eye movements: A new psychotherapeutic tool. *American Journal of Nursing, 92* (5), 18.

Hersen, M., & Detre, T. (1994). The behavioral psychotherapy of anorexia nervosa. In T. B. Karasu & L. Bellak (eds.), *Specialized Techniques for Specific Clinical Problems in Psychotherapy* (pp. 295–304). Northvale, NJ: Jason Aronson, Inc.

Kaplan, H. I., Sadock, B. J., & Grebb, J. A. (1994). *Kaplan and Sadock's Synopsis of Psychiatry* (7th ed.). Baltimore: Williams & Wilkins.

Kellner, R., Neidhardt, J., Krakow, B., & Pathak, D. (1992). Changes in chronic nightmare after one session of desensitization or rehearsal instructions. *American Journal of Psychiatry, 149* (5), 659–663.

Kleinknecht, R. A. (1993). Rapid treatment of blood and injection phobias with eye movement desensitization. *Journal of Behavioral Therapy and Experimental Psychiatry, 24,* 211–217.

Levin, C. (July/Aug. 1993). The enigma of EMDR. *Family Therapy Networker,* 75–83.

Lipke, H., & Botkin, A. (1992). Brief case studies of eye movement desensitization and reprocessing with chronic post-traumatic stress disorder. *Psychotherapy, 29,* 591–595.

Loomis, M., & Horsely, J. A. (1974). *Interpersonal Change: A Behavioral Approach to Nursing Practice.* New York: McGraw Hill.

Maletzky, B. M. (1990). *Treating the Sexual Offender.* Newbury Park, CA: Sage Publications.

Marks, I. M. (1987). *Fears, Phobias and Rituals.* New York: Oxford University Press.

Martin, G., & Pear, J. (1992). *Behavioral Modification: What It Is and How to Do It* (4th ed.). Englewood Cliffs, NJ: Prentice Hall.

Masters, W. H., & Johnson, V. E. (1970). *Human Sexual Inadequacy.* Boston: Little Brown.

O'Brien, E. (Nov./Dec. 1993). Pushing the panic button. *Family Therapy Networker, 75–83.*

Shapiro, F., Vogelmann-Sine, S., & Sine, L. (1994). Eye movement desensitization and reprocessing: Treating trauma and substance abuse. *Journal of Psychoactive Drugs, 26,* 379–391.

Thomas, R., & Gafner, G. (1993). PTSD in an elderly male: Treatment with eye movement desensitization and reprocessing (EMDR). *Clinical Gerontologist, 14,* 57–59.

Wernik, V. (1993). The rate of the traumatic component in the etiology of sexual dysfunctions and its treatment with eye movement desensitization procedure. *Journal of Sex Education and Therapy, 19,* 212–222.

Young, W. (1994). EMDR treatment of phobic symptoms in multiple personality. *Dissociation, 7,* 129–133.

THIRTEEN

13 Cognitive Therapy

Bonnie S. Joyce

DESCRIPTION

Cognitive therapy is an active, time-limited, structured form of therapy used to treat a variety of psychopathological states. It has been proven remarkably successful in treating depression, anxiety, and phobias, and is one of the first forms of psychotherapy that has withstood the test of rigorous scientific research (Burns, 1980). Cognitive therapy differs from traditional psychotherapy in that it is short-term, problem-oriented, and deals in the here and now. There is a strong emphasis on the empirical investigation of a client's cognitions and attitudes (Beck, Rush, Shaw, & Emery, 1979). Incorporating a set of interrelated techniques that are applied within the cognitive therapy of depression framework (Beck, 1976), the therapy is based on the general assumption that individuals continuously and actively experience and perceive stimuli that are organized into cognitions. These cognitions constitute stream of consciousness, reflecting how we view ourselves, the world, and the future. It is these cognitions that affect our emotional state and subsequent behavioral patterns (Beck et al., 1979). In other words, our thoughts and feelings influence the manner in which we behave.

Cognitive therapy employs the use of varied therapeutic techniques aimed at identifying distorted cognitions and modifying the underlying beliefs supporting the cognitions. Once a client is able to recognize and correct faulty cognitions, symptoms are reduced (Beck et al., 1979). Cognitive theory is employed in:

1. Individual therapy
2. Group therapy
3. Inpatient milieu therapy

KEY CONCEPTS

The cognitive model of depression postulates three concepts that are critical to understanding the theory and practice of cognitive therapy: cognitive triad (see Figure 13-1), schemas, and cognitive errors.

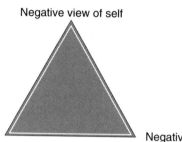

FIGURE 13-1   Cognitive Triad

COGNITIVE TRIAD

The cognitive triad consists of three negative cognitive patterns, reflecting how clients view themselves, the world, and the future (Beck et al., 1979). These negative thoughts lead to maladaptive behaviors. Table 13-1 lists the three cognitive patterns, thoughts associated with each, and the resulting maladaptive behaviors.

TABLE 13-1
Cognitive Patterns, Thoughts, and Maladaptive Behaviors

COGNITIVE PATTERN		THOUGHTS		MALADAPTIVE BEHAVIORS
Negative view of self	→	Inadequate, worthless	→	Avoidance
Negative view of the world	→	Helpless, unfair	→	Giving up
Negative view of the future	→	Failure, hopeless	→	Suicidal ideation

SCHEMAS

Schemas can be referred to as blueprints for living, as they determine how an individual conceptualizes and structures a situation (Beck et al., 1979). The structural organization that forms the core of cognitive therapy is illustrated below.

Beliefs   →   Attitudes/Personal Rules   →   Coping Strategies

1. *Beliefs* begin forming around age 2 and are present throughout childhood.
2. *Personal rules* are the rules individuals create for themselves to live by.
3. *Coping strategies* are the mechanisms individuals engage in to cope with the rules and attitudes they have created.

Beliefs influence the attitudes and personal rules we follow and these factors influence the style or pattern of coping strategies we use. Table 13-2 lists common beliefs and common dysfunctional attitudes.

TABLE 13-2
Common Negative Beliefs and Common Dysfunctional Attitudes

BELIEFS	DYSFUNCTIONAL ATTITUDES
I'm bad	Must be good to be valuable
I'm unlovable	Can't live without another person
I'm inferior	Must excel in all aspects of life
Others will hurt me	Avoid embarrassment at all costs
Others will take advantage of me	Must hide real self from others
The world is unfair	Must be accepted to be happy
I'm a failure	Must succeed to be worthwhile

COGNITIVE ERRORS

Errors in thinking represent the process and content of cognitive therapy. We are continuously involved in a series of positive, neutral, and negative events and situations. These events and situations are interpreted and processed through a series of thoughts that continuously influence mental processing. These thoughts or cognitions create an emotional response or feeling (Beck et al., 1979). The following diagram illustrates the situation, thought, and feeling process:

Situation/Event	$\rightarrow$	*Thought*	$\rightarrow$	*Feeling*
Breakup with spouse		Nobody will ever love me		Sadness

Situations and events begin the distortion process, producing automatic negative thoughts or cognitive distortions. The automatic negative thoughts and cognitive distortions occur spontaneously and on the surface are specific to a situation, but in actuality are representative of a schema, or one's belief structure. Box 13-1 lists 10 cognitive distortions and their definitions.

Thoughts and feelings often lead to maladaptive behaviors. For example:

Thought	$\rightarrow$	*Feeling*	$\rightarrow$	*Behavior*
Nobody will ever love me		Sadness		Withdraw from others

GOALS

Cognitive therapy is based on the idea that negative thoughts lead to negative emotions, which lead to behavioral problems. Thus, the goal of cognitive therapy is to identify and change negative thoughts to more realistic ones. The initial phase of cognitive therapy aims to identify and change negative thoughts, which will provide the client with symptom reduction. The second half of therapy aims to identify and modify beliefs and attitudes, which will provide the client with prophylaxis.

BEGINNING STAGE

1. Establishing a specific, concrete problem list and setting mutual realistic, achievable goals
2. Maintaining client safety
3. Finding solutions for solvable problems

MIDDLE STAGE

1. Understanding the relationship between thoughts, feelings, and behaviors

BOX 13-1: Definitions of Cognitive Distortions

1. *All-or-nothing thinking:* You see things in black-and-white categories. If your performance falls short of perfect, you see yourself as a total failure.

2. *Overgeneralization:* You see a single negative event as a never-ending pattern of defeat.

3. *Mental filter:* You pick out a single negative detail and dwell on it exclusively so that your vision of all reality becomes darkened, like the drop of ink that discolors the entire beaker of water.

4. *Disqualifying the positive:* You reject positive experiences by insisting they "don't count" for some reason or other. In this way you can maintain a negative belief that is contradicted by your everyday experiences.

5. *Jumping to conclusions:* You make a negative interpretation even though there are no definite facts that convincingly support your conclusion.

    a. *Mind reading.* You arbitrarily conclude that someone is reacting negatively to you, and you don't bother to check this out.

    b. *The fortune-teller error.* You anticipate that things will turn out badly, and you feel convinced that your prediction is an already established fact.

6. *Magnification (catastrophizing) or minimization:* You exaggerate the importance of things (such as your goof-up or someone else's achievement), or you inappropriately shrink things until they appear tiny (your own desirable qualities or the other person's imperfections). This is also called the "binocular trick."

7. *Emotional reasoning:* You assume that your negative emotions necessarily reflect the way things really are: "I feel it; therefore it must be true."

8. *Should statements:* You try to motivate yourself with "shoulds" and "shouldn'ts," as if you had to be whipped and punished before you could be expected to do anything. "Musts" and "oughts" are also offenders. The emotional consequence is guilt. When you direct "should" statements toward others, you feel anger, frustration, and resentment.

9. *Labeling and mislabeling:* This is an extreme form of overgeneralization. Instead of describing your error, you attach a negative label to yourself: "I'm a loser." When someone else's behavior rubs you the wrong way, you attach a negative label to him: "He's a goddamn louse." Mislabeling involves describing an event with language that is highly colored and emotionally loaded.

10. *Personalization:* You see yourself as the cause of some negative external event, which in fact you were not primarily responsible for.

From Burns, D. D. (1980). *Feeling Good* (pp. 40–41). New York: Signet. Copyright 1980 by David D. Burns, M.D.

2. Applying cognitive and behavioral techniques
3. Reducing symptoms

END STAGE

1. Preparing clients to be their own therapists
2. Identifying and modifying self-defeating behaviors
3. Changing and forming new beliefs

GENERAL TECHNIQUES

Cognitive therapy uses seven techniques: collaborative emphasis, agenda-setting, summarizing, hypothesis-testing, guided discovery, feedback, and homework (Beck et al., 1979).

Collaborative Emphasis Constant, active interaction between therapist and client. Both collaborate to form a therapeutic alliance in which both are working to solve the client's problems. There is a strong emphasis on empirical investigation of the client's dysfunctional ideas and beliefs (Beck et al., 1979). The therapist and client set up a series of experiments in which the client can test hypotheses. This approach minimizes client resistance and increases efficacy.

Agenda-Setting The systematic and methodical way of structuring each session, ensuring the judicious use of time. The agenda is concrete and precise and includes the client's experiences since the last session and feedback on assignments. The agenda helps ensure that the client and therapist together decide which topics to cover and their relative importance.

Summarizing A periodic review by therapist and client about each session. The review provides the therapist with the opportunity to explain the theory and rationale for specific techniques and identify and reinforce progress.

Hypothesis-Testing The process by which a client views an automatic negative thought as a hypothesis and then conducts an experiment to seek evidence that either validates or invalidates the thought. Hypothesis-testing allows the client to actively acquire new conclusions, rather than debating and arguing with the therapist.

Guided Discovery The use of hypothesis-testing and questioning to arrive at a new conclusion. After conducting an empirical test, the therapist leads the client through a series of Socratic questioning that will help the client identify and correct cognitive errors and dysfunctional beliefs. Socratic questioning is inductive questioning that leads the client to a conclusion.

Feedback A process that permits the client to express perceptions and feelings regarding the therapy, homework, and therapist, and provides the therapist with a method to evaluate the client's understanding of the therapy and its rationale. It is equally important that the therapist provide the clients with feedback about their progress and the therapist's thoughts or concerns about the clients.

Homework Homework assignments are given each session and reviewed the following session. These assignments reinforce and supplement the educational aspects of the therapy. The therapist gives specific instructions and therapeutic rationale for homework assignments, and investigates the client's attitude toward the homework, exploring reasons when the client does not complete assignments.

SPECIFIC BEHAVIORAL TECHNIQUES

Activity Scheduling Used to counteract a client's loss of motivation and inactivity. The schedule not only structures the client's day, but provides the client with information to assess daily activities.

Mastery And Pleasure Ratings Allows clients to readily view their progress and highlight their feelings of enjoyment and fun.

Box 13-2 is an example of a daily activity schedule that incorporates the use of mastery and pleasure ratings.

BOX 13-2: Daily Activity Schedule

DATE: _____	Prospective Plan your activities on an hour-by-hour basis at the start of the day.	Retrospective At the end of the day, record what you actually did and rate each activity with an M for mastery or a P for pleasure.*
TIME		
8–9		
9–10		
10–11		
11–12		
12–1		
1–2		
2–3		
3–4		
4–5		
5–6		
6–7		
7–8		
8–9		
9–12		

*Mastery and pleasure activities must be rated from 0 to 5: The higher the number, the greater the sense of satisfaction.

From Burns, D. D. (1980). *Feeling Good* (p. 88). New York: Signet. Copyright 1980 by David D. Burns, M.D.

Graded Task Assignment Illustrates to clients that they can complete a series of tasks and as a result experience some improvement in mood. This technique helps the client break down an activity into steps and permits the client to complete a task that was once seen as impossible or overwhelming.

Cognitive Rehearsal Used when a client has difficulty concentrating on routine tasks and carrying out habitual behaviors. This technique has clients imagine each step in completing a task, helping them pay attention to the task at hand and preventing distraction.

SPECIFIC COGNITIVE TECHNIQUES

Recording Dysfunctional Thoughts Involves a five-column thought recording. The client selects a situation, recognizes automatic negative thoughts, identifies emotions, forms a new thought, and identifies a new emotion. Box 13-3 illustrates a five-column thought recording.

BOX 13-3: Daily Record of Dysfunctional Thoughts

DATE	Situation	Emotion(s)	Automatic Thoughts(s)	Rational Response	Outcome
	Describe: 1. Actual event leading up to unpleasant emotion or 2. Stream of thoughts, daydream, or recollection, leading to unpleasant emotion.	1. Specify sad, anxious, angry, etc. 2. Rate degree of emotion 1–100%.	1. Write automatic thought(s) that preceded emotion(s). 2. Rate belief in automatic thought(s) 0–100%.	1. Write rational response to automatic thought(s). 2. Rate belief in rational response 0–100%.	1. Re-rate belief in automatic thought(s). 2. Specify and rate subsequent emotions 0–100%.

Explanation: When you experience an unpleasant emotion, note the situation that seemed to stimulate the emotion. (If the emotion occurred while you were thinking, daydreaming, etc., please note this.) Then note the automatic thought associated with the emotion. Record the degree to which you believe this thought: 0% = not at all, 100% = completely. In rating degree of emotion, 1 = a trace, 100 = the most intense possible.

From Beck, A. T., et al. (1979). *Cognitive Therapy of Depression* (p. 403). New York: Guilford Press. Copyright 1979 by Aaron T. Beck, A. John Rush, Brian F. Shaw, and Gary Emery.

Reattribution Techniques   Used when a client unrealistically attributes negative events or bad occurrences to a personal deficiency. The therapist helps the client review the event or situation, apply the laws of logic, and make a new assignment of responsibility.

Problem-Solving   Helps the client find acceptable solutions to problems that were once thought to be unsolvable. An example of the problem-solving steps is outlined:

Identify the problem.
Develop a list of alternatives.
Examine the pros and cons of the alternatives.
Choose and plan out a solution.
Evaluate.

Semantic Method Emphasizes the identification of "should statements" about oneself, others, and the world. Once these rigid, coercive rules are identified, they can be realistically examined and replaced with a revised version, such as "It would be nice," or "It would be preferable" (Burns, 1989).

Cost–Benefit Analysis Focuses on the client's motivation for accepting a negative thought or belief. Once the negative thought or belief is identified, the client evaluates the advantages and disadvantages of the negative thought or belief. The goal is then to modify the negative thoughts or beliefs that have more disadvantages than advantages (Burns, 1989).

EVALUATION

Cognitive therapy is considered successful when:

1. The client can independently recognize distorted thoughts, successfully challenge these thoughts, and form a more realistic thought.
2. The client is able to experience a reduction in symptoms and an elevation of mood.
3. The client can identify dysfunctional beliefs and attitudes that influence inappropriate coping strategies.
4. The client can abandon maladaptive behaviors and demonstrate adaptive behavior patterns.

REFERENCES

Beck, A. T. (1976). *Cognitive Therapy and the Emotional Disorders.* New York: International Universities Press.
Beck, A. T., Rush, A. J., Shaw, B. F., & Emery G. (1979). *Cognitive Therapy of Depression: A Treatment Manual.* New York: Guilford Press.
Burns, D. D. (1980). *Feeling Good.* New York: Signet.
Burns, D. D. (1989). *The Feeling Good Handbook.* New York: Penguin Books.

BIBLIOGRAPHY

Davis, M. H., & Casey, D. A. (1990). Utilizing cognitive therapy on the short-term psychiatric inpatient unit. *General Hospital Psychiatry, 12* (3), 170–176.
McDermott, S. P., & Wright, F. D. (1992). Cognitive therapy: Long-term outlook for a short-term psychotherapy. In J. S. Rutan (ed.), *Psychotherapy for the 1990's* (pp. 61–102). New York: Guilford Press.
Persons, J. B. (1989). *Cognitive Therapy in Practice.* New York: W. W. Norton & Company.
Rush, A. J. (1983). Cognitive therapy of depression: Rationale, techniques and efficacy. *Psychiatric Clinics of North America, 6* (1), 105–127.
Thase, M. E., & Wright, J. H. (1991). Cognitive behavior therapy manual for depressed inpatients: A treatment protocol outline. *Behavior Therapy, 22,* 579–595.
Wright, J. H., & Beck, A. T. (1983). Cognitive therapy of depression: Theory and practice. *Hospital and Community Psychiatry, 34* (12), 1119–1127.

14
FOURTEEN

Brief Solution-Focused Therapy

Carolyn V. Billings

DESCRIPTION

Brief therapy is a carefully circumscribed and time-confined modality that focuses on working with the client on the client's goals. It is not the traditional approach to treatment done in a hurry, but rather represents an entirely fresh way of approaching the therapeutic project. Brief therapy is shorter and therefore demands tight organization and focus. Brief means time-effective, not inferior.

For the most part, brief therapy is solution-focused, rather than illness-focused or problem-focused, and it is not confined to a particular type of problem. This is not "formula therapy" but rather is a model for therapy, supported by specific assumptions (see Box 14-1). Brief, solution-focused therapy is used with individuals, couples, and families (the client) for any presenting problem. In brief therapy, a problem is defined as any client complaint within the power of the client and the therapist to solve.

APPROACH

Solution-focused therapy dictates that once the client's complaint is clearly specified, attention is devoted to ways to help the client produce the desired results or solution. Because the therapy is solution-focused, little if any time is spent gathering detailed information about the problem and its origins and little value is placed on understanding *why* the problem occurred. Attention to past patterns or historical data is likely to concentrate on previous successes. In solution-focused therapy the therapist's understanding of dynamics is used primarily to help the client use the dynamic forces to promote desired change. The strategies employed in solution-focused therapy are designed to

BOX 14-1: Basic Assumptions Supporting Solution-Focused Therapy

Therapy is a cooperative venture.

There is no such thing as resistance.

The therapist co-creates the problem with the client.

The initial approach to a problem sets the course for the therapy.

Complicated problems do not require complicated solutions.

There are exceptions to every problem.

Exceptions to a problem defy the pervasiveness of the problem.

Exceptions to the identified problem are the best clue to solving it.

Past successes are the best clue to future ones.

The better the focus, the clearer the picture.

The clearer the goal, the straighter the path.

The goal belongs to the client.

The best intervention is the simplest possible one that has the desired effect.

Things seen differently become different.

There are solutions.

There is more than one solution.

Solutions are constructed, not discovered.

Change is an everyday event.

Change is not only possible, but inevitable.

Change occurs in an instant; readiness for change is what takes the time.

One small change leads to more change.

Theories and explanations are irrelevant to the process of change.

enter the realm of dynamic action. The bottom line to this approach to therapy is to create change.

The "brief therapy" of de Shazer (1985), the "possibility therapy" of O'Hanlon (1994), and the "divorce-busting therapy" of Weiner-Davis (1992) are examples of various approaches using the brief, solution-focused model.

THE NURSING PROCESS

Although it is possible to identify the elements of the nurse–client relationship and to specify aspects of the nursing process, in brief therapy these occur concurrently and simultaneously. Any division into phases or parts of the process would be artificial. By its very nature, brief therapy dictates that the orientation, working, and termination phases of the therapeutic relationship be integrated and ongoing throughout the course of treatment and, similarly, that the processes of assessment, planning, intervention, and evaluation be components of each and every therapeutic contact.

TECHNIQUES

The following techniques are employed in brief, solution-focused therapy.

INITIATE AND MAINTAIN THE NURSE–CLIENT RELATIONSHIP

○ Establish and maintain professional boundaries.
○ Use empathic responses.
○ Synchronize your style with the client's (volume, pace, posturing, language).
○ Validate the client's emotional responses.
○ Affirm the client's personal resources.
○ Join with the client in a partnership to resolve the problem.
○ Convey optimism. Use "possibility" talk.
○ Offer genuine compliments and expressions of admiration for the client's work.
○ Stay one step *behind* the client's progress and observe it out loud.
○ Treat clients as the experts they are.
○ Be solicitous, polite, and respectful.

FOCUS THE ASSESSMENT

○ Emphasize the client's strengths.
○ Construct a clear complaint.
○ Negotiate a solvable problem.
○ Immediately begin framing a solution.

CLARIFY THE EXPECTED OUTCOME

1. *Action realm:* "What are you *doing* now?" "What would you like to be *doing* differently?"
2. *Solution realm:* "What exactly are you planning to accomplish?"
3. *Goal talk:* "What small change would have to happen for you to believe that things were getting better?"
4. *Video talk:* "What will it look and sound like? What could I see now and what will I see when you succeed?" "When these changes occur, how will your (neighbor, spouse, family, friend) be able to tell that the situation is better?"
5. *Quantification:* Establish a baseline. How often? How many times per . . . ?
   "On a scale of 1 to 10 (with 1 being *x* and 10 being *y*) what rating would you give things presently? How will you get to (the next number)? What will it take to get to a ⸺ (next number)?"

EVALUATE THE READINESS FOR CHANGE

1. Assess external supports for nonchange.
   "When you accomplish these changes, whose life will be affected besides your own?"
2. Assess internal supports for nonchange.
   "Every change involves gains and losses. When your situation changes, what will you gain? What will you lose?"
3. Resist the change (paradoxically).
   "It's important not to make too many changes too quickly. Take your time and evaluate the effects of the changes you make as you go."

IDENTIFY STRENGTHS AND PAST SUCCESSES

"Remember a similar time when you had a situation that seemed impossible but you came through, and tell me about it."

CONTRACT WELL-DEFINED GOALS

1. Construct goal statements that are clear and measurable.

    Begin by getting a clear "video talk" of what the problem looks like and sounds like. Then focus on how it will look and sound when the problem is gone. Help the client to be as precise as possible. Keep reflecting and clarifying until the goal is crystal-clear and possible to measure.

2. Identify ways to measure progress.

    "What will be the very first thing you notice when things start to get better for you?"

    "If I were your closest friend, how would I be able to tell, without you telling me, that you were feeling better?"

3. Construct goal statements that are clear pathways toward solutions.

    Miracle Question: "Suppose there was a miracle and overnight this problem was solved. How would you know? What would be different?" (de Shazer, 1987)

IDENTIFY EXCEPTIONS TO THE PROBLEM

1. Discover the most recent time when the problem did *not* occur, or occurred with less frequency, duration, or intensity (exceptions).

    "Think back to a time when you and your wife had a disagreement and handled it without an argument (or when the argument was pretty minor; or when the argument was especially short). Tell me about it."

2. Listen for times when the problem isn't happening and it should be.

    "What are you doing that's good for you?"

    "Tell me about what you did when you overcame the temptation to . . ."

3. Emphasize strengths.

    "You're really clear about what you want to accomplish here. Not everyone can focus in so well on the changes they want to make."

    "You two are in agreement about more things than you are in disagreement about. You're working together in lots of ways. That's a good start."

4. Be persistent in going after exceptions.

    "Your daughter has *never* been cooperative about *anything*?"

    "Okay, so he wets the bed *every* night. When is the bed soaking wet, and when is it just damp?"

5. Express intense interest in the exceptions.

    "That's fascinating. Your friends wanted you to 'party' and you turned them down. That's a switch, isn't it?"

    "Wait a minute! You just said that things have been better in the last few days. I'm really interested in how you managed that."

6. Express wonderment about the exceptions.

    "You're amazing! How did you do that?"

    "So you've already begun the process of change. I'm really impressed."

7. Analyze with the client exactly how the exceptions occur.

    "Tell me about a typical day when you do binge eating and compare that with a day when you eat normally."

    "Just what was different about the way you handled that situation compared with how you would have dealt with it, say, last month?"

ASSIGN SOLUTION TRIALS AS HOMEWORK

1. Assign activities that represent small changes.

   "If it works, don't fix it. Once you know what works, do more of it. If it doesn't work, don't do it again: Do something different" (de Shazer, 1987).

2. Design pattern interventions.

   Change the frequency, intensity, time, or some other feature of the problem itself or of the pattern around the problem.

3. Focus on what works.

   First Session Formula Task: "Between now and our next visit observe so that you can describe what happens that you would like to continue to happen" (de Shazer, 1985).

4. Study what maintains the problem and what creates the context for change.

   "So this rule you have in your head: 'If you can't say anything nice, don't say anything at all,' is a good rule in principle, but it's not working for you."

5. Keep it simple.

   Start with encouraging small changes and work your way along:

   "Keeping your goal in mind, what is the first tiny step you can take that will let you know you are moving in the right direction?"

6. Use exceptions and successes.

   Exceptions (times when the problem doesn't occur when it normally would) and successes (when the problem is overcome) are the "keys" to solutions. Building on these can crowd the problem out of existence.

   "Think of an example of a time when you stated what you wanted or needed rather than feeling angry and upset because you weren't getting it."

   "How is it that you managed to be at the party and resist the temptation to drink?"

DESIGN DYNAMIC STRATEGIES

1. Reframe the problem.

   Present another, more positive way of looking at the problem and how it has "served" the client until now.

2. Use possibility language (O'Hanlon, 1994).

   "When these changes occur . . ." "You will . . ."

   "You can expect, watch for . . ."

   "How will your life be different when . . . ?" "Who will be the first to notice these new changes?"

3. Encourage the client to reconsider basic assumptions.

   "It is time to reconsider the beliefs that shape our lives. You have been holding on to the belief that if you get something because you ask for it, it is somehow not as good as if you hadn't had to ask. You may want to think about whether or not you still want to think that way, since now you are discovering that if you ask for something you stand a better chance of getting it."

4. Issue directives.

   Tell the client to *do* something.

   "This week, instead of going right home after work, get a babysitter and meet together for dinner out on a weeknight."

   Tell the client to *stop doing* something.

"Try turning the TV off every other evening this week and let me know what else you do with that time."

5. Employ paradoxical interventions.

Paradoxical interventions are used when straightforward approaches are not successful in helping to create change. In paradox, you "go with" the problem to get more information about it.

Prescribe the symptom—"Sometimes it's important to worry a little. I'd hate to see you give up worrying altogether. Worry can serve an important function. For one thing, it prevents us from making too many mistakes. Just so you don't forget how to worry, try this: each evening set the oven timer for 15 minutes and spend that time worrying about everything on your mind. When the timer goes off, get up and go about your usual activities."

Express helplessness—"I feel like I'm not being as helpful as I'd like to be, but this is a tough problem to solve. I'll admit, I'm stumped. What do you think we should try next?"

Restrain progress—"When you're ready, it will come more easily. We're not there yet. Don't move too quickly. Take your time."

Predict relapse—"It wouldn't surprise me if at this point you temporarily went back to where we started. Folks sometimes do that after they've made important changes. It helps to remind themselves of just how bad it used to be."

6. Use metaphors, metadramas, fables, and stories.

Stories with a therapeutic message can bypass conscious thinking and leave a seed for a solution planted in the "back" of the client's mind. The best metaphor re-creates the client's reality and then illustrates possibilities for successful resolution.

7. Initiate trance experience.

It can be very helpful to stimulate the use of nonconscious information available to the client in the form of previous learnings. When a person is in a trancelike state it is more possible to access unconscious resources, evoke involuntary skills, create an expectancy of change, and "aid in the recall of experiences that can serve as references to resolve the present difficulty" (O'Hanlon & Weiner-Davis, 1989).

OFFER POSITIVE FEEDBACK AND ENCOURAGEMENT

1. Take responsibility for failures; give credit for successes.

The solution belongs to the client, not to the therapist. The job of the therapist is to help the client access the success.

2. If things get stuck, revisit the goal.

KNOW WHEN TO STOP

1. Stay on track in pursuit of solutions.

It's easy to get distracted. There are so many interesting trails to explore. Solution-focused means to take issues one at a time, not all together.

2. Be alert for when the goal is met.

There's no need to stay on the train after you've reached the station.

3. Celebrate success.

   The energy generated by the satisfaction of a job well done is good for every-one concerned.

4. Treat every session as if it were the last.

   "Sometimes, the best thing therapists can do, once change is initiated, is to get out of their client's way!" (Weiner-Davis, 1985)

CONCLUSION

Brief solution-focused therapy is not only a crisp, pragmatic, cost-effective modality but also is very compatible with the philosophical underpinnings of the nursing profession. It is an optimistic, client-centered, nonnormative, health-focused, respectful approach that fits well within the nursing process and with nursing's strong commitment to the inclusion of clients as full partners in their health care.

REFERENCES

de Shazer, S. (1985). *Keys to Solution in Brief Therapy.* New York:Norton.

de Shazer, S. (1987). Minimal elegance. *Family Therapy Networker,* September/October, p. 59.

de Shazer, S. (1988). *Clues: Investigating Solutions in Brief Therapy.* New York: Norton.

O'Hanlon, W. H. (1994). *A Field Guide to Possibility Land: A Possibility Therapy Method Book.* Omaha: Possibility Press.

O'Hanlon, W. H., & Weiner-Davis, M. (1989). *In Search of Solutions: A New Direction in Psychotherapy.* New York: Norton.

Weiner-Davis, M. (1985). Dancing the waltz to rock and roll music. *Family Therapy Networker, 9* (4), 56.

Weiner-Davis, M. (1992). *Divorce Busting.* New York: Simon & Schuster.

BIBLIOGRAPHY

Billings, C. V. (1991). Therapeutic use of metaphors. *Issues in Mental Health Nursing, 12* (1), 1–8.

Budman, S. H., Hoyt, M. F., & Friedman, S. (1992). *The First Session in Brief Therapy.* New York: Guilford Press.

Cade, B., & O'Hanlon, W. H. (1993). *A Brief Guide to Brief Therapy.* New York: Norton.

Haley, J. (1990). Interminable therapy. *Family Therapy Networker, 14* (2), 32.

Lankton, R. R., & Erickson, K. K. (1993). *The Essence of a Single Session Success.* New York: Brunner/Mazel.

Montgomery, C., & Webster, D. (1994). Caring, curing, and brief therapy: A model for nurse psycho-therapy. *Archives of Psychiatric Nursing, 8* (5), 291–297.

Pesut, D. (1991). The art, science, and techniques of reframing in psychiatric–mental health nursing. *Issues in Mental Health Nursing, 12* (1), 9–18.

Talmon, M. (1991). *Single-Session Therapy.* San Francisco: Jossey-Bass.

Tuyn, L. (1992). Solution-oriented therapy and Rogerian nursing science: An integrated approach. *Archives of Psychiatric Nursing, 5* (2), 83–89.

Walter, J. L., & Peller, J. (1992). *Becoming Solution-Focused in Brief Therapy.* New York: Brunner/Mazel.

Webster, D. C., Vaughn, K., & Martinez, R. (1994). Introducing solution-focused approaches to staff in in-patient psychiatric settings. *Archives of Psychiatric Nursing, 8* (4), 254–261.

Weiner-Davis, M. (1990). In praise of solutions. *Family Therapy Networker,* March/April, 42–48.

FIFTEEN

Clinical Hypnosis/
Therapeutic Suggestion

Rothlyn P. Zahourek

OVERVIEW:

Introduction

Trance Phenomena

Hypnosis as a Therapeutic Intervention

    Uses

    Basic Hypnotic Approaches

    Susceptibility Scales

    Guidelines for Use

Induction Techniques

Suggestion

Direct Versus Indirect Suggestion

Factors Influencing Success

Side Effects and Precautions

INTRODUCTION

Hypnosis (often synonymous with *trance*) is a state and an intervention. Recent definitions emphasize that trance is an *expanded,* rather than altered, state of focused awareness in which the individual is receptive to new perceptions and ideas and hence is likely to initiate new behaviors (Zahourek, 1987). In the hypnotic experience the individual can easily suspend usual frames of reference and beliefs and subsequently solve problems more creatively (Erickson & Rossi, 1979, p. 3).

    The hypnotic state occurs on a continuum between sleep and wakefulness, with electroencephalogram patterns resembling more closely the waking state. Trance may occur naturally and spontaneously (driving a familiar route), be induced by another person (listening to a boring lecture), or be self-induced (meditation, relaxation techniques). This state varies in depth from a light, wakeful trance to a very deep, somnambulist trance in which amnesia and hallucinations occur. Depth is not necessarily correlated with therapeutic effectiveness. See Table 15-1 for common myths about hypnosis and corresponding facts.

TRANCE PHENOMENA

Trance phenomena include: selective inattention, dissociation, increased response to suggestion, literal interpretation, trance logic (the ability to accept illogical presentations of reality), amnesia, motoric and verbal inhibition, time distortion, age progression and regression, altered perceptions, analgesia and anesthesia, hallucinations, fluctuations in degree of involvement, willingness to experiment, lethargy and relaxation (Yapko, 1990).

TABLE 15-1
Myths and Facts About Hypnosis

MYTHS	FACTS
Only a select few can be hypnotized.	Most can respond therapeutically to hypnotic suggestion. Considering normal adults, 5% cannot go into trance at all; 95% can attain light trance; 55% can obtain medium trance; 20% are capable of deep trance (American Society of Clinical Hypnosis, 1973).
Hypnosis occurs only when clients allow themselves to be hypnotized.	Hypnosis usually involves concentration and willingness to relax. People are capable of resisting even indirect suggestions. People can also be hypnotized without conscious awareness.
Hypnosis is sleep.	Hypnosis is not sleep but an expanded or altered level of consciousness.
A hypnotherapist must possess a certain charisma or mystique.	The personality and the presence of the therapist has little to do with hypnotic responsiveness.
Hypnotherapists project their ability and skill onto the client.	The hypnotherapist merely guides clients in using their own abilities.
Under hypnosis people will behave in ways counter to their value system.	Some believe it is possible in circumstances of extreme stress and trauma or with a highly hypnotizable person under stress that individuals will perform acts counter to their values. This is debated and controversial.
Hypnotizability is a sign of mental weakness.	Research has shown the contrary; creative, bright individuals do well with hypnosis; psychopathology can impair concentration and hamper hypnotizability.
Hypnosis can create false memories.	Memories are stored in the unconscious through suppression and repression. False memories can be created by a therapist's suggestion with a vulnerable client with or without hypnosis.

Trance produces the following observable physical characteristics: muscle twitching; lacrimation; eye closure and eye flutter; change in breathing rate; relaxed jaw; pulse rate change; catalepsy, a state of little movement related to the absorption of the trance state (Yapko, 1990).

HYPNOSIS AS A THERAPEUTIC INTERVENTION

Hypnosis is a therapeutic adjunct to other forms of therapy. It may be used as a pattern of influential communication (indirect) or directly for a specific problem. The heart of intervention is the therapeutic use of suggestion following the induction.

USES

Hypnosis is used by psychiatric nurses for (Yapko, 1990; Zahourek, 1990; Spiegel & Spiegel, 1978):
1. Managing stress
2. Reducing anxiety
3. Resolving phobias

4. Changing a depressive cognitive stance
5. Enhancing the therapeutic process
6. Resolving a therapeutic impasse
7. Creating a safe mental space for working on problems
8. Resolving conflicts and making decisions
9. Retrieving memory
10. Resolving trauma

BASIC HYPNOTIC APPROACHES

Hypnosis interventions vary and usually are integrated with an overall therapeutic plan. The two basic approaches may be used in pure form or mixed either in the same induction or during the course of treatment. They are:

1. *Standard/traditional* hypnosis: characterized by direct suggestion, suggestibility tests, scripted approaches, and specific problem-orientation rather than process-orientation. Traditional hypnosis is seen as more authoritative or authoritarian than Ericksonian hypnosis (Spiegel & Spiegel, 1978; Hilgard, 1979; Kroger & Fezler, 1976; Kroger, 1977).
2. *Ericksonian* approaches: characterized by the use of indirect suggestion; utilization of individual characteristics, styles, and strengths. The Ericksonian approach is process-oriented and democratic (Erickson & Rossi, 1979; Zeig, 1985).

SUSCEPTIBILITY SCALES

Formal measurement scales have been designed to evaluate a person's responsiveness to hypnosis. The tests do *not* necessarily predict success of the intervention since they are directive and many clients respond to more individualized and permissive approaches. Susceptibility scales may help the clinician learn about hypnotic phenomena and how to phrase suggestion. See Box 15-1 for a list of susceptibility scales.

BOX 15-1: Susceptibility Scales

The Stanford Hypnotic Clinical Scale for Adults and Children

The Hypnotic Induction Profile

The Harvard Group Scale of Hypnotic Susceptibility

The Stanford Hypnotic Susceptibility Scale, Forms A, B, C

The Children's Hypnotic Susceptibility Scale

Stanford Profile Scales of Hypnotic Susceptibility

The Barber Suggestibility Scale

The Creative Imagination Scale

The Wexler-Alman Indirect Hypnotic Susceptibility Scale

The Waterloo-Stanford C Scale of Hypnotic Susceptibility

GUIDELINES FOR USE

Guidelines for practice set by the American Society of Clinical Hypnosis (Hammond & Elkins, 1994) include:

1. Clinicians do not use hypnosis for entertainment purposes.
2. Clinicians discuss ethical and legal guidelines as peers and with clients.

3. Clinicians consider written, informed consent and adhere to guidelines and precautions in using hypnosis to explore memories.

4. Clinicians use hypnosis only for treating conditions they are qualified to treat using *nonhypnotic* approaches.

5. Clinicians are cautious about maintaining professional boundaries and cautious about the potential imbalance of power in the hypnotherapy relationship.

INDUCTION TECHNIQUES

1. *Relaxation:* Any standard guided relaxation techniques such as progressive muscle relaxation can induce a trance state. Talking with clients about experiencing pleasant feelings and how this is beneficial for well-being enhances induction. Clients can remain relaxed for a period of time, then return to the usual waking state feeling relaxed, rested, and alert (Kennedy, 1984) (see Chapter 16).

2. *Imagery:* Any technique that helps the client develop an imagined mental experience can induce a trance. Imagery might involve sight, hearing, touch, smell, and taste. The more vividly the imagery is described, the greater potential for individual involvement and subsequent trance.

3. *Confusion:* When an individual experiences a large amount of confusing information a self-induced trance is often a good defense.

4. *Boredom:* When experiences are not interesting or are so common they do not require full attention, a trance state may result.

5. *Repetitive or rhythmic experiences:* Many forms of music and nonmodulating speech can induce a trance, i.e., shamanic drumming or a lecture given in the same tone and cadence.

6. *Specific instructions to do a task when the expectation is that a trance will result:* e.g., falling into another person's arms; arm levitation.

7. *Eye roll induction* (Spiegel & Spiegel, 1978): Following a relaxation technique, the client is instructed in a quiet tone, "While looking straight ahead roll your eyes up to the top of your head. Keeping your eyes up, take a deep breath. Hold your breath and slowly bring your eyelids down over your eyes. Keep looking upward and let your eyes close. Now let your breath out as slowly as you let your eyes relax. Take some deep breaths, breathing slowly and comfortably. Now imagine your body is light and buoyant and restful. You can feel relaxed and pleasant. Let all parts of your body relax. Let your head and neck and face feel loose and relaxed; your arms hang limply and your back muscles are soft; your leg muscles are completely relaxed and restful."

SUGGESTION

Suggestion is the "process by which sensory impressions are conveyed in a meaningful manner to evoke altered psychophysiological responses" (Kroger, 1977). Traditionally, suggestion was defined as a stimulus that evokes an uncritical acceptance of an idea. This, however, implies that the client is a passive recipient, unable to use cognitive reason (Sarbin & Coe, 1972). Suggestions are given in various ways and are, in essence, communication styles.

Types of suggestion include (Kroger & Fezler, 1976):

1. *Verbal:* the use of words.

2. *Nonverbal:* body language and gestures.

3. *Intraverbal:* the intonation of words (e.g., "You *will* feel comfort" (*will* emphasized and spoken more loudly).

4. *Extraverbal:* the implications of words (e.g., words such as *abuse, loose, soft, hard,* and *care* all have various implications depending on context, person, and cultural background).

Other classifications of suggestions include (Yapko, 1990):
1. *Positive suggestion:* "You can accomplish . . ."
2. *Negative suggestion:* "You cannot accomplish . . ."
3. *Direct suggestion:* "You can do . . . You will experience . . ."
4. *Indirect suggestion:* "You might do . . . Sometime in the near future you might . . ."
5. *Process suggestion:* "You can take the following steps . . ."
6. *Content suggestion:* "You can remember a pleasant birthday experience . . ."
7. *Permissive style:* "You can allow yourself to feel relaxed . . ."
8. *Authoritarian:* "I want you to . . . and then you will . . ."
9. *Posthypnotic suggestion:* "When you experience that feeling later you will be able to . . ."

DIRECT VERSUS INDIRECT SUGGESTION

1. A *direct* suggestion is usually more authoritative. The expected results are made clear. They are often associated with a formal trance induction and might be phrased, "You will open your eyes and feel more rested and comfortable." (The eye roll induction is phrased as a direct suggestion.)
2. An *indirect* suggestion is more subtle, and generally more permissive. It may or may not be associated with a formal induction and may be a part of any conversation. The above statement phrased indirectly might be, "When you feel ready, you can open your eyes and notice how different you feel; you might even be much more comfortable."

These techniques are general tools of therapeutic communication and are an essential part of Milton Erickson's utilization approach. They can be used with or without formal hypnosis. Indirect suggestions invite the client's participation and are built on empathy for their own experience and worldview. Indirect suggestions often include preliminary permissive phrases such as: "Perhaps you have already noticed that relaxation is increasing in your body" and "You might find as you take the next deep breath that you might increase the comfort and relaxation even more. . . . You might be surprised to discover how those feelings can help you to be more comfortable." These phrases encourage the client to "notice relaxation," and "change feelings toward comfort." Their permissive nature communicates choice, and often has the client wondering on a conscious level what you are talking about (Yapko, 1990), thus avoiding the potential resistance that can develop from direct suggestions.

Specific forms of indirect suggestion include such techniques as jokes and puns, stories and metaphors, reframing, assigning homework, establishing a "yes set," conversational postulates, conjunctive and contingent suggestion, embedded metaphor, dissociative suggestions, interspersed suggestions, and generalized referential index (Erickson, Rossi, & Rossi, 1976; Larkin, 1990; O'Hanlon, 1987; Yapko, 1990).

Direct and *indirect* suggestions are often incorporated into the same interaction. For example, "Relax your body by taking three deep breaths and go into the relaxed state that has become familiar to you; *as you encourage your unconscious mind to work for you, you might find that you have solved the problem and made a decision in the next few days.*" (The first suggestion is the direct approach; the *italicized* suggestion is the indirect approach.)

Theoretically, indirect approaches bypass resistance set up by more authoritarian directives, enable the individual various responses, and enlist unconscious processes that enable perceptual, cognitive, emotional, and behavioral changes. Lynn, Neufeld, and Mare (1993) reviewed the literature on direct and indirect suggestion and concluded:

1. Style minimally affects the individual's response to hypnotizability tests.
2. Subjective experiences such as pain yield contradictory results.
3. Controlled studies do not indicate that indirect suggestions are superior.

Szabo (1993) reported no difference in effect of direct and indirect suggestions on 44 subjects' subjective experiences, except the low and medium hypnotizable, measured by the Stanford Hypnotizability Scale, Form B, reported deeper hypnotic response with indirect suggestion.

Clinicians may use various approaches according to the clinical situation. In psychotherapy, for example, the indirect methods of telling stories and using metaphors help individuals reframe experiences. In contrast, in an emergency situation, instructing clients to breathe deeply and imagine themselves someplace far away may be more appropriate.

FACTORS INFLUENCING SUCCESS

Factors that influence acceptance and realization of suggestion and a successful induction are:

1. The emotional rapport and trust between the client and clinician
2. Motivation
3. Ability to follow directions
4. The effect created by the idea once it has been incorporated into the personality (Jones, 1948)
5. Expectancy
6. Ability to relax
7. Ability to imagine
8. Ability to concentrate
9. Acceptability and congruence with the client's psychological makeup, background, and life experience
10. The frequency with which a suggestion is given

Individuals respond to suggestions in two ways (Weitzenhoffer, 1980): with voluntary and conscious participation and involuntary, less conscious participation. When suggestions bypass higher cortical processes and elicit nonvoluntary response, it can be presumed that unconscious participation acceptance has occurred.

SIDE EFFECTS AND PRECAUTIONS

Side effects of hypnosis are rare but include psychotic decompensation, symptom substitution, anxiety, overdependency, depression, actual or attempted suicide, acting out, sexual seduction, conversion symptoms, masking organic disorders, posttrance headache, general distress, depersonalization, derealization, dissociation, regressions, confusion, and obsessive preoccupation (MacHovec, 1988). MacHovec (p. 46) suggests that to prevent side effects there should be consideration of: the *client* (careful screening, a good history, and informed consent), the *therapist* (assuring competent diagnostic, observational, and therapeutic skills), and the *environment* (providing physically comfortable, emotionally safe, stable, and supportive unobtrusive surroundings).

Nurses at all levels of practice can implement hypnotic approaches including relaxation therapy, imagery techniques, indirect suggestion, and use of positive suggestions during naturalistic waking trance. When using more formal hypnosis in either psycho-therapy or general practice, nurses should function only to the extent of their education and additional training in hypnosis. Maintaining regular supervision and consultation is highly recommended.

REFERENCES

American Society of Clinical Hypnosis, Education and Research Foundation (1973). *A Syllabus on Hypnosis and a Handbook of Therapeutic Suggestion.* Des Plaines, IL: American Society of Clinical Hypnosis.

Erickson, M., & Rossi, E. L. (1979). *Hypnotherapy: An Exploratory Casebook.* New York: Irvington Press.

Erickson, M., & Rossi E. L. (1980). *The Collected Papers of Milton H. Erickson, Vol. 1. The Nature of Hypnosis and Suggestion.* New York: Irvington Publications.

Erickson, M., Rossi, E. L., & Rossi, S. I. (1976). *Hypnotic Realities: The Induction of Clinical Hypnosis and Forms of Suggestion.* New York: Irvington Press.

Hammond, D. C., & Elkins, G. R. (1994). *Standards of Training in Clinical Hypnosis.* Des Plaines, IL: American Society of Clinical Hypnosis.

Hilgard, E. (1979). Divided consciousness in hypnosis: The implications of the hidden observer. In E. Fromm & R. E. Shor (eds.), *Hypnosis: Developments in Research and New Perspectives* (pp. 45–81). New York: Aldine Publishing.

Jones, E. (1948). *The Nature of Autosuggestion in Papers on Psychoanalysis* (5th ed.) Baltimore: Williams & Wilkins.

Kennedy, M. S. (1984). Hypnosis. In S. Lego (ed.), *American Handbook of Psychiatric Nursing* (pp. 319–326). Philadelphia: J. B. Lippincott.

Kroger, W. S. (1977). *Clinical and Experimental Hypnosis* (2nd ed.). Philadelphia: J. B. Lippincott.

Kroger, W. S., & Fezler, W. D. (1976). *Hypnosis and Behavior Modification: Imagery Conditioning.* Philadelphia: J. B. Lippincott.

Larkin, D. (1990). Therapeutic suggestion. In R. P. Zahourek (ed.), *Clinical Hypnosis and Therapeutic Suggestion in Patient Care* (pp. 43–55). New York: Brunner Mazel.

Lynn, S. J., Neufeld, V., & Mare C. (1993). Direct versus indirect suggestion: A conceptual and methodological review. *International Journal of Clinical and Experimental Hypnosis 41* (2), 124–152

MacHovec, F. (1988). Hypnosis complications, risk factors and prevention. *American Journal of Clinical Hypnosis, 31* (1), 40–46.

O'Hanlon, W. H. (1987). *Taproots: Underlying Principles of Milton Erickson's Therapy and Hypnosis.* New York: W. W. Norton Co.

Sarbin, T., & Coe W. (1972). *Hypnosis: A Social Psychological Analysis of Influence Communication.* New York: Holt, Reinhardt & Winston.

Spiegel, H., & Spiegel, D. (1978). *Trance and Treatment.* New York: Basic Books.

Szabo, C. (1993). The phenomenology of the experiences and depth of hypnosis: Comparison of direct and indirect induction techniques. *International Journal of Clinical and Experimental Hypnosis, 41,* 225–233.

Weitzenhoffer, A. M. (1980). Hypnotic susceptibility revisited. *American Journal of Clinical Hypnosis, 22,* 130–146.

Yapko, M. D. (1990). *Trancework: An Introduction to the Practice of Clinical Hypnosis.* New York: Brunner Mazel.

Zahourek, R. P. (November 1987). Clinical hypnosis in holistic nursing practice. *Holistic Nursing Practice Journal,* 15–24.

Zahourek, R. P. (1990). *Clinical Hypnosis and Therapeutic Suggestion in Patient Care.* New York: Brunner Mazel.

Zeig, J. (1985). *Ericksonian Psychotherapy: Vol. 1: Structures.* New York: Brunner Mazel.

BIBLIOGRAPHY

Edgette, J. H., & Edgette J. S. (1994). *The Handbook of Hypnotic Phenomena in Psychotherapy.* New York: Brunner Mazel.

Hammond, D. C. (ed.) (1994). *Hypnotic Induction and Suggestion: An Introductory Manual.* Des Plaines, IL: American Society of Clinical Hypnosis.

Havens, R. A., & Walters, C. (1989). *Hypnotherapy Scripts: A Neo-Ericksonian Approach to Persuasive Healing.* New York: Brunner Mazel.

Hunter, M. E. (1994). *Creative Scripts for Hypnotherapy.* New York: Brunner Mazel.

Yapko, M. D. (1994). *Essentials of Hypnosis.* New York: Brunner Mazel.

16
SIXTEEN

Relaxation

Elizabeth M. Varcarolis

OVERVIEW:

INTRODUCTION

It is well established that the body's emotional and physical health are interwoven. Selye (1956) identified the general adaptation syndrome (GAS), the body's reaction to physical insult. Now it is believed that Selye's general adaptation syndrome occurs in two stages: (1) an initial adaptive response and (2) the eventual maladaptive consequences of the prolonged psychobiological arousal known as the body's stress response (Rossi, 1993). See Box 16-1 for the reaction to stress over time.

Stress becomes pathogenic when it persists over time because we lose the capacity to turn off the mind–body's response signals that regulate the body's psychobiological response to stress. The body reacts physiologically in the same manner, whether the stress (real or perceived) is of a physical, psychological, or social nature. In the early 1970s, research demonstrated that clusters of certain life events (that is, death of spouse, marriage, job promotion, and so forth) can be, in themselves, stressful and can render one susceptible to illness (Holmes & Rahe, 1970).

EFFECTS OF PROLONGED STRESS

The body's physiologic stress response to emotional, environmental, and physical stressors is complex, involving both the hypothalamus–pituitary–adrenal cortex and a sympatho-adreno-medulla response. Chemicals produced by the stress response such as cortisol, adrenaline, and other catecholamines can have a profound effect on the systems of the body (Brigham, 1994). See Figure 16-1 for the stress response. Thus, the results of prolonged stress over long periods of time can precipitate or potentiate a

BOX 16-1: Reactions to Stress Over Time

Initial Adaptive Response			Prolonged Stress Response		
SECONDS	MINUTES	HOURS	DAYS	WEEKS	YEARS/DECADES
• Cannon's "Fight or Flight" Response	• **Complex Adaptive Response:** Mind–body messengers: Epinephrine, cortisol, etc.		• **Prolonged Stress Response:** Mind–body messengers:	↑ Addictions	
	↑ Energy mobilization & use		↑ Fatigue	↑ Myopathy	↑ Steroid diabetes
	↑ Cognition & performance		↕ Sleep	↑ Depression	↓ Memory & learning
	↑ Cardiovascular tone		↑ Stress hypertension		
	↑ Cardiopulmonary tone		↑ Respiratory problems		
	↑ Stress analgesia		↑ Opportunistic infections		
	↓ Immune system		↑ Psychogenic ulcers		
	↓ Digestion		↓ Libido	↑ Impotence, anovulation	
	↓ Sexuality				
	↓ Growth				

Adapted from Rossi, E. L. (1993). *The Physiology of Mind-Body Healing.* New York: W. W. Norton & Company; Sapolsky, R. (1990). Stress in the wild, *Scientific American,* Jan., 116–163.

wide variety of emotional and physical problems such as (Brigham, 1994; Moskowitz, 1992):

1. Essential hypertension
2. Heart disease/attack
3. Atherosclerosis
4. Diabetes
5. Cancer
6. Ulcers
7. Chronic gastrointestinal problems
8. Chronic fatigue
9. Allergies, eczema
10. Arthritis
11. Headaches
12. Immune compromise
13. Kidney and liver disease
14. Depression
15. Eating disorders (obesity, anorexia, bulimia)

STRESS REDUCTION

The effects of stress on the body depend on:

1. Inherited genetic predispositions
2. The way one perceives and handles stress

Stress can be reduced by relaxation techniques that usher in the relaxation response, a host of body-wide physical changes producing low physiological arousal (Dossey, 1993). Altering one's responses to stress through relaxation techniques can (Benson &

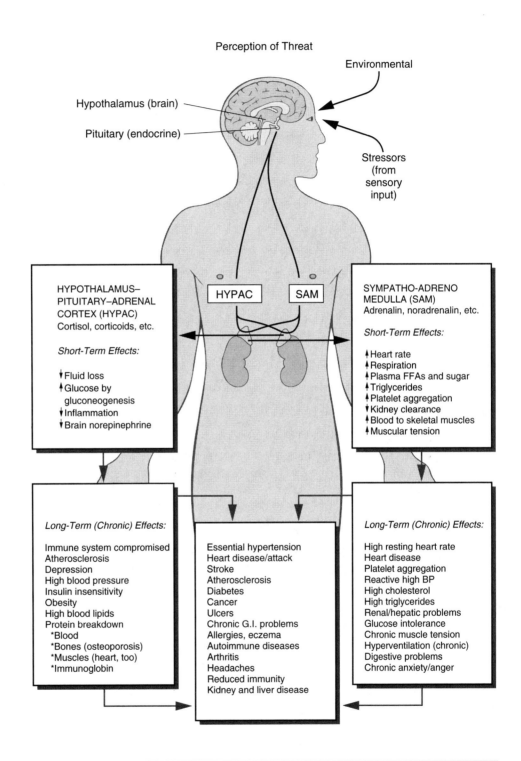

FIGURE 16-1   The Stress Response

From Brigham, D. D. (1994). *Imagery for Getting Well: Clinical Applications in Behavioral Medicine.* New York: W. W. Norton & Company.

Proctor, 1985; Rossi, 1993; Brigham, 1994; Moskowitz, 1992; Aron & Aron, 1980; Pilletteri, 1981; Heidt, 1981):

1. Alter the course of certain medical conditions such as high blood pressure, arrhythmias, arthritis, cancer, peptic ulcers, and more
2. Decrease the need for medications such as insulin, analgesics, and antihypertensives
3. Diminish or eliminate the need for unhealthy and destructive behaviors such as smoking, addictions to drugs, insomnia, and overeating
4. Increase cognitive functions such as learning, concentration, and improved study habits
5. Facilitate the Lamaze method of childbirth
6. Enhance the effectiveness of therapeutic touch
7. Break up static patterns of thinking and allow fresh and creative ways of perceiving things
8. Increase sense of well-being through endorphin release

NURSING CONSIDERATIONS

The nurse who uses relaxation techniques with clients keeps in mind that:

1. The relaxation response is a learned response that can be elicited in almost anyone.
   a. It should not be used with people who are psychotic or those who have weak ego boundaries. Symptoms, e.g., delusions and hallucinations, may become intensified.
   b. For those who are unable to use the relaxation techniques, biofeedback can obtain the same results.
2. There are many avenues toward achieving the relaxation response, and these are adapted to each client according to individual preference.
3. These techniques are not a panacea. They are tools to help people develop alternative responses to stress.
4. People have control over their actions and levels of relaxation.
5. Although deeply relaxed, the mind is alert and can respond to any sudden emergency in the environment.

PREPARING THE CLIENT

Before teaching clients the relaxation response, the nurse tells them that (Benson & Proctor, 1985; Dossey, 1993; LeShan, 1974):

1. Motivation and receptiveness greatly enhance the process of learning relaxation techniques.
2. Relaxation is a skill. Learning it requires practice and work.
3. Once learned, relaxation techniques are simple to employ.
4. Some days it will be easier to practice than others.
5. Fifteen to 20 minutes, once or twice a day, should bring desired results.
6. It may take weeks or months for results to appear.
7. Morning, midday, or evening are all good times to practice. Daily consistency is important.
8. Practicing at night might cause sleep. If that is not the desired goal, choose a time when you are alert and not fatigued.
9. The goal is improvement and not perfection.

STAGES OF THE RELAXATION RESPONSE

Initial Stage

In this stage, concentration is usually extremely difficult. There are a number of resistances that are common and expected. These resistances and ways to combat them are shown in Table 16-1.

Relaxation Stage

Eventually another phase begins in which concentration is accompanied by a sense of calm stillness, a sense of energy and vitality, and letting go of old frameworks of static thinking.

TABLE 16-1
Resistances to Relaxation and Nursing Actions

RESISTANCE TO RELAXATION	ACTION
1. Mind wandering.	The client is urged to: 1. Calmly and repeatedly bring self back to chosen word or phrase. If the mind wanders a million times, bring it back a million times.
2. Need to solve problems that have been a concern for weeks or months.	2. Understand this as a resistance. Bring self back to chosen word or phrase.
3. Feelings of boredom and unproductivity.	3. Recognize this as an expected part of the process. Stay with it and work harder, and it will eventually go away.
4. Need to change position, scratch, sneeze, etc.	4. Change position, scratch, sneeze, etc., and then continue to focus on relaxation technique.
5. Immediate urgency to carry out some task, such as cleaning the stove, going through bills, or calling a friend.	5. Calmly observe this manner of resistance and bring self back to the practice.

Toward the end of the initial stage, there is usually a feeling of pleasant self-immersion, increased feelings of well-being, and greater ease with concentration. It is often at this time that another form of resistance may arise.

6. Interest in existing and dramatic phenomena, such as colors, images, and so forth. This experience may be met with anxiety or exhilaration.	6. Discontinue practice at this moment if it is uncomfortable; return later or observe what is happening until it passes. Do not get caught up in this phenomenon for it is a form of resistance and will hamper the arrival of the second stage. Avoid the temptation to focus on these phenomena to avoid "giving in" to relaxation.

Data from Benson, H., & Proctor, W. (1985). *Beyond the Relaxation Response.* New York: Berkeley Books; LeShan, L. (1974). *How to Meditate.* Boston: Little, Brown & Co.; Moyers, B. (1993). *Healing and the Mind.* New York: Doubleday.

CRITERIA FOR ELICITING THE RELAXATION RESPONSE

Criteria essential for eliciting the relaxation response include (Benson & Proctor, 1985):

1. A quiet environment with as few distractions as possible.
2. Conscious relaxation of the body's muscles.
3. A mental device including visual, auditory, or body sensations, used to shift the mind from logical, externally oriented thought. This device should be a constant stimulus, for example, a word repeated over and over.
4. A passive attitude toward intrusive thoughts.

TECHNIQUES

BENSON'S RELAXATION RESPONSE

The nurse instructs the client as follows (Benson & Proctor, 1985):

1. Choose any word or brief phrase that reflects your belief system, such as "love," "unity in faith and love," "joy," "Shalom," "one God," "peace."
2. Sit in a comfortable position.
3. Close your eyes.
4. Deeply relax all your muscles, beginning at your feet and progressing up to your face. Keep them relaxed.
5. Breathe through your nose. Become aware of your breathing. As you breathe out, say your word or phrase silently to yourself. For example, breathe IN . . . OUT, "phrase" IN . . . OUT, "phrase," etc. Breathe easily and naturally.
6. Continue for 10 or 20 minutes. You may open your eyes and check the time, but do not use an alarm. When you finish, sit quietly for several minutes, at first with your eyes closed, then with your eyes open. Do not stand up for a few minutes.
7. Do not worry about whether you are successful in achieving a deep level of relaxation. Maintain a passive attitude and permit relaxation to occur at its own pace. When distracting thoughts occur, try to ignore them by not dwelling on them and return to repeating your word or phrase. With practice, the response should come with little effort. Practice the technique once or twice daily, but not within 2 hours after any meal, since the digestive process seems to interfere with the elicitation of the relaxation response.

MEDITATION

Meditations follow the basic guidelines described for relaxation response. Meditation is a discipline for training the mind to develop greater calm and to use that calm. It can help people access deep inner resources for healing, operate more effectively in the world, cope with stress, feel more engaged in life, and more (Moyers, 1993). Several studies have shown that meditation may induce profound change, far beyond simple relaxation, relieving stress, or reducing blood pressure (Chopra, 1989). Mental exercises the nurse may suggest to the client are described next.

Using Visual Cues

Look at a candle, flower, vase, seashell, spot on the wall, etc. The purpose is to learn to concentrate. Neither analyze the object, think a series of thoughts about the object, nor associate thoughts about the object, but rather see the object as it exists in itself, without connection to other things. Allow the perception of the object to fill all your awareness.

Using Auditory Cues

Choose a word or group of words that may or may not have special meaning, such as *peace, serenity,* or *love.* Repeat the word(s) aloud or to yourself, allowing the mind to focus inside and drown out external stimuli.

Using Body Sensations (e.g., Breathing)

Concentrate on the breathing going in and out. Feel the chest expanding and count as you inhale and then exhale. Do not allow extraneous thoughts to pull your attention away from your concentration on breathing. Accept whatever thoughts or sensations arise, and redirect your attention back to your breathing.

IMAGERY

Imagery is a very effective means of deepening relaxation and desensitizing a real-life situation that is ordinarily met with undue stress and tension (for example, test-taking). The client is encouraged to choose an image that involves all the senses (sight, sound, taste, smell, touch) and at the same time experience deep relaxation. The client is instructed as follows:

1. Relax yourself in your own usual way.
2. Take several deep breaths, slowly feeling your whole body becoming more and more relaxed.
3. See the tension drain from your feet; feel your calf muscles relaxing. Experience the tension leaving your thighs and your stomach becoming loose and comfortable. Feel your chest relax as you take a deep breath and feel all the tension drain from your shoulders, and out your head.
4. Spend some time feeling the warm, tingling sensation of being so very relaxed. It is nice to feel relaxed. Being relaxed feels good.
5. Now picture yourself in your favorite place, one in which you find joy and peace. If you do not know of a place, then imagine your own personal haven. For example, if you choose the seashore, see the waves with their frothy whitecaps, *smell* the tang in the air, *feel* the sea breeze on your arms and the warm sand under your feet. *Hear* the roaring of the waves and the cry of the gulls. *Taste* the salty spray on your lips. Let the feeling of quiet joy and peace embrace your whole being. Experience the beauty of the scene with all your senses. Spend 3 to 5 minutes feeling more and more relaxed and refreshed by the experience.

MEDITATION AND IMAGERY FOR PEOPLE WITH CANCER

The stress chemicals (cortisol, adrenaline, catecholamine) in chronic high doses help reduce the immune system needed to fight cancer (Brigham, 1994). Meditation with imagery reduces stress, reducing these chemicals so the immune system can do its job. Patients are asked to visualize the disease, the treatment, and the body's immune systems. They then picture the cancer being torn apart, erased, devoured, or in some form rendered ineffective, at the same time experiencing the immune system becoming strong and dominant. For example: "See white tigers (white blood cells) eating plums (cancer cells)," or "Imagine fish (white blood cells) eating bread (cancer cells)." A positive and optimistic attitude is encouraged while the client begins visually fighting the cancer, for the client's attitude seems to play a significant role in the course of the disease. Studies show significant positive responses for many individuals using these techniques (Dossey, 1993).

SYSTEMATIC DESENSITIZATION

Meditation can be used with imagery to desensitize any situation that causes stress. The following illustration applies to test-taking anxiety. The nurse suggests that the individual:

1. Isolate the irrational thoughts that surround the situation. Irrational thoughts or goals set up conflicts that are experienced as anxiety. Rewrite the irrational thoughts into rational thoughts in which the goals or results implied can be met comfortably by the individual. Table 16-2 shows how this is done.

TABLE 16-2
Conversion of Irrational Thoughts to Rational Thoughts in Desensitization with Test Anxiety

IRRATIONAL THOUGHT	DISCUSSION	RATIONAL THOUGHT
1. I have to study.	1. No one has to study. No one is forcing you to study. You have chosen this course of study to meet your own goal. To be successful, it is in your best interest to study.	1. Since I have chosen nursing as my career, I choose to do what is necessary to achieve my goal.
2. I have to get a 90 to pass this course.	2. You have no control over the numerical grade, but you do have control over how to prepare for the exam and to do your best.	2. I chose the time and the amount that I studied. Now I will do my best.
3. This exam is going to be tricky. They want you to fail.	3. "They" most likely do not care one way or the other. This thinking puts the focus on something you cannot control, which will only raise anxiety. You have no control over how the exam will be written. You do have control over the answers you choose.	3. I cannot control the exam. I can control the answers I choose.
4. I am going to fail this test.	4. This is a very clear negative message. You have no way of seeing into the future. If you choose not to study, you may reduce your chances of passing.	4. If I choose to study, I can increase my chances of passing the exam.
5. I will never find time to study.	5. This is true. There is no time to find. Nowhere will you "find" an extra hour. You will have to make time to study. We make time for those things that have the highest priority for us.	5. If it is important for me to be successful, I will give myself every opportunity to understand the material.

Adapted from a tape recording on test-taking anxiety using rational behavioral techniques by Maxie Maultzy.

2. Write down two or three rational thoughts and commit them to memory. These thoughts should be clear and the goals comfortably obtainable, for example, "If I choose to study, then I can increase my chances of passing the exam."
3. Follow the steps used for visualization.
4. In this relaxed state visualize going through your usual routine the morning of an exam. Experience the scene with all five senses, feeling peaceful and optimistic. Calmly repeat your rational thoughts.
5. Experience the incidents that usually cause you tension, for example, missing the train or being spoken to rudely. See yourself meeting these situations with calm acceptance. Focus on your feelings of relaxation and the knowledge that you will be doing your best on the exam.

6. Continue to visualize yourself going into the exam: Feel yourself sitting down and feel the pencil in your hand. Experience yourself relaxed and mentally alert. You see the first question and you read it. Give yourself time to read question #1. Looking now at the distracters, feeling calm and confident, you make a choice. You are concentrating on the exam. Read question #2. You see the distracters, but at this time you do not find an answer. Calmly make a mark by the question and go on to question #3. Come back to #2 when you have finished. Continue the exam in this manner, feeling relaxed and confident that you have done the best you could do.

7. Practice this daily after eliciting the relaxation response. It is helpful to tape record the scenario or to have someone run through it with you. Eventually it will come easily, and the anxiety will be reduced. A person may use this technique with almost any tense situation.

PROGRESSIVE RELAXATION

Progressive muscle relaxation is based on systematically tensing and relaxing various muscle groups as a way of combating tension and anxiety. This method of relaxation is based on the idea that anxiety and muscle relaxation produce opposite physical states and cannot exist together. The basic procedure is as follows (Jacobsen, 1974):

1. Elicit the relaxation response.
2. Tighten each muscle group for a period of 5 to 7 seconds, but not to the point of discomfort (see Box 16-2 for muscle group and suggestions). Abruptly release and

---

BOX 16-2: Muscle Groups and Suggestions for Progressive Relaxation

1. *Right/left hand and forearm*—(Begin with your dominant side.) Make a very tight fist.

2. *Right/left upper arm*—Press your elbow down into the armrest. While pressing down, try to move your upper arm toward your rib cage.

3. *Right/left hand and forearm*—Same as #1.

4. *Right/left upper arm*—Same as #2.

5. *Forehead*—Raise your eyebrows as high as you can. If this does not cause tension, make a deep frown.

6. *Middle face*—Wrinkle your nose and shut your eyelids tightly together.

7. *Jaws*—Clench your teeth and pull back the corners of your mouth. At the same time, press your tongue against the roof of your mouth.

8. *Neck*—Pull your chin toward your chest with the muscles in the front of your neck while pulling your head back with the muscles in the rear of your neck.

9. *Shoulders and upper back*—Pull your shoulders back as though you were trying to touch your shoulder blades together. An alternative movement is to shrug your shoulders. Raise your shoulders as though you were trying to touch your ears with the tops of your shoulders.

10. *Stomach*—Pull the muscles of your stomach inward while pressing them downward. This makes your stomach hard, as you would if you were preparing to be hit in the stomach.

11. *Right/left thigh*—Try to bend your knee forward with the muscles of the back of your thigh while bending in the opposite direction with the muscles on the top of your thigh.

12. *Right/left calf*—Bend your foot toward your shin as though you were trying to touch your shin with your toes. (This is the opposite movement from pointing your toes.)

13. *Right/left thigh*—Same as #11.

14. *Right/left calf*—Same as #12.

Adapted from Jacobsen, E. (1974). *Progressive Relaxation* (3rd ed.). Chicago: University of Chicago Press.

relax that muscle group for about 20 seconds, concentrating on the feeling of relaxation and warmth.

3. During the tensing, focus on the tension, study it, and be very much aware of it. During the relaxing period, tell yourself how relaxed and pleasant these sensations are and how enjoyable it is to feel so relaxed. From time to time, take slow, deep breaths, letting yourself feel more and more relaxed and peaceful.

4. At the end of the exercise, which will take from 20 to 30 minutes, let yourself relax for a short while and feel the pleasantness of such a relaxed state of mind and body.

It is helpful for the nurse to verbally take the client through this process. If this is not possible, the client can use a tape that guides the client through the whole session, starting with the steps in relaxation through the muscle tensing, giving each muscle group the proper timing and instruction.

AUTOGENIC TRAINING

In this technique, autosuggestion is taught, the main focus being passive attention to the body. This technique is useful for people with gastrointestinal problems, cardiovascular problems, pain sleep disorder, pain, and much more. When used for medical conditions the client should be medically evaluated and under the supervision of a health care provider. Autogenic training requires that the nurse be trained in this technique before leading the client through the training. It may take from 4 to 10 months before optimal benefits are realized. The process of learning goes through six steps:

1. Inducing sensations of heaviness of limbs: "My right arm is heavy, my left arm is heavy," and so forth.

2. Inducing sensations of warmth in the limbs: "My right arm is warm, my left arm is warm."

3. Cardiac regulation: "My heartbeat is calm and regular, my heartbeat is calm and regular."

4. Respiratory regulation: "My body breathes itself, my body breathes itself."

5. Induction of a sense of upper abdominal warmth: "My solar plexus is warm."

6. Induction of a sense of coolness in the forehead: "My forehead is cool."

As the individual gains control over the various musculature and internal functioning, suggested fantasy is introduced, which then progresses to focusing on problems of living and psychological conflicts (Coe, 1980).

EVALUATION

Relaxation is considered successful when the client experiences:

1. A decrease in symptoms
2. A feeling of well-being
3. Increased energy
4. Increased clarity of thinking
5. Increased ability to solve problems

REFERENCES

Aron, A., & Aron, E. (1980). The transcendental meditations' program effect on addictive behavior. *Addictive Behavior, 5* (1), 3–12.

Benson, H., & Proctor, W. (1985). *Beyond the Relaxation Response.* New York: Berkeley Books.

Brigham, D. D. (1994). *Imagery for Getting Well: Clinical Applications of Behavioral Medicine.* New York: W. W. Norton & Company.

Chopra, D. (1989). *Quantum Healing. Exploring the Frontiers of Mind/Body Medicine.* New York: Bantam Books.

Coe, W. (1980). Expectation, hypnosis and suggestion. In F. Kemler & A. Goldstein (eds.), *Behavior Change: Helping People Change* (2nd ed.). New York: Pergamon Press.

Dossey, L. (1993). *Healing Words: The Power of Prayer and the Practice of Medicine*. New York: Harper-Collins.

Heidt, P. (1981). Effects of therapeutic touch on anxiety level of hospitalized patients. *Nursing Research, 30* (1), 32–37.

Holmes, T. H., & Rahe, R. H. (1970). The social readjustment scale. *Journal of Psychosomatic Medicine, 14* (4), 391–400.

Jacobsen, E. (1974). *Progressive Relaxation* (3rd ed.). Chicago: University of Chicago Press.

LeShan, L. (1974). *How to Meditate*. Boston: Little, Brown & Co.

Maultzy, M. (1981). Adapted from a tape recording on Test Taking Anxiety Using Rational Behavior Techniques. Private teaching tape.

Moskowitz, R. C. (1992). *Your Healing Mind*. New York: Avon Books.

Moyers, B. (1993). *Healing and the Mind*. New York: Doubleday.

Pilletteri, A. (1981). *Maternal–Newborn Nursing* (2nd ed.). Boston: Little, Brown & Co.

Rossi, E. L. (1993). *The Psychobiology of Mind–Body Healing*. New York: W. W. Norton & Company.

Sapolsky, R. (1990). Stress in the wild. *Scientific American*, Jan., 116–123.

Selye, H. (1956). *Stress Without Distress*. New York: McGraw-Hill.

Spiegel, H., & Spiegel, D. (1978). *Trance and Treatment*. New York: Basic Books.

BIBLIOGRAPHY

Achterberg, J. (1986). *Imagery in Healing*. Boston: New Science Library.

Krieger, D. (1981). *Foundations of Holistic Health: Nursing Practices*. Philadelphia: J. B. Lippincott.

Krieger, D. (1993). *Accepting Your Power to Heal*. Santa Fe, NM: Bear & Company Publishing.

LeShan, L. (1977). *You Can Fight for Your Life*. New York: Wans & Co.

Locke, S., & Collgan, D. (1986). *The Healer Within: The New Medicine of Mind and Body*. New York: E. P. Dutton.

Shorr, J., Sobel, G., Robin, P., & Connella, J. (1980). *Imagery: Its Many Dimensions and Applications*. New York: Plenum.

Weil, A. (1995). *Spontaneous Healing*. New York: Knopf.

17
SEVENTEEN

Nutrition and Nutritional Supplements

Anne Gallenstein

OVERVIEW:

INTRODUCTION

As holistic health care has gained acceptance in the United States and side effects of drugs have become less acceptable, mental health nurses are beginning to include nutrition and nutritional supplements in their plan of care. Diet is not intended to replace psychotherapy or psychopharmacology but rather to enhance traditional treatments.

HISTORY

1. In 1937 the disease pellagra and concomitant pellagra dementia were found to be controlled by the administration of niacin.
2. From 1939 to 1941, Cleckley, Sydenstricker, and Geeslin (1939) reported some success in treating 48 subjects suffering with several types of acute mental illness by administering 300 mg to 1500 mg of niacin daily.
3. In 1952, Hoffer and Osmond (1961) reported improvement in hundreds of schizophrenics given megavitamin therapy in several longitudinal double-blind studies.
4. In 1973, Ananth, Ban, and Lehmann reported that vitamin B_6 potentiated the therapeutic effects of niacin in schizophrenics.
5. In 1973, the American Psychiatric Association issued a report finding evidence for megavitamin treatment as inconclusive and criticized the orthomolecular movement leaders for propagation of an unproved theory to the lay public (Kunin, 1987).

REQUIRED NUTRIENTS

Orthomolecular practitioners posit that the following nutrients are necessary and function as a "team" working in each cell:

1. Carbohydrates
2. Proteins
3. Fats
4. Minerals
5. Vitamins
6. Water

DEFICIENCIES ASSOCIATED WITH MENTAL ILLNESS

Deficiencies of certain vitamins and minerals are associated with symptoms of mental illness. These nutrients include (Young, 1993; Philpott & Kalita, 1987):

1. Thiamine (B_1)
2. Niacin (B_3)
3. Pyridoxine (B_6)
4. Hydroxocobalamin (B_{12})
5. Pantothenic acid (B_5)
6. Folic acid
7. Ascorbic acid (C)
8. Magnesium
9. Calcium
10. Potassium
11. Manganese
12. Amino acids: tyrosine, phenylalanine, and tryptophan and methionine

See Table 17-1 for nutrients, symptoms of deficiency, and food sources.

NUTRITIONAL TREATMENTS

In addition to knowledge about behavioral symptoms owing to deficiencies, a body of literature is developing about treatment of symptoms with nutritional supplements and diet.

DEPRESSION

It has been found that high carbohydrate consumption increases brain serotonin by making tryptophan more able than other competing amino acids to cross the blood–brain barrier, thereby ameliorating negative affect (Lieberman, Corkin, Spring, Growden, & Wurtman, 1983; Kunin, 1976). Some research has found this effect to be short-lived. Simple carbohydrate consumption creates a vicious cycle, and following temporary relief, it contributes to and maintains depression (Wurtman & Wurtman, 1988).

Caffeine has been related to depression as well. It has been documented that psychiatric patients frequently abuse caffeine, apparently in an attempt to combat dysphoria and lack of energy. Although caffeine seems to provide depressed persons with a transient improvement in concentration, energy, and performance, it may create a vicious cycle, as it has been revealed that caffeine may be a factor contributing to depression (Christensen & Burrows, 1990). Christensen and Burrows (1990) and Krietsch, Christensen, and White (1988) found that a diet free of caffeine and refined sucrose ameliorates depression and other symptoms such as anxiety and fatigue in certain individuals.

ADDICTIONS

Because clients who abuse alcohol and drugs often have poor nutrition, it is recommended that they receive a nutrition assessment, education, and supplements.

TABLE 17-1
Nutrients, Symptoms of Deficiency, and Food Sources

NUTRIENT	SYMPTOMS OF DEFICIENCY	FOOD SOURCE
Vitamin B_1	Depression, difficulty concentrating, fatigue, tension, hyperactivity, confusion, disorientation, hallucinations, insomnia, anorexia, weight loss (Gross, 1987)	Wheat, yeast, rice, eggs, hams, beans, soy, liver, peanuts, red snapper, trout, flounder, cashews
Vitamin B_3	Anxiety, depression, nervousness, emotional lability, poor concentration, weakness, anorexia, weight loss (Gross, 1987)	Yeast, liver, tuna, turkey, halibut, swordfish, peanuts
Vitamin B_5	Irritability, depression, dizziness (Gross, 1987)	Liver, chicken, eggs, watermelon, pineapple, soy, apple, peanuts, sardines, lentils
Vitamin B_6	Confusion, depression, irritability; B_6 deficit is rare (Gross, 1987)	Yeast, liver, avocado, brown rice, chicken, peas, prunes, tuna, lima beans, salmon
Vitamin B_{12}	Poor memory, anorexia, weight loss, confusion, dementia, depression, weakness (Gross, 1987)	Yogurt, liver, egg yolk, salmon, clams, oysters, prunes
Folic acid	Depression, nervousness, fatigue, organic psychosis (Gross, 1987)	Grains, legumes, dates, barley, liver, raisins, pecans, dark green leafy vegetables
Vitamin C	No specific psychiatric symptoms (Gross, 1987)	Greens, cabbage, cauliflower, parsley, citrus and other fresh fruits
Magnesium	Depression, irritability, paranoia with severe deficit (Gross, 1987)	Beef, milk, rice, sunflower seeds, chicken, barley, dried apricots
Calcium	Nervousness, insomnia (Gross, 1987)	Yogurt, sardines, milk products, liver, shrimp, salmon
Potassium	Extreme fatigue, indifference, lack of feeling (Gross, 1987)	Bananas, apricots, papaya, almonds, soy, turkey, salmon, pork, oranges, clams
Manganese	No specific psychiatric symptoms (Gross, 1987)	Nuts, grains, egg yolk, pineapple
Tryptophan	No specific psychiatric symptoms (Balch & Balch, 1990)	Turkey, bananas, figs, yogurt, tuna, dates

Food sources from Mindell, E. (1991). *Vitamin Bible.* New York: Warner Books.

NUTRITION PROBLEMS

1. Alcoholics may develop obesity; protein–energy malnutrition; deficiencies of thiamine, folate, and other vitamins; and depletion of magnesium and zinc (Roe, 1981). Thiamine deficiency can induce Werner-Korsakoff syndrome. Alcoholics may also suffer from cognitive changes such as dementia associated with cerebral atrophy. Such deficits may be reversible with abstinence and adequate nutrition (Gray, 1989).
2. The use of addictive drugs, such as marijuana, cocaine, nicotine, and heroin, can also interfere with nutrient status and metabolism. For example, heroin addiction can cause hyperkalemia (Mohs, Watson, & Leonard-Green, 1990).

TREATMENT

1. Several studies have shown favorable responses to amino acid loading to enhance neurotransmitter availability (Blum, Trachtenberg, Williams, & Loeblich, 1988; Brown, Blum & Trachtenberg, 1990). The amino acid compounds are nontoxic and do not create a dependence. To this end specialized formulations with high levels of minerals, vitamins, and the amino acids D-phenylalanine, L-phenylalanine, L-tryptophan, and L-glutamine decrease drug craving and thereby increase compli-

ance with withdrawal. There was a much higher percentage of compliance for those patients taking the neuronutrients (Mohs, Watson, & Leonard-Green, 1990).

ANXIETY AND PANIC DISORDER

Lactate metabolism may be altered in panic disorder. Maddock, Carter, and Gietzen (1991) found an alteration in lactic acid metabolism leading to an exaggerated increase in serum lactate following glucose loading and hyperventilation. Serum lactate elevations have also been associated with the ingestion of caffeine (480 mg orally). Patients who panicked in response to caffeine had significantly greater increases in serum lactate than those who did not panic (Uhde & Boulenger, 1989). See Table 17-2 for caffeine amounts in beverages.

TABLE 17-2
Amount of Caffeine Found in Common Beverages

BEVERAGE	AMOUNT OF CAFFEINE
Per serving (12 oz.)	
Soft drinks	
Coca-Cola	64.7 mg
Dr Pepper	60.9 mg
Mountain Dew	54.7 mg
Pepsi	43.1 mg
Diet Dr Pepper	54.2 mg
Per serving (6 oz.)	
Coffee	
Instant	66.0 mg
Percolated	110.0 mg
Drip	146.0 mg
Tea	
Black, 5-min. brew	46.0 mg
Black, 1-min. brew	28.0 mg
Cocoa	13.0 mg

From Bruce, M. S. (1990). The anxiogenic effects of caffeine. *Postgraduate Medical Journal, 66* (suppl. 2), s18–s24.

Another study found a decrease in anxiety with cessation of caffeine in 6 of 24 patients (Bruce, 1990).

SCHIZOPHRENIA

Orthomolecular practitioners view schizophrenia not as a single disease but as a combination of disorders including genetic errors, nutritional deficiencies, and acquired metabolic disorders (especially disordered carbohydrate metabolism). Also of special significance are food allergies, addictions, toxicities, metabolic errors, and unexplained hypersensitivities (Philpott & Kalita, 1987).

ORTHOMOLECULAR RESEARCH

1. Dohan (1966) examined the effects of a diet free of milk and cereal grain products based on reports of correlations between schizophrenia and celiac disease. A highly significant increased rate of release from the hospital was found in those schizophrenic patients on milk-free and grain-free diets. This study was supported by Singh and Kay's (1976) double-blind wheat gluten challenge of schizophrenic

patients being maintained on a cereal grain-free and milk-free diet. The gluten challenge interrupted or reversed therapeutic progress.

2. It is hypothesized that schizophrenics have a higher metabolic requirement for vitamin C than the suggested optimal ascorbic acid requirement for healthy humans (Pauling, 1968). Schizophrenics compared with a control group had lower fasting plasma vitamin C and a lower urinary excretion of surplus vitamin C, implying that they metabolically use and therefore need greater amounts.

3. As there is evidence of increased serotonin in schizophrenia, optimal psychopharmacotherapy involves attenuating both tryptophan and dopamine. A low-tryptophan diet improved behavioral symptomatology and performance on the Stroop Color and Word Test (i.e., word, color, color-word naming) in a group of 11 schizophrenics (Rosse, Schwartz, Zlotolow, Banay-Schwartz, Trinidad, Peace, & Deutsch, 1992). Interestingly, the decrease in plasma tryptophan did not precipitate depression. It is thought that schizophrenia or the antipsychotic medications might offer some protection against the depressive effects of the diet.

ALZHEIMER'S DISEASE

Research indicates that Alzheimer's patients have abnormalities in the metabolism of acetylcholine, a major neurotransmitter in the memory system. Other neurotransmitter systems may also be involved in this disorder.

ORTHOMOLECULAR RESEARCH

1. Vitamin C has been found to enhance the release of acetylcholine and norepinephrine in the brain (Agbayewa, Bruce, & Siemens, 1992).

2. Studies imply that Alzheimer's disease patients have a changed carbohydrate metabolism, leading to hypoglycemia and a resultant decrease in neuronal functioning including the cholinergic (memory and cognition), serotonergic (mood), dopaminergic (thought organization), and noradrenergic systems. Dietary choline, found in egg yolks, whole grains, legumes, meat, and milk, is necessary to make acetylcholine along the cholinergic pathway (Bucht & Sandman, 1990).

3. Research has shown that patients with Alzheimer's disease had lower thiamine (B_1) levels than members of a control group having the same intake. It is hypothesized that patients with Alzheimer's may suffer an abnormality in the bioavailability or metabolism of vitamin B_1, which is necessary in the synthesis of acetylcholine (Agbayewa, Bruce, & Siemens, 1992).

SLEEP DISORDERS

Interrupted sleep is often a symptom of psychiatric and various physical disorders, some of which are nutritionally linked, such as hypoglycemia and poor nutritional habits. Nutritional supplements that promote sleep include calcium, magnesium, vitamins B_6 and B_5, and tryptophan (Balch & Balch, 1990).

DISORDERED WATER BALANCE SYNDROME

Some severely ill psychiatric patients have been noted to have problems with fluid osmoregulation owing to compulsive water drinking. For these patients intake must be carefully monitored (Ribble & Thelander, 1994).

Symptoms include (Ribble & Thelander, 1994):
Polydipsia
Polyuria
Significant variation in pattern of excretion

Abnormal diurnal weight gain
Behavioral changes
Slurred speech
Confusion
Disorientation
Increased irritability
Agitated behavior
Delusions
Compulsion to drink
Hoarding/carrying cups

Possible Causes include (Ribble & Thelander, 1994):
Psychogenic polydipsia
Hypothalamic lesions
Compulsive behavior owing to emotional needs
Hippocampal degeneration
Inappropriate antidiuretic hormone induced by psychoactive medications
Dysfunction of thirst and osmoregulatory centers

The nurse intervenes by (Ribble & Thelander, 1994):
1. Monitoring the client daily for excess fluid intake or water-seeking behavior
2. Monitoring the client for physical status changes such as headaches, GI symptoms, nausea, vomiting, diarrhea
3. Monitoring changes in medication that may cause symptoms of dry mouth or increased thirst
4. Contracting with the client to maintain weight and serum sodium levels with an agreed-on range
5. Assessing weight
6. Teaching client to report increased thirst or fluid consumption
7. Providing highly structured activities that divert water-seeking behavior
8. Providing an environment with controlled access to fluids
9. Weighing client twice daily
10. Assessing and monitoring serum electrolytes
11. Providing hard candy with medications
12. Spending time with the client exploring reasons for excess water intake

FOOD ALLERGIES AND SENSITIVITIES

A summary of the literature suggests that food can produce a variety of untoward responses, though most of the evidence comes through uncontrolled case studies or correlational studies with a few experimental studies. There is also evidence, although controversial, for behavioral manifestations in children with food sensitivities (Christensen, Krietsch, White, & Stagner, 1985).

CONTROVERSY

Detractors from orthomolecular therapy claim inability to replicate the positive findings of the megavitamin studies. They also urge research to ascertain the safety of these methods. Protection of the lay public from ineffective therapies is also listed as an argument against nutritional medicine.

Orthomolecular proponents complain that the 1973 American Psychiatric Association task force report (Kunin, 1987) was biased and therefore omitted or negatively interpreted many studies reporting positive results with vitamin treatment. They further object to the double-blind method as the only credible method of determining further study and treatment efficacy, especially since funding for research of nonpatentable entities is very limited. Advocates also protest that nutritional substances are naturally occurring and toxicities of most are already known and side effects are few (Pauling, 1968; Philpott & Kalita, 1987).

Currently, the health care community remains polarized. Nutritional treatments are given limited credence in orthodox psychiatry. However, research in nutrition for psychotropic purposes continues. There are numerous anecdotal reports of success with nutritional methods including diet and supplementation to diet. A survey in the *New England Journal of Medicine* (Eisenberg, Kessler, Foster, Norlock, Calkins, & Delbanco, 1993) found that one in three Americans had used alternative treatments, which along with many other modalities included nutrition and vitamin therapy. Consumers are showing a growing interest in the role of nutrition in mind–body interaction.

REFERENCES

Agbayewa, M. O., Bruce, V., & Siemens, V. (1992). Pyridoxine, ascorbic acid and thiamine in Alzheimer's and comparison subjects. *Canadian Journal of Psychiatry, 37,* 661–662.

Ananth, J. V., Ban, T. A., & Lehmann, H. E. (1973). Potentiation of therapeutic effects of nicotinic acid by pyridoxine in chronic schizophrenics. *Canadian Psychiatric Association Journal, 18,* 377–382.

Balch, J. F., & Balch, P. A. (1990). *Prescription for Nutritional Healing.* Garden City Park, NY: Avery Publishing Group.

Blum, K., Trachtenberg, M. C., Williams, R. W., & Loeblich, L. A. (1988). Reduction of both drug hunger and withdrawal against advice rate of cocaine abusers in a 30-day inpatient treatment program by the neuronutrient tropamine. *Current Therapeutic Research, 43,* 1204–1214.

Brown, R. J., Blum, K., & Trachtenberg, M. C. (1990). Neurodynamics of relapse prevention: A neuro-nutrient approach to outpatient DUI offenders. *Journal of Psychoactive Drugs, 22* (2), 173–186.

Bruce, M. S. (1990). The anxiogenic effects of caffeine. *Postgraduate Medical Journal, 66* (suppl. 2), s18–s24.

Bucht, G., & Sandman, P. O. (1990). Nutritional aspects of dementia especially Alzheimer's disease. *Age and Aging, 19,* s32–36.

Christensen, L., & Burrows, R. (1990). Dietary treatment of depression. *Behavior Therapy, 21,* 183–193.

Christensen, L., Krietsch, K., White, B., & Stagner, B. (1985). The impact of a dietary change on emotional distress. *Journal of Abnormal Psychology, 94,* 565–579.

Cleckley, H. M., Sydenstriker, V. P., & Geeslin, L. E. (1939). Nicotinic acid and the treatment of atypical psychotic states. *Journal of the American Medical Association, 112* (21).

Dohan, F. C. (1966). Cereals and schizophrenia: Data and hypothesis. *Acta Psychiatrica of Scandinavia, 42,* 125–152.

Eisenberg, D. M., Kessler, R. C., Foster, C., Norlock, F., Calkins, D. R., & Delbanco, T. L. (1993). Unconventional medicine in the United States. *New England Journal of Medicine, 328* (10), 246–252.

Gray, G. E. (1989). Nutritional aspects of psychiatric disorders. *Perspectives in Practice, 89* (10), 1492–1498.

Gross, L. (1987). Neuropsychiatric aspects of vitamin deficiency states. In R. E. Hale & S. C. Yudofsky (eds.), *The American Psychiatric Press Textbook of Neuropsychiatry* (pp. 327–338). Washington, DC: American Psychiatric Press.

Hoffer, A., & Osmond, H. (1961). Double blind clinical trials. *Journal of Neuropsychiatry, 2* (5), 221–227.

Krietsch, K., Christensen, L., & White, B. (1988). Prevalence, presenting symptoms and psychological characteristics of individuals experiencing a diet related mood disturbance. *Behavior Therapy, 19,* 593–604.

Kunin, R. A. (1976). Ketosis and the orthocarbohydrate diet: A basic factor in orthomolecular psychiatry. *Journal of Orthomolecular Psychiatry, 5,* 203–211.

Kunin, R. A. (1987). Orthomolecular psychiatry. In R. P. Huemer (ed.), *The Roots of Molecular Medicine* (pp. 180–213). New York: W. H. Freeman and Co.

Lieberman, H. R., Corkin, S., Spring, B., Growden, J. H., & Wurtman, R. J. (1983). Mood, performance and sensitivity: Changes induced by food constituents. *Journal of Psychiatric Research, 17,* 135–145.

Maddock, R. J., Carter, S. C., & Glietzen, D. W. (1991). Elevated serum lactate associated with panic attacks induced by hyperventilation. *Psychiatric Research, 38,* 301–311.

Mindell, E. (1991). *Vitamin Bible.* New York: Warner Books.

Mohs, M. E., Watson, R. R., & Leonard-Green, T. (1990). Nutritional effects of marijuana, heroin, cocaine and nicotine. *Journal of the American Dietetic Association, 90* (9), 1261–1267.

Pauling, L. (1968). Orthomolecular psychiatry: Varying the concentrations of substances normally present in the human body may control mental disease. *Science, 160,* 265–271.

Philpott, W. H., & Kalita, D. K. (1987). *Brain Allergies: The Psychonutrient Connection*. New Canaan, CT: Keats Publishing, Inc.

Ribble, D. J., & Thelander, B. (1994). Patients with disordered water balance: Innovative psychiatric nursing strategies. *Journal of Psychosocial Nursing, 32* (10), 35–42.

Roe, D. A. (1981). Nutritional concerns in the alcoholic. *Journal of the American Dietetic Association, 78* (17), 17–21.

Rosse, R. B., Schwartz, B. L., Zlotolow, R. D., Banay-Schwartz, M., Trinidad, A., Peace, T., & Deutsch, S. (1992). The effect of a low tryptophan diet as adjuvant to conventional neuroleptic therapy in schizophrenia. *Clinical Neuropharmacology, 15* (2), 129–141.

Singh, M. M., & Kay, S. R. (1976). Wheat gluten as a pathogenic factor in schizophrenia. *Science, 191*, 401–402.

Uhde, T. W., & Boulenger, J. P. (1989). Caffeine model of panic. In B. Lerer & S. Gershon (eds.), *New Directions in Affective Disorders* (pp. 410–413). New York: Springer-Verlag.

Wurtman, R. J., & Wurtman, J. J. (1988). Do carbohydrates affect food intake via neurotransmitter activity? *Appetite, 11* (suppl. 1), 42–47.

Young, S. N. (1993). The use of diet and dietary components in the study of factors controlling affect in humans: A review. *Journal of Psychiatry and Neuroscience, 18* (5), 235–241.

18
EIGHTEEN

Telephone Therapy

Suzanne Lego

OVERVIEW:

Introduction
Uses
Advantages
Disadvantages

Logistics
Differences from Face-to-Face Therapy
The Future of Telephone Therapy

INTRODUCTION

In this age of the "information highway" the telephone has come to play a part in psychotherapy for those who cannot leave home, those who live in isolated rural areas or dangerous urban areas, and those who simply want the convenience of therapy at home.

USES

The telephone has been used successfully to intervene with a number of mental health problems including:

1. Suicide prevention
2. General crisis intervention
3. Counseling high-risk teens (Tolmach, 1985; Tolchin, 1987)
4. Abortion counseling
5. Rape counseling
6. Counseling parents who abuse their children
7. Counseling drug users who are on a "bad trip"
8. Counseling people who fear they are HIV-infected, or infected persons who are anxious
9. Treating sexual problems (Crenshaw, 1985)
10. Follow-up of discharged alcoholics (Catanzaro & Green, 1970)
11. Clinical supervision
12. Reinforcement of behavior modification
13. Hypnosis following dental work
14. Psychotherapy with cancer patients (Mermelstein & Holland, 1991)
15. Integration of hospitalized schizophrenics into their families (Beebe, 1968)
16. Psychiatric rehabilitation following discharge (Meyersberg, 1985)
17. Family therapy with college students (DeSalvo, 1988)
18. Psychotherapy of the unreachable client (Ranan & Blodgett, 1983; Grumet, 1979)
19. Cognitive therapy with disabled elderly clients (Evans, Haler, & Smith, 1985)

20. Counseling by disabled therapists for disabled clients (Melton & Smoyak, 1992)
21. Supportive therapy (Shepard, 1987)
22. Psychoanalysis (Robertiello, 1972)

ADVANTAGES

Telephone therapy offers the following advantages (Lester, 1979):

1. Clients can be treated who might otherwise be unreachable owing to their emotional problems, physical disabilities, the danger of travel in cities, lack of transportation, or long distances as in rural areas.
2. Clients and therapists are on equal ground, as opposed to therapy in the office or client's home, where one is on familiar terrain and the other is a visitor.
3. Clients can terminate the session without a scene or confrontation.
4. Clients feel freer without eye contact and are able to regress by the same principle as lying on the couch. Clients who are very dependent learn to express themselves without benefit of verbal cues from the therapist.
5. Clients can go on with weekly sessions even if they are traveling or the therapist is away. They have the convenience of calling from home or work.
6. Therapy can be continued if either the client or therapist relocates to a new area.
7. Clients and therapists can be casually dressed and comfortable.

DISADVANTAGES

Telephone therapy offers the following disadvantages:

1. Nonverbal cues are missed by both client and therapist.
2. It is easier for the therapist to slip into a conversation mode (Brockopp, in Lester, 1977).
3. Some clients are untreatable, for example, paranoid patients who must see the therapist to feel safe or who fear others are listening.

LOGISTICS

1. The client calls the therapist at the appointed hour and pays for the call. On Saturdays or after 6 P.M. the cost of the call may be less than transportation back and forth to the office.
2. The usual time boundaries are maintained. The session begins and ends on time.
3. The client is billed in the usual way.

DIFFERENCES FROM FACE-TO-FACE THERAPY

A study of clients who experienced both face-to-face and telephone therapy with the same therapist found that clients described the following differences with telephone therapy (Lego, 1993):

1. Clients were more comfortable slipping into silence, which they believed sparked more introspection.
2. Clients were more uncomfortable with the therapist's silence, which then sparked more productive talk based on the introspection.
3. Clients felt more comfortable discussing difficult or embarrassing matters.
4. Clients reported no difference in the transference they felt.
5. Clients reported no difference in their perceptions of the therapists' reactions to them.

THE FUTURE OF TELEPHONE THERAPY

Telephone therapy will probably increase in use because:

1. As our society is becoming more mobile, people move from state to state more easily than in the past.
2. The elderly are increasing in number, and people are living longer with chronic illnesses, increasing the number of homebound.
3. Travel is becoming more inconvenient and dangerous in urban areas.
4. There is a trend toward people working at home and remaining at home owing to advances in technological communication.
5. Telephone use in general is increasing.
6. Videophones will eliminate the disadvantage of missing nonverbal communication.

REFERENCES

Beebe, J. E. (1968). Allowing the patient to call home: A therapy of acute schizophrenia. *Psychotherapy: Theory, Research and Practice, 3* (1), 18–20.

Catanzaro, R. J., & Green, W. G. (1970). WATS telephone therapy: New follow-up technique for alcoholics. *American Journal of Psychiatry, 126* (7), 148–151.

Crenshaw, T. L. (1985). Resolution of ejaculatory incompetence through telephone therapy. *Medical Aspects of Human Sexuality, 19* (10), 113–117.

DeSalvo, F. J. (1988). Family phone therapy in university counseling and psychological service centers: A family systems approach. *Journal of American College Health, 37* (2), 71–76.

Evans, R. L., Haler, E. M., & Smith, K. M. (1985). Cognitive therapy to achieve personal goals: Results of telephone group counseling with disabled adults. *Archives of Physical Medicine and Rehabilitation, 66* (10), 693–696.

Grumet, G. W. (1979). Telephone therapy: A review and case report. *American Journal of Orthopsychiatry, 49* (4), 574–589.

Lego, S. (1992). Patient's reactions to telephone therapy. Presented at Medical College of Pennsylvania, Continuing Nursing Education, Feb., 1992.

Lester, D. (1977). *The Use of Alternate Modem for Communication in Psychotherapy: The Computer, the Book, the Telephone, the Television, the Tape Recorder.* Springfield, IL: Thomas.

Lester, D. (1979). The unique qualities of telephone therapy. *Psychotherapy: Theory, Research and Practice, 11* (3), 219–221.

Melton, M. C., & Smoyak, S. A. (1992). Telephone therapy. Call for help. *Journal of Psychosocial Nursing, 30* (4), 29–32.

Mermelstein, H. T., & Holland, J. C. (1991). Psychotherapy by telephone: A therapeutic tool for cancer patients. *Psychosomatics, 32* (4), 407–412.

Meyersberg, G. (1985). The use of the telephone in psychiatric rehabilitation. *Nordisk Psykiatrisk Tidsskrift, 39* (3), 185–188.

Ranan, W., & Blodgett, A. (1983). Using telephone therapy for "unreachable" clients. *Social Casework, 64* (1), 39–44.

Robertiello, R. C. (1972). Telephone sessions. *Psychoanalytic Review, 59* (4), 633–634.

Shepard, P. (1987). Telephone therapy: An alternate to isolation. *Clinical Social Work Journal, 15* (1), 56–65.

Tolchin, J. (1987). Telephone psychotherapy with adolescents. *Adolescent Psychiatry, 14* (6), 332–341.

Tolmach, J. (1985). There ain't nobody on my "side": A new day treatment program for black urban youth. *Journal of Clinical Child Psychology, 14* (3), 214–219.

BIBLIOGRAPHY

Noy, B. (1992). The open line for students in the Gulf War in Israel. *School Psychology International, 13* (3), 207–227.

Spiro, R. H., & Devenis, L. (1991). Telephone therapy: Enhancement of the psychotherapeutic process. *Psychotherapy in Private Practice, 9* (4), 31–55.

NINETEEN

Gerontological Counseling

Donna Felber Neff

OVERVIEW:

INTRODUCTION

The elderly, 65 years of age and older, represent 12% of the U.S. population (McBride & Burgener, 1994). By the year 2025, their numbers will increase to 20% of the population (Cassetta, 1993; Mikulencak, 1993). Mental health problems in the elderly differ in symptoms and etiologies from the younger adult (Abraham et al., 1991). The interface of physical, social, and mental illness among the elderly poses a challenge for the psychiatric nurse. Therefore, the following considerations are critical for the psychiatric nurse caring for this cohort:

1. One-fifth of older adults have a mental illness (American Psychological Association, 1993).
2. The highest rate of mental illness is found among older adults in institutional settings (Cassetta, 1993; Mikulencak, 1993).
3. Three to 4 million elderly are affected by cognitive, behavioral losses (American Psychological Association, 1993).
4. The elderly account for 21% of suicides (American Psychological Association, 1993).

5. Those over 85, known as the oldest old, suffer from chronic illnesses and frailties (Gatz, 1989).
6. The majority of oldest old are women. Forty-three percent live alone (Gatz, 1989).
7. The older ethnic minority population is increasing more rapidly than the older population as a whole (Cassetta, 1993; Mikulencak, 1993).
8. Eighty-five percent of older adults with mental illnesses are underserved owing to ageism, negative stereotypes, stigma, and reluctance to use mental health services (Dellasega, 1991).
9. Mental health professionals often misdiagnose mental illness in older adults (Dellasega, 1991).
10. Psychotropic medications are used four times more frequently than psychotherapy/counseling for the elderly (Harper & Grau, 1994).
11. Ninety-one percent of nursing home residents have mental health needs that are not met (Harper & Grau, 1994).
12. There is a disproportionate number of homeless over age 50 (American Psychological Association, 1993).

SETTINGS

Settings in which the psychiatric nurse might work with aged clients include the following.

GENERAL HEALTH CARE FACILITIES

1. Acute care facilities (hospitals)
2. Community mental health centers
3. State and county mental hospitals
4. Veterans administration hospitals
5. Alcohol treatment programs
6. The client's home

SPECIALIZED AGENCIES FOR THE ELDERLY

1. Nursing homes or health-related facilities
2. Geriatric day-care centers
3. Senior citizens' programs
4. Geriatric assessment centers

PSYCHODYNAMICS OF AGING

Erickson (1963) has described the last stage of psychological development as "ego integrity versus despair." The developmental task of the elderly person is to develop a sense of satisfaction with life and its meaning, and a belief that life is fulfilling and successful. When this task of ego integrity is attained, the individual adapts to the changing environment and strives toward personhood (Haight & Burnside, 1993; Lappe, 1987; Schmidt & Burnside, 1994). To do this, the elderly client must adjust to and overcome a number of losses that may include (Sadavoy & Leszcz, 1987):

1. Loss of strength
2. Loss of power
3. Loss of prestige
4. Loss of recognition
5. Loss of physical ability
6. Loss of beauty
7. Loss of friends and affiliations

8. Loss of material wealth
9. Loss of intimacy
10. Loss of sexual opportunities
11. Loss of occupation
12. Loss of opportunity or possibility

MYTHS ABOUT TREATING THE ELDERLY

Sadavoy and Leszcz (1987) list a number of myths about treating the elderly in psychotherapy. They are shown along with facts in Table 19-1.

TABLE 19-1
Myths and Facts About Treating the Elderly with Psychotherapy

MYTH	FACT
1. The elderly are untreatable as they are rigid and inelastic.	1. The elderly are integrated, vigorous, capable of learning new things, and never lose their capacity for psychological growth (Miller, 1990).
2. The elderly must be babied.	2. A person's emotional style remains similar throughout the life cycle. Approximately 90% of elderly manage their own affairs (Edinberg, 1985).
3. Therapy with the aged is the same as therapy at any age.	3. The therapist who works with the elderly must consider the following: a. "Antecedent psychopathology, either latent or manifest" (Pollock, 1987, p. 17). b. "Situational crisis, acute or chronic, that strains the ego's ability to maintain equilibrium" (Pollock, 1987, p. 17). c. "Organic illness, which can increase reactive symptoms such as depression and psychosocial ills. . . . There can be regressions to earlier fixations which may become chronic and return the individual to infantile levels of functioning" (Pollock, 1987, p. 17). d. Functional limitations are prevalent in the elderly. e. Older persons wish to be useful and to preserve their dignity (Pollock, 1987).
4. Emotional disturbance, depression, disengagement, and demoralization in the elderly are inevitable and immutable.	4. The elderly have great powers of survival (Pollock, 1987). How a person will adjust to being old is reflective of how that person adjusted to changes throughout life.
5. The elderly lack the availability of new love objects.	5. Although the frequency of sexual activity gradually declines with age, the level of sexual interest and competence of the elderly does not decline (Miller, 1990).
6. The elderly have reduced motivation toward relationships.	6. The elderly have motivation to change and make new social relationships or restructure those of the past in more positive ways (Pollock, 1987).
7. The elderly have reduced motivation toward insight.	7. The elderly have the capacity for and utilization of insight, the capacity to dream and fantasize, and the ability to relate these fantasies and dreams to the therapeutic process as well as to their past (Pollock, 1987).

ASSESSMENT

Table 19-2 presents a comprehensive nursing assessment tool adapted from the *Psychogeriatric Nursing Assessment Protocol* (Abraham et al., 1990). This protocol takes into consideration the complexity of the multifaceted problems of older clients and provides a guide for holistic assessment by the psychiatric nurse. Demographic and health–illness data collection will complete the comprehensive assessment of the older adult.

TABLE 19-2
Psychogeriatric Nursing Assessment

ASSESSMENT AREA	GUIDELINES FOR NURSING ASSESSMENT
Functional Assessment	
Physical activities of daily living	Assess basic skill capabilities: eating, toileting, ambulation, dressing, bathing, and grooming (see OARS Physical ADL items, Duke University Center for the Study of Aging and Human Development, 1978).
Instrumental activities of daily living	Assess more complex activity: using transportation, shopping, housekeeping, doing laundry, cooking, managing money, taking medication, and using the telephone (see OARS).
Nutritional status	Assess general nutritional appearance, habits, appetite. What food is available to the client? Is the client on a special diet? Is the client compliant? Is the client hydrated?
Mobility	Assess need for assistance, loss of mobility and extent, range of motion, posture, gait, and endurance. Does the client take medications that impede mobility? Is there paralysis? Does the client have a prosthesis?
Sleep	Assess sleep–wake pattern. Has this changed? Is medication altering the pattern?
Hearing	Assess for hearing impairment. Assess use of hearing aid and client's response to hearing aid.
Vision	Assess visual status and client's use of glasses/contacts.
Medication behavior	Assess medications, prescribed and over the counter. Does the client take medications independently or with assistance?
Mental Assessment	
General appearance	Assess the client's appearance. Assess gait and posture. Are abnormal involuntary movements present? Assess hygiene, clothing, and facial expression.
Involvement in interview	Is client cooperative, friendly, evasive, indifferent, passive, dependent, hostile during interview?
Comprehension of interview	Assess client's comprehension of the interview. Does the client attempt to cover up cognitive deficits with humor, sarcasm, avoidance, evasiveness, confabulation? Assess thought content, language expression, and speech.
Speech	Assess speech for speed, tone, level, and articulation. Is there congruence of verbal and nonverbal?
Cognitive status	Assess client's cognitive status by administration of a mental status instrument—i.e., Folstein Mini–Mental State Examination (Folstein, Folstein, & McHugh, 1975).
Memory	Assess recent and remote memory. Observe client in daily activities and during interview.
Delirium (acute confusional state)	Assess for evidence of global cognition/attention disorder meeting criteria for delirium/acute confusional state (see Chapter 33).
Insight	Assess insight to condition/situation using Folstein Mini–Mental State Examination (Folstein, Folstein, & McHugh, 1995).
Affect	Assess nonverbal and verbal congruence. Are the client's expressions consistent with a recent problematic external event? Assess meaning of event for client. Consider cultural/gender norms of clients.
Mood	Assess mood and nonverbal cues/behaviors. Ask client, "How would you describe your usual mood?" Use formalized tools to assess for depression—i.e., Beck Depression Inventory (Beck & Steer, 1993).
Suicide potential	Assess suicide risk. Is client at risk for hurting self? Does client describe suicidal ideation? Assess extent of planning, follow through, and history of suicidal thoughts/attempts.

TABLE 19-2 *(continued)*

ASSESSMENT AREA	GUIDELINES FOR NURSING ASSESSMENT
Behavioral Assessment	
Dress	Assess appropriateness in dressing. Does the client have episodes or patterns of inappropriate undressing?
Hallucinations/delusions	Assess nature of hallucinations/delusions. Are these symptoms effects of medications, alcohol, physiological or environmental disturbances? Observe client for clues such as social isolation, withdrawal, or gesture. Are the client's perceptions based in reality? Ask client, "Have you heard voices when nobody was there, or seen something that no one else could see?"
Cooperation/resistance	Assess response to caregiving.
Aggressive behavior	Assess for aggressive behavior. Has the client physically attacked, threatened others, or been verbally abusive?
Sexual behavior	Assess for evidence of inappropriate sexual behavior, sexual advances, exposing.
Repetitive behavior	Assess for evidence of repetitive behaviors.
Family and Social Functioning Assessment	
Family/social dynamics	Assess family and social environment. Assess perceptions of own status and self-respect. Assess for factors that interfere with current relationships between client, family, and significant others. What are client's strengths? Is there agreement between client and family? How does the client accomplish day-to-day tasks? Identify persons who help with tasks. Ask client, "On whom in the family do you rely for help?" Does the client have a confidential relationship with anyone? Are there unreasonable expectations of family and significant others? How has the client and family incorporated the chronic physical, cognitive, and mental conditions into daily living?
Social functioning	Assess the home environment. Is it conducive to maximum functional abilities? What are the client's daily, weekly, and regular contacts? Assess community integration of client and family, church, social, recreational clubs, and civic organizations. Whom does the client rely on for help? Does the client verbalize insight into needs for services? Assess transportation. Ask the client, "What do you do in a typical day?"
Financial resources	Assess financial resources. Has there been a change in income? Is client able to meet basic needs of food, shelter, and clothing? Do finances allow for extras such as recreation or trips? Assess housing for quality, space, security, and privacy. How does the client perceive the home environment?

LIFE REVIEW THERAPY

DEFINITION

Life review therapy (Fitzpatrick, 1984) is a mental process through which past experiences are progressively returned to consciousness for review, assessment, and resolution. It is often initiated by the realization of approaching death.

GOALS

The goals of life review therapy are to:
1. Review unresolved conflicts
2. Increase hopefulness about the rest of life
3. Increase flexibility in meeting current or future conflicts and frustrations
4. Enhance purpose in life by providing meaningful activity
5. Enhance personal integrity and life satisfaction through a review of past accomplishments and satisfactions

6. Provide opportunity to make amends and restore harmony with friends and relatives
7. Gain self-understanding

PURPOSE OF NURSING INTERVENTION

The nurse enhances the process by helping clients to review their lives consciously, deliberately, efficiently, thoughtfully, and emotionally. The therapist may work with individuals or groups.

METHODS OF INTERVENTION

The nurse:
1. Encourages
   a. Written or taped autobiographies, diaries, journals
   b. Attending reunions
   c. Tracing geneology
   d. Visiting hometown
   e. Visiting relatives
   f. Preserving/exploring ethnic identity
   g. Reading literature (e.g., novels, poetry) evocative of the client's life or being (e.g., the journals of May Sarton, 1984, 1988, 1992, 1993, 1995)
2. Reviews and discusses scrapbooks and photographs with the client
3. Reviews work accomplishments
4. Enhances and encourages:
   a. Creativity
   b. Sharing favorite foods
   c. Discussion of family traditions
   d. Intergenerational groups
   e. Groups with contemporaries
   f. Oral histories
   g. Visits to museums
5. Emphasizes the quality of the present life rather than quantity
6. Discusses fears, answers questions about death
7. Helps client deal with present conflicts, in light of past accomplishments
8. Listens actively and sensitively

REMINISCENCE

DEFINITION

Reminiscence (Fitzpatrick, 1984) is the therapeutic process of sharing memories of past experiences and events (especially those considered personally significant), conscious recall of these experiences, and purposeful seeking of memories.

GOALS

The goals of reminiscence are to:
1. Maintain a sense of familiarity about life and the world
2. Develop increasing understanding and integration of life experiences
3. Increase self-esteem
4. Enhance interpersonal relations
5. Improve cognitive activity
6. Exercise memory
7. Maintain a unique identity

8. Bridge the generation gap through memories of past events similar to current activities of young people
9. Entertain others

PURPOSE OF NURSING INTERVENTION

The nurse encourages and enhances the process by structuring the environment so as to facilitate the process either with individuals or groups.

METHODS OF INTERVENTION

The same as for life review process.

REALITY ORIENTATION

DEFINITION

Reality orientation (Fitzpatrick, 1984) is a specific remotivation process that trains individuals to recall recent and remote memory (experiences, ideas, facts, and general information such as time and place).

GOALS

The goals of reality orientation are to:
1. Evaluate contact with the environment
2. Increase contact with the environment
3. Improve social and cognitive functioning
4. Increase self-esteem

PURPOSE OF NURSING INTERVENTION

The nurse helps the client to reverse or halt confusion, disorientation, social withdrawal, and apathy in a group setting.

METHODS OF INTERVENTION

The nurse:
1. Questions reality contact: "Can you tell us what day today is?"
2. Rewards positive behavior: "Good! Your memory is improving."
3. Focuses on behaviors: "Show us how you use your comb."
4. Confirms what clients see and hear: "Yes, there is a lot of noise on the unit today."
5. Does not give false reassurance.
6. Uses touch.

GRIEF WORK

DEFINITION

Grief work (Fitzpatrick, 1984) is employed when the client is experiencing an acute state of despair and anguish caused by the loss of a person or object.

GOALS

The goals of grief work are to:
1. Express grief with a view toward resolution and acceptance
2. Prevent social isolation and withdrawal
3. Prevent physical illnesses
4. Prevent depression and suicide

PURPOSE OF NURSING INTERVENTION

The nurse helps the client accept the loss, express feelings, and learn and grow from the experience. Usually the nurse intervenes with individuals, but may lead a group of clients who have suffered recent loss.

METHODS OF INTERVENTION

1. Help client work through grief: "Tell me what you're feeling today."
2. Accept ambivalence: "Sometimes we feel angry at people who die and leave us."
3. Anticipate somatic complaints: "Do you sometimes feel like not even eating?"
4. Prevent isolation and loneliness: "Why not join the others for lunch today?"
5. Prevent self-destruction: "Please call me when you feel really down."

PSYCHODYNAMIC PSYCHOTHERAPY

DEFINITION

Psychodynamic psychotherapy is a form of treatment provided in individual or group settings to help elderly clients make more of their inner lives available to themselves for present and future creative and satisfying life experiences (Pollock, 1987).

GOALS

The goals of psychodynamic therapy are to:

1. Help clients be in touch with parts of themselves that have been forgotten, neglected, or pushed away and yet continue to exert important influences (Pollock, 1987)
2. Reawaken in clients old emotional allegiances, passions, rages, and "overgrown paths" (Pollock, 1987)
3. Help clients mourn the past through self-investigation

PURPOSE OF NURSING INTERVENTION

The nurse helps clients to confront the inevitable traumas of later life, resolve alienations, and work through private experiences that may lie in the past but are still alive. Energy is released for new investments in both inner life and outer life.

METHODS OF INTERVENTION

The nurse:

1. Encourages clients to talk about their lives, eliciting much description of the past and present: "Tell me more about what happened. Start at the beginning."
2. Facilitates description of abandonment experiences such as hospitalizations, death of parents, death of children, immigration experiences, retirement: "Tell me about the day your mother died."
3. Discusses symptomatic acts: "Tell me what you thought/felt just before you yelled at your daughter."
4. Interprets fantasies and dreams: "Tell me what happened the day you dreamed your husband was alive again."
5. Helps the client discuss and work through feelings of anger, depression, resistance, envy, and jealousy.
6. Interprets acting out and helps client to verbalize instead.
7. Establishes and works through transference: "So, you were wishing last night your son was as attentive as I am? Say more about that."
8. Investigates with another professional any intense countertransference.

EVALUATION

Success in the work with elderly clients is measured by a heightened sense of self-worth, overall improvement in morale, and a sense of having made a contribution to others based on one's life experiences (Fitzpatrick, 1984). Clients have been able to mourn the past states of the self and be liberated from the past, so they can move forward (Pollock, 1987).

REFERENCES

Abraham, I. L., Fox, J. M., Harrington, D. P., Snustad, D. G., Steiner, D. A., Abraham, L. H., & Brashear, H. R. (1990). A psychogeriatric nursing assessment protocol for use in multidisciplinary practice. *Archives of Psychiatric Nursing, 4,* 242–259.

Abraham, I. L., Thompson-Heisterman, A. A., Harrington, D. P., Smullen, D. E., Onega, L. L., Droney, E. G., Westerman, P. S., Manning, C. A., & Lichtenberg, P. A. (1991). Outpatient psychogeriatric nursing services: An integrative model. *Archives of Psychiatric Nursing, 3,* 151–164.

American Psychological Association (1993). *Vitality for Life: Psychological Research for Productive Aging.* Washington, DC: American Psychological Association.

Beck, A. T., & Steer, R. A. (1993). *Beck Depression Inventory Manual.* San Antonio, TX: Psychological Corporation.

Cassetta, R. A. (1993). Opportunities on the rise in long-term care. *American Nurse, 25* (7), 13–14.

Dellasega, C. (1991). Meeting the mental health needs of elderly clients. *Journal of Psychosocial Nursing, 29* (2), 10–14.

Duke University Center for the Study of Aging and Human Development (1978). *Multidimensional Functional Assessment: The OARS Methodology* (2nd ed.). Durham, NC: Duke University.

Edinberg, M. A. (1985). *Mental Health Practice with the Elderly.* Englewood Cliffs, NJ: Prentice-Hall.

Erickson, E. H. (1963). *Childhood and Society* (2nd ed.). New York: W. W. Norton.

Fitzpatrick, J. (1984). Gerontological counseling. In S. Lego (ed.), *The American Handbook of Psychiatric Nursing* (pp. 357–364). Philadelphia: J. B. Lippincott.

Folstein, M. F., Folstein, S. E., & McHugh, P. R. (1975). Minimental state: A practical method for grading the cognitive state of patients for the clinician. *Journal of Psychiatric Research, 12,* 189–198.

Gatz, M. (1989). Clinical psychology and aging. In P. T. Costa, M. Gatz, B. L. Neugarten, T. A. Salthouse, & I. C. Siegler (eds.), *The Adult Years: Continuity and Change* (pp. 83–115). Washington, DC: American Psychological Association.

Haight, B. K., & Burnside, I. (1993). Reminiscence and life review: Explaining the differences. *Archives of Psychiatric Nursing, 7* (2), 91–98.

Harper, M., & Grau, L. (1994). State of the art in geropsychiatric nursing. *Journal of Psychosocial Nursing, 32* (4), 7–12.

Lappe, J. M. (1987). Reminiscing: The life review therapy. *Journal of Gerontological Nursing, 13* (4), 12–16.

McBride, A. B., & Burgener, S. (1994). Strategies to implement geropsychiatric nursing curricula content. *Journal of Psychosocial Nursing, 32* (4), 13–18.

Mikulencak, M. (1993). The "graying of America"—Changing what nurses need to know. *American Nurse, 25* (7), 1, 12.

Miller, C. A. (1990). *Nursing Care of Older Adults: Theory and Practice.* Glenview, IL: Scott, Foresman/Little, Brown Higher Education.

Pollock, G. (1987). The mourning-liberation process: Ideas on the inner life of the older adult. In J. Sadavoy & M. Leszcz (eds.), *Treating the Elderly with Psychotherapy: The Scope for Change in Later Life* (pp. 3–30). Madison, CT: International Universities Press.

Sadavoy, J., & Leszcz, M. (1987). *Treating the Elderly with Psychotherapy: The Scope of Change in Later Life.* Madison, CT: International Universities Press.

Sarton, M. (1984). *At Seventy.* New York: W. W. Norton.

Sarton, M. (1988). *After the Stroke: A Journal.* New York: W. W. Norton.

Sarton, M. (1992). *End Game: A Journal of the Seventy-Ninth Year.* New York: W. W. Norton.

Sarton, M. (1993). *Encore: A Journal of the Eightieth Year.* New York: W. W. Norton.

Sarton, M. (1995). *At Eighty-Two: A Journal.* New York: W. W. Norton.

Schmidt, M. G., & Burnside, I. (1994). Demographic and psychological aspects of aging. In I. Burnside & M. G. Schmidt (eds.), *Working with Older Adults: Group Process and Techniques* (pp. 8–23). Boston: Jones and Bartlett Publishers.

BIBLIOGRAPHY

Abraham, I. L., & Buckwalter, K. C. (1994). Geropsychiatric nursing: A clinical knowledge base in community and institutional settings. *Journal of Psychosocial Nursing, 32* (4), 20–26.

Agostinelli, B., Kemers, K., Garrigan, D., & Waszynski, C. (1994). Targeted interventions: Use of the mini–mental state exam. *Journal of Gerontological Nursing, 20* (8), 15–23.

Beckingham, A. C., & Baumann, A. (1990). The ageing family in crisis: Assessment and decision-making models. *Journal of Advanced Nursing, 15,* 782–787.

Birren, J. E., Sloane, R. B., & Cohen, G. D. (eds.) (1992). *Handbook of Mental Health and Aging.* New York: Academic Press.

Blazer, D. G. (1993). *Depression in Late Life* (2nd ed.). Philadelphia: Mosby.

Burnside, I. (1990). A scarce professional: The geropsychiatric clinical nurse specialist. *Clinical Nurse Specialist, 4* (3), 122–127.

Burnside, I. (1990). Reminiscence: An independent nursing intervention for the elderly. *Issues in Mental Health Nursing, 11,* 22–48.

Cataldo, J. K. (1994). Hardiness and death attitudes: Predictors of depression in the institutionalized elderly. *Archives of Psychiatric Nursing, 8* (5), 320–325.

Conn, D. K., Herrmann, N., Kaye, A., Rewilak, D., Robinson, A., & Schogt, R. (1992). *Practical Psychiatry in the Nursing Home: A Handbook for Staff.* Toronto: Hogrege & Huber.

Davidhizar, R., & Bowen, M. (1992). The dynamics of laughter. *Archives of Psychiatric Nursing, 6* (2), 127–132.

Fopma-Loy, J. (1989). Geropsychiatric nursing: Focus and setting. *Archives of Psychiatric Nursing, 3* (4), 183–190.

Friedan, B. (1993). *The Fountain of Age.* New York: Simon & Schuster.

Hamilton, G. (1990). Promotion of mental health in older adults. In M. O. Hogstel (ed.), *Geropsychiatric Nursing* (pp. 38–69). Philadelphia: C. V. Mosby.

Hirst, S. P., & Miller, J. (1986). The abused elderly. *Journal of Psychosocial Nursing, 24* (10), 28–34.

Hogstel, M. O. (1990). *Geropsychiatric Nursing.* Philadelphia: C. V. Mosby.

Hummert, M. L., Wieman, J. M., & Nussbaum, J. (1994). *Interpersonal Communication in Older Adulthood.* Newbury Park, CA: Sage Publications.

Johnsow, J., & Slater, R. (1994). *Aging and Late Life.* Newbury Park, CA: Sage Publications.

Keith, J. (1994). *Age and Culture: Diversity and Commonality in Experience of Aging.* Newbury Park, CA: Sage Publications.

Kovach, C. R. (1991). Reminiscence: A closer look at content. *Issues in Mental Health Nursing, 12,* 193–204.

Kurlowicz, L. H. (1993). Social factors and depression in late life. *Archives of Psychiatric Nursing, 7* (1), 30–36.

Mellick, E., Buckwalter, K. C., & Stolley, J. M. (1992). Suicide among elderly white men: Development of a profile. *Journal of Psychosocial Nursing, 30* (2), 29–34.

Midlarsky, E., & Kahana, E. (1994). *Altruism and Helping by the Elderly.* Newbury Park, CA: Sage Publications.

Newboern, V. B. (1992). Sharing the memories: The value of reminiscence as a research tool. *Journal of Gerontological Nursing, 18* (5), 13–18.

Pearlman, I. R. (1993). Group psychotherapy with the elderly. *Journal of Psychosocial Nursing, 31* (7), 7–10.

Sarton, M. (1973). *As We Are Now* (novel). New York: W. W. Norton.

Simon, J. M. (1990). Humor and its relationship to perceived health, life satisfaction, and morale in older adults. *Issues in Mental Health Nursing, 11,* 17–31.

Thobaben, M. (1990). Depression in the medically ill homebound patient. *Journal of Home Health Care Practice, 2* (3), 33–38.

Wallsten, S. M. (1992). Geriatric mental health: A portrait of homelessness. *Journal of Psychosocial Nursing, 30* (9), 20–24.

Walter, K. (1992). That was then: Elderly survivors of incest. *Journal of Psychosocial Nursing, 30* (1), 14–16.

Whall, A. L. (1990). Nursing approaches to the mental health of the elderly: A position paper. *Issues in Mental Health Nursing, 11,* 71–77.

20
TWENTY

Counseling Dying Adults and Their Significant Others

Edith Brogan de la Fuente

OVERVIEW:

INTRODUCTION

Dying is an inevitable part of living. Though expected universally it is never anticipated individually. The dying process contains many moments that, if recognized, allow the patient, family members, friends, and caretakers to achieve closure with the dying person. Caring for a dying family member or friend can also initiate the grieving process for those who remain, as they help the individual realize a "good" death.

Dying is a family process. The attempt to encapsulate it as an individual experience prevents the sharing, caring, and dignity that should be associated with life's ending. The sharing allows for patients to undertake a life review with a multiperson perspective, to reexamine the meaning in their lives, and hence confront death with a feeling of fullness. Deception, whether well meaning or not, destroys the bond of trust between patient, significant others, and health caregivers.

Psychiatric nurses are often called upon to help with the dying process as they are experts in interpreting and clarifying human responses. However, nurses, like others in the health care professions, may feel inadequate for this role, or they may view death as an affront to their healing profession. This is especially true when death is sudden or unexpected, or when the patient is a young adult or a child. Nurses will benefit by an examination of their own feelings, personal views, and values about death.

SUDDEN DEATH OR UNEXPECTED DEATH

Sudden death may occur as a result of cardiac arrest, stroke, accidents, trauma, or violence and extract a high toll on significant others. Health care workers who witness this devastation may experience frustration and grief. The survivors, especially those dealing with traumatic or violent deaths, are at risk for pathological grief. Notifying significant others is an important process, and initiates the grieving process.

Borrowing from Collins (1989), Box 20-1 is a sudden death counseling protocol.

BOX 20-1: Sudden or Unexpected Death Counseling Protocol

Phone Contact—Local
1. Ask for survivor or next of kin by name if known.
2. Introduce yourself by name, title, and hospital.
3. Inform the survivor of the accident or the reason the patient was brought to the hospital.
4. Ask for the survivor to come to the hospital with family or friends and give the location of the hospital.
5. Do not inform of death on phone, but if asked do not lie.

Phone Contact—Long Distance
1. Identify yourself by name, title, and hospital.
2. Establish the next of kin.
3. Using a progressive approach, share the information regarding the accident or cause of death, including the resuscitative methods used and the patient's response.
4. Using the word *death,* give time for questions.
5. Repeat your name and give a phone number for further contact.
6. Ask for organ donation or follow protocol as set up by your agency or state.

Meeting the Survivors
1. Introduce yourself and lead survivors into a private room.
2. Sit close to the member who seems to be in the most distress, and maintaining eye contact, start to tell about the accident or the cause of death, giving time and place.
3. Describe any injuries sustained, any lifesaving measures that were taken, and the patient's response.
4. Use the word *death* and provide time for questions.
5. Provide emotional and physical support.

Viewing the Body
1. Offer to take survivors to where the patient is, and inform them about any equipment at the bedside and the condition of the body.
2. Encourage them to look, touch, or hold the body.
3. Offer them a chaplain or prayer at the bedside.
4. If possible, allow them to go between the waiting room and the patient's room for individual or consecutive viewings.

Follow-Up Support
Send a condolence letter within 2–3 weeks, including your professional card and information about local bereavement groups.

Adapted from Collins, S. (1989). Sudden death counseling protocol. *Dimensions of Critical Care Nursing, 8* (6), 375–382. Copyright 1989, Hall Johnson Communications, Inc. Reproduced with permission. For further use, contact the publisher at 9737 West Ohio Avenue, Lakewood, CO 80226.

**DYING PERSON'S
BILL OF RIGHTS**

Before counseling persons who are dying, it is important for the nurse to consider the rights of these patients. Box 20-2 lists the dying person's Bill of Rights.

BOX 20-2: The Dying Person's Bill of Rights

1. I have the right to be treated as a living human being until I die.

2. I have the right to maintain a sense of hopefulness, however changing its focus may be.

3. I have the right to be cared for by those who can maintain a sense of hopefulness, however changing this might be.

4. I have the right to express my feelings and emotions about my approaching death in my own way.

5. I have the right to participate in decisions concerning my care.

6. I have the right to expect continuing medical and nursing attention even though "cure" goals must be changed to "comfort" goals.

7. I have the right not to die alone.

8. I have the right to be free from pain.

9. I have the right to have my questions answered honestly.

10. I have the right not to be deceived.

11. I have the right to have help from and for my family in accepting my death.

12. I have the right to die in peace and dignity.

13. I have the right to retain my individuality and not be judged for my decisions, which may be contrary to beliefs of others.

14. I have the right to discuss and enlarge my religious or spiritual experiences, whatever these may mean to others.

15. I have the right to expect that the sanctity of the human body will be respected after death.

16. I have the right to be cared for by caring, sensitive, knowledgeable people who will attempt to understand my needs and will be able to gain some satisfaction in helping me face my death.

Donovan, M. I., & Pierce, S. G. (1984). *Cancer Care Nursing*. New York: Appleton Century Crofts.

**STAGES OF DEATH
AND DYING AND
NURSING
INTERVENTIONS**

Table 20-1 lists Kubler-Ross's stages of death and dying and nursing interventions for each stage. These stages, or human responses, may not be sequential. They may be experienced at any point in the illness, or all at the end.

TABLE 20-1
Stages of Death and Dying and Nursing Interventions

STAGES	NURSING INTERVENTION
Stage 1: Shock and Denial Shock is often the first response to receiving a terminal diagnosis. Denying or refusing to accept the diagnosis or the prognosis may lead patients and families to pursue various doctors and experimental treatments.	Encourage the patient, family, and friends to share what they think is going on. Asking how the nurse might help may elicit the family's true knowledge. Some patients need to deny to the end. This should be accepted without aiding or encouraging this deception.
Stage 2: Anger Anger or the "Why me?" and "Why now?" reaction is almost universally felt. Peplau (1991, pp. 83–97) defines anger as destructive feelings and thoughts that arise in response to a frustrating situation.	Listen as the patient expresses anger over possible changes in body image and function, the loss of future dreams and goals, or over past regrets. Rather than express anger openly, the patient may displace it for fear of retaliation, rejection, or abandonment. Help the patient to express the anger openly. Remain nonjudgmental and open to those who use anger as a coping mechanism throughout the illness.
Stage 3: Bargaining Patients negotiate with God, life, or the doctor to change the diagnosis, prognosis, or alter the trajectory of the illness.	Listen nonjudgmentally to hear the underlying pleas and fears of patients not wanting to disconnect with life and those they love. Nurses can help by reflecting their patients' sense of loss and frustration, letting them know that this is a normal and expected response.
Stage 4: Depression In the reactive depression phase patients mourn past losses. They often feel sad, lonely, tearful, have a lack of energy, changes in sleep patterns, and may have periods marked by despair. The anticipatory grieving phase or the grieving for the future is what Kubler Ross calls the "silent phase." It is often hard for family and friends to accept patients' withdrawal from all but a few people.	Using interpersonal and cognitive therapy, help patients modify negative thoughts, work through problem relationships, and set short-term goals. Be alert to suicidal feelings. When they are expressed, ask if the patient has a plan. Evaluate for antidepressants (see Chapter 69) as well as psychotherapy (see Chapter 23). Clarify to the family that in the anticipatory grief phase, the patient's withdrawal is natural and expected.
Stage 5: Acceptance Patients accept that life is limited and enjoy each day with a sense of inner peace.	Reinforce this attitude, making sure the patient is accepting death rather than merely becoming resigned to escape because life is empty and meaningless. Help patients find meaning in their final phase of life.

NEARING DEATH AWARENESS

"Nearing death awareness" is a phenomenon described by Callanan and Kelley (1992) as a special knowledge and sometimes control patients have over the dying process. Nurses and family should keep an open mind to the language dying patients use as they may be (1) sharing what they are experiencing or (2) asking for something they need to die peacefully.

Callanan and Kelley (1992, pp. 213–215) describe four phenomena that occur as the person nears death. These include (Lego, 1994; reproduced with permission):

1. *Preparing for travel or change.* Dying people are aware of impending death. They communicate this to loved ones using travel metaphors. Examples are asking for a map, asking how the tide is, asking for passports, and so forth. The nurse can be helpful in "translating" this message to loved ones.

2. *Being in the presence of someone not alive.* The authors give several examples of dying persons seeing and talking with loved ones who have already died. This may be upsetting to family, friends, and caretakers who do not understand, but it is comforting to the dying person. Nurses can be helpful by explaining why the dying person is gesturing, waving, or talking to persons unseen by others in the room. Occasionally others think the dying person is hallucinating or is receiving too much pain medication, or is losing intellectual function. The nurse can help by answering the patient's questions honestly, for example, "Do you know where my mother is?" The nurse replies, "Your mother died years ago." When the dying person says, "She was just here," rather than argue or humor the person, the nurse replies, "Yes, I understand that you saw her." Often dying persons are visited by someone they do not know has died. In such instances it is important the dying person be told the truth. The truth can help the person feel comfort at the thought of reunion with the loved one. Lying about the death only leads to discomfort and anxiety.

3. *Seeing a place not visible to anyone else.* Often the dying person mentions a place no one else can see. It is usually described as lovely, peaceful, and may contain a "light." Often the words "home" or "going home" are mentioned. When this happens the nurse gently asks about that other place or home. "Would you like to tell me about the other place?" "Which home?" "Are you telling us you are ready to leave?" Dying persons are sometimes found on the floor near their beds, perhaps because they have gotten out of bed to follow someone they have seen to the new place.

4. *Knowing when death will occur.* The dying person often knows when death will occur and communicates this to others. For example, she may say, "I won't be here on Sunday." This uncanny awareness, which the authors call "nearing death awareness," is a signal to the nurse and others that loved ones should be called to the bedside for final partings. It is important, therefore, that the nurse hear and understand this message. However, some persons prefer to die alone. They may ask loved ones to go home and rest or go for a walk. They can then die peacefully. Callanan and Kelley (1992, pp. 213–215) offer a number of practical suggestions for recognizing, understanding, and responding to nearing death awareness:

   a. Pay attention to *everything* the dying person says. You might want to keep pens and a spiral notebook beside the bed so that anyone can jot down notes about gestures, conversations, or anything out of the ordinary said by the dying person. Talk with one another about these comments and gestures.

   b. Remember that there may be important messages in any communication, however vague or garbled. Not every statement made by a dying person has significance, but heed them all so as not to miss the ones that do.

   c. Watch for key signs: a glassy-eyed look; the appearance of staring through you; distractedness or secretiveness; seemingly inappropriate smiles or gestures, such as pointing, reaching toward someone or something unseen, or waving when no one is there; efforts to pick at the covers or get out of bed for no apparent reason; agitation or distress at your inability to comprehend something the dying person has tried to say. Respond to anything you don't understand with gentle inquiries. "Can you tell me what's happening?" is sometimes a helpful way to initiate this kind of conversation. You might also try saying, "You seem different today. Can you tell me why?"

d. Pose questions in open-ended, encouraging terms. For example, if a dying person whose mother is long dead says, "My mother's waiting for me," turn that comment into a question: "Mother's waiting for you?" or "I'm so glad she's close to you. Can you tell me about it?" Accept and validate what the dying person tells you. If he says, "I see a beautiful place!" say, "That's wonderful! Can you tell me more about it?" or "I'm so pleased. I can see that it makes you happy," or "I'm so glad you're telling me this. I really want to understand what's happening to you. Can you tell me more?" Don't argue or challenge. By saying something like "You couldn't possibly have seen Mother, she's been dead for 10 years," you increase the dying person's frustration and isolation, and run the risk of putting an end to further attempts at communicating.

e. Remember that a dying person may employ images from life experiences like work or hobbies. A pilot may talk about getting ready to go for a flight; carry the metaphor forward: "Do you know when it leaves?" or "Is there anyone on the plane you know?" or "Is there anything I can do to help you get ready for takeoff?"

f. Be honest about having trouble understanding. One way is to say, "I think you're trying to tell me something important and I'm trying very hard, but I'm just not getting it. I'll keep on trying. Please don't give up on me."

g. Don't push. Let the dying control the breadth of the conversation; they may not be able to put their experiences into words; insisting on more talk may frustrate or overwhelm them.

h. Avoid instilling a sense of failure in the dying person. If the information is garbled or the delivery impossibly vague, show that you appreciate the effort by saying, "I can see that this is hard for you; I appreciate your trying to share it with me," or "I can see you're getting tired/angry/frustrated. Would it be easier if we talked about this later?" or "Don't worry. We'll keep trying and maybe it will come."

i. If you don't know what to say, don't say anything. Sometimes the best response is simply to touch the dying person's hand, or smile and stroke her forehead. Touching gives the very important message "I'm with you." Or you could say, "That's interesting. Let me think about it."

j. Remember that sometimes the dying person picks an unlikely confidant. Dying people often try to communicate important information to someone who makes them feel safe—who won't get upset or be taken aback by such confidences. If you're an outsider chosen for this role, share the information as gently and completely as possible with the appropriate family members or friends. They may be more familiar with innuendos in a message because they know the person well.

RATIONAL SUICIDE

Psychiatric nurses are encountering more and more patients who want to plan in advance a "death with dignity." This is very different from the situation when a patient is actively suicidal. When patients tell the nurse they want to control their own death, the nurse performs the following assessments.

RATIONALITY ASSESSMENT

1. Asking the patient's rationale for a planned death
2. Assessing the patient's knowledge of the consequences of rational suicide to the self and significant others

3. Assessing the patient's awareness of the consequence of a failed attempt

SYMPTOM CONTROL ASSESSMENT

Determining everything is being done that can be done to alleviate the symptoms that make the disease or dying process unbearable

ASSESSMENT OF THE PATIENT'S AND FAMILY'S FINANCIAL AND HUMAN RESOURCES

Obtaining a social service evaluation to determine that everything is being done that can be done to provide community resources, such as hospice, support groups, and so forth

ASSESSMENT OF THE PATIENT'S MORAL OR RELIGIOUS BELIEFS

Offering the opportunity to talk to a clergy member (See Chapter 71 regarding the psychiatric nurse's consideration of the ethics of rational suicide.)

BEREAVEMENT

Bereavement occurs during the year following the death of a loved one. It is important for nurses to realize and to communicate to the bereaved that the length of time for mourning varies with individuals. Time needed may be influenced by the cause of death, age of the deceased, relationship to the deceased and degree of emotional attachment, for example, positive, negative, or ambivalent. Bereavement is harder when the relationship was negative or ambivalent. Grief experiences include the following.

PHYSICAL SYMPTOMS

1. Tightness in the throat or in the muscles
2. Heaviness or pressure in the chest
3. Inability to sleep
4. Periods of nervousness or even panic
5. Lack of desire to eat (or)
6. Desire to overeat
7. Visual or auditory hallucinations of the deceased
8. Headaches or stomach/intestinal disorders
9. Lack of energy
10. Inability to concentrate

EMOTIONAL SYMPTOMS

1. Sadness or depression
2. Forgetfulness
3. Guilt or anger about things that happened or didn't happen in the relationship with the deceased
4. Unexpected anger toward others, God, or the deceased
5. Tearfulness, sometimes unexpectedly
6. Mood swings
7. Discomfort around other people but disinclination to be alone
8. Sensation of the death being unreal, that it didn't actually happen
9. Feelings of emptiness, or having been cheated
10. Thoughts like "If only things had happened differently"
11. Fear of what will happen next
12. Doubts or questions concerning why the death occurred
13. Desire to run away, or to become very busy, to avoid the pain of loss
14. Experience of "going crazy" when overwhelmed with intensity of feelings

**NURSING
INTERVENTIONS
WITH THE BEREAVED**

The nurse can be helpful to those going through bereavement by:

1. Listening, since through talking the death will become a reality, and the pain will be shared. The bereaved can over time become liberated from the pain of losing the loved one by reviewing both positive and negative aspects of the relationship.
2. Offering practical help to guide the bereaved back into reality, perhaps learning new skills, such as balancing a checkbook, paying bills, and so forth.
3. Helping the bereaved reconnect with others by reconnecting with old friends or starting new relationships. Box 20-3 contains guidelines for families and friends experiencing bereavement.

BOX 20-3: Guidelines for Families and Friends Experiencing Bereavement

What to do for physical relief and healing:

1. Take care of yourself by having a physical checkup.
2. In early stages of grief, don't force yourself to eat more than you want. As your appetite returns, eat a healthy, well-balanced diet.
3. Get some exercise—even a peaceful, quiet walk. Physical exercise helps you to relax.
4. It may be helpful to give up caffeine as a way to relieve nervousness. Beware of alcohol, which is a depressant. Some findings indicate that alcohol interrupts normal sleep patterns.
5. Check frequently that you have balance in your life: rest, recreation, prayer/meditation, and work.

What to do for emotional relief and healing:

1. Be gentle with yourself. Although you may often feel overwhelmed, remind yourself that what you are going through is normal.
2. Reach out to others. It is important to find friends with whom you can talk. Sharing with someone who's "been there" can be especially helpful.
3. Tell and retell what happened, remembering things about the loved one and the experience of his or her death. Good memories are also very important.
4. Be aware that people grieve in different ways. Don't measure your progress in handling grief against others.
5. You may or may not cry often, but when you do, realize it is therapeutic. Don't fight the tears. As the author Jean G. Jones says: "Cry when you have to—and laugh when you can."
6. Confront guilt by realizing you did the best you could.
7. Become familiar with the normal experiences of grieving and be willing to engage in your own grief work.
8. Remember that grieving takes time, and that experiences and emotions can recur. Be patient with yourself, and allow yourself to heal at your own pace.
9. Beware of being critical of yourself, either consciously or unconsciously, owing to unrealistic expectations.

BOX 20-3 *(continued)*

10. Other events in your life may also be causing anxiety (trouble with spouse, children, work, or friends). Realize this happens to many grieving people, and these situations can complicate the grieving process.

11. Find support from both inside and outside your family. But don't expect your family to meet all of your needs. Remember that they, too, have their grief.

12. Many of us have been brought up to be independent: "I'm going to handle this on my own." We find it difficult to ask for help. Yet, we all need support. Take the risk of joining a support group. Asking for help from caring people can make a big difference in your working through your grief.

13. It may be time to struggle with new life patterns. In the past, you may have handled grief by overactivity. If your previous style of grieving has not been helpful, be willing to try new approaches, such as becoming active in a support group; finding telephone friends; reading and learning about grief; developing new coping skills; reaching out and helping others; holding on to hope.

REFERENCES

Callanan, M., & Kelley, P. (1992). *Final Gifts.* New York: Poseidon Press.

Collins, S. (1989). Sudden death counseling protocol. *Dimensions of Critical Care Nursing, 8* (6), 375–382.

Donovan, M. I., & Pierce, S. G. (1984). *Cancer Care Nursing.* New York: Appleton Century Crofts.

Kubler-Ross, E. (1969). *On Death and Dying.* New York: Macmillan.

Lego, S. (1994). *Fear and AIDS/HIV: Empathy and Communication.* Albany, NY: Delmar.

Peplau, H. E. (1991). *Interpersonal Relations in Nursing.* New York: Springer.

BIBLIOGRAPHY

Broyard, A. (1992). *Intoxicated by My Illness.* New York: Fawcett Columbine.

Crenshaw D. (1990). *Bereavement.* New York: Continuum.

Humphry, D. (1991). *Final Exit.* Eugene, OR: The Hemlock Society.

Kirchberg, T. M., & Neimeyer, R. (1991). Reactions of beginning counselors to situations involving death and dying. *Death Studies, 15,* 603–610.

Kubler-Ross, E. (1974). *Questions and Answers on Death and Dying.* New York: Collier Books.

Kubler-Ross, E. (1981). *Living with Death and Dying.* New York: Collier Books.

Kubler-Ross, E. (1982). *Working It Through.* New York: Collier Books.

Kubler-Ross, E. (1987). *AIDS: The Ultimate Challenge.* New York: Collier Books.

Leliaert, R. M. (1989). Spiritual side of "Good Grief": What happened to Holy Saturday? *Death Studies, 13,* 103–117.

Lewis, C. S. (1989). *A Grief Observed.* San Francisco: Harper.

MacIntyre, R. (1992). Point/counterpoint: Nurse-assisted suicide. *Journal of the Association of Nurses in AIDS Care, 3* (1) 23–24.

Morse, M., & Perry, P. (1990). *Closer to the Light.* New York: Villard Books.

Nuland, S. B. (1994). *How We Die.* New York: Alfred A. Knopf.

Pickrel, J. (1989). "Tell me your story": Using life review in counseling the terminally ill. *Death Studies, 13,* 127–135.

Saunders, J. M., & Valente, S. M. (1994). Nurses' grief. *Cancer Nursing, 17* (4), 318–325.

Serdahely, W. J. (1992). The near-death experience and caregivers. *Caring, 11* (1) 8–11.

Staucacher, C. (1987). *Beyond Grief.* Oakland, CA: New Harbinger.

Stoddard, S. (1992). *The Hospice Movement.* New York: Vintage.

Wyatt, P. (1993). The role of nurses in counseling the terminally ill patient. *British Journal of Nursing, 2* (14) 701–704.

TWENTY ONE

Bereavement Counseling of Children and Their Families

Donna A. Gaffney

OVERVIEW:

INTRODUCTION

Nurses often intervene in situations with children and adolescents who have experienced a loss, or children who are anticipating and fearing their own death. Effective intervention requires accurate assessment of the young person's cognitive development and the nature and impact of the loss, both real and perceived. It is the responsibility of the nurse to determine the impact of these related factors on both the child and family.

NURSES' PREPARATION

Nurses who work with bereaved children and their families have:
1. Knowledge of normal growth and development
2. Awareness of children's understanding of death and dying
3. Clinical expertise in child therapy and grief work
4. Supervision by a professional who is familiar with issues related to loss and bereavement during childhood
5. Knowledge of their own feelings about loss and death

GOALS

Nurses who work with bereaved children have the following goals:
1. Assessing the child's emotional response to the loss
2. Helping the child express feelings about the loss
3. Supporting the child's movement through the bereavement process
4. Providing information and guidance to the child regarding bereavement

5. Preventing or modifying behaviors not conducive to the integration of loss into the child's life
6. Helping the child identify other sources of support

ASSESSMENT

To determine the most appropriate treatment plan nurses assess:
1. The children's conceptions of death based on age (see Box 21-1)
2. The nature of the child's loss from the child's perspective as well as the family's
3. Cultural, religious/spiritual, or social customs that may influence the child's bereavement experience

---

BOX 21-1: Children's Conceptions of Death According to Age

1–3 Years
No concept of death exists.
Death is the absence of the person.

4 Years
The concept of death is somewhat limited.
Death is associated with absence or sleep.
Death is a continuation of life but in a different way (living underground in the coffin).
There is some sense of reversibility.

5 Years
The concept of death expands and includes some knowledge of cessation of body functioning.
Death is associated with violence or disaster.
The child is intrigued by and curious about dead "living things."
The child may still believe death is reversible.

6 Years
The child understands death is not reversible and that body functions cease.
Death is associated with violence, accidents, and disaster.
There is some preoccupation with graves, funerals, and cemeteries.
Death is associated with separation.
The child believes death only happens to other, older people.

7 Years
The concept of death becomes further detailed and realistic but causation is still unclear.
The child is unable to understand why death cannot be prevented.
The child believes death may occur in self, but not for a very long time.
There is curiosity about cemeteries, bogeymen, "scary" things.

8–10 Years
The concept of death expands to include the body's functioning after death.
Causation of death becomes clearer and relates to physical causes.
The child accepts that all people die when they are older.

11–13 Years
The concept of death is nearly like that of an adult.
The cause of death may be understood to have multiple reasons.
The child is able to articulate outcomes of death, for example, bodily response.

Adapted from Giblin, M., & Ryan, F. (1991). Reading the child's perception of death. In J. Morgan (ed.), *Young People and Death* (pp. 3–4). Philadelphia: The Charles Press.

4. Previous experience in the child's life or in the family's history that may influence the child's response to the loss and the subsequent bereavement experience including any physical illnesses, prolonged separations, mental illnesses, catastrophic events such as disasters, fires, or accidents
5. Availability of support systems in the child's and family members' lives

FACTS ABOUT CHILDREN'S GRIEF

Nurses work best with bereaved children when they bear in mind that:
1. Children are capable of grieving.
2. Children understand loss, death, and the finality of life in age-appropriate ways.
3. Children will almost always remember a loss, even if they don't talk about it. They will remember images and feelings even when they are very young.
4. Children cannot and *should* not be protected from emotional pain. Adults often protect themselves through their children, though the children know what is happening and should be allowed to share their own feelings.
5. Helping children with grief involves more than confronting the child with reality. Patience, understanding, love, and support are needed as well.
6. There is no right or wrong way to grieve. Children grieve differently than adults (even their parents). They may express less sadness, talk and cry less. This doesn't mean that they aren't grieving; they're doing it in their own way.
7. Grief work is not always a time of devastating sadness and tears. There are moments of sweetness, as members of the family remember joyous moments.
8. Children experience the same losses as adults. A parent's loss affects the children.
9. Parents may not always be aware of losses in their children's lives (a pet in school, a friend's grandparent).
10. If a child's grief wasn't addressed at the time of the loss, there is always a second chance to work through those earlier feelings.
11. Grief work is an opportunity for growth, a time for finding new strengths and sharing feelings with significant others.

PHASES OF THE BEREAVEMENT EXPERIENCE

Table 21-1 shows the "seasons" of grief, the time frame, family tasks, and the nurse's tasks.

METHODS

Working with children and adolescents during such painful times requires a flexible and patient approach. Methods used include the following.

PLAY AND ACTIVITY TECHNIQUES

Use of dolls, toy animals, and dollhouse equipment is often helpful in exploring the child's perception of loss. Children will reenact their understanding of the loss event or what they anticipate will happen. Paper, paints, and other art materials allow children to draw or paint their images of the people and events involved. The nurse encourages the child to "tell the story" of the loss. This retelling of the event will occur several times during the therapeutic process, facilitating the integration of death in the child's life. Children will often dramatize or illustrate the events most challenging or intriguing; for example, an accident scene, the hospital room, funeral, religious or burial scenes. It is important for the nurse to remember that the information children share may not be the reality of the event but their perceptions or interpretations of the event based on the verbal and nonverbal communication of others. It is important to correct miscon-

TABLE 21-1
The "Season," Time Frame, Tasks, and Clinical Goals of the
Nurse During Children's Bereavement

"SEASON"	TIME FRAME	TASKS	CLINICAL GOALS
Beginnings (returning the news)	First 24–48 hours after loss	Understanding the loss Acknowledging the turmoil of crisis, denial, and anger	Identify support systems Explain/acknowledge feelings of grief and bereavement Clarify and reinforce understanding of death and circumstances in age-appropriate ways Guide decision-making
Sharing grief (public and private rituals and ceremonies of bereavement	First week to 10 days after loss	Participation in formal services with family Appreciation of cultural and religious practices	Guide decision-making Prepare/clarify/reinterpret rituals to child Facilitate open communication between parent and child
Reentering (returning to occupational and social activities)	First 2–4 weeks after loss	Rejoining familiar activities Establishing mutual support between child and parent Acknowledging that things are different	Guide decision-making Assess readiness of child to rejoin activities Prepare child for difficult situations
Living through the first year (a year of "firsts")	Months 2–12 of the first year after loss	Integrating the impact of loss in the child's life Maintaining supports and communication with family and peers Experiencing significant events during the year and revisiting loss during those times Commemorating loss	Facilitate open communication between parent and child Help the child work through and anticipate holidays and important occasions during the year
Future grief work	After the first anniversary of loss	Revisiting loss as the child moves through each developmental stage Exploring loss and its significant aftermath as milestones are reached	Address the impact and meaning of change over time Help the child move through different levels of understanding and emotional experiences

ceptions in a nonthreatening way and explore how children came to understand the experience.

BIBLIOTHERAPY

There are many children's books dealing with issues of loss, death, and dying. It is critical for the nurse to read any book before recommending it to a child or family. Some are "advisement" books that tend to focus primarily on the loss and the immediate time period following the death. Compared to traditional children's literature, these books are shorter and involve fewer characters. Young children benefit from the nurse or a family member reading the advisement books with the child. Older children find the longer, more literary books useful during the months following the loss. When using books with children in groups, the nurse serves not only as group leader but storyteller as well. When the nurse reads aloud to the group, children can listen to the story rather than focus on their own word pronunciation and reading skills. The content of the story can be provocative and precipitate a group response quite easily. In one group of third-grade girls, the nurse was reading the book *Sarah, Plain and Tall*. At the beginning of the story a mother dies in childbirth, leaving three small children and her husband alone. This situation stimulated discussion among the group members about losses in their own lives. One young girl even told of her own mother's death. The experience of the fictional character helps children to address their own circumstances (Lovrin, 1995).

USE OF FILM AND DRAMA

Commercial films, videotapes, and plays can also be used to help children explore their feelings of loss. Animated features such as *Bambi, Snow White, Dumbo,* and *The Lion King* (all by Walt Disney Studios) depict significant loss in a child's life, namely that of the parent. It is very important that grieving children do not view these films alone. An adult can provide nonverbal comfort and observe the child's response to the events on screen. The nurse should address the nature of the loss, the fictional character's response, and how the story relates to the child's own experience. *Corrina, Corrina* (1994) is a commercial film dealing with a young girl's reaction to her mother's death and her own subsequent relationship with her father. *Stand By Me,* a classic from the 1980s, focuses on how a group of young boys are intrigued by finding a body in the woods while trying to manage their fears of death.

THE MEMORY BOOK

1. Introduce the "idea" of the Memory Book one or two weeks after therapy is initiated. Actual work on the book varies according to the needs of the children. Two to 4 months after the death is usually a good time to begin.
2. Have children select their own scrapbook, notebook, or photo album. They can decorate it or label it anyway they wish. Reintroduce the topic of the "book" the week before beginning work in it; then make special preparations to buy and decorate the book.
3. Prior to starting work on the memory book, talk about what the book means and the guidelines:
   "First of all, let's talk about rules—there are no rules. This is your book of memories of your Dad. You can put anything you want in the book: pictures, letters, drawings, anything at all."
   "This is your book. Keep it in a safe place—only you can look at it unless you give another person permission."
   "This book is for *your* memories and words. You can put in newspaper clippings if it was something that you really wanted to remember (or a special event or award in honor of the person who died)."
   This is also the time to bring up fears some children may have related to grieving the dead person—that is, forgetting what the person looked like, sounded like, and so forth. "I'm wondering if you've ever worried you might forget." Reassure children that those fears are not unusual and that memories are important. The memory book helps to keep mental images "fresh."
4. For younger children, a word game may help initiate work.
   "We're going to start with a word game. Think of five words that describe your dad, for example, funny, supportive, a good coach." After the children take time to write the words, have them tell how the words describe their father.
   "Tell me one time your dad was a good coach. What is the first thing that comes into your mind . . . when was it, where did it occur, who was there, what was said?"

When the scenario is complete, ask the children to say how they will put the word and the event in the Memory Book.

"You can write a few sentences about this special time, paste in a photograph, draw a picture, anything you like." This makes an appropriate homework assignment.

As an assignment have the child choose the second word on the list. This will be the topic for the next time. The child is asked to find a picture or some other memento that will help to visualize the person. When used with a group or sibling this discussion generates a great deal of sharing. Each child contributes recollections of the person who died and experiences positive feelings with the other children.

5. For future times allow for discussion and exploration of the book. Other things to add to the book are:
   ○ The person's favorite holiday
   ○ The person's favorite place to visit
   ○ The person's favorite food
   ○ Favorite or important photographs from the family album
   ○ Jokes or stories associated with the person
6. Special occasions such as graduations, change of seasons, holidays, and so forth are opportunities for children to add significant mementos to their books. In addition, a letter, poem, or story expressing their feelings at this important time might be encouraged.
7. Working on the Memory Book can take place on a regular basis but should not be forced. Brothers and sisters can share this time together. Adults can use information learned during the book time to talk with each child individually.

USE OF STORIES AND METAPHORS

Children will have to cope again with their early losses during significant turning points or milestones later in their lives, for example, entering a new school, graduating from high school, getting married, moving, and having a child. These events involve change and can have a negative or positive influence on behavior. Adults have already experienced many of these milestones; children look forward to these events in their futures. Stories and metaphors may help illustrate how the loss will be a part of a child's life. The following two examples are easy to understand and reassuring to families.

FOR PARENTS

"We all carry emotional baggage, echoes of past events that influence the present and the future. Children have to carry their baggage for a longer distance than adults, so it is important to pack the contents with care from the beginning. During those early days and weeks of grief work children are 'packing' their emotional suitcases. Unconsciously they weigh each thought and feeling before putting it away. Some children don't want to look at what they have to carry. They stuff all their emotions into the suitcase and try to shut it as soon as possible. If they're not careful, feelings hang out, caught between the sides. These children may appear to have coped, but soon we see those caught emotions: anger, aggression, frustration, and loneliness. Other children succeed in shutting all of their thoughts and feelings in the bag. They push the top down and force those emotions to stay inside. Eventually, however, they will have to reopen that suitcase, maybe at another time of loss, maybe at an important turning point in their lives. When they do open it, the suitcase bursts open, and all of those feelings tumble out. Sometimes the suitcase will spring open even when its owner wants to keep it shut.

These are the times when children least expect to deal with their grief. Their burden becomes heavier as they grow older, and, as a result, they have difficulty with all emotional aspects of their lives.

"Adults cannot pack children's bags for them, but they can be there to supervise and give support. We can help children load their feelings and thoughts so they can be carried comfortably. We can let children know the nature of their burden because that makes it easier to carry. We can tell children that there will be other times in their lives when these feelings will have to be unpacked, unfolded, and put away again."

FOR CHILDREN

"Grief is like a butterfly. Before the butterfly is ready to go free in the world, it has to go through changes. While all these changes are taking place the caterpillar is very vulnerable and most safe in a cocoon. When we are grieving, we are much the same. When someone we love dies it hurts us. Sometimes the only way we can feel better is to stay in our own little cocoon. We stay in that cocoon for a while, experiencing different thoughts and feelings about the person who has died. That is what grieving is all about: having those thoughts and feelings, sharing them with other people, and protecting ourselves a little bit, as if we were in a safe cocoon. As time goes by we don't need the protective cocoon as much. We want to spread our wings. There is something different, we have grown and changed. We now have beautiful colors and the ability to soar."

A GUIDE FOR FAMILIES

The nurse can be helpful to families of bereaved children by advising families to (Gaffney, 1988):

1. Recognize and admit what is happening.
2. Try to express their own feelings to their child.
3. Include their children in what is happening and the feelings surrounding those events.
4. Remember that although the situation may be painful, the passage of time will help everyone become acclimated to new situations and roles.
5. Accept the help and support (both physical and emotional) offered by others, since they would want *your* friendship and caring during their time of loss.
6. Try to be flexible about demands on all family members; difficult times call for modifying standards.
7. Break down the problem into manageable pieces rather than view it as an overwhelming whole.
8. Avoid making hasty decisions or major changes too soon; the security of familiarity is important and time may alter viewpoints.
9. Not expect too much of other family members. At the time of loss, nonessentials can be delayed.
10. Consider seeking professional help if, after a reasonable period of time, their efforts seem inadequate.
11. Try to remain hopeful and patient; working through bereavement takes time.

ADVOCACY IN THE COMMUNITY

The nurse serves as an advocate for those at risk and can be instrumental in designing, implementing, and referring to programs for those who are grieving. For children and their families such interventions could include:

1. Referral to educational programs that teach adults to help children deal with loss.
2. Consultation services with schools, social and religious organizations.

3. Publication of articles in lay magazines with local, religious, or national circulation.

4. Networking with other clinicians and school systems to identify children and adolescents who may be at risk for untoward sequelae of early losses.

5. Identification, evaluation, and compilation of support services and groups for children, adolescents, and their parents in hospitals, funeral homes, hospice programs, and community resource centers. Establishment of links with personnel and clinicians at the involved agencies.

6. Networking with librarians and bookstore owners to identify literature that is therapeutic and supportive to children and their families. (See Bibliography.) After reading these, development of reference lists for agency distribution.

7. Development of personal, children's, and professional libraries that address the issues of death, dying, and counseling children and their families. These books should include both fiction and nonfiction.

8. Identification and evaluation of appropriate community self-help groups. There are many self-help groups in churches, hospitals, resource centers, as well as those freestanding groups created at the national level such as the Compassionate Friends. Nurses may caution family members that not every group is for every person and may talk to clients after they have attended the groups to assess their reaction, comfort level, and the competency of leadership. Nurses do not recommend a group unless they are comfortable with the purpose and organization of the group as well as the leadership and professional resources.

EVALUATION

The child and family have successfully moved through the bereavement when they:

1. Acknowledge and value different grieving styles in family members
2. Talk openly to each other and yet respect the need for private moments as well
3. Share the joyful moments of their relationship with the deceased as well as the more painful times
4. Move forward with their own lives and make appropriate choices driven by self-awareness, not by what they believe the deceased would want them to do

REFERENCES

Gaffney, D. (1988). *The Seasons of Grief: Helping Children Grow Through Loss.* New York: New American Library.
Giblin, M., & Ryan, F. (1991). Reading the child's perception of death. In J. Morgan (ed.), *Young People and Death.* Philadelphia: The Charles Press.
Lovrin, M. (1995). Interpersonal support among eight year old girls who have lost their parents or siblings to AIDS. *Archives of Psychiatric Nursing, 9* (2), 92–98.

BIBLIOGRAPHY

Aliki. (1987). *The Two of Them.* New York: William Morrow.
Baker, L. S. (1991). *You and HIV: A Day at a Time.* Philadelphia: W. B. Saunders.
Buscalglia, L. (1982). *The Fall of Freddie the Leaf.* New York: Henry Holt.
Clifton, L. (1983). *Everett Anderson's Goodbye.* New York: Henry Holt.
Gaffney, D. (1988). Death in the classroom: A lesson in life. *Holistic Nursing Practice, 2* (2), 20–26.
Hausherr, R. (1989). *Children and the AIDS Virus.* New York: Houghton Mifflin.
Hazen, B. S. (1985). *Why Did Grandpa Die?* New York: Golden Books.
Hoffman, A. (1988). *At Risk.* New York: Bantam Books.
Krementz, J. (1989). *How It Feels to Fight for Your Life.* Boston: Little Brown.
LeShan, E. (1976). *Learning to Say Goodbye.* New York: Macmillan.
LeShan, E. (1986). *When a Parent Is Very Sick.* Boston: Little Brown.
Mayer, M. (1968). *There's a Nightmare in My Closet.* New York: Dial Books.
Merrifield, M. (1990). *Come Sit by Me.* Toronto: Women's Press.
Morgan, J. (1991). *Young People and Death.* Philadelphia: The Charles Press.

Rosenberg, L. (1995). *The Carousel*. New York: Harcourt Brace.

Rudman, M. (1984). *Children's Literature. An Issues Approach* (2nd ed.). New York: Longman Press.

Sims, A. M. (1986). *Am I Still a Sister?* Albuquerque: Big A & Co.

Stein, S. B. (1974). *About Dying*. New York: Walker.

Viorst, J. (1971). *The Tenth Good Thing About Barney*. New York: Macmillan.

Wilhelm, H. (1988). *I'll Always Love You*. New York: Crown Publishers.

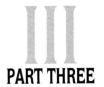

PART THREE

Counseling Specific Clients

TWENTY TWO

The Client Who Is Anxious

Marie C. Smith-Alnimer

DESCRIPTION

Anxiety is experienced by everyone at one time or another. Extreme forms of anxiety early in life lead to the development of defense mechanisms, personality traits, and interpersonal behaviors intended to make the person feel relatively secure. When these overall defense mechanisms fail, the client can suffer intense emotional and physical discomfort. Box 22-1 lists the subjective and objective (physiologic) symptoms of anxiety (American Psychiatric Association, 1994; Mathew, 1982; Selye, 1965).

DEFINITION

Anxiety occurs when a severe, unexpected threat to one's feeling of self-esteem or well-being occurs. It has been noted that anxiety often takes place when a person expects one thing and is suddenly confronted with something quite different (Peplau, 1989). This process has been operationalized in Table 22-1.

RELIEF BEHAVIORS

Anxiety may be directly felt or, more characteristically, may not be felt at all. That is, as soon as the client senses a threat, a relief behavior occurs automatically. Over time, the individual develops a characteristic pattern of relief behaviors intended to provide comfort and protection in the face of anxiety. Four major conversion patterns for anxiety have been identified (Peplau, 1989).

ACTING-OUT BEHAVIOR

There may be overt expressions of anger and aggression, or covert expressions of resentment.

BOX 22-1: Symptoms of Anxiety

Subjective (Reported by Clients)	Objective (Observed by the Nurse)
Intense apprehension	Increased heart rate
Fear, terror	Increased rate and depth of respiration
Feelings of impending doom	Shifts in body temperature
Dyspnea	Alternating blood pressure from norm
Palpitations	Abnormal or absent menstrual flow
Chest pain or discomfort	Urinary urgency or retention
Choking, smothering sensations	Dryness of the mouth
Dizziness	Loss or increase in appetite
Vertigo	Cold, clammy skin
Unsteady feelings	Dilation of pupils
Numbness and tingling of fingers/toes	Release of sugar by the liver
Hot and cold flashes	Retention of sodium (aldosteronism)
Sweating, particularly in palms	
Faintness	
Trembling or shaking	
Fear of dying	
Fear of going crazy	
Fear of loss of self-control	
Apprehensive expectation	
Motor tension with hyperactivity	
Vigilance and scanning	
Phobias	
Hallucinations	
Delusions	
Ringing in the ears	
Visual disturbances	
Anger or hostility	
Increased irritability	

Sources: American Psychiatric Association (1994). *Diagnostic and Statistical Manual of Mental Disorders* (4th ed). Washington, DC: American Psychiatric Association; Mathew, R. J. (1982). *The Biology of Anxiety*. New York: Brunner-Mazel; Selye, H. (1974). *Stress Without Distress*. New York: New American Library.

TABLE 22-1
A Concept of Anxiety

DEFINITION: SEQUENCE OF STEPS IN DEVELOPMENT OF ANXIETY	INFORMATION NEEDED TO UNDERSTAND A PERSON'S EXPERIENCE OF ANXIETY
1. Expectations are held, up front, in mind.	What expectations? Origins? How long held?
2. Expectations held are not met.	What interfered? What happened instead? Who was to meet the expectation, when, how, what evidence?
3. Discomfort is felt.	Experienced in what part of the body? What degree? What was noticed by patient?
4. Relief behaviors are used.	What behavioral act or acts related to what pattern?
5. The relief behaviors are justified and rationalized.	

From Peplau, H. E. (1989). Anxiety, self and hallucinations. In A. W. O'Toole & S. R. Welt (eds.), *Interpersonal Theory in Nursing Practice*. New York: Springer. Used with permission.

SOMATIZING

Somatizing includes a number of "psychosomatic" disorders. The automatic nervous system quickly converts anxiety to an organ function. Rather than the client having the felt experience of anxiety, the organ takes the stress and strain.

FREEZING-TO-THE-SPOT BEHAVIOR

Withdrawal into depression or schizophrenia may be seen.

USING THE ANXIETY IN THE SERVICE OF LEARNING

The nurse encourages the client to tolerate the anxiety while helping the client figure out the cause of the anxiety.

LEVELS OF ANXIETY

Four levels of anxiety have been identified. It is important for the nurse to assess the client's anxiety level, since the intervention is based on the level. In mild (+) or moderate (+ +) anxiety, the nurse intervenes by helping the client to figure out what is causing the anxiety. In severe anxiety (+ + +) or panic (+ + + +), the nurse helps the client through nonverbal means (walking with the client, or just remaining quiet) or by offering medication to reduce the anxiety. (See Chapter 69.)

Table 22-2 shows the effect of the degrees of anxiety on the client's ability to observe, focus, and learn, and observable behaviors.

TABLE 22-2
Degrees of Anxiety, Effect on Perceptual Field, and Observable Behavior

DEGREE OF ANXIETY	EFFECTS ON PERCEPTUAL FIELD AND ON ABILITY TO FOCUS ATTENTION	OBSERVABLE BEHAVIOR
+ Mild	Perceptual field widens slightly. Able to observe more than before and to see relations (make connections among data).	Aware, alerted, sees, hears, and grasps more than before. Usually able to recognize and name anxiety easily.
+ + Moderate	Perceptual field narrows slightly. Selective inattention: does not notice what goes on peripheral to the immediate focus but can do so if attention is directed there by another observer.	Sees, hears, and grasps less than previously. Can attend to more if directed to do so. Able to sustain attention on a particular focus; selectively attends to content outside the focal area. Usually able to state "I am anxious now."
+ + + Severe	Perceptual field is greatly reduced. Tendency toward dissociation: to not notice what is going on outside the current reduced focus of attention; largely unable to do so when another observer suggests it.	Sees, hears, and grasps far less than previously. Attention is focused on a small area of a given event. Inferences drawn may be distorted due to inadequacy of observed data. May be unaware of and unable to name anxiety. Relief behaviors generally used.
+ + + + Panic (terror, horror, dread, uncanniness, awe)	Perceptual field is reduced to a detail, which is usually "blown up," i.e., elaborated by distortion (exaggeration), or the focus is on scattered details. The speed of the scattering tends to increase. Massive dissociation especially of contents of self-system. Felt as enormous threat to survival.	Says, "I'm in a million pieces." "I'm gone." "What is happening to me?" Perplexity, self-absorption. Feelings of unreality. "Flight of ideas" or confusion. Fear. Repeats a detail. Many relief behaviors used automatically (without thought). The enormous energy produced by panic must be used and may be mobilized as rage. May pace, run, or fight violently. With dissociation of contents of self-system, there may be very rapid reorganization of the self, usually along pathological lines, e.g., a "psychotic break" is usually preceded by panic.

From Peplau, H. E. (1989). Anxiety, self and hallucinations. In A. W. O'Toole & S. R. Welt (eds)., *Interpersonal Theory in Nursing Practice*. New York: Springer. Used with permission.

Table 22-3 outlines nursing interventions for each level of anxiety.

TABLE 22-3
Nursing Interventions Related to Degree of Anxiety

DEGREE OF ANXIETY	NURSING INTERVENTIONS
+ Mild	Learning is possible. Nurse assists patient to use the energy that anxiety provides to encourage learning. See Table 22-4 to apply in nurse–patient interaction.
+ + Moderate	Nurse checks own anxiety so patient does not empathize with it. Encourages patient to talk: to focus on one experience, to describe it fully, then to formulate the patient's generalizations about that experience.
+ + + Severe	Learning is less possible. Allows relief behaviors to be used but does not ask about them. See Table 22-4 to apply in nurse–patient interaction. Encourages the patient to talk: Ventilation of random ideas is likely to reduce anxiety to moderate level. When this is observed by the nurse, proceeds as above.
+ + + + Panic	Learning is impossible. Thereness: nurse stays with the patient. Allows pacing and walks with the patient. No content inputs to the patient's thinking should be made by the nurse. (They burden the patient, who will distort them.) Uses instrumental inputs only, the fewest possible, and the least number of words: e.g., "Drink this" (give liquids to replace lost fluids and to relieve dry mouth); "Say what's happening to you," "Talk about yourself," or "Tell what you feel now" (to encourage ventilation and externalization of inner, frightening experience). Picks up on what the patient says: e.g., Pt: "I'm in a million pieces," N: "Talk about that," or Pt: "What's happening to me—how did I get here?" N: "Say what you notice." Short phrases by the nurse—direct, to the point of the patient's comment, and investigative—match the current attention span of the patient in panic and therefore are more likely to be heard, grasped, and acted upon with the patient's responses gradually reducing the anxiety in a helpful way. Does not touch the patient; patients experiencing panic are very concerned about survival, experiencing grave threat to the self, and usually distort the intentions of all invasions of their personal space. When the patient's anxiety is very obviously greatly reduced, then apply Table 22-4.

From Peplau, H. E. (1989). Anxiety, self and hallucinations. In A. W. O'Toole & S. R. Welt (eds.), *Interpersonal Theory in Nursing Practice.* New York: Springer. Used with permission.

NURSING INTERVENTION

Table 22-4 describes nursing interventions and begins at the step where anxiety is manifest.

PANIC DISORDERS

The American Psychiatric Association has addressed a number of anxiety disorders that involve panic-level anxiety. They are (American Psychiatric Association, 1994):
1. Panic Attack
2. Agoraphobia
3. Panic Disorder Without Agoraphobia
4. Panic Disorder With Agoraphobia
5. Panic Disorder Without History of Panic Disorder
6. Specific Phobia
7. Social Phobia
8. Obsessive-Compulsive Disorder
9. Posttraumatic Stress Disorder
10. Acute Stress Disorder
11. Generalized Anxiety Disorder
12. Anxiety Disorder Due to a General Medical Condition
13. Substance-Induced Anxiety Disorder
14. Anxiety Disorder Not Otherwise Specified

TABLE 22-4
Nursing Intervention Related to Steps in the Development of Anxiety

NURSING AIM	NURSING VERBAL INTERVENTIONS
3.* Get the operative expectations formulated and stated by patient.	3. After the patient is clearly aware of the relation between #1 and #2 below, then ask, "What were you thinking about before you felt upset?"
4. Get a formulation and recognition of the connection between expectations held and what happened instead.	4. When the patient has clearly formulated an expectation, then ask, "What happened instead?"
5. Consider which factors in the sequence are amenable to control.	5. Discuss what change in #3 or #4 above might be possible.
1. Get patient to become aware of and name anxiety.	1. Ask the patient, "Are you anxious?" "Are you nervous?" "Are you upset?" "Are you tense now?"
2. Get the patient to become aware of and state the connection between the named anxiety and the behavior used to relieve it.	2. When a yes answer has been obtained to #1, ask the patient, "What are you doing now to relieve being nervous?"

*Note that the sequence of steps here is different from those in the definition in Table 22-1. Vary the language, not the message.

From Peplau, H. E. (1989). Anxiety, self and hallucinations. In A. W. O'Toole & S. R. Welt (eds.), *Interpersonal Theory in Nursing Practice.* New York: Springer. Used with permission.

Box 22-2 lists the diagnostic criteria for panic attack. Treatment of panic attack includes the talking interventions of the nurse (see Tables 22-1, 22-3, 22-4) and the addition of antianxiety medication as needed. (See Chapter 69.)

Box 22-2: Criteria for Panic Attack

Note: A panic attack is not a codable disorder. Code the specific diagnosis in which the panic attack occurs (e.g., 300.21 Panic Disorder With Agoraphobia).

A discrete period of intense fear or discomfort, in which four (or more) of the following symptoms developed abruptly and reached a peak within 10 minutes:

1. Palpitations, pounding heart, or accelerated heart rate
2. Sweating
3. Trembling or shaking
4. Sensations of shortness of breath or smothering
5. Feeling of choking
6. Chest pain or discomfort
7. Nausea or abdominal distress
8. Feeling dizzy, unsteady, lightheaded, or faint
9. Derealization (feelings or unreality) or depersonalization (being detached from oneself)
10. Fear of losing control or going crazy
11. Fear of dying
12. Paresthesia (numbness or tingling sensations)
13. Chills or hot flushes

From American Psychiatric Association (1994). *Diagnostic and Statistical Manual of Mental Disorders* (4th ed.). Washington, DC: American Psychiatric Association. Used with permission.

REFERENCES

American Psychiatric Association (1994). *Diagnostic and Statistical Manual of Mental Disorders* (4th ed). Washington, DC: American Psychiatric Association.

Mathew, R. J. (1982). *The Biology of Anxiety*. New York: Brunner-Mazel.

Peplau, H. E. (1989). Anxiety, self and hallucinations. In A. W. O'Toole & S. R. Welt (eds.), *Interpersonal Theory in Nursing Practice* (pp. 270–326). New York: Springer.

Selye, H. (1965). *The Stress of Life*. New York: McGraw-Hill.

BIBLIOGRAPHY

Asnis, G. M., & Van Praag, H. M. (eds.) (1995). *Panic Disorder: Clinical, Biological, and Treatment Aspects.* New York: John Wiley & Sons.

Badger, J. M. (1994). Calming the anxious patient. *American Journal of Nursing, 94,* 46–50.

Ballenger, J. C. (1990). *Clinical Aspects of Panic Disorder.* Somerset, NJ: John Wiley & Sons.

Beeber, L., Anderson, C. A., & Sills, G. M. (1990). Peplau's theory in practice. *Nursing Science Quarterly, 3* (1), 6–8.

Carroll, P., & Maher, V. F. (1991). Legal issues in the care of patients with anxiety. *Advances in Clinical Care, 6* (5), 16–17.

Childs-Clark, A., & Shapiro, J. (1991). Keeping the faith: Religion in the healing of phobic anxiety. *Journal of Psychosocial Nursing and Mental Health Services, 29* (2), 40–43.

Curtis, G. C., & Glitz, D. A. (1991). Neuroendocrine findings in anxiety disorders. *Endocrinology Metabolic Clinics of North America, 17,* 131.

Frederici, C. M., & Tommasine, N. R. (1992). The assessment and management of panic disorder. *Nurse Practitioner, 17* (3), 20, 22, 27–28.

Frederickson, K. (1993). Using a nursing model to manage symptoms: Anxiety and the Roy adaptation model. *Holistic Nursing Practice, 7* (2), 36–43.

Gourray, K. J. M. (1991). The failure of exposure treatment in agoraphobia: Implications for the practice of nurse therapists and community psychiatric nurses. *Journal of Advanced Nursing, 16,* 1099–1109.

Kneisl, C. R. (1990). Combating anxiety, *RN, 53*(8), 50–54.

Laria, M. T. (1991). Biological correlates of panic disorder with agoraphobia: Practice perspectives for nurses. *Archives of Psychiatric Nursing, 5,* 373–381.

Lesse, S. (1994). Psychotherapy of ambulatory patients with severe anxiety. In T. Karasu & L. Bellak (eds.), *Specialized Techniques for Specific Clinical Problems in Psychotherapy* (pp. 220–235). Northvale, NJ: Jason Aronson.

Roy-Byrne, P. (1993). Psychopharmacologic treatment of panic anxiety disorder and social phobia. *Psychiatric Clinics of North America, 16,* 719–735.

Sadow, D., & Ryder, M. (1990). Anxiety reduction: Lessons that benefit students and patients. *Journal of Psychosocial Nursing and Mental Health Services, 28* (9), 29–30.

Selye, H. (1974). *Stress Without Distress.* New York: New American Library.

Waddell, K. L., & Demi, A. S. (1993). Effectiveness of an intensive partial hospitalization program for the treatment of anxiety disorders. *Archives of Psychiatric Nursing, 7* (1), 2–10.

Whitley, G. G. (1992). Concept analysis of anxiety. *Nursing Diagnosis, 3,* 107–116.

23
TWENTY THREE

The Client Who Is Depressed

Linda S. Beeber

OVERVIEW:

Definition
Symptoms
Theories of Etiology
Effective Therapies
Risk Factors
Coexisting Conditions
Rating Scales Used in Assessment
Assessing Symptoms

Assessing Stressors
Assessing Resources
Tasks of Psychotherapy
    Loneliness and Emptiness
    Guilt
    Inadequacy
Nursing Intervention

DEFINITION

Depression is a disorder of mood with accompanying difficulties in cognition, motivation, interpersonal relations, and physiological processes.

SYMPTOMS

The classic symptoms of depression are (American Psychiatric Association, 1994):
1. Feeling of intense sadness
2. Anhedonia
3. Lack of appetite and weight loss
4. Insomnia or hypersomnia
5. Psychomotor retardation or agitation
6. Fatigue or loss of energy
7. Feelings of worthlessness or excessive guilt
8. Inability to concentrate or make decisions
9. Thoughts about death or suicide

THEORIES OF ETIOLOGY

The major theories about depressions are:
1. *Psychodynamic:* See Box 23-1 for an operational definition of the psychodynamic theory.
2. *Interpersonal:* Depression is the manifestation of patterns in the self-system that exist to protect against interpersonal anxiety resulting from loss, including those situations when the client disavows the self (Beeber, 1989b).
3. *Cognitive:* Depression arises from habitual negative cognitive appraisals (Helm, 1984; Campbell, 1992).

BOX 23-1: Operational Definition of Depression from a Psychodynamic Perspective

1. As a child, client experienced one or more of the following:

    a. A highly significant loss, e.g., of a parent (Arieti, 1978)

    b. The belief that love was dependent on performance that pleased significant others (Arieti, 1978)

2. The child develops a "poorly integrated, aggressively cathected and inadequately differentiated self-image" (Mendelson, 1994).

3. As an adult, the client experiences a loss, or an interruption in object relations.

4. The client relives the feelings connected with the earlier loss or interpersonal deprivation, including anger.

5. The client turns this anger toward the self, intensifying the feelings of low self-worth and guilt.

Courtesy of Suzanne Lego.

---

4. *Self-in-relation:* Depression arises as an outcome of irreconcilable strains between self-identity derived from connectedness to others and striving for achievement that separates self from others (Jack, 1987; Chodorow, 1978; Miller, 1976).

5. *Social:* Depression arises out of an interaction between stressful events and disrupted social resources (Beeber, 1989a).

6. *Biological:* Depression arises as a result of stress-related biological dysregulatory processes (Siever & Davis, 1985). Some psychiatric nurses believe this biological process is triggered by loss (Lego, 1992).

EFFECTIVE THERAPIES

Therapies found to be effective alone or in combination with antidepressant drugs include (Agency for Health Care Policy and Research, 1993):
1. Behavioral therapy
2. Brief dynamic psychotherapy
3. Cognitive therapy
4. Interpersonal psychotherapy
5. Marital therapy

RISK FACTORS

See Table 23-1 for risk factors associated with depression and explanations.

COEXISTING CONDITIONS

Some physical disorders are often associated with depression including:
1. Hypothyroidism
2. Cushing's syndrome
3. Cerebral and pancreatic neoplasms
4. Cerebral vascular accidents
5. Huntington's chorea
6. Arteritis
7. Malnutrition and vitamin deficiencies (e.g., folate deficiency)

TABLE 23-1
Risk Factors Associated with Depression and Explanations

RISK FACTOR	EXPLANATION
1. Client lost a parent or close significant other in childhood (Arieti, 1978).	1. The inevitable losses in adulthood arouse feelings from the earlier loss, triggering depression.
2. Client had a childhood characterized by high expectations for performance (Arieti, 1978).	2. The inevitable failures in adulthood arouse feelings about childhood experience, triggering depression.
3. Client is a female.	3. Females develop a sense of self-in-relation to interpersonal connectedness (Chodorow, 1978; Miller, 1976). The inevitable separations and losses of adulthood threaten self-definition and self-worth, and trigger depression.
4. Client is a female born since 1970.	4. Explanation is unclear at this time. Possible factors include increased incidence of divorce after 1970 and rapidly changing roles and expectations for women.
5. Client's parents have suffered depression.	5. The experience of growing up with depressed adults produces a feeling of loss and separation in childhood. The inevitable losses and separations in adulthood arouse earlier feelings, triggering depression. Those who favor biological theories believe this relationship to be genetic in origin.
6. Client has had previous depressions.	6. Approximately 75% of clients who seek treatment experience subsequent episodes even if medication and psychotherapy are used.
7. Client has given birth.	7. Major stressors in postpartum depression are lack of support and help (Tavris, 1992), biological dysregulatory processes, and the increased stress of parenting.

8. Lupus erythematosus
9. Electrolyte imbalances
10. Dementias including AIDS-related dementia
11. Cardiac insufficiency

RATING SCALES USED IN ASSESSMENT

Several scales are used to determine the existence and extent of depression. These include:
1. Hamilton Rating Scale for Depression (HRSD) (Hamilton, 1960)
2. Raskin Severity of Depression Scale (Raskin, Schulterbrandt, Reatig, & McKeon, 1969)
3. Global Assessment of Functioning (American Psychiatric Association, 1994)
4. Beck Depression Inventory (Beck & Steer, 1984)

ASSESSING SYMPTOMS

The client is asked about the:
1. Intensity of symptoms (e.g., "I wish I would die"). For suicide assessment, see Chapter 24.
2. Duration of symptoms (e.g., "This started a month ago when Dad died").
3. Meaning attached (e.g., "I guess this means I'll have to quit school").

Clients who are chronically depressed are asked to graph a "life map" of symptoms going back as far as they can recall.

ASSESSING STRESSORS

The nurse assesses stressors by asking about:
1. Marital status and marital satisfaction
2. Number and ages of children
3. Health of self and significant others
4. Economic status
5. Cultural/ethnic/sexual identity
6. Life interests and recreational pursuits

ASSESSING RESOURCES

The nurse assesses resources by asking about:
1. Emotional and physical availability of significant others
2. Community ties
3. Spiritual framework and worldview

TASKS OF PSYCHOTHERAPY

Therapy involves one or more of the following tasks (Mendelson, 1994, pp. 159–160).

LONELINESS AND EMPTINESS

When clients feel empty and lonely, the nurse helps them uncover the factors that prevent them from achieving the kind of object relationships necessary for adequate self-esteem. This may lead into the following areas:
1. Helping clients identify their needs, for not every person is consciously aware of interpersonal and affectional needs
2. Examining defensive maneuvers that tend to isolate the client

Achieving these goals often requires a long period of intensive therapy, especially if clients have evolved complex or stubborn defenses or personality patterns that interfere with the gratification of needs.

GUILT

Where the problem is one of guilt, the therapeutic task may involve the modification of an unrealistically harsh conscience, that is, of a superego retaining much of its early un-modulated punitiveness, somehow insufficiently affected by the usually softening influence of the developmental process. Although guilt is probably more characteristic of psychotic depressions, it is by no means unusual in the dysthymic depressive reaction.

INADEQUACY

When clients' reduced self-esteem is a consequence of an unrealistic feeling of inadequacy, the therapeutic goal, whether accomplished by cognitive or other modes of treatment, is to help them acquire a more realistic perspective of their abilities and talents. This usually includes the modification of an unrealistic ego-ideal in the direction of a more reasonable level of aspiration.

NURSING INTERVENTION

Depression is characterized by interpersonal phenomena involving both the client and the nurse. Table 23-2 lists some of these phenomena and nursing interventions. Table 23-3 lists nursing interventions and their theoretical rationale for working with depressed clients.

TABLE 23-2
Interpersonal Phenomena with the Depressed Client and Nursing Interventions

INTERPERSONAL PHENOMENA	NURSING INTERVENTIONS
Disrupted self-worth Presentation of self as unlovable; challenges the nurse's ability to be caring in the face of rejections.	Maintenance of "presence without expectations" and keeping caring responses to a steady minimum will help client tolerate the anxiety of the relationship. Maintenance of an antagonistic or oppositional relation ("self-loathing—intolerance of self-loathing"), or a mutual relation of disrupted self-worth, is ineffective (Peplau, 1989b).
Disrupted self-efficacy Presentation of self as immobile, helpless, and over-whelmed; challenges the nurse's ability to keep the focus on the client's capability to resolve difficulties.	Maintenance of the focus on the client's experience, helping the client to name and link anxiety to interpersonal situations, and use of the shared interactions as "laboratories" to understand the immobilization are therapeutic. Complementary ("helpless and helpful") or mutual ("helpless and helpless") relations are nontherapeutic (Peplau, 1989b).
Disconnection Presentation of self as actively hostile and rejecting or passively uninvolved; both patterns are not reciprocal and protect the client from anxiety generated by needs for security from significant others.	Maintenance of "caring neutrality" in response to hostility, continual focus on the client, identification of anxiety, and linkage to interpersonal situations including those experienced in the therapeutic relationship are helpful. Complementary ("I'm mean—kick me"), mutual ("hostile and hostile"), and alternating ("First I'll be hostile, then you be hostile") are nontherapeutic (Peplau, 1989b).

TABLE 23-3
Nursing Interventions and Rationales for Working with Depressed Clients

NURSING INTERVENTION	THEORETICAL RATIONALE
1. Assess and intervene in suicidal crises. (See Chapter 24.)	1. Suicidal potential is associated with depression. Fifteen percent of clients with major depression kill themselves. Assess suicide directly, e.g., "Are you intending to hurt or kill yourself?"
2. Engage the client in contracting to stop self-injurious acts.	2. Self-injurious processes must be interrupted to relay the message to clients that they are valued by the nurse.
3. Encourage the client to reverse self-neglect by gradually engaging in self-nurturing activities.	3. Disrupted self-worth manifests as self-neglect. Behavioral changes (e.g., scheduling self-nurturing activities) will not change the valuation of the self, but will provide new experiences that can be examined in the therapeutic relationship with the nurse.
4. Engage the client in health-seeking activities by providing examples and opportunities in a neutral fashion and avoid investing in whether the client accepts the intervention.	4. See rationale for intervention 3. Examples include balanced nourishment, self-soothing behaviors, exercise, pleasurable activities, and aesthetic pursuits. Client may resist health promotion because self-nurturance conflicts with low self-worth and guilt.
5. Document symptoms to create a baseline against which to measure progress of nursing interventions; choose symptoms central to depression and symptoms the client finds bothersome.	5. Client-derived baselines are the most accurate standard. "Central symptoms of depression include anhedonia, thought and behavioral sluggishness, loss of energy, sleep changes, and appetite changes (Costello, 1993).
6. Document patterns of interpersonal and social interactions with the nurse and others in the milieu.	6. Validate the patterns the client has identified as creating difficulties in living.

(Continued)

TABLE 23-3 *(continued)*

NURSING INTERVENTION	THEORETICAL RATIONALE
7. Establish and maintain a therapeutic relationship with the client that includes a clear contract for meeting times, clarity of expectations for the respective roles of client and nurse, and consensual validation of the work to be done.	7. The relationship provides the structure for provision of care.
8. If clients are severely symptomatic, the nurse cares for them until they are able to contract to collaborate in their own care (Loomis, 1985). The nurse will need to "be" with the client in a nurturing, accepting manner until symptoms abate. Use short, frequent contacts, paying attention to consistency between the nurse's words and actions.	8. Matching expectations for client participation with capabilities prevents "failures" the depressed person will use to validate low self-worth. Short contacts reduce pressure in the very depressed client.
9. Use an investigative approach where the nurse guides the client in understanding anxiety and the patterns developed to avoid it. When the client is ready, contract for change. Focus the work on consensually validated patterns that create life problems for clients such as immobilization, withdrawal, and anxiety.	9. In this role, the client, not the nurse, does the work of understanding and change (Peplau, 1989a).

9a. Interventions focused on immobilization include:
  a. observation by the nurse and acknowledgment by the client
  b. empathic reflection by the nurse
  c. division of tasks into small, incremental steps
  d. consistent encouragement to try without expectations by the nurse of success
  e. investigation of the experience by the client
	9a. Incremental steps lead to incremental successes, providing new experiences for the client to examine with the nurse. Simply experiencing the change is not enough; examination and learning must occur for the client to change.

9b. Interventions focused on withdrawal include:
  a. short, systematic contacts with the nurse
  b. contract for short, self-generated contacts with others
  c. reflection about experiences with others, especially when the client is self-critical
	9b. Slow, increasing contact with others and examination of these contacts provides a learning opportunity for the client.

9c. Interventions focused on anxiety include:
  a. observing and asking clients if they are anxious
  b. encouraging clients to observe and name anxiety when it occurs
  c. helping clients observe external and internal experiences such as feeling inferior to others, emphasizing self-perceived deficits, imagining failures before any have occurred
  d. offering the nurse's observation about these issues
  e. encouraging clients to reflect on differences between nurse's observations and client's self-observations
	9c. Observation, naming, and understanding the context of anxiety provides an opportunity for the client to understand low self-worth and self-criticism as well as focusing on identifying needs and expectations.

10. Monitor antidepressant therapy if used; intervene in side effects; provide education for the client and family; monitor for increasing suicidal risk as energy returns.	10. Sensitive, immediate responses to medication-related problems enhance client's sense of control and engagement in treatment.
11. Encourage client's participation in other therapy modalities, e.g., group therapy.	11. Specific approaches for depression have demonstrated effectiveness (Gordon, Matwychuk, Sachs, & Canedy, 1988; Maynard, 1993).
12. Engage significant others in understanding and changing the stressful elements of life; support existing strengths and resources; help clients engage in therapy with family and significant others; engage clients and family in community supports.	12. Engagement of family and significant others in treatment provides a bridge to ongoing support structures.

REFERENCES

Agency for Health Care Policy and Research (1993). *Depression in Primary Care: Volume 2. Treatment of Major Depression*. Washington, DC: U.S. Department of Health and Human Services.

American Psychiatric Association (1994). *Diagnostic and Statistical Manual of Mental Disorders* (4th ed.). Washington, DC: American Psychiatric Association.

Arieti, S. (1978). Psychodynamics of severe depression. In S. Arieti & J. Bemporad (eds)., *Severe and Mild Depression: The Psychoanalytic Approach* (pp. 129–155). New York: Basic Books.

Beck, A., & Steer, R. (1984). Internal consistencies of the original and revised Beck Depression Inventory. *Journal of Clinical Psychology, 40,* 1365–1367.

Beeber, L. S. (1989a). The role of social resources in depression: A woman's perspective. In L. Beeber (ed.), *Depression: Old Problems, New Perspectives in Nursing Care* (pp. 1–13). Thorofare, NJ: Slack.

Beeber, L. S. (1989b). Enacting corrective interpersonal experiences with the depressed client: An intervention model. *Archives of Psychiatric Nursing, 3,* 211–217.

Campbell, J. M. (1992). Treating depression in well older adults: Use of diaries in cognitive therapy. *Issues in Mental Health Nursing, 13,* 19–29.

Chodorow, N. (1978). *The Reproduction of Mothering*. Berkeley, CA: University of California Press.

Costello, C. Q. (ed.) (1993). *Symptoms of Depression*. New York: Wiley.

Gordon, V., Matwychuk, A., Sachs, E., & Canedy, B. (1988). A 3-year follow-up of a cognitive–behavioral therapy intervention. *Archives of Psychiatric Nursing, 2,* 218–226.

Hamilton, M. (1960). A rating scale for depression. *Journal of Neurology, Neurosurgery, and Psychiatry, 12,* 56–62.

Helm, S. (1984). Nursing care of the depressed patient: A cognitive approach. *Perspectives in Psychiatric Care, 22,* 100–107.

Jack, D. (1987). Self-in-relation theory. In R. Formanek & A. Gurian (eds.), *Women and Depression: A Lifespan Perspective*. New York: Springer.

Lego, S. (1992). Biological psychiatry and psychiatric nursing in America. *Archives of Psychiatric Nursing, 6,* (3) 147–150.

Loomis, M. E. (1985). Levels of contracting. *Journal of Psychosocial Nursing, 23* (3), 9–14.

Maynard, C. K. (1993). Comparison of effectiveness of group interventions for depression in women. *Archives of Psychiatric Nursing, 8,* 277–283.

Mendelson, M. (1994). The psychotherapy of the depressed patient. In T. B. Karasu & L. Bellak (eds.), *Specialized Techniques for Specific Clinical Problems in Psychotherapy* (pp. 143–161). Northvale, NJ: Jason Aronson.

Miller, J. B. (1976). *Toward a New Psychology of Women*. Boston: Beacon Press.

Peplau, H. (1989a). General application of theory and techniques of psychotherapy in nursing situations. In A. O'Toole & S. Welt (eds.), *Interpersonal Theory in Nursing Practice* (pp. 99–107). New York: Springer.

Peplau, H. (1989b). Pattern interactions. In A. O'Toole & S. Welt (eds.), *Interpersonal Theory in Nursing Practice* (pp. 108–119). New York: Springer.

Raskin, A., Schulterbrandt, J., Reatig, N., & McKeon, J. J. (1969). Replication of factors of psychopathology. *Journal of Nervous and Mental Disorders, 148,* 87–98.

Siever, L., & Davis, K. (1985). Overview: Toward a dysregulation hypothesis of depression. *American Journal of Psychiatry, 142,* 1017–1031.

Tavris, C. (1992). *The Mismeasurement of Women*. New York: Simon and Schuster.

BIBLIOGRAPHY

Beck, C. T. (1992). The lived experience of post-partum depression: A phenomenological study. *Nursing Research, 41* (3), 166–170.

Maynard, C. (1993). Psychoeducational approach to depression in women. *Journal of Psychosocial Nursing, 31* (12), 9–14.

Styron, W. (1990). *Darkness Visible*. New York: Random House.

TWENTY FOUR

The Client Who Is Suicidal

Linda S. Beeber*

OVERVIEW:

Definition	Risk
Prevalence	Assessment
Theories of Origin	Nursing Interventions

DEFINITION

Suicide, or the intentional taking of one's own life, is the irreversible outcome of a spectrum of self-destructive acts including self-neglect, accident proneness, and deliberate self-injury (Valente, 1991). Suicide as a negative act is presently challenged by the heightened visibility of persons choosing death to end their suffering and elevation of public debates about the right of people to make this choice.

PREVALENCE

Approximately 30,000 persons die by suicide annually in the United States, making it the eighth leading cause of death; approximately 500,000 persons attempt suicide annually (Berman, 1990; Susser, 1993). Adolescent suicide has increased threefold over the last 25 years to 10 per 100,000 deaths per year (Rotheram-Borus, 1993).

THEORIES OF ORIGIN

Classical theories of suicide were Durkheim's (1963) 1897 view of suicide as the product of disrupted integration into society, and Freud's (1985) theory in which the ego objectifies the self and directs murderous hostility against it. These have been challenged by empirical findings (Baumeister, 1993). Newer theories thought to have greater predictive power and applicability include:

1. *Beck's theory* proposes that suicide originates when depression is linked to lethal action by hopelessness (persistent negative cognitive expectations) (Beck, Steer, Beck, & Newman, 1993; Lester, 1994).
2. *Leenaars's theory* proposes that suicide requires unendurable psychological pain, helplessness and hopelessness, poor relationships, limited coping and communication capabilities, and a narrow range of problem-solving abilities (Lester, 1994; Leenaars, 1988).
3. *Maris's theory* proposes that knowledge of lethal methods, previous self-destructive adaptations, ambivalence, severe life stressors, and a lack of deep religious convictions create lethality (Lester, 1994; Maris, 1981).

*The author would like to acknowledge the assistance of Ms. Kerryanna Kershner in the preparation of this chapter.

4. *Baumeister's theory* of escape proposes that sequential decisions begin with disappointment and culminate in mental narrowing, which removes meaningful evaluations, and with those, inhibitions against suicide (Baumeister, 1993).

RISK

Certain demographic characteristics place clients at greater risk than those in the general population. These characteristics are shown in Table 24-1. Table 24-2 shows comorbid conditions that increase the risk for suicide.

TABLE 24-1
Assessment of Suicidal Risk

CHARACTERISTIC	RISK FACTOR
Age	Adolescents and persons over 45 years of age are at higher risk.
Gender	Women make more attempts than men; men kill themselves more often; some shift may be anticipated as women become more familiar with firearms.
Race/ethnicity	Native Americans and whites kill themselves more frequently than African Americans.
Marital status	Widowed and separated/divorced persons are at higher risk than never-married and married persons.
Relations	Socially isolated persons, especially those who have just cut off ties with others, are at high risk.
Occupation	Police officers and physicians are in high-risk groups; unemployed persons are at higher risk than employed persons.
Contextual factors	Presence of a plan; availability of highly lethal means with skill at using them and previous attempts place client at high risk.
Comorbid conditions	See Table 24-2.

TABLE 24-2
Comorbid Conditions That Increase Risk for Suicide

CATEGORY	DESCRIPTION
1. Substance use disorder	The combination of depression and impulsivity may account for the high incidence of suicide in this disorder; suicide often occurs within 1 year (Fawcett et al., 1990).
2. Schizophrenia	There is a high suicide risk if the client is experiencing command hallucinations and delusions of grandeur.
3. Mood disorders • Bipolar disorders • Major depressive episode	Suicide is always of major concern with depressed clients. If depressive symptoms are severe or if suicide assessment shows high lethality, there is reason for extreme concern. Manic depressive clients in the depressed phase are usually highly suicidal.
4. Organic mental disorders	Suicide may be a risk in this disorder if the client is experiencing severe depressive symptoms, is impulsive, confused, hallucinating, or delusional, or is using alcohol or drugs.
5. Personality disorder • Histrionic • Antisocial • Borderline	The impulsive, demanding, and manipulative behavior coupled with depression may indicate suicidal risk.
6. Anxiety disorders • Posttraumatic stress disorder	PTSD accompanied by grief increases risk for suicide (Berman, 1990).

Adapted from Barile, L. (1984). The client who is suicidal. In S. Lego (ed.), *The American Handbook of Psychiatric Nursing*. Philadelphia: J. B. Lippincott, p. 399.

ASSESSMENT	See Chapter 1 for assessment of suicidal potential.
NURSING INTERVENTIONS	Table 24-3 shows guidelines, nursing interventions, and theoretical rationales for suicidal clients.

TABLE 24-3
Guidelines for Care of the Suicidal Client

GUIDELINE	NURSING INTERVENTION	THEORETICAL RATIONALE
Acute Presuicidal Crisis		
Establish contact.	Relay empathy for the client and a willingness to understand the dilemma; do not participate in the pressure to solve things immediately; relay an attitude of unhurried patience; share personal thoughts and experiences if these establish a bond of mutual understanding; avoid reactivity to hostility and distancing stances of the client; expect ambivalence and emphasize the will-to-live side of the ambivalence by strategic reflection, e.g.: Client: "They'll regret it when I'm gone tomorrow." Nurse: "So you can envision a tomorrow?"	Ambivalence is generally the reason for making contact prior to an attempt; clients will respond to hearing their own reasons for wanting to stay alive, and these are the foundation for an alliance with the nurse for survival.
Separate from the means of destruction.	Ask the client to throw the gun out of the window, flush pills down the toilet, drop the car keys down the heat register. Elicit identifying data in case police must be notified.	Increases distance between the urge and the means; allows rescuers to intervene if the interaction deteriorates before a contract is established.
Build an alliance and develop a contract.	Do this in an incremental way—do not push too hard, too soon, e.g.: Client: "I don't want your help." Nurse: "You don't need to decide that now. Can you just continue talking to me for now?" Emphasize areas where the client is taking control and making choices by strategic reflection, e.g.: Client: "I think about suicide all the time." Nurse: "So you are being thoughtful about this decision?"	Rejecting help is usually evidence of the client's energy toward maintaining control, which is a force that needs to be protected as it can operate to control the urge for self-destruction; as such, a slow, patient approach allows the client to choose and decide to align, which will ultimately strengthen the alliance.
Ongoing Care		
Extend contract and secure ongoing safety.	Arrange for client to be in a safe place; this can be a community setting with others in attendance, a crisis evaluation center, or an inpatient facility. Establish a consistent, safe environment with policies and observational methods as necessary, e.g., removal of potential weapons, intensified observation, secure windows, etc. Treat and monitor sequelae of any injuries sustained during the crisis period.	Continuing care can be best done in a contained environment where the client's energy can be focused on understanding the crisis without the possibility of acting on self-destructive urges. Be watchful for delayed consequences of drug overdoses. Changes in intent will be noticed if staff doing observations is kept consistent.

TABLE 24-3 *(continued)*

GUIDELINE	NURSING INTERVENTION	THEORETICAL RATIONALE
Contract for resolution of ongoing conditions producing the crisis.	Support the client's right to decide how crisis might be resolved (Loomis, 1985).	Mutual expectations and shared objectives create structure (Loomis, 1985).
Treat comorbid conditions.	Collaborate to engage client in pharmaco-therapy, psychotherapy, or specialized treatment for chemical dependency.	Treatment of comorbid conditions will lower future risk.
Focus on the experience of the suicidal crisis.	Elicit contextual variables such as feelings pre-ceding the crisis, supports sought, problem-solving attempts, factors in close relationships, life stressors, operative life strengths, and resources.	Contextual information gives a picture of the whole person who is often missing from narrow theories of suicide; nursing care can augment and extend these narrow views by constructing additional areas in which the client may engage.
Establish a therapeutic relationship; within the theoretical framework for nursing care; engage clients in changing the aspects of their lives that cause pain.	For example, elicit the whole/part self-represen-tations, the feelings of rage associated with these, and historical sources of these (psycho-analytic approach); automatic thoughts and negative attributions (cognitive approach) tracked by the client (Beck, Rush, Shaw, & Emery, 1979); feelings of helplessness, hope-lessness, sources of pain, relationship ele-ments, and problem-solving are addressed using the therapeutic relationship (Leenaars, 1988).	The nurse–patient relationship provides a context for catharsis, reevaluation, and a reconsidera-tion of approaches to life dilemmas.
Help client engage in additional treatment modalities.	Encourage client to attend group therapy. Encourage client to engage in therapy with sig-nificant others (couples and family therapy).	Multiple modalities can bring different information to the client and enhance resolution.
Involve client and signif-icant others in educative experiences about crises and suicide.	Focus learning on precursors to the crisis, re-sources, focused problem-solving skills.	Cognitive learning and written resources can enhance recognition and coping if crisis recurs.
Establish long-term plan-ning and contracting in the event of future crises.	Develop a written list of recognized precursors to the present crisis. Develop a contingency plan if precursors reappear. Engage client in sharing the plan and developing a contract with significant others/community resource providers.	Clear communication with client and significant others will facilitate the ongoing and future safety of the client. A protective "envelope" will possibly reduce risk or future crises.

Prevention and Community Intervention

Activate and advocate for community prevention resources.	Offer ongoing suicide prevention education. Develop crisis management plans with target agencies (e.g., school crisis teams to do follow-up interventions postsuicide). Advocate for changes in "popular" suicide landmarks, e.g., bridges that are repeated sites of suicidal acts (Berman, 1990).	Increasing community awareness and supports and reducing attractive sites will increase the safety of all members.

(Continued)

TABLE 24-3 *(continued)*

GUIDELINE	NURSING INTERVENTION	THEORETICAL RATIONALE
Advocate for resources and method to offer follow-up for significant others of persons who die by suicide; provide system for sharing information with vulnerable persons and families.	Develop nonintrusive but effective means of information; make these available to persons at critical points of contact, e.g., emergency departments, funeral homes, medical examiner's office. Develop support groups and intervention teams for individuals seeking care following a suicide of a significant other or of particularly significant figures. Develop resources for follow-up with nurses who lose clients to suicide; make these available to inpatient units, to individual nurse-therapists, and to nursing organizations.	Offers a means to reduce the risk for "contagion" or "pact" suicides particularly among adolescents (Berman, 1990). Offers a means of preventing suicide of significant others, particularly children of persons who commit suicide.

REFERENCES

Barile, L. (1984). The client who is suicidal. In S. Lego (ed.), *The American Handbook of Psychiatric Nursing*. Philadelphia: J. B. Lippincott.

Baumeister, R. F. (1993). Suicide attempts. In C. G. Costello (ed.), *Symptoms of Depression* (pp. 259–289). New York: Wiley.

Beck, A. T., Rush, A., Shaw, B., & Emery, G. (1979). *Cognitive Therapy of Depression*. New York: Guilford Press.

Beck, A. T., Steer, R. A., Beck, J. S., & Newman, C. F. (1993). Hopelessness, depression, suicidal ideation, and clinical diagnosis of depression. *Suicide and Life-Threatening Behavior, 23* (2), 139–145.

Berman, A. L. (1990). *Suicide Prevention: Case Consultations*. New York: Springer.

Durkheim, E. (1963). *Suicide*. New York: Free Press.

Fawcett, J., Scheftner, W. A., Fogg, L., Clark, D. C., Young, M. A., Hedeker, D., & Gibbons, R. (1990). Time-related predictors of suicide in major affective disorder. *American Journal of Psychiatry, 147* (9), 1189–1194.

Freud, S. (1985). Mourning and melancholia. In J. C. Coyne (ed.), *Essential Papers on Depression*. New York: New York University Press.

Leenaars, A. A. (1988). *Suicide Notes*. New York: Human Sciences Press.

Lester, D. (1994). A comparison of 15 theories of suicide. *Suicide and Life-Threatening Behavior, 24* (1), 80–88.

Loomis, M. E. (1985). Levels of contracting. *Journal of Psychosocial Nursing, 23* (3), 9–14.

Maris, R. W. (1981). *Pathways to Suicide*. Baltimore: Johns Hopkins University Press.

Rotheram-Borus, M. J. (1993). Suicidal behavior and risk factors among runaway youths. *American Journal of Psychiatry, 150* (1), 103–107.

Susser, M. (1993). Suicide: Risk factors and the public health. *American Journal of Public Health, 83* (2), 171–172.

Valente, S. M. (1991). Deliberate self-injury: Management in the psychiatric setting. *Journal of Psychosocial Nursing, 29* (12), 19–25.

BIBLIOGRAPHY

Shneidman, E. J. (1994). Psychotherapy with suicidal patients. In T. B. Karasu & L. Bellak (eds.), *Specialized Techniques for Specific Clinical Problems in Psychotherapy* (pp. 305–313). Northvale, NJ: Jason Aronson.

TWENTY FIVE

The Client Who Is Diagnosed Bipolar

Suzanne Lego

OVERVIEW:

INTRODUCTION

Bipolar I disorder affects approximately 8% of the adult population, and bipolar II disorder affects approximately 0.5% over the course of a lifetime (APA, 1994b). The mean age of onset is 21 years of age. The first episode in males is usually a manic episode, and in females a depressed episode.

ETIOLOGY

Epidemiological and twin study data have suggested bipolar disorder is inherited. If bipolar disorder is inherited, the mode of inheritance remains unknown, and the magnitude of the role played by environmental stressors also remains uncertain (APA, 1994b). Clients with bipolar disorder often have relatives with the same disorder, but it is still not clear whether "nature" or "nurture" is responsible (Ross & Pam, 1995).

DIAGNOSTIC CRITERIA

Bipolar disorders vary as follows:
    Bipolar I—One manic episode by history or presentation
    Bipolar II—One hypomanic episode and one major depressive episode

The APA Practice Guidelines for the Treatment of Patients with Bipolar Disorder (1994b) note that clients may present a mixed picture of affective states or may present during a depressive episode. It is crucial that there be another person who has a consistent relationship with the client to provide an adequate history. Further, it is important for clinicians to rule out another medication or treatment, a general medical condition, or substance abuse as causative factors. The manic or hypomanic client may exhibit the following characteristics (American Psychiatric Association, 1994a).

EMOTIONAL MANIFESTATIONS

1. Mood swings from elevated, euphoric, elated to irritable, angry, or paranoid rage with marked lability
2. Affect shifting from happy, hilarious to depressed, negative, or hostile
3. Uncritical self-confidence
4. Wishes to be gratified and unrestrained in endeavors

COGNITIVE MANIFESTATIONS

1. Reports racing thoughts
2. Is distractable; attention easily drawn to irrelevant stimuli; hyperalert
3. Demonstrates pressured speech; speech that is rapid, loud, and difficult to interrupt
4. Manifests flight of ideas leading to disorganized, incoherent speech
5. Acts impractical; shows impaired judgment with poor insight
6. Has ideas of reference; delusional thoughts of grandiosity, persecution, or religiosity, and hallucinations

BEHAVIORAL MANIFESTATIONS

1. Displays dramatic mannerisms, flamboyant dress and makeup
2. Increases goal-directed activities
3. Is intrusive, domineering, demanding, physically threatening to others
4. Resists efforts to be treated
5. Dislikes having wishes thwarted
6. Displays impulsive, extravagant behavior
7. Acts out sexual behavior unusual to the person or hypersexuality

PHYSICAL MANIFESTATIONS

1. Awakens full of energy and does not become fatigued easily
2. Displays extreme motor activity, which may lead to exhaustion
3. Has insomnia with decreased need for sleep
4. May have increased or decreased appetite
5. Does not attend to personal hygiene, grooming, and general health

See Chapter 23 for a description of depressive symptoms.

NURSING INTERVENTIONS ON AN INPATIENT UNIT

Clients diagnosed bipolar are very sensitive to the environment and responsive to others. Staff members may find the behaviors engaging and encourage the client to "perform" and act out the staff's unconscious feelings. Such encouragement could lead to uncontrolled behavior, requiring seclusion or restraints.

Table 25-1 describes nursing interventions and theoretical rationales for working with the bipolar client during a manic or hypomanic episode on an inpatient unit.

TABLE 25-1
Nursing Interventions and Theoretical Rationales with the
Manic or Hypomanic Client on an Inpatient Unit

NURSING INTERVENTION	THEORETICAL RATIONALE
1. Provide for adequate nutrition; offer easy-to-eat foods and drinks.	1–2. Extreme motor activity and inadequate nutrition can lead to physical exhaustion.
2. Modify environment to decrease stimulation; provide time out in quiet room or client's room.	
3. Assess fluid and electrolyte status.	3. Lithium toxicity can occur if the client is dehydrated.
4. Teach the client and significant others the signs and symptoms of lithium toxicity; side effects of mood stabilizers, such as valproate (Depakote) and carbamazepine (Tegretol).	4. Knowledge is necessary to differentiate therapeutic effects and untoward effects and toxicity.
5. Monitor client during electroconvulsive therapy. (See Chapter 61.)	5. Therapeutic effects occur along with adverse effects.
6. Help with personal hygiene and encourage client to initiate grooming.	6. Good hygiene and grooming preserve the client's dignity and influence attitude.
7. Assess for suicidal and homicidal ideation and elopement risk.	7. Careful assessment and monitoring will allow early intervention and prevention of injury and death.
8. Encourage client to approach staff when feeling agitated or hostile.	8. Redirection of negative feelings through talking and exercising can help prevent acting-out episodes.
9. Administer PRN medications.	9. Medications help to calm the client and prevent aggressive, destructive episodes.
10. Praise client for efforts to express anger constructively.	10. Reinforcement of positive behavior will help client adapt to acceptable norms.
11. Seclude and restrain client as necessary.	11. Such interventions are necessary if less restrictive means are not effective.
12. Listen for expressions of thoughts and feelings that client is beginning to trust.	12. Establishment of a therapeutic alliance will improve client outcome.
13. Focus on the meaning of delusions to the client, rather than the content.	13. Confrontation of the content may increase the client's aggression. Accepting the client's need to express such beliefs preserves self-esteem.
14. Encourage client when beginning to distinguish delusional content from nonreality-based thoughts.	14. Reinforcement of reality is possible when the client's perceptions are less delusional.
15. Encourage client to express thoughts and feelings just before the delusion began.	15. Connecting thoughts and feelings to the delusion will help to diminish need for the delusion and help client feel understood.
16. Continue to encourage client to express feelings appropriately.	16. Verbalizing feelings helps to discharge negative emotions and retain impulse control.
17. Monitor the client's ability to tolerate increased interactions in the milieu, for example, starting group therapy.	17. Successful interaction is dependent on client's tolerance for interpersonal relations.
18. Offer feedback regarding the client's inappropriate expression of feelings.	18. Awareness of the effect of client's behavior provides incentive to modify the behavior.
19. Keep one-to-one contacts brief and frequent.	19. The client is not able to tolerate long interactions.
20. Educate the client and significant others to signs and symptoms of hypomania and mania.	20. Early intervention will help the client maintain control and may prevent rehospitalization.
21. Educate the client and significant others to action, dosage, side effects of medication.	21. Knowledge of the medication regimen will enable the client to maintain therapeutic levels and encourage compliance.

(Continued)

TABLE 25-1 *(continued)*

NURSING INTERVENTION	THEORETICAL RATIONALE
22. Provide psychotherapy to client when sufficiently stabilized.	22. Psychotherapy is necessary to address the consequences of the client's impulsive and risk-taking behaviors that cause emotional distress and further problems.
23. Prepare the client for discharge through knowledge of self-management.	23. Clients will be able to manage their daily lives and relationships if they understand the illness.
24. Carefully assess the client for the most appropriate site for follow-up and choice of therapies.	24. The presence of psychotic symptoms, risk of harm to self or others, or history of substance abuse influences follow-up treatment decisions.
25. Reinforce to the client and significant others the necessity of follow-up treatment.	25. Bipolar disorder is a chronic, recurrent, fluctuating illness that has a profound effect on clients and their relationships.

Adapted from Fortinash, K., & Holoday-Worret, P. (1991). *Psychiatric Nursing Care Plans.* St. Louis: Mosby–Year Book, Inc.; and American Psychiatric Association (1994b). Practice guidelines for the treatment of patients with bipolar disorder. *American Journal of Psychiatry 151* (12), supplement.

INTERVENTIONS OF THE ADVANCED PRACTICE PSYCHIATRIC–MENTAL HEALTH NURSE

Table 25-2 is taken from the APA practice guidelines, but is adapted to fit advanced practice nursing models.

TABLE 25-2
Interventions of the Advanced Practice Nurse and Theoretical Rationales
When Treating Outpatient Clients Diagnosed Bipolar

NURSING INTERVENTION	THEORETICAL RATIONALE
1. Provide psychotherapy or refer clients for psychotherapy.	1. Psychotherapy helps client to manage manic or depressive episodes and to prevent future episodes by: • increasing insight • improving self-esteem • providing catharsis
2. Provide education regarding bipolar disorder to the client and significant others. (See Bibliography for education materials.)	2. As clients and significant others learn more about the illness, they will be able to recognize signs of an oncoming episode and learn to "increase or decrease medications with the waxing and waning of the illness" (APA, 1994b, p. 4).
3. Encourage clients to take their medications regardless of how they feel.	3. There is often a reluctance to take medication during a manic episode, as the client enjoys the increased energy and euphoria, and denies or minimizes the self-destructive aspects of the manic episode.
4. Encourage clients to adopt a regular sleep and waking schedule.	4. If a sleep pattern is established, other aspects of life are also regulated.
5. Help clients avoid embarrassing or self-destructive behavior during a manic episode by: • encouraging them to take time off from work or to get child care help • discouraging major life changes	5. Behavior during manic episodes can have far-reaching consequences, e.g., loss of job or custody of children.
6. Prescribe medication as indicated. (See Chapter 68 for psychopharmacological treatment of bipolar disorder.)	6. Medications have been shown to be effective in the treatment of acute episodes and in preventing future episodes (APA, 1994b, p. 5).

REFERENCES

American Psychiatric Association (1994a). *Diagnostic and Statistical Manual of Mental Disorders* (4th ed.). Washington, DC: American Psychiatric Association.

American Psychiatric Association (1994b). Practice guidelines for the treatment of patients with bipolar disorder. *American Journal of Psychiatry, 151* (12), supplement.

Fortinash, K., & Holiday-Worret, P. (1991). *Psychiatric Nursing Care Plans.* St. Louis: Mosby–Year Book.

Ross, C. A., & Pam, A. (1995). *Pseudoscience in Biological Psychiatry: Blaming the Body.* New York: John Wiley & Sons.

BIBLIOGRAPHY

Pollack, L. E. (1990). Improving relationships: Groups for inpatients with bipolar disorder. *Journal of Psychosocial Nursing and Mental Health Services, 28* (5), 17–22.

Pollack, L. E. (1993). How do patients with bipolar disorder evaluate diagnostically homogeneous groups? *Journal of Psychosocial Nursing and Mental Health Services, 31* (10), 26–32.

Pollack, L. E. (1995). Treatment of inpatients with bipolar disorders: A role for self-management groups. *Journal of Psychosocial Nursing and Mental Health Services, 33* (1), 11–16.

EDUCATIONAL MATERIALS

Bohn, J., & Jefferson, J. W. (1993). *Lithium and Manic Depression: A Guide* (2nd ed.). Madison, WI: Lithium Information Center, Dean Foundation.

Jefferson, J. W., & Greist, J. H. (1993). *Valproate and Manic Depression: A Guide* (2nd ed.). Madison, WI: Lithium Information Center, Dean Foundation.

Medenwald, J. R., Greist, J. H., & Jefferson, J. W. (1993). *Carbamazepine and Manic Depression: A Guide* (2nd ed.). Madison, WI: Lithium Information Center, Dean Foundation.

Schou, M. (1993). *Lithium Treatment of Manic-Depressive Illness* (5th ed.). New York: S. Karger.

TWENTY SIX

The Client Who Exhibits Passive-Aggressive Behavior

Marie C. Smith-Alnimer

OVERVIEW:

Description	Workplace Dynamics
Etiology	Nurses' Nonproductive Reactions
Psychodynamics	Nursing Interventions
Characteristic Behaviors	Supervisory Interventions

DESCRIPTION

Passive-aggressive behavior may be seen as an isolated personality trait disturbance or it may occur in conjunction with more severe psychopathologic conditions such as depression, alcoholism, obsessive-compulsive personality, borderline personality, psychosomatic disorder, and many others (APA, 1994; Mahler, Pine, & Bergman, 1975; Mullahy, 1970).

Passive-aggressive behavior is defined as behavior intended to mask anger and anxiety from the self and significant others (Mullahy, 1970). It is shown in subtle resistance to demands for adequate performance in both work and social environments (APA, 1994). The person with this disorder sidetracks or channels anger into passive measures, which consciously and more frequently unconsciously obstruct growth in love and work relationships. Typically, resentment is expressed through procrastination, dawdling, stubbornness, intentional inefficiency, and forgetfulness (APA, 1994).

ETIOLOGY

Early experiences of the child who is to become passive-aggressive as an adult include dependency on adults who are hypercritical, demanding, unloving, and sometimes punitive. Punishment may have been physically violent or psychologically threatening, causing fears of abandonment and rejection (Mullahy, 1970). The early gratification of needs for nurturance and physical protection are essential to the growing child, and as the child grows, anxiety and helplessness become masked by anger. Anger in the child becomes as frightening as the initial anxiety and is seen by the child's mind as destructive. The perception of destruction of those upon whom one is dependent is equal to self-destruction, a predicament unacceptable to the child's growing ego. The compromise that is struck by the growing ego is to unconsciously channel anger and aggression very quietly into passive resistance and passive-aggressive behaviors (Mahler, Pine, & Bergman, 1975).

PSYCHODYNAMICS

Adults or children who are passive-aggressive have difficulty trusting normal dependency on others; they may become overdependent and compliant and will not tolerate normal anger or anxiety in the self or others without intense discomfort (Mahler, Pine, & Bergman, 1975). Failure to express anger constructively, over time, causes its covert or passive expression in a manner that causes the least discomfort to the client. Surprisingly, passive-aggressive behaviors are unconscious to the client but have a demoralizing effect on others (Trimpey & Davidson, 1994). The behavior of others toward the client becomes unrewarding and the client experiences isolation and loss of affection and attention. Significant others experience frustration and anger and may deny that a problem exists, but withhold warmth and affection, something the client also does all too frequently. As a result, the client becomes unhappy and sullen and eventually sulks and verbalizes a variety of complaints that become chronic. The person may suffer psychosomatic illness and may be clinically depressed (APA, 1994).

CHARACTERISTIC BEHAVIORS

Research criteria for passive-aggressive personality disorder appear in Box 26-1. In addition to the DSM-IV criteria, other observations have been made of the typical and everyday behavior of persons who are passive-aggressive (Shives, 1994; Trimpey & Davidson, 1994). They are:

1. Failure to meet deadlines
2. Inability to compromise, appears to agree but will take no action
3. Whining, pessimism, and chronic complaining
4. Verbal and nonverbal oppositional behavior
5. Externalization of responsibility by blaming "the Establishment" or other authority figures
6. Resentment of persons and situations that don't meet the client's needs
7. Ambivalence toward supervisors and fear of authority
8. Failure to express doubt or disagreement with subsequent sabotage of family or group goals

---

BOX 26-1: Research Criteria for Passive-Aggressive Personality Disorder

A. A pervasive pattern of negativistic attitudes and passive resistance to demands for adequate performance, beginning by early adulthood and present in a variety of contexts as indicated by four (or more) of the following:

(1) Passively resists fulfilling routine social and occupational tasks

(2) Complains of being misunderstood and unappreciated by others

(3) Is sullen and argumentative

(4) Unreasonably criticizes and scorns authority

(5) Expresses envy and resentment toward those apparently more fortunate

(6) Voices exaggerated and persistent complaints of personal misfortune

(7) Alternates between hostile defiance and contrition

B. Does not occur exclusively during major depressive episodes and is not better accounted for by dysthymic disorder.

From American Psychiatric Association (1994). *Diagnostic and Statistical Manual of Mental Disorders* (4th ed.). Washington, DC: American Psychiatric Association. Used with permission.

9. Avoidance of any discussion where anger might "come out," or falling asleep as passions rise
10. Unconscious comfort with the victim role
11. Helplessness when action is called for
12. Expressions of ignorance and lack of understanding when others show frustration and ask for behavior change
13. Other socially annoying behavior and lack of courtesy toward others

WORKPLACE DYNAMICS

"The passive-aggressive disorder is considered the most common maladaptive behavior or psychiatric disorder" (Shives, 1994, p. 322). It is not surprising then to find a high incidence of passive-aggressive behavior in the work setting (Trimpey & Davidson, 1994). Many people with these traits work in public agencies, social service agencies, and hospitals. While passive-aggressive behavior has its origins in early personality development, its manifestations can be influences of the work setting (Kernberg, 1980). According to Kernberg, the functioning of employees is influenced by (a) the predisposing personality of the employee; (b) the work environment; and (c) the exertion of power and authority beyond the amount needed for the organizational task (Kernberg, 1980). Others have observed that work in public or human service positions, where agency goals include service to others and employee altruism, contribute to a high incidence of burnout and job dissatisfaction (Mulhern, 1983).

Mulhern has found that professionals with unmet dependency needs and separation-individuation conflicts are drawn to careers in the social service area. In general, such places offer covertly to take care of the employee by overtly promoting many benefits, permanence, and early retirement. Often, work expectations are not challenging and the termination of employment is unlikely. The additional benefit for the employee with unmet dependency needs, including the passive-aggressive employee, is that partial gratification of dependency needs is met vicariously while giving care to others (Mulhern, 1983). In reality, traditional authoritarian and bureaucratic management is most common in social service agencies and institutions, and staff needs for resources, recognition, and gratification of dependency needs will be frustrated. This frustration leaves the employee with much to complain about, from the boss to the establishment. Often these employees do just enough work to get a decent evaluation, and superiors are unable to "pin" anything on the employee. If confronted with inadequate performance, the employee may be able to "shape up" for a time. The supervisor may be exhausted after lengthy counseling with the employee, who needs excessive explanation and reassurance. If employees are faced with a deadline attached to a task, they will not be able to "produce" and will blame the person who set the deadline for the failure. At this point, a negative evaluation becomes a reality (Trimpey & Davidson, 1994).

NURSES' NONPRODUCTIVE REACTIONS

Initially, the well-meaning clinician may not notice the passive-aggressive behavior as abnormal or provocative in view of the client's good reality testing. Nurses may even support it through their own passivity and mistakenly think that the client's complaints are valid, that this point of view warrants consideration, and that this behavior is "semi-normal." Sooner or later, depending on the degree of the client's pathology, others catch on to the pattern of passive-aggressiveness, feel angry or resentful themselves, and defend against it as the client does. Initially, oversolicitousness of the client may be seen with well-meaning efforts at being empathetic to cover up the direct expression of exasperation and hopelessness. Genuine empathy for the client's anger is lacking. As time goes on, it becomes clear that these clients really do not know why or how they frustrate others, as their behavior is not deliberate or intentional. As the pathology becomes clearer, there is an emergence of new rules and regulations aimed at stopping the "slippery" passive-aggressive client. Typically, nurses themselves experience passive-aggressive, passive-dependent, and aggressive-aggressive responses to the client, including:

1. Moodiness and feelings of demoralization
2. Ambivalence toward the client
3. Feelings of discouragement and helplessness
4. Avoidance and withdrawal (may "work around" the client)
5. Excessive sympathy and "understanding"
6. Compliance to client's suggestions

Over time, when the client is an inpatient, anger, frustration, and ultimate exasperation may lead to acting out through:

1. Argumentativeness
2. Excessive rules and regulations, which tend to be punitive
3. Severe confrontations of the behavior without exploration of its meaning (to make the client see the "light")
4. Care plans designed to artificially induce open anger and hostility in the client
5. Excessive labeling with psychiatric nomenclature
6. Assertiveness training for staff and client
7. Sadistic joking and humoring of the client
8. Threats of discharge from treatment or the less direct quiet transfer of the client

NURSING INTERVENTIONS

Table 26-1 shows the nursing interventions and theoretical rationale in work with passive-aggressive clients.

TABLE 26-1
Nursing Interventions and Theoretical Rationale with the Passive-Aggressive Client

NURSING INTERVENTION	THEORETICAL RATIONALE
1. Define responsibilities of both parties and avoid authoritarian attitudes.	1. Discourages artificially compliant behavior and resentment and guards against duplication of early pathologic relationships in which excessive demands were made with critical attitudes.
2. Provide a spontaneous, flexible attitude with a sense of humor.	2. Encourages genuineness in the client, who will be more likely to give up passive-aggressive behavior when the atmosphere is open and the nurse is not sitting in judgment.
3. Present active, directive approaches, rather than passive listening and nondirective approaches.	3. Encourages clients to be curious about themselves and diminishes indecisiveness and passivity.
4. Assist the client to identify and clarify feelings of irritation and resentment.	4. Unacknowledged and unexpressed anger is at the root of the client's difficulties in living.
5. Assist the client to express hostility openly when it is being shown passively.	5. Hostility that arises naturally in the relationship reduces the need for passive-aggressive responses over time, and more appropriate expressions of anger can be applied to the client's life. Artificially induced hostility will cause too much anxiety and may drive the client away.
6. Avoid arguments and driving interpretations when the client offers excuses for passive-aggressive behavior. Instead, explore feelings.	6. Arguments that force the client to "see the light" induce stubbornness, passive resistance, and more passive-aggressive behavior.

SUPERVISORY INTERVENTIONS

When the passive-aggressive person is an employee, the boss/supervisor may experience nonproductive reactions and responses similar to those of the clinician. It is important that interventions for the passive-aggressive person be appropriate for the context of the relationship. For example, a clinician is interested in helping the passive-aggressive client with the recognition and expression of angry feelings. The work supervisor, on the other hand, is interested in helping the employee with improved task initiation and completion. Discussion of the employee's anger would not be appropriate or facilitative of work performance. Table 26-2 identifies supervisory interventions and rationales for use when working with passive-aggressive employees.

TABLE 26-2
Supervisory Interventions and Rationale for the Passive-Aggressive Employee

INTERVENTION	RATIONALE
1. Use task-specific job descriptions.	1. Concrete direction minimizes dawdling and procrastination.
2. Never accept silence as agreement; ask employees their thoughts about a task.	2. Brings responses that would ordinarily be hidden, and verbal commitment or an explanation of why the person can't comply will occur.
3. Allow time for extra conferences.	3. These employees have difficulty following through and need help with problems.
4. Provide prompt feedback.	4. Offers support for positive behavior change and stops resistance early if it is occurring.
5. Avoid defending or justifying leader behavior and limit time listening to grievances.	5. Communicates that the issue is the completion of tasks correctly and in a timely fashion.
6. Avoid asking why a task is not done.	6. Passive-aggressive staff are experts at blame and rationalization.
7. Interrupt passivity and redirect responsibility back to the employee.	7. Reinforces self-reliance and encourages goal-directed behavior.
8. Avoid "trapping" employee with confrontation.	8. Power struggles waste energy on both sides and can prompt litigation.

From Trimpey, M., & Davidson, S. (1994). Chaos, perfectionism, and sabotage: Personality disorders in the workplace. *Issues in Mental Health Nursing, 15* (1), 27–36.

REFERENCES

American Psychiatric Association (1994). *Diagnostic and Statistical Manual of Mental Disorders* (4th ed.). Washington, DC: American Psychiatric Association.

Kernberg, O. (1980). *Internal World and External Reality: Object Relations Theory Applied.* New York: Aronson.

Mahler, M. S., Pine, F., & Bergman, A. (1975). *The Psychological Birth of the Human Infant: Symbiosis and Individuation.* New York: Basic Books.

Mulhern, T. J. (1983). Burnout and dependency: Awakening in the arm of the wire frame surrogate. *Journal of the Association of Mental Health Administration, 2,* 27–30.

Mullahy, P. (1970). *Psychoanalysis and Interpersonal Psychiatry: The Contributions of Harry Stack Sullivan.* New York: Science House.

Shives, L. R. (1994). *Basic Concepts of Psychiatric–Mental Health Nursing* (3rd ed.). Philadelphia: J. B. Lippincott.

Trimpey, M., & Davidson, S. (1994). Chaos, perfectionism, and sabotage: Personality disorders in the workplace. *Issues in Mental Health Nursing, 15* (1), 27–36.

BIBLIOGRAPHY

Alexander, G. R., (1989). Personality styles. *Nurse Manager's Bookshelf, 2* (3), 71–83.

Maier, W., Lichtermann, D., Klinger, T., Heun R., & Hallmayer, J. (1992). Prevalence of personality disorders in the community. *Journal of Personality Disorders, 6,* 187–196.

McCann, J. T. (1988). Passive-aggressive personality disorders: A review: *Journal of Personality Disorders, 2,* 170–179.

Perry, J. C., & Vallant, G. E. (1989). Personality disorders. In H. I. Kaplan & B. J. Sadock (eds.), *Comprehensive Textbook of Psychiatry* (vol. 2, pp. 1352–1395). Baltimore: Williams and Wilkins.

Wagner, C. M. (1991). Five problem personalities and how to manage them. *Nursing '91, 21* (6), 32W, 32Z.

Widell, J. (1990). Coping with problem personalities. *Nursing '90, 20* (9), 102, 104, 106.

Widiger, T. A., & Frances, A. J. (1988). Personality disorders. In J. A. Talbott, R. E. Hales, & S. C. Yudofsky (eds.), *Text of Psychiatry* (pp. 621–648). Washington, DC: American Psychiatric Press.

27
TWENTY SEVEN

The Client with an Eating Disorder

Michelle Conant

OVERVIEW:

INTRODUCTION

Though anorexia nervosa was identified nearly 100 years ago, in the past two decades it and bulimia nervosa have become prominent disorders among young women. (The female pronoun will be used for clients, as most eating-disorder clients are female.) Table 27-1 contrasts these two disorders.

DIAGNOSTIC CRITERIA

Boxes 27-1 and 27-2 show the DSM-IV criteria for anorexia and bulimia.

ASSESSMENT

An assessment guide for anorexia and bulimia is shown in Table 27-2.

ETIOLOGY

PSYCHODYNAMIC

Primary issues are separation–individuation, control, shame, assumed helplessness, and sexual abuse.

1. Parents display anxiety, overprotectiveness, negative judgments, or overt abuse when the child seeks to form a separate identity.
2. These responses are consistent and the child's overt attempts to individuate become bound to shameful feelings.
3. Shameful feelings are split off by denying needs that are considered shameful.

TABLE 27-1
Contrasting Characteristics of Anorexics and Bulimics

ANOREXIA	BULIMIA
Appearance Underweight; 25% below normal weight.	Normal or overweight.
Age Ages 13–22, average 18 years. Often younger than bulimics.	Ages range: 20s to 30s; often older than anorexics.
Signs Cachexia, hair loss, yellowish skin, lanugo, cyanosis of extremities, peripheral edema, amenorrhea.	Chipmunk faces (enlarged parotid glands), chronic hoarseness, dental caries, dehydration, electrolyte imbalance.
Family Environment Rigid and controlled; less overt evidence of marital discord than with bulimics.	More conflicts and fighting than anorexics, chaotic, poor impulse control among family members, i.e., violence, drugs, alcohol.
Clinical Characteristics Introverted; more socially isolated than bulimics.	Extroverted, sexually active, high incidence of compulsive behaviors, i.e., promiscuity, drugs, stealing, suicide attempts.
Awareness of Disorder Denies hunger more often than bulimics. More denial of problem than in bulimics.	More aware of own eating disorder than anorexics. More distressed by symptoms than anorexics.

From Varcarolis, E. (1994). *Foundations of Psychiatric Mental Health Nursing.* Philadelphia: W. B. Saunders Company, 1994. Reprinted with permission.

BOX 27-1: 307.1—DSM-IV Criteria for Anorexia Nervosa

A. Refusal to maintain body weight at or above a minimally normal weight for age and height (e.g., weight loss leading to maintenance of body weight less than 85% of that expected; or failure to make expected weight gain during period of growth, leading to body weight less than 85% of that expected).

B. Intense fear of gaining weight or becoming fat, even though underweight.

C. Disturbance in the way in which one's body weight or shape is experienced, undue influence of body weight or shape on self-evaluation, or denial of the seriousness of the current low body weight.

D. In postmenarcheal females, amenorrhea, i.e., the absence of at least three consecutive menstrual cycles. (A woman is considered to have amenorrhea if her periods occur only following hormone, e.g., estrogen, administration.)

Specify type:
   Restricting Type: During the current episode of Anorexia Nervosa, the person has not regularly engaged in binge-eating or purging behavior (i.e., self-induced vomiting or the misuse of laxatives, diuretics, or enemas).
   Binge-Eating/Purging Type: During the current episode of Anorexia Nervosa, the person has regularly engaged in binge-eating or purging behavior (i.e., self-induced vomiting or the misuse of laxatives, diuretics, or enemas).

From American Psychiatric Association (1994). *Diagnostic and Statistical Manual of Mental Disorders* (4th ed.). Washington, DC: American Psychiatric Association.

---

4. Bingeing, purging, and fasting behaviors serve the functions of:
   - providing covert forms of rebellion
   - allowing some individuation
   - temporarily relieving pervasive feelings of emptiness by producing a "high"
   - engendering more shame, which reinforces the eating disorder

(Text continues on page 228)

BOX 27-2: 307.51—DSM-IV Criteria for Bulimia Nervosa

A. Recurrent episodes of binge eating. An episode of binge eating is characterized by both of the following:

   (1) Eating, in a discrete period of time (e.g., within any 2-hour period), an amount of food that is definitely larger than most people would eat during a similar period of time and under similar circumstances.

   (2) A sense of lack of control over eating during the episode (e.g., a feeling that one cannot stop eating or control what or how much one is eating).

B. Recurrent inappropriate compensatory behavior in order to prevent weight gain, such as self-induced vomiting, misuse of laxatives, diuretics, enemas, or other medications; fasting; or excessive exercise.

C. The binge eating and inappropriate compensatory behaviors both occur, on average, at least twice a week for 3 months.

D. Self-evaluation is unduly influenced by body shape and weight.

E. The disturbance does not occur exclusively during episodes of Anorexia Nervosa.

Specify type:

   Purging Type During the current episode of Bulimia Nervosa, the person has regularly engaged in self-induced vomiting or the misuse of laxatives, diuretics, or enemas.

   Nonpurging Type During the current episode of Bulimia Nervosa, the person has used other inappropriate compensatory behaviors, such as fasting or excessive exercise, but has not regularly engaged in self-induced vomiting or the misuse of laxatives, diuretics, or enemas.

From American Psychiatric Association (1994). *Diagnostic and Statistical Manual of Mental Disorders* (4th ed.). Washington, DC: American Psychiatric Association.

TABLE 27-2
Assessment Guide for Eating Disorders

TO DETERMINE	SAMPLE QUESTIONS
Weight	
1. Presence of distortion/delusions about body image.	1a. What do you consider your ideal weight? 1b. Do you often "feel fat"?
2. Influence of moods or events on weight.	2a. How do you feel when you gain weight? 2b. What happens just before you decide to lose weight? 2c. (If purging) Would you be able to tolerate gaining 10 pounds if you could stop purging?
3. Feelings about current weight.	3. What do you think about your present weight?
4. Fluctuations in weight over time.	4a. Have you recently lost weight? 4b. How much? In what period of time?
5. Past treatment history and response to past treatment.	5. Have you ever been treated for a weight disorder? Was it successful?
Eating	
1. Exact eating patterns, i.e., amounts and types of food eaten normally and during binges and mealtimes.	1a. What do you eat in a typical day? How much? When and where? 1b. What do you eat when you binge? How much? When and where? Why do you terminate binges? 1c. Do you ever induce vomiting after you have eaten? 1d. Do you ever fast? How long? How often?
2. Signs of "secret" eating or shame associated with bingeing.	2a. Do you prefer eating alone? 2b. How does your eating change when you are around people?

TABLE 27-2 *(continued)*

TO DETERMINE	SAMPLE QUESTIONS
3. Perception of eating as a problem behavior.	3. Do you think your eating pattern is normal?
4. Degree of disabling effects on activities of daily living.	4a. How does eating (or not eating) interfere with your life? 4b. Do you find yourself thinking about food and calories often?
5. Anxieties precipitating bingeing and purging.	5a. Do you ever fear losing control over your eating? 5b. Do you feel you have any control over purging?
6. Function of the bingeing, purging, and fasting behaviors.	6a. How do you feel after you binge eat? How do you feel after you purge? 6b. How do you feel when you can fast?

Activity

1. Presence of compulsive exercise as a form of purging.	1. Do you exercise? What type and how much each day?
2. Function exercise serves both physically and emotionally.	2a. How do you feel physically after exercising? Emotionally? 2b. How do you feel physically if you cannot/do not exercise? Emotionally?

Family (In the context of presenting problem)

1. Presence of marital conflict in parents' marriage or with spouse if client is married.	1a. Do your parents appear to be happy? 1b. How would you describe your marriage?
2. Parental response to emotional needs of children, to separation/independence of children.	2a. How do members of your family express anger? 2b. Does your family show affection? How? Sadness? How? 2c. Describe a situation when you brought a problem to your mother/father. What did they do? How did you feel? 2d. How did you feel about expressing opinions that differ from those of your parents? 2e. How did your parents react when you finished high school? Left home for college?
3. Feelings and reactions of each family member, spouse, or significant person concerning client's eating behavior and weight.	3. What does your mother (father, sibling) do when you refuse meals? Eat too much? Purge?
4. Presence of poor impulse control, i.e., drug/alcohol abuse or excessive tempers in family members.	4. Does anyone in your family abuse alcohol? Drugs?
5. Presence of overcontrol of appetites and feelings by family.	5. What do your mother, father, siblings do when they are upset, angry, happy, hungry, sad? How do you know when they are angry? Sad? Hungry? Happy?
6. Eating patterns of the family unit.	6a. Who plans the family meals? Who does the food shopping? Who pays for the food? 6b. Does your family eat meals together? 6c. Do you speak to each other at these times? 6d. How does it feel for you to eat meals with your family? 6e. How long does it take you to eat a meal?

Physical

1. Signs and symptoms often associated with *anorexia nervosa.*	1. Is there presence of • cachexia/emaciation; • decreased body temperature; • peripheral edema; • cyanosis of the extremities; • constipation; • atrophic dry skin; • slow pulse; • yellowish skin; • amenorrhea;

(Continued)

TABLE 27-2 *(continued)*

TO DETERMINE	SAMPLE QUESTIONS
	• hair loss; • lanugo on skin; • anemia/malnutrition.
2. Signs and symptoms often associated with *bulimia*.	2. Is there presence of • parotid gland enlargement (chipmunk facies); • dehydration; • chronic hoarseness/sore throat; • dental caries—loss of enamel on teeth; • rebound water retention (when purging stops); • anemia; • irregular menses/amenorrhea; • electrolyte imbalance, i.e., hypokalemia.
3. Presence of abuse of substances used for "purging."	3a. Do you use laxatives or diuretics to lose weight? How many? How often? 3b. Do you ever take amphetamines, caffeine/diet pills? How many? How often?

From Valcarolis, E. (1994). *Foundations of Psychiatric Mental Health Nursing.* Philadelphia: W. B. Saunders Company, 1994. Reprinted with permission.

5. Simultaneously, the client learns that anticipating and meeting the needs of others, even at the expense of her own, allows her to present an acceptable image in relationship with the other. This often leads to a pattern of exploitative or abusive relationships in the future.

6. When separation or loss is experienced during any of life's crises or transitions, such as puberty, leaving home, first sexual expression, death, or childbirth, an onset or exacerbation of the eating disorder occurs.

7. "Assumed" helplessness is adopted. This is an unrealistic perception of one's own capabilities as a defense against separation–individuation. "Assumed" helplessness is subjectively experienced as a feeling of inadequacy or incompetence.

8. The primary issues, especially shame reduction, should be the foci of treatment to avoid symptom substitution and to facilitate separation–individuation.

See Figure 27-1 for the role of shame in the development of eating disorders.

SOCIOCULTURAL

1. As gender roles become blurred, conflicting messages are transmitted by society through family, friends, lovers, institutions of learning, and the workplace, as well as the media regarding expectations for the roles, behavior, and image of the modern woman.

2. These messages lead to the development of a double "self" whereby the woman who is achievement-oriented and is in situations where assertiveness is required must also refine her social skills in such a way as to avoid seeming aggressive.

3. The average woman in the United States is 5'4" and weighs 130 lbs. This average is far from the "ideal" beauty-pageant contestant, who averages 5'7" and weighs 120 lbs.

4. Eating disorders may be the result of the desperate attempt of women who lack a strong identity to define their own criteria for success.

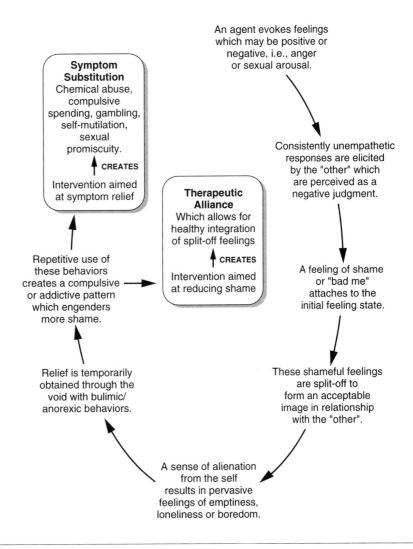

FIGURE 27-1   Development of Bulimic/Anorexic Behaviors as a Response to Shame

GENETIC

1. There is a higher incidence of anorexia in siblings of anorexics than in control groups.
2. There is a higher incidence of anorexia in monozygotic twins than in dizygotic twins.
3. Addictions and mood disorders are more common among first-degree relatives of bulimics than in control groups. It must be noted that these similarities may relate to family dynamics in relatives raised together, rather than a genetic explanation (Kaplan & Sadock, 1991).

NEUROCHEMICAL

1. Anorexics and bulimics have been found to have lower than normal concentrations of norepinephrine. Again, it must be noted that the client's thoughts, feelings, and actions may cause the decrease in norepinephrine rather than the reverse.

2. This may explain the successful use with these clients of some antidepressant drugs that affect the neurotransmitter system (Fava et al., 1989).

RELATED DISORDERS
1. Major Depressive Disorder
2. Obsessive-Compulsive Disorder
3. Agoraphobia/Social Phobia
4. Substance Abuse
5. Impulse Control Disorders
6. Borderline Personality Disorder

RELATED NURSING DIAGNOSES
1. Altered growth and development related to starvation/overexercise
2. Altered nutrition; more than body requirements or high risk for obesity related to bingeing/compulsive eating
3. Altered nutrition; less than body requirements related to starvation/purging
4. Sleep pattern disturbance; insomnia related to hunger
5. High risk for altered body temperature; hypothermia related to starvation/fat loss
6. Impaired thought processes related to physiological effects of starvation or concentration or obsessions with food
7. Severe anxiety related to weight gain
8. Impaired social interaction related to shame over physical appearance
9. Altered family processes related to preoccupation with physical status of child
10. Body image disturbance related to feelings of shame about womanly aspects of the body
11. Powerlessness related to fears about separation–individuation
12. Sexual dysfunction; frigidity/painful intercourse related to fear of losing control with concurrent feelings of shame

CRITERIA FOR HOSPITALIZATION
Clients are hospitalized when the following is present:
1. Suicidal ideation
2. Severely purging or self-destructive behavior that is out of control
3. Psychosis
4. Any life-threatening physical condition (based on laboratory data)

NURSING INTERVENTIONS
Table 27-3 shows nursing interventions and examples.

PHARMACOLOGICAL TREATMENT
Table 27-4 shows the medications prescribed for clients with anorexia and bulimia and their effect.

OBESITY
Obesity is a physical condition resulting from:
1. A medical condition
2. Diet
3. Side effect of medications, for example, steroids
4. Compulsive eating that is psychogenic in origin:
   - Developmental obesity begins in childhood with overfeeding.
   - Reactive obesity occurs in later life, when compulsive eating is used to cope with stress.

TABLE 27-3
Nursing Interventions and Examples

NURSING INTERVENTION	EXAMPLE
1. Avoid statements that indicate shock, disbelief, or disgust at the eating or purging behaviors. Instead communicate empathy.	"It must be frightening for you to feel so out of control when you binge."
2. In collaboration with the client devise an eating plan, using a liquid diet if there is a morbid fear of solid food.	"Let's plan a way for you to eat with as little anxiety as possible."
3. Provide tube feedings if the client is unable to maintain or increase weight.	"We will have to help you maintain your weight until you are able to do this yourself."
4. Provide intravenous hyperalimentation if there is guilt about eating or to restore electrolyte balance in severe cases.	"We will have to help you with this because your health is at serious risk."
5. Maintain a slow weight gain toward a range of weight that is acceptable to the client and compatible with life.	"We will help you slowly gain weight until you reach a weight you can tolerate emotionally and physically."
6. Assess for suicidal thoughts and other signs of depression as weight gain or behavioral changes occur.	"You have been bingeing and purging much less, and gaining some weight. What are your thoughts about that? Your feelings?"
7. Avoid discussions of diets or food unless these issues are linked with feelings.	"What did you feel when you fasted for several days?"
8. Explore the possibility of symptom substitution when the client reports cessation of bingeing, purging, or fasting.	"How were you able to handle that confrontation with your boss without purging?"
9. Encourage any behaviors or statements that indicate separation–individuation, unless self-destructive.	"Your plan to get a job so you can move into your own apartment sounds realistic. Let's see if we can figure out a way for you to take some first steps."
10. Encourage identification of similarities in feeling states experienced in different situations.	"The shame you describe feeling when you ate that food sounds similar to your feelings when your father teased you about gaining weight."
11. Provide family therapy to help resolve family conflicts.	"Let's spend some time today talking about things that happen in the family that have nothing to do with Mary's eating disorder. What do you two (parents) argue about?"
12. Provide individual therapy designed to help the client discover inner thoughts, feelings, and conflicts with the goal of separation/individuation.	"When you thought you might like to leave home and live in a dorm, what feelings did you have?"

TABLE 27-4
Pharmacological Treatment of Eating Disorders

MEDICATIONS	ACTION
1. Cyproheptadine (Periactin) Amitriptyline (Elavil) (Maxmen, 1991)	1. Enables weight gain and antidepressant
2. Chlorpromazine (Thorazine) Clomipramine (Anafranil) Fenfluramine (Pondimin)	2. Reduces obsessive-compulsive symptoms
3. Imipramine (Tofranil) Fluoxetine (Prozac) Sertraline (Zoloft) Phenelzine (Nardil) Opiate antagonist (naltrexone) (Pope et al., 1983, Maxmen, 1991)	3. Reduces intensity of binges

TABLE 27-5
Nursing Interventions and Rationales: Psychotherapeutic
Needs of a Person Who Compulsively Eats

INTERVENTION	RATIONALE
Nursing Diagnosis: Ineffective individual coping related to low self-esteem and unmet emotional needs, as evidenced by compulsive overeating	
1. Assess suicidal risk.	1. Feelings of hopelessness and poor self-concept indicate high risk factors.
2. Assess for depression.	2. Compulsive eating can be a way of handling depression and internalizing aggression.
3. Provide or refer to psychotherapy.	3. Opportunities to verbalize and understand feelings can diminish acting out through compulsive eating.
4. Provide or refer for medications.	4. Need for psychopharmacology, i.e., antianxiety or antidepression medication, must be evaluated.
5. Evaluate personal strengths and significant supports with client.	5. Present situation should be assessed realistically. Strengths must be emphasized and need for support evaluated.
6. Provide structured activities.	6. Structured activities help use empty time and control compulsive eating.
7. Provide group activities.	7. Group activities provide feedback, aid development of a realistic self-image, and allow outlets to relieve tension and aggression.
8. Encourage physical evaluation.	8. Abnormalities resulting from obesity should be evaluated and treated.

Adapted from Conant, M. (1990). People who defend against anxiety through eating disorders. In E. Varcarolis (ed.), *Foundations of Psychiatric Mental Health Nursing*. Philadelphia: W. B. Saunders.

PSYCHODYNAMICS

Bruch (1985) proposed that compulsive eating and obesity are defenses against feelings of depression or more unacceptable acting-out behaviors and that the premature removal of the eating behaviors and subsequent weight loss may allow these feared feelings and behaviors to surface.

If viewed in this way, compulsive eating and "being fat" may serve a similar function for the obese person that fasting and "being thin" serve for the anorexic. For example, a woman, when in an obese state is withdrawn and isolated, blames her lack of close relationships on "being fat." If she were slim, she believes, she would be more physically attractive and would become outgoing. Although this change is desirable, it is also feared because obesity is, for her, a protection from the risks of intimacy. She believes her "fat" is controlling her fate and, subsequently, denies responsibility for her own isolation. Like the anorexic, she believes that "if I were thin, all my problems would be solved." By holding onto this belief, she avoids the painful process of examining her own participation in her problems.

Like the anorexic and the bulimic, a person who uses food to maintain obesity may be experiencing conflicts about independence, autonomy, separation, and intimacy. Although there are many obese men, the current literature seems to focus on obese women, children, and adolescents. The reason for this is that these populations seek professional counseling for weight-related problems more often than adult males. Although there is a social stigma placed on "fat people" in general, obese women, children, and adolescents feel society's disapproval more acutely. Self-esteem is more dependent on body image among these populations. Feelings of shame and guilt, with subsequent depression, are frequent complaints. These feelings may be suppressed through an escalation of the compulsive eating and denial of the obesity. Obesity is denied when an obese person sees only her "better" parts in a mirror or avoids the mirror altogether. (Conant, 1994, pp. 733–734)

NURSING INTERVENTION

Table 27-5 shows nursing interventions and the theoretical rationale with clients who are compulsive eaters.

REFERENCES

American Psychiatric Association (1994). *Diagnostic and Statistical Manual of Mental Disorders* (4th ed.). Washington, DC: American Psychiatric Association.

Bruch, H. (1985). Four decades of eating disorders. In D. M. Garner & P. E. Garfinkel (eds.), *Handbook of Psychotherapy for Anorexia Nervosa and Bulimia*. New York: Guilford Press.

Conant, M. (1994). People who defend against anxiety through eating disorders. In E. Varcarolis (ed.), *Foundations of Psychiatric Mental Health Nursing*. Philadelphia: W. B. Saunders.

Fava, M., et al. (1989). Neurochemical abnormalities of anorexia nervosa and bulimia nervosa. *American Journal of Psychiatry, 146* (8), 963.

Kaplan, H. I., & Sadock, B. J. (1991). *Synopsis of Psychiatry* (6th ed.). Baltimore: Williams and Wilkins.

Maxmen, J. S. (1991). *Psychotropic Drugs: Fast Facts*. New York: W. W. Norton.

Pope, H. G., et al. (1983). Bulimia treated with imipramine: A placebo controlled, double-blind study. *American Journal of Psychiatry, 140,* 554.

BIBLIOGRAPHY

Hersen, M., & Detre, T. (1994). The behavioral psychotherapy of anorexia nervosa. In T. Karasu & L. Bellak (eds.), *Specialized Techniques for Specific Clinical Problems in Psychotherapy*. Northvale, NJ: Jason Aronson.

Staples, N., & Schwartz, M. (1990). Anorexia nervosa support group: Providing transitional support. *Journal of Psychosocial Nursing. 28* (2) 6–10.

Van Den Bergh, N. (ed.) (1991). *Feminist Perspectives on Addictions*. New York: Springer.

TWENTY EIGHT

The Client with Borderline Personality Disorder

Suzanne Lego

OVERVIEW:

DEFINITION

The DSM-IV defines borderline personality disorder (BPD) as "a pervasive pattern of instability of mood, interpersonal relationships and self-image, beginning in early adulthood and present in a variety of contexts" (American Psychiatric Association, 1994, pp. 280–281). See Box 28-1 for the diagnostic criteria for BPD.

ETIOLOGY

BIOLOGICAL THEORY

There is some speculation that genetic and constitutional variations in affect activation play a part in etiology. "Abnormalities in the adrenergic and cholinergic system, for example, may be related to general affective instability; deficits in the dopaminergic system may relate to the disposition toward transient psychotic symptoms in borderline patients; and impulsive, aggressive, self-destructive behavior may be facilitated by a lowered function of the serotonergic system." These theories are "still tentative and open to varying interpretations" (Kernberg, 1994, p. 703).

DEVELOPMENTAL THEORY

1. Otto Kernberg hypothesizes that these clients perceived their mothers in infancy as strongly nurturing, loving, and protective, as well as hateful, depriving, and punish-

---

BOX 28-1: Diagnostic Criteria for Borderline Personality Disorder

DSM-IV 301.83: Borderline Personality Disorder

A pervasive pattern of instability of interpersonal relationships, self-image, and affects, and marked impulsivity beginning by early adulthood and present in a variety of contexts, as indicated by five (or more) of the following:

(1) Frantic efforts to avoid real or imagined abandonment. *Note:* Do not include suicidal or self-mutilating behavior covered in Criterion 5.

(2) A pattern of unstable and intense interpersonal relationships characterized by alternating between extremes of idealization and devaluation.

(3) Identity disturbance: markedly and persistently unstable self-image or sense of self.

(4) Impulsivity in at least two areas that are potentially self-damaging (e.g., spending, sex, substance abuse, reckless driving, binge eating). *Note:* Do not include suicidal or self-mutilating behavior covered in Criterion 5.

(5) Recurrent suicidal behavior, gestures, or threats, or self-mutilating behavior.

(6) Affective instability due to a marked reactivity of mood (e.g., intense episodic dysphoria, irritability, or anxiety usually lasting a few hours and only rarely more than a few days).

(7) Chronic feelings of emptiness.

(8) Inappropriate, intense anger or difficulty controlling anger (e.g., frequent displays of temper, constant anger, recurrent physical fights).

(9) Transient, stress-related paranoid ideation or severe dissociative symptoms.

From American Psychiatric Association. *Diagnostic and Statistical Manual of Mental Disorders* (4th ed.). Washington, DC: American Psychiatric Association. Reprinted with permission.

---

ing without warning. These mothers let needs go unmet for long periods of time and abandoned the infants unpredictably. The infant perceived *both* contradictory views of the mother, and became highly anxious. To reduce the anxiety, the mother was "split" into a "good" and "bad" mother. This primitive defense is carried into adult life, and others are seen as strongly nurturant and objects of inordinate attachment or hateful, mean, and sadistic. The "good" person is idealized and the "bad" is devalued. The client can feel good only by a flight into omnipotence. Both hating the other person and feelings of extreme dependence on the other lead to a disowning of the feelings through the use of projective identification and denial (Kernberg, 1975).

2. James Masterson has described the borderline client's problems as beginning during Mahler's rapprochement subphase of the separation individuation process of development, between 18 and 36 months of age. At this time the toddler begins to move away from the mother, but returns from time to time for "emotional refueling," reassurance that the mother will not disappear and that separation is acceptable and rewarding. The mothers of these clients do not reward separation but rather discourage it by emotionally abandoning the child. That is, the child is punished for autonomous behavior, and rewarded for crying, clinging, dependent behavior. This clinging behavior leads to an "emotional reunion" with the mother that comes to be longed for and repeated throughout life. By the same token, moves toward independence and autonomy lead the patient to experience what Masterson calls "abandonment depression" (Masterson, 1976).

TRAUMA

Physical and sexual abuse in early childhood appear to play a large part in the development of BPD. "Unconsciously identifying with both victim and victimizer, they tend to reproduce the traumatic relationship again and again in an effort to free themselves from their uncontrollable hatred and to overcome the fear of being a victim by unconsciously identifying with the aggressor" (Kernberg, 1994, p. 710; see also Herman & van der Kolk, 1987; Marziali, 1992; Perry & Herman, 1993).

INCIDENCE

BPD is the most common personality disorder in the United States. Several explanations have been offered regarding its prevalence in the 1990s:

1. *The medicalization of deviant behavior:* There is a tendency in the United States to give a medical or psychiatric label to behavior that is considered deviant.
2. *New diagnostic terms:* BPD used to fall under the categories of "as-if personality," "pseudoneurosis," and "undifferentiated schizophrenia."
3. *The "virus" of psychiatry:* In physical symptomatology, when health care practitioners are not sure what to call a disorder, it may be attributed to a "virus." BPD has become a label used to cover a variety of symptoms (Kreisman & Straus, 1989).
4. *Symbol of today's society:* Just as hysteria was a symbol of repression and sexual conflicts in Freud's Vienna, BPD is a symbol of the lack of structure leading to identity conflicts in the United States.

GENDER DIFFERENCES

There are far more females than males with BPD. Some reasons are:

1. Identity problems in males are considered "normal." Females are still held to stricter role expectations than are males.
2. Females are more likely than males to receive diagnoses implying neediness and dependency. Anger in females is more likely to be labeled "sick."
3. While females enter the health care system, males with BPD are more likely to end up in jails or prisons. In fact, in a long-term study of mostly middle-class to upper-class clients with BPD, about one-quarter of the males either killed themselves, killed someone else, or were killed by another person (Stone, 1994).
4. Separation and individuation, thought to be important in the etiology, is more difficult for females than males in American society (Simmons, 1992).

DESCRIPTION

The person with BPD often presents the following characteristics (Perry & Klerman, 1980):

APPEARANCE AND BEHAVIOR

1. Appears less attractive than those of other diagnostic categories
2. Behavior is not adaptive to interview
3. Expresses angry feelings at variety of targets
4. Is argumentative
5. Devalues others
6. Is overtly manipulative
7. Is demanding
8. Acts entitled
9. Acts special
10. Does inappropriate things
11. Is irritable
12. Is sarcastic

MOOD

1. Reports feeling angry
2. Reports feeling lonely
3. Reports anhedonia

SPEECH CONTENT

1. Lacks anxiety tolerance
2. Has episodic depersonalization (feels strange or unreal)
3. Has episodic derealization (the environment seems strange or unreal)
4. Has chronic feelings of emptiness

COGNITIVE PROCESSES

1. Reality testing is intact
2. Seems bright, intelligent
3. Demonstrates poor judgment
4. Makes arbitrary or doubtful inferences from one thing to another

PERSONAL HISTORY

1. Has had limited, transient psychotic episodes, which sometimes developed during psychotherapy or following intoxication
2. Is generally impulsive and displays highly unpredictable behavior
3. Has slashed wrists or mutilated self in other ways
4. Abuses alcohol habitually or is addicted
5. Reports unusual sexual behavior
6. Lacks creative achievement, given ability
7. Lacks creative enjoyment or recreation
8. Has good scholastic abilities or potential, whether used or not
9. Has one or several repetitive impulses that periodically erupt
10. Has made suicide attempts that were deemed manipulative
11. Displays regressed behavior during hospitalization
12. Has a history of discrete depressive episodes, hypomanic episodes, or undue elations
13. Has been destructive to property or things

INTERPERSONAL RELATIONSHIPS

1. Is manipulative, clinging, demanding, hostile, angry, ambivalent, controlling, exploitative, intense, unstable, sadistic, or masochistic in close relationships
2. Seeks out others to *avoid* being alone rather than to *be* with the other
3. Shows a lack of real concern or regard for others
4. Has little capacity to evaluate others realistically
5. Close relationships are typically transient and brief
6. Has promiscuous sexual relationships

DEFENSE MECHANISMS

1. Externalizes and acts out anger
2. Acts impulsively when tensions from any source build up
3. Sees others as hostile and dangerous
4. When feeling hostile, accuses others of hostile feelings (projection)
5. Expresses contradictory and unreconciled ideas of others, talking about them as all good or bad (splitting)

6. Uses bland denial when faced with contradictions in feelings or actions
7. Denies relevance of past feelings when opposite to current ones
8. Denies relevance of a sector of life that is obviously important
9. Talks as if omnipotent
10. Seems gratified by talking of alleged relationships with idealized people
11. Has distorted ideas and perceptions of others

OTHER ASPECTS OF PERSONALITY

1. Is emotionally shallow
2. Lacks a sense of own identity
3. Is not usually psychotic
4. Suggests grossly inappropriate treatment for self
5. Overreacts to minor external stressors
6. Is narcissistic, preoccupied with self
7. Is deficient in empathy for others
8. Has underlying feelings of inferiority and insecurity

PRIMITIVE DEFENSES AND CLINICAL EXAMPLES

The anger, acting out, and self-destructive behavior seen in borderline clients are related to primitive defenses. Table 28-1 shows these defenses and gives clinical examples of each.

TABLE 28-1
Primitive Defenses and Clinical Examples

DEFENSE	DEFINITION	CLINICAL EXAMPLE
Splitting	Active separation of affects of opposite quality so that one does not contaminate the other. Is differentiated from repression, ambivalence, and reaction formation in which one affect is kept unconscious. In splitting, opposite affects remain conscious but separate (Kernberg, 1975).	The client displays a clinging attitude toward one nurse and stormy, aggressive behavior with another. The client may plead to talk to only one person: "You're much nicer than those people on nights," or "You're the only nurse who really understands." Nurses are seen as all good or all bad. The same nurse may be seen alternately as good or bad.
Projective identification	Disowning of unwanted feelings by placing or infusing them into others (Tansey & Burke, 1989).	The client who is very frightened approaches a nurse who is calm. After an interchange the nurse feels frightened.
Primitive idealization	Archaic form of intense idealization to protect the client from recognizing strong, aggressive, angry tendencies toward one on whom the client is dependent.	The client expresses strong, exaggerated positive feelings toward the nurse. "You're a wonderful person. Your children are sure lucky."
Omnipotence	Fantasies of greatness, which lead these clients to believe they need not adhere to the conventions others follow, and that they cannot be touched by illness, death, or the passing of time.	When the client is confronted with impulsive or unconventional behavior just displayed, he replies, "That's ridiculous! You don't know what you're talking about!" These clients often abuse drugs or make suicide attempts.
Devaluation	Consistent, exaggerated criticism designed to deflect the client and others from the client's strong feelings of inadequacy and insecurity.	"You've made me much worse since I came here. Does anybody ever get well here?"
Denial	Unconscious shutting out of aspects of an experience, particularly feelings.	"I was bored, so I took a bottle of Valium, drank some whiskey, and cut my wrists." Feelings that preceded the self-destructive behavior are not consciously available to the client.

**NURSES'
NONPRODUCTIVE
REACTIONS**

INDIVIDUAL REACTIONS

The emotional intensity of the borderline client as well as the ability to intuitively strike at each staff member's "weak spots" have a profound effect on the nurse's treatment of the client. Some of the reactions of the nurse include (Smith & Lego, 1984):

1. Feelings of massive responsibility for the client's welfare
2. Feelings of guilt because of failure to help the client
3. Omnipotent urges to rescue the client from the mishandling of others
4. Feelings of intense love and attachment to the client
5. Promises to keep secrets for the client as a token of trust and esteem
6. Feeling honored that the client "finally opened up"
7. Feeling highly confirmed in professional identity
8. Feeling highly repudiated in professional identity
9. Experiencing a need for excessively firm limits on the amount and quality of attention given to the client
10. Guilt by association with some value or person viewed as hostile by the client
11. Feelings of disappointment in one's work
12. Feelings of being emotionally drained to the extent that one's personal relationships suffer
13. Manifestations of the nurse's latent personality difficulties
14. Hostile acting out toward the clients by discharging them or resigning from the setting
15. Contempt, jealousy, and envy of the seeming "normal" client who manages to get considerable attention
16. Feelings of general paranoia and fear of the client's "next" projection
17. Feeling emotionally exposed and vulnerable because of the client's "part-true" projections
18. Defensiveness, counterattacking, rejection, and appeasement of the client

In addition to setting off irrational reactions in individual nurses, these clients often set in motion group dynamics that are unusual and potentially destructive. The staff members may find that they begin to idealize the head nurse or clinical coordinator, become dependent, compete with one another, develop coalitions and even sexual involvements with one another. This is because the daily intense bombardment of primitive material and behavior leads to regression and the eruption of primitive feelings in the staff.

GROUP REACTIONS

Specifically, the splitting and massive projections from clients may lead to the following group behaviors (Kernberg, 1978):

1. Diagnostic uncertainty with contradictory evaluations of clients occur.
2. Groups of staff members may feel emotionally isolated from one another.
3. Two or more staff members may become suspicious of the motives and behavior of other staff members toward the client.
4. Lunch-hour and coffee-break time may be dominated by discussion of specific clients.
5. The nucleus of an in-group may believe that they are the only ones who can help the client.
6. Loss of morale and confusion may be seen in the "out-group."
7. Staff cleavage with excessive clash of opinions is seen by outside observers.

8. Blurring of staff–client role boundaries is seen in many forms (for example, client and staff discuss another staff member, or staff share personal information with the client).
9. Split in- and out-groups make the following accusations:
   a. "Ins" accuse "outs" of being cold and insensitive.
   b. "Outs" accuse "ins" of being too permissive and gullible and of spoiling the client.
10. Splits between departments in a hospital structure may be seen.
11. Administrative decisions to change the client's therapist occur when the therapist is part of the "bad" split.

INTERVENTIONS DURING HOSPITALIZATION

Intervention with these clients involves concerted efforts to deal effectively with splitting and projection, to diminish the acting out of anger and self-destructive behavior, and to promote the beginning of new, more mature, and genuinely independent ways of relating with others. Table 28-2 lists problems, interventions, and rationales with the hospital client (Smith & Lego, 1984).

TABLE 28-2
Problems, Interventions, and Rationales with Borderline Clients

PROBLEM	INTERVENTION	RATIONALE
Splitting	1. The nurse recognizes the behavior as defensive, rather than feeling flattered by the positive feelings or destroyed by the negative, and remains neutral. The nurse does not attempt to stop the behavior outright, but rather explores the underlying feelings. *Client:* I'm so glad you're here today! or God, not you today! *Nurse:* You feel like you need a friend today?	1. Splitting is a major defense against the client's intense aggressive and needy feelings. Prevention of the use of the defense would make the underlying feelings less available for exploration. When nurses become aware of the process and understand the meaning of splitting, the client becomes more comfortable with the intense underlying feelings.
	2. The nurse or therapist assigned to the client should not be changed according to the client's whim.	2. Firm limits are set so that the client is forced to face the feelings rather than run from them.
	3. Regularly scheduled staff meetings are held.	3. Each member brings a different experience of the client to the attention of the total group. When combined, these pieces of information help provide a total picture of the client that is more comprehensive than a picture given by a single staff member. The nurse's sense of having private knowledge and responsibility for the client is lessened so that individual nurses are relieved of the burden of being the "only" viable helper. The need to "rescue" the client from the other staff is diminished, as well as guilt resulting from not meeting the client's insatiable demands. Blaming of colleagues is diminished, and increased tolerance of the opinions of others emerges. Comprehensive treatment approaches are developed, individual members having full knowledge of their roles in the care of the client. Administrators and clinicians are less likely to work at cross-purposes. A split staff is detrimental to clients who have part identity and splitting problems.

TABLE 28-2 *(continued)*

PROBLEM	INTERVENTION	RATIONALE
Projection	1. The nurse recognizes the part of the client's accusation that is a projection, notes the underlying feeling, and questions that: *Client:* You certainly are an angry person. How'd they ever let you into the nursing profession? *Nurse:* How come you're so mad at me today? 2. The nurse recognizes the part of the accusation that is a half-truth and acknowledges it: *Client:* You treat me differently from the others: You're more strict with me and you get mad. *Nurse:* You're right. I think you need to know exactly what we expect of you. Sometimes your behavior does make me mad. 3. The nurse encourages the client to explore feelings and experiences instead of making interpretations of the client's behavior.	1. Rather than engage the client in a power struggle over who was angry first, the nurse moves straight to the client's feeling. Over time, as the nurse readily accepts the client's anger, the client is able to do the same and to explore it further. 2. As the nurse is able to acknowledge and accept responsibility for her own behavior and feelings, the client will do the same. The client can see anger communicated in a nondestructive way, rather than acted out destructively. 3. Correct interpretations tend to create a feeling of distance, inferiority, and unconscious envy of the nurse.
Anger and acting out	1. In a nonpunitive way, the nurse a. Tells the client to stop the behavior and to talk about the feeling b. Offers empathic statements c. Clarifies what has happened d. Provides safety for all clients 2. If these measures fail, the nurse provides medication, restraint, or seclusion. Once these measures are started, they are followed to completion. 3. Secluded or restrained clients are observed at all times.	1. Provides temporary ego boundaries, assists with impulse control, helps client delay gratification, inhibits self-destruction and violence, helps client to talk about feelings, helps client to work cooperatively and to gain self-understanding. 2. Helps the client regain control, prevents violence, provides safety. Premature release from restraint or seclusion causes anxiety and may lead to a sudden escalation of violent behavior. The implicit message of ambivalent use of restraint or seclusion is that the nurse is insecure and not in control. This terrifies the client. 3. The client often suffers remorse and humiliation over having lost control. The incidence of suicide is great following a violent act.
Self-mutilation	1. The nurse provides first aid. 2. The nurse encourages discussion of thoughts and feelings that preceded the act. 3. The nurse avoids elaborate focusing on the injury itself.	1. Prevents further loss of function and treats the injury. 2. Most self-destructive behavior follows a real or fantasied disappointment. All disappointments must be discussed because these clients are chronically disappointed with life. 3. Once the injury is treated, avoidance of discussing it prevents unnecessary development of secondary gains. When self-mutilation is deemed manipulative, healthier ways of getting attention are encouraged. Discussion and oversolicitous care of the wound serve as a defense against what the client was actually thinking and feeling.
Serious suicide attempts	Interventions are the same for all suicidal clients (see Chapter 24).	

INTERVENTIONS IN OUTPATIENT THERAPY

Table 28-3 shows the major clinical problems presented by clients with BPD in outpatient therapy, the psychodynamics of each problem, and suggested interventions.

TABLE 28-3
Clinical Problems with BPD Patients in Outpatient Therapy, Psychodynamics, and Interventions

PROBLEM	PSYCHODYNAMICS	INTERVENTION
Substance abuse	Owing to faulty ego development, these clients have trouble tolerating anxiety. They often turn to alcohol or drugs to find instant relief. When the client is also an addictive personality, the prognosis is poor. However, when the substance is used to act out only, the prognosis is better, and the client's substance abuse can be controlled through limit setting. Alcohol and drugs are used for a primitive sense of goodness, happiness, fulfillment, and well-being (Kernberg, 1984).	Clients are treated as adults who will assume responsibility for themselves. They should not be seen on the same day they use alcohol or drugs. Instead they are told they may not stay for the session, as is the rule on any day they use alcohol or drugs, and that they must pay for the session. In the next session the therapist and client investigate the reasons for the alcohol or drug use. Was it used for anxiety relief, as acting out, and was it related to transference?
Phone calls to the therapist	Any separation from the therapist causes anxiety and even panic. Object constancy is often absent. The client is unable to sustain the image of the relationship without the physical presence of the other. Also, the patient fears the therapist will be destroyed because of the rage engendered by separation.	The call is kept as short as possible. If therapists are busy when the call comes through, they say so, reminding the client of the time of the next session. Most importantly, the client is encouraged to confront thoughts and feelings when they occur in sessions. "Are you angry now? Talk about it here; don't phone me about it later." The client is confronted with the underlying anger and fear of abandonment and the attached feelings are explored.
Self-mutilation	Self-mutilation has been seen as: 1. A way to act out rage over rejection toward the self, or the introjected rejector 2. A way to gain control over therapists who feel worried, fearful, impotent (Kernberg, 1984) 3. An expression of guilt 4. A sadistic act toward the therapist 5. A way to cover and avoid envy 6. A way for the client to feel alive through the production of pain 7. A way of identifying with the aggressor in clients who were abused as children	Some therapists take a tough stand from the beginning, saying they will help clients get emergency care but will terminate therapy if self-mutilation persists. The disadvantage to this method is that clients may push the limit a little more each time to test the therapist. Another approach is to analyze each episode in great detail, conveying that behavior has meaning, exploring which theories apply.
Suicidal behavior	Suicidal behavior represents: 1. The desire for the "magical reunion" through rescue or joining a dead parent in heaven 2. Identification with the aggressor whom the client hates, loves, and fears 3. A challenge to the therapist to stand up to such massive aggression (Kernberg, 1984) 4. Freedom from longing, frustration, and intimacy (Kernberg, 1984), responsibility, and concern	If the client leaves the office threatening suicide, the therapist may need to notify the family or police. This may prompt in the client extreme rage at the therapist, which is then explored in future sessions along with the wishes underlying the suicidal behavior. Some therapists use nonsuicidal contracts.
Desire for hospitalization	Hospitalization represents a fantasized reunion with an early significant other, a desire to be cared for, an escape from the frustrations of everyday life.	Hospitalization is avoided if at all possible, as it confirms the clients' view of themselves as defective. Inpatients who are diagnosed with BPD are stigmatized by mental health professionals (Gallop, Lancee, & Garfinkel, 1982), further decreasing the value of hospitalization. Occasionally long-term hospitalization is used as respite for families.

TABLE 28-3 *(continued)*

PROBLEM	PSYCHODYNAMICS	INTERVENTION
Intense positive or negative transference	Clinging idealization represents a projection of the idealized self, and covers envy and paranoia (Kernberg, 1984). The devaluing transference is a protection against rage at rejection, wishes for nurturance, envy, projected anger, low self-esteem, feelings toward significant others who they believe have devalued or rejected them (Adler, 1973).	The therapist is careful not to stifle transference by being too "nice" or too rigid. The therapist interprets the introjects and interacts as a real person. This leads to new, healthier introjects. Care is taken to avoid struggles over how much of the client's reaction is based on past relationships and how much is triggered by the here and now (Kernberg, 1984).
Counter-transference	Much of the countertransference is caused by the therapist's introjection of the client's projections through projective identification. In this process the client infuses the therapist with self-representations (feelings clients have themselves) or other representations (feelings others have had about them). The therapist allows these feelings to be introjected and then experiences irrational or exaggerated feelings toward the client (Tansey & Burke, 1989).	The therapist tries to avoid these introjections and stands back to examine the situation. By exploring the self-representations and other representations with the client, empathy can take place. Sharing countertransference with clients can be helpful, as they are very tuned in to the therapist anyway, and can benefit by learning about their impact on others.

THE CLIENT'S EXPERIENCE

Often nurses know little about the experience with psychiatric illness. This is especially true in the case of BPD, as nurses tend to avoid these clients. A recent book by a client with BPD describes her experience in a hospital for over 2 years (Kaysen, 1993; Lego, 1994). Box 28-2 shows part of the findings in a study of the client's perspective. "Reports of their experience differed markedly from clinical descriptions of the disorder" (Miller, 1994).

BOX 28-2: Statements Reflecting Estrangement, Inadequacy, and Despair by a Patient with Borderline Personality Disorder

Estrangement
I had a lot of friends, but I never felt part of the group.
Even when very young, taking the bus to kindergarten, feeling like I wasn't part of the people on the bus.
I felt . . . separated in a way, not quite in there with the rest.
I think it is because I already feel I'm different, so I feel I should separate myself from everyone else in some way.

Inadequacy
What has always been there, for as long as I can remember, even back in school, even in middle school . . . is like a rating scale. . . . I don't give people numbers. I just rate them against me and I never met anyone that I was equal to or better than, no matter what. . . . Even if it is a bum on the street, there is something that makes him better than me. It is not that I have done anything bad; it is like what I was born with.
I have such low esteem of myself. I am constantly comparing. . . . I feel that everyone is superior to me. Everyone. And I am not worthy.

(Continued)

BOX 28-2 *(continued)*

I feel like I am not up to standard for something. . . . I always feel there is something lacking and so I look at other people to see if they feel the same way and they don't. . . . So I compare myself with other people. . . . There is this constant civil war going on inside my head—who I want to be and who I'm stuck with.

I can't explain it, but . . . you feel you're useless, you're worthless.

I am already bad enough. [By bad, you mean?] Not worthy, not meeting society's standards.

Despair

The main thing is that you want to die. You want to be out of this life, out of the pain. I don't think there is anything anyone can do to make me feel differently.

I wouldn't wish this upon someone else. If someone said you could get rid of it by giving it to someone else, I don't think I would do it knowing what I have been through.

I don't know if I would have the nerve to kill myself. I feel like it a lot, and I think about it a lot, at least once a week.

From Miller, S. G. (1994). Borderline personality disorder from the patient's perspective. *Hospital and Community Psychiatry, 45* (12), 1215–1219.

REFERENCES

Adler, G. (1973). Hospital treatment of borderline patients. *American Journal of Psychiatry, 130,* 32–35.

American Psychiatric Association (1994). *Diagnostic and Statistical Manual of Mental Disorders* (4th ed.). Washington, DC: American Psychiatric Association.

Gallop, R., Lancee, W. J., & Garfinkel, P. (1982). How nursing staff respond to the label "borderline personality disorder." *Hospital and Community Psychiatry, 40,* 815–819.

Herman, J. L., & van der Kolk, B. A. (1987). Traumatic antecedents of borderline personality disorder. In B. A. van der Kolk (ed.), *Psychological Trauma* (pp. 111–126). Washington, DC: American Psychiatric Press.

Kaysen, S. (1993). *Girl, Interrupted.* New York: Turtle Bay Books.

Kernberg, O. F. (1975). *Borderline Conditions and Pathological Narcissism.* New York: Jason Aronson.

Kernberg, O. F. (1978). Leadership and organizational functioning. Organization regression. *International Journal of Group Psychotherapy, 28* (1), 11–19.

Kernberg, O. F. (1984). Severe personality disorders. *Psychotherapeutic Strategies.* New Haven, CT: Yale University Press.

Kernberg, O. F. (1994). Aggression, trauma, and hatred in the treatment of borderline patients. *Psychiatric Clinics of North America, 17* (4), 701–714.

Kreisman, J. J., & Straus, H. (1989). *I Hate You—Don't Leave Me.* New York: Avon Books.

Lego, S. (1994). Book review: Girl, interrupted. *Archives of Psychiatric Nursing, 8* (3), 210–211.

Marziali, E. (1992). The etiology of borderline personality disorder: Developmental factors. In J. F. Clarkin, E. Marziali, & H. Munroe-Blum (eds.), *Borderline Personality Disorder* (pp. 27–44). New York: Guilford Press.

Masterson, J. (1976). *Psychotherapy of the Borderline Adult.* New York: Brunner/Mazel.

Miller, S. G. (1994). Borderline personality disorder from the patient's perspective. *Hospital and Community Psychiatry, 45* (12), 1215–1219.

Perry, J. C., & Herman, J. L. (1993). Trauma and defense in the etiology of borderline personality disorder. In J. Paris (ed.), *Borderline Personality Disorder* (pp. 123–139). Washington, DC: American Psychiatric Press.

Perry, C., & Klerman, G. L. (1980). Clinical features of the borderline personality disorder. *American Journal of Psychiatry, 137* (2), 238–349.

Simmons, D. (1992). Gender issues and borderline personality disorder: Why do females dominate the diagnosis? *Archives of Psychiatric Nursing, 6* (4), 219–223.

Smith, M. C., & Lego, S. (1984). The client who has a borderline personality disorder. In S. Lego (ed.), *The American Handbook of Psychiatric Nursing* (pp. 415–422). Philadelphia: J. B. Lippincott.

Stone, M. H. (1994). Characterologic subtypes of the borderline personality disorder. With a note on prognostic factors. *Psychiatric Clinics of North America, 17* (4), 773–784.

Tansey, M. J., & Burke, W. F. (1989). *Understanding Countertransference: From Projective Identification to Empathy.* Hillsdale, NJ: The Analytic Press.

BIBLIOGRAPHY

Goldstein, W. (1991). Clarification of projective identification. *American Journal of Psychiatry, 148* (2), 153–161.

Kernberg, O. F., et al. (1989). *Psychodynamic Psychotherapy of Borderline Patients.* New York: Basic Books.

Lego, S. (1987). The borderline patient: The psychoanalytic approach. *Archives of Psychiatric Nursing, 1* (5), 318–321.

Lego, S. (1994). The borderline personality disorder. In E. M. Varcarolis (ed.), *Psychiatric Mental Health Nursing* (2nd ed., pp. 397–406). Philadelphia: W. B. Saunders Co.

Lego, S. (1995). Borderline personality disorder and post-traumatic stress disorder in Vietnam veterans. *Journal of the American Psychiatric Nurses Association, 1* (1), 6–11.

Masterson, J. F. (1988). *The Search for the Real Self.* New York: Free Press.

Masterson, J. F., & Klein, R. (1989). *Psychotherapy of Disorders of the Self.* New York: Brunner/Mazel.

Nehls, N. (1991). Borderline personality disorder and group therapy. *Archives of Psychiatric Nursing, 5* (3), 137–146.

Nehls, N. (1992). Group therapy for people with borderline personality disorder: Interventions associated with positive outcomes. *Issues in Mental Health Nursing, 13* (3), 255–269.

Nehls, N. (1994). Brief hospital treatment plans for persons with borderline personality disorder: Perspectives of inpatient psychiatric nurses and community mental health clinicians. *Archives of Psychiatric Nursing, 8* (5), 303–311.

Ogden, T. H. (1991). *Projective Identification and Psychotherapeutic Technique.* Northvale, NJ: Jason Aronson.

Scharff, J. S. (1992). *Projective and Introjective Identification and the Use of the Therapist's Self.* Northvale, NJ: Jason Aronson.

Vaccani, J. M. (1989). Borderline personality disorder and alcohol abuse. *Archives of Psychiatric Nursing, 3* (2), 113–119.

Volkan, V. (1995). *Six Steps in the Treatment of Borderline Personality Organization.* Northvale, NJ: Jason Arsonson. Master Work Series.

TWENTY NINE

The Client with Dissociative Identity Disorder

Suzanne Lego

OVERVIEW:

Introduction
Diagnostic Criteria
Differential Diagnosis
Etiology

Examples of Alternates
Relationships Among Alternates
Initial Interview
Nursing Interventions

INTRODUCTION

Dissociative identity disorder (DID) has become a diagnostic category fraught with controversy. From the time it first appeared in the literature, mental health professionals have been reluctant to accept its validity. Skepticism has been fueled by a number of factors:

1. Psychotherapists who are awed and intrigued by the dissociative phenomenon have exploited clients by furthering their dissociations and raising doubts about the existence of the clients' alternative personalities (sometimes called *alternates* or *alters*).
2. People with borderline personality disorder who are vulnerable and suggestible have taken on these symptoms, also causing mental health workers to wonder if DID actually exists.
3. Unscrupulous attorneys have attempted to use DID as a legal defense when its existence in the defendant is questionable.
4. DID has sometimes been thought to be associated with adults who spent time in cults in their childhood. Many people are skeptical about the existence of cults, especially those who have had no firsthand experience with them.

In addition to these social factors, the nurse's first encounter with a client with DID sparks incredulity, as the behavior is so bizarre. In fact, countertransference with these clients tends to be profound. Some countertransference reactions include:

1. Awe at the power of dissociation
2. Shock at the histories of abuse, sadism, and terror of these clients as children
3. Embarrassment when the nurse does not know what to say to various alternate personalities in the same person
4. Fear that an angry alter will appear and express uncontrollable rage
5. Anxiety over identification with the patient's various emotions

6. Fear of loss of control, as the nurse never knows "who" will appear next and what will happen next
7. Grandiosity as the nurse wishes to take over and save or rescue the client
8. Burnout owing to the neediness of the clients, who drain nurses' energy

DIAGNOSTIC CRITERIA

Box 29-1 shows the American Psychiatric Association's DSM-IV criteria for dissociative identity disorder.

BOX 29-1: 300.14—DSM-IV Diagnostic Criteria for Dissociative Identity Disorder (formerly Multiple Personality Disorder)

A. The presence of two or more distinct identities or personality states (each with its own relatively enduring pattern of perceiving, relating to, and thinking about the environment and self).

B. At least two of these identities or personality states recurrently take control of the person's behavior.

C. Inability to recall important personal information that is too extensive to be explained by ordinary forgetfulness.

D. The disturbance is not due to the direct physiological effects of a substance (e.g., blackouts or chaotic behavior during Alcohol Intoxication) or a general medical condition (e.g., complex partial seizures). *Note:* In children, the symptoms are not attributable to imaginary play.

American Psychiatric Association (1994). *Diagnostic and Statistical Manual of Mental Disorders* (4th ed.). Washington, DC: American Psychiatric Association. Reprinted with permission.

DIFFERENTIAL DIAGNOSIS

DID is often difficult to differentiate from other dissociative states, psychotic states, and personality disorders such as:
1. Borderline personality disorder
2. Histrionic personality
3. Drug and alcohol abuse
4. Epilepsy
5. Nonpsychotic dissociative states
6. Malingering
7. Conversion and somatization disorders
8. Depression
9. Psychosexual disorders such as impotence, frigidity, transsexualism, and transvestism

In fact, some of these occur with DID. In addition, these clients often report headaches, hysterical conversion symptoms, drug and alcohol abuse, suicidal gestures, self-mutilation, and stormy relationships.

ETIOLOGY

The development of dissociative identity disorder can be summarized in the following operational steps (Lego, 1988):
1. The individual has the potential to dissociate.
2. The individual experiences overwhelming life events.

3. The individual is not provided with soothing, restorative experiences.
4. The individual dissociates the traumatic experiences.
5. The dissociated experiences or aspects of them, that is, feeling states, later appear in personality formations.

EXAMPLES OF ALTERNATES

A prototype of the constellation of personalities, also called alternates or alters, is as follows:

1. The host: This personality is typically depressed, anxious, anhedonic, rigid, frigid, compulsively good, conscious-stricken, masochistic, and suffers from a variety of somatic symptoms, particularly headaches (Kluft, 1984). Clients report feeling overwhelmed and powerless, at the mercy of forces beyond their control or comprehension. Two-thirds in an NIMH sample did not know about the existence of other personalities (Putnam, 1989).
2. A prim, proper alternate.
3. A sexually promiscuous "id" alternate.
4. An angry alternate, prone to violence.
5. Fragments of personalities may also appear who serve the function of carrying out some behavior for the host personality. For example, a fragment may accept enemas, or quickly remove clothes for a prostitute alter (Lego, 1988).

RELATIONSHIPS AMONG ALTERNATES

There is great variety in the relations among alternates (Confer & Ables, 1983):

1. The host personality may have no knowledge of alternates.
2. The host personality may know of some alternates but not others.
3. The alternates may have knowledge of the host when the host knows nothing of the alternates.
4. The alternates may know of one another and work cooperatively.
5. The alternates may be antagonistic toward one another and torment or injure one another.

INITIAL INTERVIEW

Usually the initial history is taken from the host personality, that with the least access to the early history and current experience. Therefore, the client may present frequent inconsistencies and a lack of a clear history. These clients often say they "can't remember." Actually they may (Putnam, 1989):

1. Not remember and say so
2. Remember but have internal pressures not to tell
3. Not remember and confabulate
4. Allude diagnosis or fear sounding crazy by lying
5. Pretend to know more than they do

Some categories of symptoms with useful questions to determine the diagnosis are included in Table 29-1. Other behaviors noted in the initial interview might include eye rolls, blinking, twitches, grimaces, and voice changes. The client may also suddenly refocus attention, signaling that a new personality has appeared and does not remember getting there.

TABLE 29-1
Symptom Categories with Useful Questions to Determine the Diagnosis of Multiple Personality Disorder*

SYMPTOM	EXAMPLES OF QUESTIONS
Time loss	1. "Do you look at the clock, for example, at 9 A.M. and the next time it's 3 P.M.? 2. "Do you ever find clothing, jewelry, or other things you'd never buy in your home?" (For men this may include weapons, tools, or vehicles.) 3. "Close your eyes. Tell me what you're wearing." 4. "Do people approach you and seem to know you, when you don't know them?" 5. "Are there events in your life you've been told about but don't remember?" 6. "Are there times you find yourself in places such as strange towns and don't remember how you got there?"
Depersonalization/ derealization	1. "Are there times you seem to be watching yourself as if in a movie?" 2. "Do you ever feel mechanical or dead?"
Common life experiences	1. "Have you been called a liar when you thought you were telling the truth?" 2. "Did you have erratic school behavior—failure one matriculating period, and A's the next?" 3. "Did you get back tests or homework you didn't recall doing?" 4. Are there grades or periods of time you don't remember?"
Flashbacks, intrusive images, dreamlike memories	1. "Do you ever remember a past event so vividly it seems to be happening again?" 2. "Do you ever have images that you see over and over again?" 3. "Do you have memories that seem like dreams or dreams that seem like memories?" 4. "Do you have nightmares or wake up frequently?"
Morning changes	"Have you awakened to find poems, drawings, letters you have written or furniture moved around?"
Unknown abilities	"Have you found or been told you can speak a foreign language or play a musical instrument you didn't know about?"
Schneider's primary symptoms	1. "Do you hear voices talking, arguing, screaming in your head?" 2. "Do you feel made to do things you would not normally do?" 3. "Do you talk to yourself and get an answer when you're alone?"

*Much of this material is adapted from Putnam, 1989.

NURSING INTERVENTIONS

Table 29-2 provides nursing interventions and their rationales. Table 29-3 provides milieu interventions and their rationales.

TABLE 29-2
Nursing Interventions and Rationales for Working with the Client Who Has DID

NURSING INTERVENTION	THEORETICAL RATIONALE AND EXAMPLES
1. Does not ask for other alternates even when the client wants others to take over.	1. Nurses must take care not to further dissociation. Instead the client is told she (more are female than male) can speak for herself.
2. Reminds alters they are part of the host personality, even though this may seem confusing to the client on a conscious level.	2. Discourages dissociation and encourages integration. "It seems to you, you are 4 years old, but you are 34 now. The things that happened then are over and can never happen again."
3. Encourages clients to experience openly the feelings that have been dissociated, rather than asking for alternates.	3. Discourages dissociation and encourages integration. "Tell me about feeling angry" is better than "Is one of you angry?" and "Is there an angry person inside who wants to talk?"
4. Emphasizes the multiplicity of feelings in all of us: nurses, clients, families.	4. Fosters integration. For example, the client says, "I bet you never get angry." Nurse: "We all get angry sometimes."
5. Helps alters to understand one another and the purpose of each by pointing out the host will one day be able to tolerate all feelings.	5. Fosters integration. For example, when one alter complains about how "good" another is: "Someday (host's name) will be able to tolerate anger." This is preferable to the more mechanistic approach: "Someday you will all merge."
6. Does not reassure calm alters that they will be protected from angry alters.	6. Tends to strengthen the angry alters. Setting alters against one another fosters and strengthens dissociation.
7. Keeps a chart of all the personalities and what they represent in the client's record. This is not discussed with or shared with the client.	7. Helps nurses recognize alters when they appear. Clients are not involved in this process, as this may be seen as encouragement to produce more alters, furthering dissociation. If all nurses know about all the alters, they will be able to offer quiet reassurance when angry alters appear.
8. Seeks supervision when countertransference leads to an "enjoyment" of certain alters or a desire to seek them out.	8. Lack of supervision can lead to unconscious encouragement of dissociation.
9. Emphasizes safety, by reassuring clients they are in a safe place. When one alter tries to hurt another, the nurse intervenes.	9. The client must feel safe to abreact. It fosters integration to say, "You are (the core) and (the core) is you. When you hurt (the core), you hurt yourself." This may confuse the client consciously, but will be reassuring on an unconscious level.
10. If the client is being secluded or restrained, and another, calmer alter appears, the nurse goes ahead with the restrictions, explaining it is for protection, not punishment.	10. Reassures that client is in a safe environment.
11. When child alters appear, the client is kept on the unit and away from others.	11. Protects client from embarrassment.
12. Avoids situations that may be seen by the client as intrusive or assaultive.	12. These clients have often been abused and are sensitive to situations where they are overpowered.
13. Avoids physical contact with client.	13. Owing to history of abuse, this can be seen as intrusive, controlling, or seductive, and may increase anxiety.
14. Helps the client combat loneliness by remaining emotionally available.	14. Because of their bizarre and sometimes unpredictable behavior, these clients are often avoided and shunned by others.
15. Avoids being overly nice or solicitous but rather remains kind and neutral.	15. Owing to emotional vulnerability, neediness, and suggestibility, clients can become extremely dependent.
16. When clients request PRN medications, helps clients explore the feelings that may have led to the symptoms, or the history that is being abreacted.	16. When clients remember or abreact abuse, they feel the same pain they felt earlier. The nurse might say, "It's okay to remember what happened without feeling the pain."

From Lego, S. (1988). Multiple personality disorder: An interpersonal approach to etiology, treatment, and nursing care. *Archives of Psychiatric Nursing, 2* (4), 231–235.

TABLE 29-3
Milieu Management of Clients with Dissociative Identity Disorder

INTERVENTION	RATIONALE
1. A contract is negotiated with the entire personality system, i.e., all alters, to cover: • the reason for admission • an agreement to cooperate with unit rules • the criteria for discharge	1. Owing to loose boundaries, these clients require very clear structure.
2. The client is given a private room if possible.	2. The room serves as a refuge from unit turmoil, a place for alters to emerge inconspicuously, and eliminates the potential for roommate problems.
3. The staff is informed about the diagnosis as soon as possible. Concerns are aired and discussed, and staff members are told they may find themselves split about how to handle the client. The therapist encourages staff to call with any concerns or during any crisis.	3. Staff members often behave differently with these clients than with others, having strong countertransference reactions. Communication across disciplines and among staff members is very important.
4. Staff members are told they need not interact with separate alters, and the client is told not to expect they will.	4. Alters must learn to deal with others who do not know about DID. This also discourages staff from behavior based on a fascination with alters, and discourages separateness.
5. A primary nurse or case manager coordinates the client's care on each shift. Alters are introduced to these persons and encouraged to call on them in a crisis.	5. Consistency and coordination are needed to avoid the potential confusion when the client has a number of alters.
6. The therapist explains the unit rules to the personality system including all alters. When unit rules are broken, nonpunitive consequences are enforced.	6. Reinforces structure and consistency.
7. Home visits and passes are restricted until the client has been stabilized on the unit.	7. Avoids elopement and suicidal risk.
8. Client is not included in group therapy.	8. These clients are disruptive and do not benefit from heterogeneous groups.
9. Client is included in therapeutic community (TC) meetings, art, music, occupational, or movement therapy.	9. These clients do benefit from TC and from nonverbal group therapies where they can express feelings about past trauma.
10. Staff members are encouraged to document the client's behavior carefully.	10. Alters unknown to the therapist may be discovered, as well as talents or abilities (for example, a neurological disability was ruled out by observations by the staff that the client could perform certain activities.)

From Putnam, R. W. (1989). *Diagnosis and Treatment of Multiple Personality Disorder.* New York: Guilford Press.

The overall goal of our work with DID clients is to help them integrate all their feelings and experiences and to prevent further dissociation. This is done by relating in an honest, open way, ever mindful of the client's tendency to dissociate to avoid pain.

REFERENCES

American Psychiatric Association (1994). *Diagnostic and Statistical Manual of Mental Disorders* (4th ed.). Washington, DC: American Psychiatric Association.

Confer, W. M., & Ables, B. S. (1983). *Multiple Personality: Etiology, Diagnosis, and Treatment.* New York: Human Sciences Press.

Kluft, R. P. (1984). An introduction to multiple personality disorder. *Psychiatric Annals, 14,* 19–24.

Lego, S. (1988). Multiple personality disorder: An interpersonal approach to etiology, treatment, and nursing care. *Archives of Psychiatric Nursing, 2* (4), 231–235.

Putnam, R. W. (1989). *Diagnosis and Treatment of Multiple Personality Disorder.* New York: Guilford Press.

BIBLIOGRAPHY

Casey, J. F., & Wilson, L. (1991). *The Flock: The Autobiography of Multiple Personality Disorder.* New York: Alfred A. Knopf.

Clark, M. H. (1992). *All Around the Town* (novel). New York: Pocket Books.

THIRTY

The Client Who Is Addicted to Alcohol

Ona Z. Riggin

OVERVIEW:

INTRODUCTION

The client is considered to be addicted to alcohol when a pattern of pathologic use occurs that impairs social, psychological, and occupational functioning. Alcoholism is characterized by chronic, progressive, and potentially fatal biogenic and psychosocial impairment. Tolerance and psychological and physical dependence lead to loss of control, distorted thinking, and other familial and social consequences.

INCIDENCE

Substance abuse is the number one health problem in the United States. The cost of substance abuse has been estimated to be $238 billion per year of which $99 billion is attributed to alcohol (Brady, 1995). It is estimated that 18 million individuals are heavy drinkers and approximately 10 million of this number are alcoholics. High school seniors and young adults ages 18–25 are at highest risk.

ETIOLOGY

Current literature on substance abuse indicates that no one theory adequately explains the etiology for alcoholism. Recent research findings place increasing emphasis on the genetic predisposition to alcoholism and biochemical causation as opposed to psychological and behavioral theories.

BIOLOGICAL THEORIES

Jellinek (1960) proposed that some individuals have a predisposition to alcoholism. He conjectured that alcoholism resulted from an addiction process that was characterized by "loss of control" over the use of alcohol. Jellinek (1977) proposed that individuals pass through progressive stages:

1. Prealcoholic symptomatic phase
2. Prodromal phase
3. Crucial phase
4. Chronic phase

Twin studies and adoption studies reinforced Jellinek's theory. Early studies that indicated a genetic component in the development of alcoholism were reported by Goodwin, Schulsinger, Hermansen, Guze, and Winokur (1973), and Goodwin, Schulsinger, Moller, Hermansen, Winoker, and Guze (1974). Schuckit (1985) reported that children of alcoholics are four times more likely to become alcoholic even when raised in nonalcoholic homes. A strong relation between a low response to alcohol and the later development of alcohol dependence or abuse was reported by Schuckit (1994).

PSYCHOLOGICAL THEORIES

Psychological explanations for the "alcoholic personality" have been sought through extensive research. To date no one personality profile has been identified.

Freud believed people used alcohol excessively to release inhibitions and express repressed urges. Other psychoanalysts emphasized the passive dependent personality traits and extreme oral needs of alcoholic clients.

Still other personality theories focus primarily on the fact that clients with alcoholism experience early childhood rejection, overprotection, or premature responsibility resulting in inadequate personalities and dependency. The individual attempts to counterbalance feelings of inadequacy and turns to alcohol and other substances to compensate for feelings of rejection. Initially alcohol provides feelings of strength, self-worth, and power. Over time increasing amounts of alcohol are required to maintain the positive effects. The individual becomes addicted to alcohol and experiences feelings of self-deprecation, guilt, shame, remorse, and self-hatred as family, peer, and social relationships deteriorate.

BEHAVIOR THEORIES

Learning theories based on operant conditioning models and modeling theory provide further explanation for alcoholism. In accordance with these theories alcohol use is reinforced through the positive effect of mood alterations that occur as the result of chemical alterations in the body. Differential reinforcement of alcohol occurs through many levels including peer group pressures, ready availability of alcohol in the home, and media portrayals of the "good times" that result from alcohol consumption. Youth frequently model behaviors of parents, extended family members, and authority figures who use alcohol on a regular basis.

FAMILY THEORIES

Most family theories incorporate biological and learning theories. Bowen's (1978) work on family systems theory concerning the role of dysfunctional family systems and lack of individual differentiation provides a potential explanation for alcoholism. Quinn, Kuehl, Thomas, Joanning, and Newfield (1989) noted that enmeshed families' interactional patterns do not permit individuals to establish "distance-regulating mechanisms." The use of alcohol requires the family's attention and may promote increased pseudocloseness of the members.

PERINATAL ALCOHOL USE

The use of alcohol during pregnancy has potentially negative consequences for the unborn infant. Since most perinatal drug users use a number of substances, e.g., cocaine, marijuana, nicotine, etc., it is difficult to predict the outcomes for a specific substance on the offspring. However, it is known that fetal alcohol syndrome and fetal alcohol effects that adversely affect the infant's, child's, and adolescent's neurological and intellectual development are completely preventable if the mother abstains from using alcohol during pregnancy. Infants born with fetal alcohol syndrome present with the following characteristics: microcephaly (head circumference below the third percentile), microthalmia, small eyes and/or short palpebral fissures, poorly developed philtrum, thin upper lip, short nose, small chin, and flattening of the maxillary area. These individuals continue to experience a variety of learning and behavioral problems throughout life (Streissguth, 1978).

DIAGNOSTIC CRITERIA

See Box 30-1 for diagnostic criteria of alcohol dependence and Box 30-2 for diagnostic criteria of alcohol abuse.

BOX 30-1: DSM-IV Criteria for Alcohol Dependence

The DSM-IV describes alcohol dependence as a maladaptive pattern of use leading to significant impairment or distress, when three or more of the following seven items occur in the same 12-month period:

1. Tolerance can be evidenced either as (a) a need for markedly increased amounts of alcohol to achieve intoxication or the desired effect, or (b) diminished effect with continued use of the same amount.
2. Withdrawal leads to (a) characteristic signs of alcohol withdrawal, or (b) the use of the same or closely related substance to relieve or avoid withdrawal.
3. Drinking occurs in larger amounts or over a longer period than was intended.
4. There is persistent desire or unsuccessful efforts to cut down or control drinking.
5. A great deal of time is spent in activities related to drinking, or recovering from drinking episodes.
6. Important social, occupational, or recreational activities are given up or reduced due to drinking.
7. Drinking continues even when it is known that physical or psychological problems are caused by or aggravated by continued use.

Adapted for alcohol from American Psychiatric Association (1994). *Diagnostic and Statistical Manual of Mental Disorders* (4th ed.). Washington, DC: American Psychiatric Association.

BOX 30-2: DSM-IV Criteria for Alcohol Abuse

The DSM-IV describes alcohol abuse as:

A. A maladaptive pattern of use leading to significant clinical impairment or distress, when one or more of the following have occurred in a 12-month period:

   1. Recurrent drinking that results in a failure to fulfill major role obligations at work, school, or home.

   2. Recurrent drinking when it is physically hazardous, such as while driving, or operating a machine when impaired by substance use.

   3. Recurrent alcohol-related legal problems.

   4. Continued drinking despite persistent social or interpersonal problems caused or exacerbated by the effects of alcohol.

B. The symptoms have never met the criteria for substance dependence for this class of substance.

Adapted for alcohol from American Psychiatric Association (1994). *Diagnostic and Statistical Manual of Mental Disorders* (4th ed.). Washington, DC: American Psychiatric Association.

ADDICTIVE BEHAVIORS

Clients addicted to alcohol display the following addictive behaviors:

1. Psychological dependence evidenced by needing alcohol to "feel good."
2. Physiological dependence evidenced by tolerance, i.e., the need to consume increasing amounts of alcohol to gain the same effect.
3. Impairment of social relationships including family, peer, and significant others.
4. Decreased social and occupational functioning, leading to disruption with family and loss of job.
5. Increased use of defense mechanisms to explain behavior including rationalization, projection, and denial, among others.
6. Increased feelings of inadequacy, leading to feelings of anxiety, guilt, shame, and remorse.
7. Protective measures to ensure an adequate supply of alcohol, such as sneaking drinks, hiding bottles, and engaging in devious and illegal behaviors to obtain alcohol.
8. Physical (bodily) alterations, i.e., sleep disturbance, eating disorders, and sexual dysfunction including impotence.
9. Secondary complications of alcohol, e.g., gastrointestinal disturbances, liver dysfunction, pancreatitis, cardiac problems, neuromuscular problems, etc.
10. Other behavioral changes: mood changes and mood variations, antisocial behavior, aggressiveness, impulsiveness, lowered frustration levels, abusive behaviors, grandiosity, omnipotence, resentments.
11. Late behavioral changes: blackouts, i.e., temporary amnesia or loss of memory for a period of time.
12. Withdrawal symptoms, including tremors, sweating, fever, rapid pulse, increased blood pressure, disorientation, delusions, and hallucinations. If untreated, toxic symptoms may lead to grand mal seizures, cardiovascular collapse, and possibly death.

ASSESSMENT

ASSESSMENT SCALES FOR PRIMARY CARE SETTINGS

Assessment for alcohol abuse should be included in all health assessments. The type and depth of assessment depends on the health care setting and the purpose of the assessment. In primary health care settings screening instruments can be used to quickly identify potential problems. When screening is positive, additional assessment of the amount, quantity, and longevity of alcohol use is required. In a clinical setting assessment data are used to make a definitive diagnosis and to outline a treatment plan.

Several instruments have been developed to screen for alcohol use, abuse, or dependence including the CAGE questionnaire, the Michigan Alcohol Screening Test (MAST), and the Alcohol Use Disorders Inventory Test (AUDIT).

The CAGE questionnaire (Box 30-3) is probably the most frequently used screening instrument. It is simple to use and has good reliability, validity, and sensitivity (Ewing, 1984). A positive response to one question indicates that the client has a potential problem with alcohol. An affirmative response to two of the CAGE questions correctly identifies 75% of clients with an alcohol problem.

BOX 30-3: CAGE Screening Test for Alcoholism

1. Have you ever felt you ought to *C*ut down on your drinking?

2. Have people *A*nnoyed you by criticizing your drinking?

3. Have you ever felt bad or *G*uilty about your drinking?

4. Have you ever had a drink first thing in the morning to steady your nerves or get rid of a hangover (*E*ye-opener)?

Source: Ewing, J. A. (1984). Detecting alcoholism: The CAGE questionnaire. *Journal of the American Medical Association, 252* (14), 1905–1907.

The Michigan Alcohol Screening Test (MAST), developed by Selzer in 1971, is another screening instrument widely used to identify alcohol use. The short MAST (SMAST) (Selzer, Vinoker, & Van Rooijen, 1975) contains 13 items and is self-administered (Box 30-4). Five or more positive responses place the individual in an "alcoholic" category. Four positive responses suggest a potential problem with alcohol and need for further follow-up. Three or fewer positive responses indicate that the individual does not have a problem with alcohol.

The Alcohol Use Disorders Identification Test (AUDIT) was developed as a part of the World Health Organization collaborative project to identify early problem drinkers (Babor, de la Fuente, Saunders, & Grant, 1989; Babor & Grant, 1989). The AUDIT is an easily administered 10-item questionnaire that assesses consumption, use, and consequences of drinking (Box 30-5). The client education brochure that accompanies the questionnaire recommends maximum safe levels of drinking for men and women in terms of standard drinks. A standard drink contains approximately 1 ounce of pure alcohol. One 12-ounce can of ordinary beer, a single shot of spirits, i.e., whiskey, gin, vodka, etc., a 6-ounce glass of wine, a 4-ounce glass of sherry, or a 4-ounce glass of liqueur constitutes a standard drink (Brown, 1992).

BOX 30-4: Short Michigan Alcoholism Screening Test (SMAST)

1. Do you feel you are a normal drinker? (By normal we mean you drink less than or as much as most other people) (No.)

2. Does your wife, husband, a parent, or other near relative ever worry or complain about your drinking? (Yes.)

3. Do you ever feel guilty about your drinking? (Yes.)

4. Do friends or relatives think you are a normal drinker? (No.)

5. Are you able to stop drinking when you want to? (No.)

6. Have you ever attended a meeting of Alcoholics Anonymous? (Yes.)

7. Has drinking ever created problems between you and your wife, husband, a parent, or other near relatives? (Yes.)

8. Have you ever gotten into trouble at work because of drinking? (Yes.)

9. Have you ever neglected your obligations, your family, or your work for 2 or more days in a row because you were drinking? (Yes.)

10. Have you ever gone to anyone for help about your drinking? (Yes.)

11. Have you ever been in a hospital because of drinking? (Yes.)

12. Have you ever been arrested for drunken driving, driving while intoxicated, or driving under the influence of alcoholic beverages? (Yes.)

13. Have you ever been arrested, even for a few hours, because of other drunken behavior? (Yes.)

From Selzer, M. L., Vinokur, A., & Van Rooijen, L. (1975). A self-administered short Michigan Alcoholism Screening Test (SMAST). *Journal of Studies on Alcohol, 36* (1), 117–126. Copyright 1975 by Alcohol Research Documentation, Inc., Rutgers Center of Alcohol Studies, Piscataway, NJ 08855.

ASSESSMENT INSTRUMENTS FOR CLINICAL SETTINGS

Two frequently used assessment instruments in clinical settings with individuals who have a problem with alcohol are:

A. The Diagnostic Interview Schedule (DIS), a broad interview schedule used for diagnostic and research purposes to determine psychiatric diagnosis. The DIS contains an alcohol dependence subscale (Robins, Helzer, Croughan, & Ratcliff, 1981).

B. The Addiction Severity Index (ASI), a semistructured interview designed to assess alcohol and drug use and the medical, psychological, and legal complications of use within the family, employment, and social setting (McLellan et al., 1992).

LABORATORY TESTS

Laboratory tests used to assess the physiological effect of alcohol on the body include liver function tests and the mean corpuscular volume. Common liver function tests are the gamma glutamyl transferase (GGT), the aspartate amino transferase (AST), and the alanine amino transferase (ALT). Of these the GGT is the most effective to determine heavy alcohol use because it is consistently elevated in heavy drinkers. The mean corpuscular volume (MCV), an index of red blood cell production, is elevated in the early stages of alcohol abuse. This occurs because alcohol suppresses bone marrow and directly affects the production of red blood cells (Brown, 1992).

BOX 30-5: The Alcohol Use Disorders Identification Test (AUDIT)

1. How often do you have a drink containing alcohol?
   (0) Never   (1) Monthly or less   (2) Two to four times a month
   (3) Two to three times a week   (4) Four or more times a week

2. How many drinks containing alcohol do you have on a typical day when you are drinking?
   (0) 1 or 2   (1) 3 or 4   (2) 5 or 6   (3) 7 or 9   (4) 10 or more

3. How often do you have six or more drinks on one occasion?
   (0) Never   (1) Less than monthly   (2) Monthly   (3) Weekly
   (4) Daily or almost daily

4. How often during the last year have you found that you were unable to stop drinking once you had started?
   (0) Never   (1) Less than monthly   (2) Monthly   (3) Weekly
   (4) Daily or almost daily

5. How often during the last year have you failed to do what was normally expected from you because of drinking?
   (0) Never   (1) Less than monthly   (2) Monthly   (3) Weekly
   (4) Daily or almost daily

6. How often during the last year have you needed a first drink in the morning to get yourself going after a heavy drinking session?
   (0) Never   (1) Less than monthly   (2) Monthly   (3) Weekly
   (4) Daily or almost daily

7. How often during the last year have you had a feeling of guilt or remorse after drinking?
   (0) Never   (1) Less than monthly   (2) Monthly   (3) Weekly
   (4) Daily or almost daily

8. How often during the last year have you been unable to remember what happened the night before because you had been drinking?
   (0) Never   (1) Less than monthly   (2) Monthly   (3) Weekly
   (4) Daily or almost daily

9. Have you or someone else been injured as the result of your drinking?
   (0) No   (2) Yes, but not in the last year   (3) Yes, during the last year

10. Has a relative, friend, or a doctor or other health worker been concerned about your drinking or suggested you cut down?
    (0) No   (2) Yes, but not in the last year   (3) Yes, during the last year

Source: *AUDIT: The Alcohol Use Disorders Identification Test,* developed by the World Health Organization, AMETHYST project, 1987. From Department of Health and Human Services (1993). *Eighth Special Report to the U.S. Congress on Alcohol and Health* (Contract No. ADM-281-91-0003). Alexandria, VA: U.S. Dept of Health and Human Services.

NURSES' ATTITUDES

It is essential that nurses evaluate their attitudes toward clients who abuse alcohol. If their own value system causes them to be judgmental or to be negative, therapeutic interventions will be difficult, if not impossible. Nurses who were reared in families where alcohol abuse occurred or nurses who have had experiences with alcoholic spouses are especially vulnerable to the manipulative and provocative behaviors these clients display.

It is helpful for nurses to:
1. View alcohol as an illness
2. Evaluate their own attitudes toward clients who abuse alcohol
3. Be open and honest with the client
4. Actively establish rapport with the client
5. Manifest an understanding attitude
6. Help the client learn new coping strategies
7. Help the client participate in diversional activities that will reinforce a new lifestyle
8. Be patient and recognize that relapses may occur
9. Set reasonable and firm limits
10. Avoid moralistic, judgmental behaviors
11. Avoid threats
12. Avoid preaching, nagging, or lecturing
13. Avoid emotional appeals
14. Avoid withdrawal from clients

NURSING INTERVENTIONS FOR INPATIENTS

Table 30-1 describes nursing interventions and theoretical rationales for clients with acute alcohol intoxication.

PSYCHOTHERAPEUTIC INTERVENTIONS

PSYCHOTHERAPY

Individual, group, and family therapy are all acceptable psychotherapeutic interventions with alcoholic clients. Clients with a high level of anxiety, poor coping skills, and a low level of tolerance or clients who have a dual diagnosis usually require individual psychotherapy before group or family therapy. Family therapy is effective, especially if the spouse and family members are supportive of the client and are interested in participating in therapy. Psychotherapy is geared toward helping clients gain a better understanding of self, learn to control anxiety, and develop more effective coping skills.

BEHAVIOR THERAPY

Aversive conditioning with disulfiram (Antabuse) can be used with clients who are in good health, are highly motivated, and need additional help to refrain from using alcohol. The client goes through a conditioning process in which the sight, smell, and odor of alcohol are paired with an emetic. Induced nausea and vomiting serves as an aversion to alcohol. A small amount of alcohol will cause severe nausea and vomiting within 15 minutes of ingestion. More severe symptoms include chest pain, hypotension, syncope, and cardiovascular effects that can lead to death if not treated (Fleming, 1992). Clients are advised to carry a card stating they are on Antabuse and require emergency medical treatment if found in a debilitated state.

12-STEP SUPPORT GROUPS

The original self-help group for alcoholics, Alcoholics Anonymous (AA), was founded in 1935 by two alcoholics. Support and encouragement from others addicted to alcohol helps members abstain from using alcohol. Members work through a 12-step program in which they acknowledge that they are powerless over alcohol. A lifetime commitment to the principles of AA is required for sobriety. Box 30-6 lists the 12 steps involved in ongoing recovery.

TABLE 30-1
Nursing Intervention and Theoretical Rationale with Clients Who Have Acute Alcohol Intoxication

NURSING INTERVENTION	THEORETICAL RATIONALE
Physiological Stability	
1. Assess safety needs and provide necessary restrictions.	Clients require supervision while they are intoxicated owing to confusion, disorientation, motor instability, and impulsive behaviors.
2. Monitor vital signs at indicated intervals.	Clients who are withdrawing from alcohol have the potential to develop elevated temperatures and tachycardia. Temperatures in excess of 100°F and pulse in excess of 100 beats per minute may indicate impending delirium tremens.
3. Assess need for fluids and food; monitor intake and output. Check mucous membranes and skin turgor to determine fluid needs. Do not force fluids if the client does not have signs of dehydration.	Clients who are withdrawing from alcohol require high-calorie diets and may be dehydrated. Since clients are already agitated, this may add to their frustration.
4. Administer medications (antianxiety medications) as ordered or per protocol. Do not undermedicate.	Careful monitoring of vital signs and administration of antianxiety medication reduces the possibility of seizures, delirium tremens, and possible death.
5. Assure adequate rest and relaxation.	Clients who are withdrawing from alcohol experience feelings of agitation and hyperactivity. Measures to induce sleep such as warm baths, darkened rooms, and a quiet environment promote relaxation and sleep.
Delirium Tremens (DTs)	
1. Ascertain as complete a drinking history as possible including amount consumed, duration of drinking episode, time and amount of last drink.	Delirium tremens may occur 24–72 hours post last drink. Prodromal symptoms may occur as early as 6–12 hours after the last drink.
2. Monitor vital signs every 15 minutes if temperature is in excess of 100°F and pulse is in excess of 100 beats per minute.	Elevation of vital signs accompanied by restlessness, tremulousness, hyperalertness, and agitation are signs of impending DTs.
3. Administer antianxiety medication as prescribed based on vital signs.	Careful monitoring of vital signs with administration of antianxiety medication is effective in providing rest and relaxation, reducing symptoms, and preventing grand mal seizures.
4. Maintain a quiet, safe, darkened environment.	Clients who experience DTs are hyperalert; any noises or quick movements are greatly exaggerated, shadows are misinterpreted, and illusions and hallucinations may occur. Clients are prone to injury if not adequately supervised.
5. Assure adequate nutrition and fluid intake.	Clients who experience DTs require small, frequent, high-carbohydrate feedings that are easily digested. Adequate fluid intake is essential; overhydration should be avoided.

Other 12-step groups have evolved to provide support for adolescents (Al-a-Teen) and spouses and significant others (Al-Anon). Likewise, support groups for Adult Children of Alcoholics (ACoA) are available for adults who were reared in alcoholic homes and need help with problems related to low self-esteem, interpersonal difficulties, and codependence.

BOX 30-6: Alcoholics Anonymous Twelve Steps

1. We admitted we were powerless over alcohol, that our lives had become unmanageable.
2. Came to believe that a Power greater than ourselves could restore us to sanity.
3. Made a decision to turn our will and our lives over to the care of God as we understood Him.
4. Made a searching and fearless moral inventory of ourselves.
5. Admitted to God, to ourselves, and to another human being the exact nature of our wrongs.
6. Were entirely ready to have God remove all these defects of character.
7. Humbly asked Him to remove our shortcomings.
8. Made a list of all persons we had harmed, and became willing to make amends to them all.
9. Made direct amends to such people wherever possible, except when to do so would injure them or others.
10. Continued to take personal inventory, and when we were wrong promptly admitted it.
11. Sought through prayer and meditation to improve our conscious contact with God as we understood Him, praying only for knowledge of His will for us and the power to carry that out.
12. Having had a spiritual awakening as the result of these steps, we tried to carry this message to alcoholics and to practice these principles in all our affairs.

The Twelve Steps are reprinted with permission of Alcoholics Anonymous World Services, Inc. Permission to reprint this material does not mean that A.A. has reviewed or approved the contents of this publication, nor that A.A. agrees with the views expressed herein. A.A. is a program of recovery from alcoholism—use of the Twelve Steps in connection with programs and activities which are patterned after A.A., but which address other problems, does not imply otherwise.

USE OF NALTREXONE

Recent clinical trials indicate that naltrexone (REVIA) given to alcoholics is approximately 50% effective in reducing craving and blocking the reinforcing effects of alcohol. Additional research is indicated to determine long-term effects of the drug for maintaining sobriety and for its effect on the individual (Gordis, 1995).

REFERENCES

AUDIT: The Alcohol Use Disorders Identification Test, developed by the World Health Organization collaborative project on identification and treatment of persons with harmful alcohol consumption: United States participation was funded by National Institute on Alcohol Abuse and Alcoholism (P50AA03510).

Babor, T. F., de la Fuente, J. R., Saunders, J, & Grant, M. (1989). AUDIT: The Alcohol Use Disorders Identification Test: Guidelines for Use in Primary Care. Geneva: World Health Organization.

Babor, T. F., & Grant, M. (1989). From clinical research to secondary prevention: International collaboration in the development of the Alcohol Use Disorders Identification Test (AUDIT). Alcohol Health and Research World, 13 (4): 371–374.

Bowen, M. (1978). Family Therapy in Clinical Practice. New York: Jason Aronson.

Brady, K. (1995). Training about alcohol and substance abuse for all primary care physicians. In D. C. Lewis (ed.), Training About Alcohol and Substance Abuse for All Primary Care Physicians. New York: Josiah Macy, Jr. Foundation

Brown, R. L. (1992). Identification and office management of alcohol and drug disorders. In M. F. Fleming & K. L. Barry (eds.), Addictive Disorders. St. Louis: C. V. Mosby Co.

Ewing, J. A. (1984). Detecting alcoholism: The CAGE questionnaire, *Journal of the American Medical Association, 252* (14), 1905–1907.

Fleming, M. F. (1992). Pharmacologic management of nicotine, alcohol and other drug dependence. In M. F. Fleming & K. L. Barry (eds.), *Addictive Disorders.* St. Louis: C. V. Mosby Co.

Goodwin D. W., Schulsinger, F., Hermansen, L., Guze, S. B., & Winokur, G. (1973). Alcohol problems in adoptees raised apart from biological parents. *Archives of General Psychiatry 28,* 228.

Goodwin, D. W., Schulsinger, F., Moller, N., Hermansen, L., Winokur, G., & Guze, S. (1974). Drinking problems in adopted and nonadopted sons of alcoholics. *Archives of General Psychiatry, 31,* 164.

Gordis, E. (February 1995). Letter to colleagues announcing preliminary research findings for supported trials at University of Pennsylvania and Yale University funded by NIAAA.

Jellinek, E. M. (1960). *The Disease Concept of Alcoholism.* New Haven, CT: Hillhouse Press.

Jellinek, E. M. (1977). Phases of alcohol addiction. *Quarterly Journal of Studies on Alcohol, 38,* 114–130.

McLellan, T. A., Kushner, H., Metzger, D., Peters, R., Smith, I., Grissom, G., Pettinati, H., & Argeriou, M. (1992). The fifth edition of the Addiction Severity Index. *Journal of Substance Abuse Treatment, 9,* 199–213.

Quinn, W. H., Kuehl, B., Thomas, F., Joanning, H., & Newfield, N. (1989). Family treatment of adolescent drug abuse: Transitions and maintenance of drug free behavior. *American Journal of Family Therapy, 17* (3), 229–243.

Robins, L. N., Helzer, J. E., Croughan, J., & Ratcliff, K. S. (1981). National Institute of Mental Health Diagnostic Interview Schedule: Its history, characteristics, and validity. *Archives of General Psychiatry, 38,* 381–389.

Schuckit, M. (1985). Genetics and the role for alcoholism. *Journal of the American Medical Association, 254* (18), 2614–2617.

Schuckit, M. A. (1994). Low level response to alcohol as a predictor of future alcoholism. *American Journal of Psychiatry, 15,* 184–189.

Selzer, M. L. (1971). The Michigan Alcoholism Screening Test: The quest for a new diagnostic instrument. *American Journal of Psychiatry, 127* (12), 1653–1658.

Selzer, M. L., Vinokur, A., & Van Rooijen, L. (1975). A self administered Short Michigan Screening Test (SMAST). *Journal of Studies on Alcohol, 36* (1), 117–126.

Streissguth, A. (1978). Fetal alcohol syndrome: An epidemiologic perspective. *American Journal of Epidemiology, 107,* 467–477.

BIBLIOGRAPHY

Beck, A. T., Wright, F. D., Newman, C. F., & Liese, B. S. (1993). *Cognitive Therapy of Substance Abuse.* New York: Guilford Press.

Bennett, G., & Woolf, D. (1991). *Substance Abuse.* Albany, NY: Delmar Publishers.

Department of Health and Human Services (1993). *Eighth Special Report to the U.S. Congress on Alcohol and Health* (Contract No. ADM-281-91-0003). Alexandria, VA: U.S. Dept of Health & Human Services.

Fitzgerald, K. W. (1993). *Alcoholism: The Genetic Inheritance.* Lake Forest, IL: Whales Tales Press.

Fleming, M. F., & Barry, K. L. (1992). *Addictive Disorders.* St. Louis: C.V. Mosby Co.

Kaij, L. (1960). *Alcoholism in Twins. Studies on the Etiology and Sequelae of Abuse of Alcohol.* Stockholm, Sweden: Alonquist and Winkell Publishers.

Kaufman, E. (1994). *Psychotherapy of Addicted Persons.* New York: Guilford Press.

Kinney, J., & Leaton, G. (1995). *Loosening the Grip: A Handbook of Alcohol Information* (5th ed.). St Louis: Mosby.

May, G. (1988). *Addictions and Grace.* San Francisco: Harper.

Robins, L. N., Helzer, J. E., Cotler, L., & Goldring, E. (1989). *NIMH Diagnostic Interview Schedule, Version III, Revised.* St. Louis: Washington University.

Sullivan, E. (1995). *Nursing Care of Clients with Substance Abuse.* St. Louis: Mosby.

Thombs, D. L. (1994). *Introduction to Addictive Behaviors.* New York: Guilford Press.

31

THIRTY ONE

The Client Who Is Abusing Substances Other Than Alcohol

Ona Z. Riggin

OVERVIEW:

Description
Amphetamines
Barbiturates
Cocaine
Inhalant-Related Disorders
Marijuana
Nicotine-Related Disorders

Opiate-Related Disorders
Methadone Treatment
Phencyclidine-Related Disorders
Caffeine
Designer Drugs
Steroids
Nursing Interventions

DESCRIPTION

Substance abuse is a maladaptive pattern of substance use that affects the central nervous system and alters the individual's perceptions. It is characterized by pathologic use and impairment in role functions, interpersonal interactions, social responsibility, and occupational functioning.

Abused substances commonly referred to as "mood-altering" substances include both natural and synthetic drugs and substances that stimulate or depress the central nervous system and affect one's mood, thought processes, and judgment.

The *Diagnostic and Statistical Manual of Mental Disorders* (American Psychiatric Association, 1994) provides diagnostic criteria for each class of substance relative to dependence, abuse, intoxication, and withdrawal in addition to criteria for substance-induced disorders relative to delirium, psychosis, mood, anxiety, sleep, and sexual dysfunction. Table 31-1 shows diagnoses associated with classes of substances. Table 31-2 provides the classifications of abused substances from the DSM-IV with symptoms of intoxication and withdrawal. Table 31-3 shows generic and street names for commonly abused substances.

(Text continues on page 268)

TABLE 31-1
Diagnoses Associated with Classes of Substances

	Depen-dence	Abuse	Intoxi-cation	With-drawal	Intoxi-cation Delirium	With-drawal Delirium	Dementia	Amnestic Disorder	Psychotic Disorders	Mood Disorders	Anxiety Disorders	Sexual Dysfunc-tions	Sleep Disorders
Alcohol	X	X	X	X	I	W	P	P	I/W	I/W	I/W	I	I/W
Amphetamines	X	X	X	X	I				I	I/W	I	I	I/W
Caffeine			X								I		I
Cannabis	X	X	X		I				I		I		
Cocaine	X	X	X	X	I				I	I/W	I/W	I	I/W
Hallucinogens	X	X	X		I				I*	I	I		
Inhalants	X	X	X		I		P		I	I	I		
Nicotine	X			X									
Opioids	X	X	X	X	I				I	I		I	I/W
Phencyclidine	X	X	X		I				I	I	I		
Sedatives, hypnotics, or anxiolytics	X	X	X	X	I	W	P	P	I/W	I/W	W	I	I/W
Polysubstance	X												
Other	X	X	X	X	I	W	P	P	I/W	I/W	I/W	I	I/W

*Also Hallucinogen Persisting Perception Disorder (Flashbacks).

Note: X, I, W, I/W, or P indicates that the category is recognized in the DSM-IV. In addition, I indicates that the specifier With Onset During Intoxication may be noted for the category (except for Intoxication Delirium); W indicates that the specifier With Onset During Withdrawal may be noted for the category (except for Withdrawal Delirium); and I/W indicates that either With Onset During Intoxication or With Onset During Withdrawal may be noted for the category. P indicates that the disorder is Persisting.

American Psychiatric Association (1994). *Diagnostic and Statistical Manual of Mental Disorders* (4th ed.). Washington, DC: American Psychiatric Association.

TABLE 31-2
Abused Substances: Symptoms of Intoxication and Withdrawal

SUBSTANCE	INTOXICATION	WITHDRAWAL
Amphetamine	1. euphoria or affective blunting 2. changes in sociability 3. hypervigilance 4. interpersonal sensitivity 5. anxiety, tension, or anger 6. stereotyped behaviors 7. impaired judgment 8. impaired social or occupational functioning 9. psychomotor agitation 10. tachycardia 11. pupillary dilation	1. dysphoric mood 2. fatigue 3. vivid, unpleasant dreams 4. insomnia or hypersomnia 5. increased appetite 6. psychomotor retardation or agitation 7. anhedonia 8. drug craving 9. lassitude 10. depression 11. weight loss
Caffeine	1. restlessness 2. nervousness 3. excitement 4. insomnia 5. flushed face 6. diuresis 7. gastrointestinal disturbance 8. muscle twitching 9. rambling flow of thought and speech 10. tachycardia or cardiac arrhythmia 11. periods of inexhaustibility 12. psychomotor agitation	1. headache 2. listlessness 3. lack of energy

(Continued)

TABLE 31-2 (continued)

SUBSTANCE	INTOXICATION	WITHDRAWAL
Cannabis (marijuana)	1. impaired motor coordination 2. euphoria (drowsiness) 3. anxiety (jitteryness) 4. sensation of slowed time 5. impaired judgment 6. disinhibition 7. conjunctival injection 8. increased appetite 9. dry mouth 10. tachycardia 11. positive urine tests 12. sinusitis, persistent cough, bronchitis	Following several weeks of high-dose use: 1. addictive craving 2. emotional lability 3. anxiety 4. restlessness 5. headache 6. insomnia 7. mild gastrointestinal upset
Cocaine	1. euphoria 2. hypervigilance 3. impaired judgment 4. interpersonal insensitivity 5. tachycardia or bradycardia 6. pupillary dilation 7. elevated or lowered blood pressure 8. perspiration or chills 9. nausea or vomiting 10. psychomotor agitation or retardation 11. muscular weakness, respiratory depression, chest pain, or cardiac arrhythmias 12. confusion, seizures, dyskinesias, dystonias, or coma	1. dysphoric mood 2. fatigue 3. vivid, unpleasant dreams 4. insomnia or hypersomnia 5. increased appetite 6. psychomotor retardation or agitation 7. anhedonia 8. drug craving Acute withdrawal symptoms—"crash": 1. intense feelings of lassitude and depression 2. suicidal ideation
Hallucinogens	Recent use or during use of hallucinogens: 1. marked anxiety or depression 2. ideas of reference 3. fear of losing one's mind 4. paranoid ideation 5. impaired judgment 6. restlessness 7. nausea 8. tachycardia 9. sweating 10. blurring of vision 11. palpitations 12. incoordination	Hallucinogen Persisting Perception Disorder, Flash-backs (reexperiencing one or more of the perceptual symptoms following cessation of use): 1. false perceptions of movement in peripheral visual field 2. flashes of color, vivid colors 3. trails of images of moving objects 4. halos
Inhalants	Recent intentional use or high-dose exposure to volatile inhalants: 1. belligerence 2. assaultiveness 3. apathy 4. impaired judgment 5. dizziness or visual disturbance 6. nystagmus 7. incoordination 8. slurred speech 9. unsteady gait 10. tremor 11. euphoria	Chronic use not associated with consistent abstinence syndrome

TABLE 31-2 *(continued)*

SUBSTANCE	INTOXICATION	WITHDRAWAL
Inhalants (continued)	Higher doses: 1. lethargy 2. psychomotor retardation 3. generalized muscle weakness 4. depressed reflexes 5. stupor and coma	
Nicotine	Secondary effects of smoking: 1. bronchitis 2. chronic obstructive lung disorder 3. cardiovascular problems 4. cancer 5. stroke	Abrupt cessation of nicotine use, or reduction in the amount of nicotine used, following daily use for several weeks: 1. dysphoric or depressed mood 2. insomnia 3. irritability, frustration, or anger 4. anxiety 5. difficulty concentrating 6. restlessness 8. decreased heart rate 8. increased appetite or weight gain 9. craving
Opioid	Recent use of an opioid: 1. initial euphoria followed by apathy 2. dysphoria 3. psychomotor agitation or retardation 4. impaired judgment Pupillary constriction (or pupillary dilation due to anoxia from severe overdose) and one (or more) of the following signs, developing during or shortly after opioid use: 1. drowsiness or coma 2. slurred speech 3. impairment in attention or memory	Cessation of opioid use or reduction in use following heavy use: 1. dysphoric mood 2. anxiety, restlessness 3. craving 4. severe muscle aches and cramps 5. lacrimation or rhinorrhea 6. pupillary dilation 7. piloerection 8. diarrhea, nausea, vomiting 9. yawning 10. fever (sweating) 11. insomnia 12. serious depression with suicidal risk
Phencyclidine	1. belligerence 2. assaultiveness 3. impulsiveness 4. unpredictability 5. psychomotor agitation 6. impaired judgment 7. confused and bizarre behavior 8. vertical or horizontal nystagmus 9. hypertension or tachycardia 10. numbness or diminished responsiveness to pain 11. ataxia, dysarthria, or muscle rigidity 12. cardiovascular and neurological seizures 13. respiratory problems	1. cold sweats 2. upset stomach 3. tremor

Adapted from American Psychiatric Association (1994). *Diagnostic and Statistical Manual of Mental Disorders* (4th ed.). Washington, DC: American Psychiatric Association; and Brust, D. M. (1993). *Neurological Aspects of Substance Abuse.* Boston: Butterworth–Heineman.

TABLE 31-3
Generic and Street or Slang Names for Frequently Abused Substances

CLASS	GENERIC OR TRADE NAME	STREET OR SLANG NAME
Amphetamines and related drugs	Amphetamine (Benzedrine)	Bennies, beans, black beauties, footballs
	Methamphetamine (Desoxy Methedrine)	Speed, crystal, meth, eye openers
	Dextroamphetamine (Dexadrine)	Dexies, hearts, Christmas trees, pep pills, uppers, wake-ups
	Ritalin	
Anxiolytics	Chlordiazepoxide (Librium)	Libs
	Diazepam (Valium)	Blues (10 mg), yellows (5 mg), whites (2 mg)
	Meprobamate (Miltown, Equanil), Oxazepam (Serax)	
Barbiturates	Amobarbital	Red and blues, rainbows, double trouble, tooies
	Phenobarbital	Yellowjackets, yellows, nembies
	Secobarbital	Reds, red devils, seggy's, downers, redbirds
Cannabinols	Cannabis, marijuana	Acapulco gold, cannabis, Colombian, grass, hemp, joint, mota, mutah, Panama, red, reefer, pot, smoke, stick, weed, yerba
	Hashish	Rope, sweet Lucy
Hallucinogens	Phencyclidine	PCP, angel dust, hog, peace pill
	Mescaline (peyote)	Big chief, cactus, half moon
	Lysergic acid diethylamide (LSD)	Acid, hawk, royal blue, sugar cubes, pearly gates, instant zen, blotter acid, purple haze
	Psilocybin	Magic mushrooms
	Dimethoxymethyl amphetamine	DOM, STP ("serenity, tranquility, peace")
	Dimethyltryptamine	DMT
Cocaine	Cocaine, crack	Coke, flake, girl, snow, dust, happy dust, gold dust, blow, "c", coca, rock, lady
Opioids and related analgesics	Heroin	Horse, smack, junk
	Morphine	Morf, white stuff, monkey
	Codeine	Lords, little D
	Hydromorphine (Dilandid)	
	Meperidine (Demerol)	Demies
	Oxycodone (Percodan)	Perkies
Inhalants	Glue	
Nicotine	Tobacco products	

AMPHETAMINES   Amphetamines were first marketed in 1932 under the trade name Benzedrine. Drugs included in this classification are central nervous system (CNS) stimulants and they comprise a family of drugs similar to catecholamines (epinephrine and norepinephrine) released by the sympathetic nervous system under stress. Amphetamines cause an increase in heart and respiration rates and blood pressure, pupil dilation, increased locomotor activity, hyperglycemia, sleeplessness, and bronchodilation (Brust, 1993).

Amphetamines are administered orally, intravenously, or through inhalation. Benzedrine, if taken orally, reaches its peak effect in 1 hour and lasts for several hours. Methamphetamine, known as "speed," has a longer half-life (6–12 hr), stronger CNS effects, and fewer peripheral effects. An immediate sense of pleasure occurs if the drug is injected intravenously or if it is inhaled in its purest form ("ice"). Individuals develop tolerance to the drug and addiction is rapid (Cho, 1990). Overdoses call for emergency measures and may be life-threatening.

BARBITURATES

Barbiturates are classified as sedative hypnotics. They were introduced in 1903 and used as hypnotics, sedatives, and anticonvulsants. Barbital (Veronal) was the first barbiturate followed by phenobarbital in 1912. Phenobarbital and barbital are long-acting drugs with a half-life of 12–24 hours. Amobarbital (Amytal) has an intermediate active half-life of 6–12 hours and pentobarbital (Nembutal) and secobarbital (Seconal) are short-acting drugs with a half-life of 3–6 hours (Kaplan & Sadock, 1991).

Barbiturates are frequently abused drugs because they are legitimately manufactured in large quantities, available in many forms, and readily obtained through black market outlets where the strength is unknown because the drug has been replaced with sugar and other substances. Secobarbital, phenobarbital, and amobarbital are the three most frequently abused barbiturates.

In 1914 barbiturates were classified as controlled substances under the Harrison Narcotic Act. Since that time, both abuse and prescriptive use has diminished (Kaplan & Sadock, 1991).

Barbiturate abuse occurs most frequently among young users who use the drug to experience a high or who substitute barbiturates for heroin or morphine because they are cheaper and more readily available. Middle-aged individuals sometimes obtain prescriptions from physicians for anxiety or insomnia and become dependent on the drug. Barbiturates have a cross-tolerance to other drugs including alcohol, benzodiazepines, and heroin. Intravenous users experience a sudden warm "rush" followed by a prolonged drowsy feeling.

Barbiturate intoxication is confirmed by blood tests (Kaplan & Sadock, 1991; Brust, 1993). Barbiturates are especially dangerous drugs because overuse leads to potentially deleterious health effects. They are a common cause of lethal overdoses through accidental ingestion by children and others and are frequently used in suicide attempts. Death occurs as a result of deep coma that progresses to respiratory arrest and cardiovascular failure. Lethal doses vary widely from individual to individual. A narrow therapeutic index exists; the therapeutic dose is very close to the lethal dose (Kaplan & Sadock, 1991).

COCAINE

Cocaine (crack) is a highly addictive alkaloid derived from *Erythroxylon coca,* a plant indigenous to Bolivia and Peru. The addictive properties of cocaine were not fully recognized until the 1980s when both the general public and physicians became aware of the problem. Peak use occurred in 1985 (Jaffe, 1990). By 1988 there were 5000 new cocaine users daily, 6 million were regular users, and nearly 1 million were "compulsive" users (Barnes, 1988).

Cocaine is ingested orally, through inhalation (snorting), subcutaneous or intravenous injections, and smoking (freebasing). Inhalation is the least dangerous and the least effective in producing a "high." The peak occurs in 30 to 160 minutes depending on the strength. For oral ingestion the peak occurs in 60 minutes. "Crack" or "rock," an extremely addictive form of freebase cocaine, appeared in 1985; it is relatively cheap and readily available through drug dealers (Jaffe, 1990).

Cocaine blocks reuptake of dopamine, serotonin, and norepinephrine. An intense feeling of euphoria occurs, which accounts for the highly addictive nature of the drug. A single dose of cocaine, especially in the form of "crack," may cause psychologic dependence. The main effect is relatively brief (30 minutes to an hour) when used intravenously or sniffed. However, cocaine remains in the brain for approximately 10 days. A period of depression occurs after the acute effect, which may precipitate suicidal ideation (Kaplan & Sadock, 1991; Brust, 1993).

Individuals who inhale while they smoke cocaine may experience swelling and inflammation of the nasal passages and ulceration of the nose. Sharing needles frequently causes infection and emboli at the injection sight and predisposes the individual to the risk of contracting human immunodeficiency virus (HIV) disease. Toxic symptoms are usually self-limiting to approximately 24 hours after which time withdrawal symptoms occur, referred to as the "crash" (Jaffe, 1990).

Treatment is multifaceted and requires cooperation by the family, employer, and health professionals. Urine testing for toxicologic analysis is an essential part of continuing treatment. Psychotherapy, family support, and support groups (Cocaine Anonymous [CA]) are useful in helping individuals remain abstinent.

INHALANT-RELATED DISORDERS

Inhalant-related disorders are induced by inhaling the aromatic hydrocarbon toluene and halogenated hydrocarbons found in gasoline, glue, paint thinners, kerazene, spray paints, typewriter correction fluid, spray can propellants, cleaning fluid, and other volatile compounds containing esters, ketones, ethers, and anesthetic gases (Brust, 1993).

Inhalants are ingested through the nasal and oral routes either by sniffing or inhaling the spray. A frequent method is to soak a rag with the substance, place it over the nose and mouth, and inhale the fumes. Individuals who use inhalants become dependent on their use. Physical symptoms resulting from recurrent use are specifically related to the abused substance. Respiratory symptoms including irritated upper and lower airway passages, coughing, sinusitis, dyspnea, rales, and rhonchi frequently occur (American Psychiatric Association, 1994, pp. 239–242).

Inhalants are readily available, cheap, and legal. Their use is most common among adolescents who use the substances in group settings to experience a "high." Solitary use occurs more frequently with long-term and heavy use. Most adolescents are not aware of long-term physical effects noted above. Some inhalants (e.g. methylene chloride) may be metabolized to carbon dioxide, causing respiratory or cardiovascular depression and possible death.

MARIJUANA

Marijuana continues to be the most frequently used illicit drug in the United States. It is obtained from the flowering portion of the hemp plant, *Cannabis sativa,* and can be refined as hashish or hashish oil. The most common route of administration is by inhalation. Marijuana is usually dried and smoked as a cigarette or in a pipe. Special pipes called "bongs" or "hookups" are used to humidify the smoke, permitting deeper inhalation. Effects begin within 10–20 minutes and last 2–3 hours. Ingested marijuana is about one-third as potent and lasts up to 12 hours (Lieberman & Lieberman, 1971).

The exact mechanism of action of the drug in humans is not known. It is believed that it combines with a variety of neurotransmitters in the brain. A brief period of euphoria followed by a sense of relaxation and somnolence occurs. Enhancement of senses, distortion of time and space, confusion, short-term memory impairment, and sexual arousal may occur. Lighter doses have a tendency to be excitatory while heavy doses are inhibitory (Czechowicz, 1991).

The long-term effects of marijuana are not fully understood, as findings from research studies conflict. Dramatic toxic symptoms similar to those observed with opioids and other illicit drugs are rarely observed. The primary concern about marijuana use is that it serves as a "gateway" drug and leads to use of more serious illicit drugs. Attempts to legalize marijuana use continue to be prevalent.

NICOTINE-RELATED DISORDERS

Nicotine is readily available in the form of several tobacco products. Cigarettes are the most commonly used tobacco product; tobacco products are responsible for a high percentage of deaths owing to secondary effects of smoking or chewing tobacco. Nicotine therapy including transcutaneous administration of nicotine via a nicotine patch is frequently used in combination with smoking cessation programs. It is essential that individuals refrain from smoking or use of other tobacco products to prevent an overdose of nicotine when and if they are receiving nicotine through transcutaneous or oral administration.

Successful outcomes of smoking cessation programs with or without prescriptive help are dependent on the individual's desire and motivation to stop smoking. Health care professionals who discuss with clients the health risks associated with smoking and who offer smoking cessation programs experience a high rate of success in helping clients stop. Box 31-1 provides suggestions for smoking cessation (Daugton, Susman, & Sitorius, 1994).

BOX 31-1: Suggestions for Smoking Cessation

1. Set a quit day and resolve that you are not going to smoke on *that* day no matter what.
2. Prepare for the quit day and the first week of quitting.
   - Purchase several packets of gum or chewy candy to be used whenever you experience an intense craving for cigarettes. Weight gain should not be a concern at this stage.
   - Schedule less demanding activities for your first 3 days of quitting.
   - If you work in a smoke-free environment, consider setting your quit day on a workday. If you work in an environment where people regularly smoke, set your quit day on a non-workday.
3. Take several preventive measures during your first 3 weeks of quitting.
   - Avoid situations where people smoke.
   - Monitor your caffeine intake. If you are already feeling extremely anxious, avoid caffeine until your anxiety subsides.
   - If you need something to do with your hands, rub on a smooth rock or use worry beads.
   - Use deep-breathing exercises to help you relax.
   - Carry around a picture of a loved one or a card reminding you of why you are quitting where you normally carry your cigarettes.
   - Be aware that drinking alcohol may weaken your willpower and lead to relapse. Monitor alcohol intake carefully.
   - Increase your level of physical activity.
   - Avoid the normal cues to smoke. For example, if you routinely sit down and light a cigarette when the phone rings, answer the phone standing up.

(Continued)

> **BOX 31-1** *(continued)*
>
> 4. Don't cheat or bum a cigarette.
>   - In doing this you only cheat yourself. Remember that if you cheat and have a single cigarette, the likelihood of quitting is negligible. The single best way to avoid cheating is to get rid of all of your cigarettes.
>   - Remember that cigarettes do not help you handle stress. They only help you fight the physical stress of withdrawal caused by smoking.
> 5. Don't smoke and wear nicotine patches at the same time.
> 6. Remind yourself that the urge to smoke will go away.
> 7. Don't let your cigarette addiction win without a battle!
>
> From Daughton, D. M., Susman, J., Sitorius, M., & Rennard, S. I. (1994). Confronting cigarette addiction: A guide to efficient clinical intervention. *IM—Internal Medicine 9*, 68–79. Copyright Medical Economics Company.

OPIATE-RELATED DISORDERS

Opiates, drugs derived from seeds of the poppy plant, include morphine, codeine, and heroin. The term *opioids* is also used to describe synthetic drugs related to opium such as fentanyl, meperidine, and methadone.

Opioids are CNS depressants that produce a sedative analgesic effect and also cause a "high" with a sense of euphoria, well-being, and sleeplessness. They are highly addictive drugs, especially when used for recreational purposes. Chronic abuse may cause apathy, anorexia, depression, and states of lethargy or anxiety. Overdoses may lead to respiratory depression, cardiovascular arrest, and possible death (Brust, 1993). Oral ingestion and intravenous injection are the two most common routes for taking opiates. They may also be consumed intranasally or by inhalation. Tolerance and dependence occur quickly, especially in individuals who seek the drug for recreational and nonmedicinal uses.

METHADONE TREATMENT

Methadone, a synthetic opioid, continues to be the treatment of choice for morphine and heroin addicts. A daily dose of 20–80 mg is usually sufficient to stabilize a patient. Methadone maintenance is continued until the patient can be withdrawn from methadone. If methadone patients become addicted, they can be withdrawn with the addition of other drugs such as clonidine, an anticonvulsant drug, 0.1–0.3 mg three to four times a day (Kaplan & Sadock, 1991).

PHENCYCLIDINE-RELATED DISORDERS

The phencyclidines or phencyclidine-like substances (PCP, Sernylan) and similar acting compounds such as ketamine (Ketalar, Ketaject) were first developed as dissociative anesthetics in the 1950s, becoming street drugs in the 1960s. Phencyclidines can be ingested orally, smoked, or used intravenously; they are sold illicitly under such names as PCP, Hog, Tranq, Angel Dust, and Peace Pill (American Psychiatric Association, 1994).

Dependence has not been demonstrated in humans, but craving is common. With intravenous use the peak effect begins almost immediately. Peak effect for oral use occurs in 2 hours and lasts 8–20 hours. The half-life for most people is approximately 21 hours, with a range of 11–51 hours (Brust, 1993). Signs and symptoms of severe intoxication may last for several days and may precipitate a phencyclidine-induced psychotic disorder that may exist for weeks (American Psychiatric Association, 1994, pp. 257–258).

CAFFEINE

Caffeine is consumed from a number of different sources. Brewed coffee contains 100 mg/6 oz, tea 40 mg/6 oz, and caffeinated soda 45 mg/12 oz. Chocolate and cocoa contain lesser amounts. Over-the-counter cold medicines and weight-loss aids contain varying amounts of caffeine. Caffeine is a central nervous system stimulant that diminishes fatigue and results in increased clarity of thought.

DESIGNER DRUGS

The label "designer drugs" refers to fentanyl analog drugs that are manufactured by clandestine laboratories and suddenly appear on the street. Most so-called designer drugs are potent reinforcers and are thus addictive. In 1979 drug users in Southern California were sold alpha-methylfentanyl, an analog of fentanyl, when they thought they were purchasing Southern Asia ("China White") heroin. A number of deaths occurred because several of the analogs of fentanyl are more than 1000 times more potent than heroin. They are usually taken intravenously, but may be snorted. Users describe a fainter "rush," longer "nod," and slower "comedown" than that experienced with heroin (LaBarbera & Wolfe, 1983). Health professionals must be cognizant of new drugs available on the street to effectively treat overdoses and prevent death.

STEROIDS

In recent years increasing attention is being given to the use of anabolic androgenic steroids by athletes and developing adolescent males who wish to enhance masculine appearance and maximize physical development. Athletes are disqualified from competitive sports if urine tests are positive for steroids or other illegal drugs.

Several types of anabolic steroids are available through black market sources. Whether they contain the male hormone testosterone or its synthetic forms, they all have similar action at the cellular level. They frequently produce adverse behavioral effects such as confusion, poor judgment, impulsiveness, psychotic symptoms, and extreme aggressiveness ("roid rage"). Some states such as New York have classified steroids as controlled substances. Individuals who abuse steroids use dosages 10 to 100 times that prescribed for therapeutic use. Withdrawal is characterized by severe depression that may continue for 3 months. No specific treatment is available (Kaplan & Sadock, 1991).

NURSING INTERVENTIONS

A nursing care plan for clients with substance use disorders is shown in Table 31-4. Programs and self-help groups for substance abusers include:
1. Betty Ford Treatment Center, Palm Desert, CA
2. Cocaine Anonymous (CA)
3. Hanley–Hazelden Center at St. Mary's, Minneapolis, MN
4. Mentally Ill Chemical Abusers (MICA)
5. Narcotics Anonymous (NA)
6. Phoenix House, New York, NY

TABLE 31-4
Nursing Care Plan for Clients with Substance Use Disorders

NURSING DIAGNOSIS	BEHAVIORS	INTERVENTION
Ineffective coping	Poor self-concept, inadequate coping skills, use of substances as a coping mechanism	• Set realistic, firm limits on manipulative behavior. • Administer consequences if limits are violated. • Help client develop skills to reduce anxiety other than use of substances. • Provide positive reinforcement for use of adaptive coping strategies and constructive behaviors.
Ineffective denial	Verbal denial of substance abuse. Statements like "I don't have a problem with drugs," "I can quit if I want to," "I only drink or smoke pot, etc., to relax," "I smoke because my wife nags me."	• Develop rapport with client, which leads to a mutual trust relationship. • Focus on the dysfunctional behavior of substance abuse, not on the client. • Do not accept the client's rationalizations for drug use or permit projection of blame on others. • Confront client's rationalizations and excuses with concrete facts, i.e., alcohol blood levels, laboratory tests, etc.

REFERENCES

American Psychiatric Association (1994). *Diagnostic and Statistical Manual of Mental Disorders* (4th ed.). Washington, DC: American Psychiatric Association.

Barnes, D. M. (1988). Drugs: Running the numbers. *Science, 240,* 1729.

Brust, J. C. (1993). *Neurological Aspects of Substance Abuse.* Boston: Butterworth–Heineman.

Cho, A. K. (1990). Ice: A new dosage form of an old drug. *Science, 249,* 631–634.

Czechowicz, D. (1991). Adolescent alcohol and drug addiction and its consequences: An overview. In N. M. Miller (ed.), *Comprehensive Handbook of Drug and Alcohol Addiction* (pp. 205–210). New York: Marcel Dekker.

Daugton, D. M., Susman, J., & Sitorius M. (September 1994). Confronting cigarette addiction: A guide to efficient clinical intervention. *IM—Internal Medicine,* 68–79.

Jaffe, J. (1990). Drug addiction and drug abuse. In A. G. Gilman, T. W. Rall, A. S. Niles, & P. Taylor (eds.), *Goodman and Gilman's The Pharmacological Basis of Therapeutics* (pp. 522–573). New York: Pergamon Press.

Kaplan, H. I., & Sadock, B. J. (1991). *Kaplan and Sadock's Synopsis of Psychiatry: Behavioral Sciences, Clinical Psychiatry* (pp. 292–319). Baltimore: Williams and Wilkins.

LaBarbera, M., & Wolfe, T. (1983). Characteristics, attitudes and implications of fentanyl use based on reports from self-identified fentanyl users. *Journal of Psychoactive Drugs, 15* (4), 293–301.

Lieberman, C. M., & Lieberman, B. W. (1971). Current concepts: Marijuana—A medical review. *New England Journal of Medicine, 284* (2), 88–91.

BIBLIOGRAPHY

American Society of Addiction Medicine (1994). *Principles of Addiction Medicine.* Chevy Chase, MD: American Society of Addiction Medicine.

Bennett, E. G., & Woolf, D. (1991). *Substance Abuse: Pharmacologic, Developmental, and Clinical Perspectives* (2nd ed.). Albany, NY: Delmar Publishers.

DuRant, R. H., Rickert, V. I., Ashworth, C. S., Newman, C., & Slavens, G. (1993). Use of multiple drugs among adolescents who use anabolic steroids. *New England Journal of Medicine, 328,* 922–926.

Fleming, M. F., & Barry K. L. (1992). *Addictive Disorders.* St. Louis: Mosby.

Frances, R. J., & Miller, S. I. (1991). *Clinical Textbook of Addictive Disorders.* New York: Guilford Press.

Institute for Health Policy (1993). *Substance Abuse: The Nation's Number One Health Problem.* Princeton, NJ: The Robert Wood Johnson Foundation.

Kaufman, E. (1994). *Psychotherapy of Addicted Persons.* New York: Guilford Press.

Lee, E. W., & D'Alonzo, G. E. (1993). Cigarette smoking, nicotine addiction, and its pharmacologic treatment. *Annals of Internal Medicine, 153,* 34–48.

Minkler, M., Roe, K. M., & Robertson-Beckley, R. J. (1994). Raising grandchildren from crack cocaine households: Effects on family and friendship ties of African-American women. *American Journal of Orthopsychiatry, 64* (1), 20–29.

Richmond, R. L., Kehoe, L. A., & Webster, I. W. (1993). Multivariate models for predicting abstention following intervention to stop smoking by general practitioners. *Addiction, 88,* 1127–1135.

Sullivan, E. J. (1995). *Nursing Care of Clients with Substance Abuse.* St. Louis: Mosby.

Thombs, D. S. (1994). *Introduction to Addictive Behaviors.* New York: Guilford Press.

THIRTY TWO

The Client with Dual Diagnosis

Rothlyn P. Zahourek

OVERVIEW:

INTRODUCTION

Dual diagnosis is used to designate clients who suffer comorbid illnesses of chemical dependency or abuse and mental illness. Examples include major depression with alcoholism, polydrug use with schizophrenia, and cocaine addiction with borderline personality disorder. Awareness and prevalence of this population has increased over the last decade as a result of several social factors:

1. Deinstitutionalization
2. Shortened hospital stays for psychiatric patients
3. High use of alcohol and drugs in American society
4. Increased lay and professional awareness of mental illness in addicted populations and substance use and abuse in psychiatric populations

Clients who have mental disorders often turn to alcohol and drugs for self-medication of psychiatric symptoms or severe environmental stress. It is also known that drug and alcohol use over extended periods of time will cause or trigger mental illness, for example, alcohol use leading to dementia, marijuana use leading to schizophrenia, and cocaine intoxication leading to psychotic symptoms. Other terms for dual diagnosis include:

1. *MICAA (mentally ill chemically abusing and addicted):* implies that the mental illness comes first or is predominant and the chemical abuse and addiction follows or is secondary.
2. *CAMI (chemical abusing and mentally ill):* implies that the chemical abuse came first, precipitating a secondary mental illness.

3. *Double trouble:* a popular term for this population, and for specialized services for them, has a pejorative stereotypic quality. A less stigmatized term is *mentally ill chemically affected* (Reis, 1994, p. 4).

Categories of chemical effects are:
1. *Chemical abuse:* the frequent, problematic misuse of prescription and nonprescription drugs and alcohol; this category can also include nicotine, caffeine, and other psychoactive chemical abuse.
2. *Chemical dependency:* as described by the DSM-IV (American Psychiatric Association, 1994), includes tolerance and withdrawal from substances as well as continued use of prescription and nonprescription drugs, alcohol, and other psychoactive substances.

DIAGNOSTIC CATEGORIES

The following diagnostic categories have been developed to describe the dually diagnosed client (Wallen & Weiner, 1989):

Category 1: Mental illness is primary and increases the risk for environmental influences resulting in substance abuse.
Category 2: Substance abuse occurs initially and results in a secondary mental illness, organic affective syndromes, organic delusional disorders, and antisocial behaviors that decrease or disappear when the substance used is discontinued.
Category 3: Substance abuse and mental illness occur simultaneously with no appar-ent etiologic interrelationship.
Category 4: Substance abuse precipitates the onset of a primary mental disorder.
Category 5: Mental illness results in substance abuse to self-medicate feelings or symptoms.

PREVALENCE RATES

Prevalence rates of addictive disorders in clinical psychiatric clients are as follows (Reiger, et al., 1990; Drake & Wallach, 1989; Brady, Casto, & Lydiard, 1991; Miller, 1994; Group for Advancement of Psychiatry, 1991):
1. 30% of patients with major depression
2. 50% of patients with schizophrenia
3. 50–75% of patients with bipolar disorders
4. 80% of patients with antisocial personality disorder
5. 30% of patients with anxiety disorder
6. 25% of patients with phobic disorders

Prevalence for psychiatric disorders with addicted clients are lower and are as follows (Helzer & Pryzbeck, 1991; Meyers, Weissman, & Tschler, 1984):
1. Depressive disorders—5.0%
2. Bipolar disorder—0.8%
3. Schizophrenic disorder—1.1%
4. Antisocial personality disorder—2.0%
5. Anxiety disorder—3.0%
6. Phobic disorder—6.0%

The ratio of prevalence rates in psychiatric to addictive disorders indicates the importance of setting in understanding reports of comorbidity (Miller, 1994). The following are those ratios of comorbid disorders psychiatric to addictive in treatment settings:
1. Depressive disorders—6.0
2. Bipolar disorders—62.5
3. Schizophrenia—45.5
4. Antisocial personality disorder—40.0

5. Anxiety disorders—10.0
6. Phobic disorders—4.2

Other epidemiological findings include (Miller, 1994, Miller, Ericksen, & Owley, 1994):
1. Because of organic sequelae from drug use, psychotic symptoms have less validity for psychiatric diagnosis in the addicted population than in the normal population (Miller, 1994).
2. The prevalence of psychiatric disorders resulting from drug and alcohol use is greater than the prevalence of coexisting independent psychiatric conditions in addicted clients.
3. When psychiatric disorders are considered independent disorders, prevalence rates are remarkably higher for combined illness in clients with schizophrenia and antisocial personality disorders.
4. Greater comorbidity is found in psychiatric settings.
5. Many epidemiological studies were completed prior to the extensive use of crack cocaine in the psychiatrically disordered population.
6. Daily marijuana use doubles the risk for psychosis.
7. Daily cocaine users have a seven times greater risk of a psychotic episode than nonusers.
8. Heavy alcohol use has no influence on psychosis but dependence doubles the risk; men are at a higher risk than women.
9. Findings are confounded in multiple drug use (Miller et al., 1994).

THEORIES OF ETIOLOGY

Two models dominate theoretical beliefs about etiology:
1. *Vulnerability model:* For example, drug use causes schizophrenia in a previously susceptible population (Miller et al., 1994).
2. *Self-medication hypothesis:* The person medicates symptoms with drug use. Some schizophrenics claim that drugs and alcohol counter the positive and negative symptoms of schizophrenia as well as the neuroleptic side effects. No study has confirmed this hypothesis. Studies demonstrate that continued use worsens symptoms and addicts, mentally ill or not, use drugs whether symptoms change or not (Miller, 1994).

CONTRASTING TREATMENT MODELS

The treatment models for mental illness versus chemical dependency are often quite different, resulting in conflict at the system level as well as the client level. Table 32-1 shows the difference in treatment philosophies and approaches.

STEREOTYPIC BELIEFS

Problems in treatment also result from the stereotypes each treatment group has about the other. These are shown in Table 32-2.

VULNERABILITIES

Clients who are dually diagnosed are at risk in many ways including:
1. Use of drugs and alcohol seriously disrupts the action of psychiatric medications, leading to irritability, depression, delusions, hallucinations, sedation, hostility, aggression, and suicidal behaviors.
2. Many have repeated relapses and institutionalizations often as much as two and a half times more than severely mentally ill patients who do not have a substance abuse history (Safer, 1987).
3. These clients require many and frequent services that are often splintered and poorly coordinated, resulting in high costs for care.

4. Many are suicidal.
5. Many are violent.
6. Many have medical problems including AIDS and tuberculosis.
7. Many are homeless and aimless.
8. Many experience decreased motivation for treatment.
9. Dually diagnosed clients are more likely to miss outpatient appointments and to discontinue treatment (Hall, Popkin, & Devalu, 1977).
10. Dually diagnosed clients are more at risk for health and medical problems (Drake & Wallach, 1989), more severe psychiatric symptoms (Barbee et al., 1989), and criminal behavior (Safer, 1987).

TREATMENT MODELS

The following models are used (Miller, 1994):
1. *Serial model:* traditional, one treatment follows another and occurs in different sites with different staff. Addiction treatment often follows psychiatric treatment. In contrast, in the Veterans Administration system for Posttraumatic Stress Disorder (PTSD), psychiatric treatment follows addiction treatment. Treatment can be fragmented; the dumping syndrome can occur—"That client belongs in your facility, not ours." The client falls through the cracks. Dropout rates and relapses are high. If staff members do not communicate across services, tensions can develop.
2. *Parallel model:* concurrent treatment for both problems in separate facilities with separate staff. Limitation and problems of the serial model apply. The parallel model works best in a situation where the staff members communicate and the programs are easily accessible to one another. Treatment might be stressful if the client has to travel between settings; the client often receives different and conflicting messages. The use of medications can be an example of these problems. High dropout rates are associated with this model.
3. *Integrated or unified model:* treatment is derived from both models and is called *dual-diagnosis* treatment; staff members are trained in both models and have experience with both groups. Denial of either problem is lessened as is splitting of staff. Diagnoses are both considered primary, each requiring specific interventions, implemented simultaneously (Minkoff, 1989, 1994). The more severely mentally ill the client, the more the need for the integrated approach. One limitation may be less aggressive treatment of the addictive disorder, and another caution is overdiagnosis of the psychiatric disorder in clients who have only an addictive disorder but who may have also sought psychiatric help for symptoms related to their drug or alcohol use, for example, depressive and anxiety symptoms (Miller, 1994) and suicidal ideation, phobias, and organic psychoses. These clients might receive medications and treatments prematurely (Minkoff, 1989).

TREATMENT MODALITIES

Types of treatment include individual, group, milieu, family, supportive, confrontational, educational, and motivational therapy. Self-help groups include Alcoholics Anonymous, Narcotics Anonymous, Rational Recovery, and Women for Sobriety.

LOCATION OF TREATMENT

Treatment is offered in inpatient psychiatric units, inpatient chemical dependency (CD) treatment units, day and evening treatment programs, respites and emergency services, outpatient CD and mental health facilities, shelters, general hospitals, and outpatient general medical units.

TABLE 32-1
Differences in Mental Health and Substance Abuse Treatment Models

MENTAL HEALTH–MEDICAL MODEL	RECOVERY–CHEMICAL DEPENDENCY MODEL
1. Syndrome concept	1. Disease concept and process
2. Biopsychosocial with some philosophical emphasis	2. Biopsychosocial with emphasis on spiritual
3. Chemical use secondary to psychiatric disorder	3. Psychiatric problems secondary to chemical use
4. Client has a reason for ineffective coping	4. Client is out of control from substance use
5. Poor insight causes problems in treatment	5. Denial causes problems in treatment
6. Stability is the primary goal	6. Abstinence is the primary goal
7. Achieving empowerment is the goal	7. Admitting powerlessness is the goal
8. Rehabilitation is the goal	8. Recovery is the goal
9. Psychotropic medications are valued	9. Mind-altering substances are avoided
10. Case managers and therapists	10. Sponsors and people to call
11. Organized clinics; psychotherapy	11. Self-help 12-step programs; step work
12. Behavior change is valued	12. Concrete action is valued
13. Positive self-talk, imagery, cognitive changes, awareness, and insight are valued	13. Slogans, stories, affirmations, self-examinations, making amends, and self-acceptance are valued
14. See self as whole person with a disorder	14. Label self as an addict/alcoholic

Adapted from Evans, K., & Sullivan, J. M. (1990). *Dual Diagnosis: Counseling the Mentally Ill Substance Abuser.* New York: Guilford Press.

TABLE 32-2
Stereotypes Held by Mental Health and Substance Abuse Workers

MENTAL HEALTH WORKERS	SUBSTANCE ABUSE WORKERS
Believe addicts and alcoholics:	*Believe the mentally ill:*
1. Are hopeless	1. Are hopeless
2. Are sociopaths, manipulators, liars, and cheats who are potentially violent	2. Are crazy, violent, and to be feared
3. Could control their behavior if they wanted to	3. Must avoid mind-altering drugs or alcohol
4. Can only be helped when they hit bottom, want help, and are drug-free	4. Can only be helped by prescribed medication

PHASES OF TREATMENT

Minkoff (1994) and Osher and Kalofed (1989) have described phases of treatment:

1. Acute stabilization
   a. Manage psychosis.
   b. Manage withdrawal.
   c. Manage personal and other safety.
2. Engagement

   This phase can be broken down into subsequent steps requiring their own treatment approaches. Each phase includes multiple interventions. Forming a therapeutic alliance with the client and family and other care providers is basic.

   a. Engagement

      Recognize the validity of the client's worldview; help clients identify ends they view as valuable; use motivational interviewing (Miller & Rollinick, 1991) to establish a sense of cognitive dissonance between current situation and goals.

   b. Persuasion (education)
      - Help clients recognize problematic behaviors and symptoms.
      - Prepare clients for active change strategies.
      - Enable clients to hope for and work toward a better psychosocial adjustment.
      - Help clients explore at their own pace the barriers to meeting goals.
      - Support development of self-efficacy.
      - Include peer group discussions.
      - Include family education.
      - Encourage social network interventions.
      - Develop social skill–building activities.
      - Help clients maintain stability with medications.
      - Support and reward abstinence.
      - Introduce self-help (12-step, rational recovery, etc.) concepts and meetings.

   c. Active treatment
      - Target specific abstinence-related strategies, e.g., coping with stress.
      - Use cognitive–behavioral approaches.
      - Work on the social network strengths and liabilities.
      - Encourage work.
      - Encourage family involvement and support.

   d. Relapse prevention
      - Teach signs and symptoms of relapse.
      - Continue identification of problems caused by drugs and alcohol.
      - Help client identify cues and triggers to use.
      - Attend to specific risk factors: dangerous people, places, things.
      - Practice and reinforce behavioral changes.
      - Teach alternative coping strategies.
      - Monitor for substance use with urine testing.
      - Encourage adoption of wellness activities: healthy diet and exercise, decreased nicotine and caffeine use.

3. Prolonged stabilization
   - Continue above activities.
   - Anticipate crises and develop stress and crisis management skills in the client and family.
4. Rehabilitation and recovery
   - Encourage a return to work; help client begin volunteer activities.

- Promote active participation in self-help groups.
- Encourage attempts to reach out to others in a giving way.

OTHER TREATMENTS

1. Medications
   - "Good drug, bad drug" confusion can occur with clients wanting to stop psychotropic medications, needing them, and using the desire to be "drug-free" as an excuse.
   - Clients must avoid addicting benzodiazepines and sleep medications and must use care with pain medications.
   - Clients are reassured about the nonaddictive healthful nature of neuroleptics and antidepressants when indicated.
2. Group treatment
   Some controversy exists over whether to mix clients with different degrees of disability and varying lengths and quality of sobriety or to form homogeneous groups based on length of sobriety or severity of psychiatric disability. It is more difficult to lead mixed groups but often necessary. Often early, middle, and late sobriety groups are offered. Clients who are quite psychotic may have difficulty in groups and in maintaining any length of sobriety.
3. Psychoeducation
   Clients, families, and other caregivers are taught how to avoid relapse, the disease concepts, the meaning of dual diagnosis, self-help resources, the importance of medications, steps to recovery, sponsors, and so forth. Clients are taught the importance of working toward sobriety and a stable mental state. Learning About Drugs and Alcohol (LADA) is an educational group for the dual-diagnosis client.
4. Self-help, 12-step programs (Alcoholics Anonymous, Narcotics Anonymous, Rational Recovery)
   - Finding groups where the severely mentally ill will be accepted and not shunned may be hard even though AA and NA tend to be accepting. These clients themselves may feel different.
   - "Double Trouble" (dual diagnosis) AA meetings are also becoming more common in many communities. AA and NA are working closely with treatment programs addressing the needs of dual-diagnosis clients.
   - Some AA or NA members will, although now less often, discourage people from taking psychotropic medications. A pamphlet is available from AA regarding medications and following the health care professional's, not AA's, orders regarding medications.
   - Rational recovery meetings are common and take a less spiritual, more cognitive/behavioral approach to sobriety than does AA or NA. These groups are a valuable alternative or supplement to AA or NA for the dual-diagnosis client.
5. Matching clients with treatment
   It is useful to match a treatment program with clients' strengths, liabilities, and specific needs and to help clients establish an ongoing support network.

NURSING INTERVENTIONS

Table 32-3 shows specific nursing interventions and theoretical rationales for problems occurring in the care of dually diagnosed patients.

TABLE 32-3
Problems, Nursing Interventions, and Theoretical Rationales with the Dually Diagnosed Client

PROBLEM	NURSING INTERVENTION	THEORETICAL RATIONALE
1. Multiple health problems	• Educate clients about effect of drugs and alcohol. • Support positive health promotion, e.g., oral hygiene, adequate diet. • Encourage prevention screening, e.g., HIV testing.	• Clients are at risk for all health problems related to self-care deficits with chronic mental illness and substance abuse.
2. Denial of mental illness and addiction	• Educate client about chemical dependency and relationship with mental illness. • Recognize consequences of substance abuse and exacerbation of mental illness. • Refer to 12-step program.	• Both illnesses are stigmatized. • Denial protects self-esteem, allows previous behavior to continue.
3. Potential for alteration in thought processes	• Stabilize client medically and psychiatrically; manage withdrawal. • Provide or refer for psychotherapy. • Teach material in small amounts, short periods of time. • Reinforce learning often. • Support reality orientation/problem solving.	• Insight, judgment, problem-solving ability, and reality testing are impaired as a result of both mental illness and substance abuse.
4. Potential for self-harm	• Assess for suicide potential. • Provide safe environment. • Involve family or significant others. • Teach caregivers, family, and client that intensive episodic treatment may be necessary. • Teach that both problems are long-term and relapse risk is high. • Anticipate crises; develop support network.	• Inhibitions and judgment are decreased in both substance abuse and mental illness. • Depression and hopeless/helpless states are common with both mental illness and substance abuse.
5. Need for long-term problem management in short-term climate	• Educate third-party payers about the need for long-term episodic care.	• Clinical reports are indicating that stabilization of both problems may take as long as 3–4 years with active caregiver involvement.
6. Potential for relapse	• Watch for warning signs of relapse. • Educate client and significant others to signs of relapse for both illnesses.	• Both illnesses are characterized by non-compliance with treatment and subsequent relapse.

PROGNOSIS

Limited data exist regarding the prognosis for the dually diagnosed client. In a 4-year study, Drake and Norsdy (1994) assessed outcomes for 18 schizophrenic outpatients in an integrated program with case managers. Sixty-one percent became abstinent from alcohol and the mean duration was 26.5 months. Jerrell and Ridgely (1995) semiannually evaluated 147 clients' responses to specialized treatment over a 2-year period. Residential stability and work was increased, alcohol and drug use diminished, use of acute and subacute services decreased, while outpatient and case management services increased. Trained observers rated their psychological improvement as dramatic.

REFERENCES

American Psychiatric Association (1994). *Diagnostic and Statistical Manual of Mental Disorders* (4th ed.). Washington, DC: American Psychiatric Association.

Barbee, R. E., Clark, P. D., & Crapanzano, M. S. (1989). Alcohol and substance abuse among schizophrenic patients presenting to an emergency service. *Journal of Nervous and Mental Disease, 177*, 400–407.

Bartels, S. J., Drake, R., & Wallach, M. A. (1995). Long term course of substance use disorders among patients with severe mental illness. *Psychiatric Services, 46*, 248–251.

Brady, K., Casto, S., & Lydiard, R. B. (1991). Substance abuse in an inpatient psychiatric sample. *American Journal of Drug and Alcohol Abuse, 17*, 389–398.

Drake, R. E., & Norsdy, D. L. (1994). Case management for people with coexisting severe mental disorder and substance use disorder. *Psychiatric Annals, 24*, 427–431.

Drake, R. E., & Wallach, M. A. (1989). Substance abuse among the chronically mentally ill. *Hospital and Community Psychiatry, 40*, 1041–1046.

Evans, K., & Sullivan, J. M. (1990). *Dual Diagnosis: Counseling the Mentally Ill Substance Abuser.* New York: Guilford Press.

Group for Advancement of Psychiatry Committee on Alcoholism and the Addictions and Substance Abuse: A Psychiatric Priority (1991). *American Journal of Psychiatry, 148*, 1291–1300.

Guebaly, N. (1990). Substance abuse and mental disorders: The dual diagnosis concept. *Canadian Journal of Psychiatry, 35*, 261.

Hall, R., Popkin, M. K., & Devalu, R, (1977). The effect of unrecognized drug abuse on diagnosis and therapeutic outcome. *American Journal of Drug and Alcohol Abuse, 4*, 455–456.

Helzer, J. E., & Pryzbeck, T. R. (1991). The co-occurrence of alcoholism with other psychiatric disorders in the general population and its impact on treatment. *Journal of Studies in Alcoholism, 49*, 219–225.

Jerrell, J. M., & Ridgely, M. S. (1995). Evaluating changes in symptoms and functioning of dually diagnosed clients in specialized treatment. *Psychiatric Services, 46* (3), 233–238.

Meyers, J. K., Weissman, M. M., & Tschler, G. L. (1984). Six month prevalence of psychiatric disorders in three communities. *Archives of General Psychiatry, 41*, 959–967.

Miller, N. (1994). Prevalence and treatment models for addiction in psychiatric populations. *Psychiatric Annals, 24*, 394–406.

Miller, N., Ericksen, A., & Owley, T. T. (1994). Psychosis and schizophrenia in alcohol and drug dependence. *Psychiatric Annals, 24*, 418–424.

Miller, W. R., & Rollinick, S. (1991). *Motivational Interviewing.* New York: Guilford Press.

Minkoff, K. (1989). An integrated treatment model for dual diagnosis of psychosis and addiction. *Hospital and Community Psychiatry, 40*, 1031–1036.

Minkoff, K. (1994). Models of addiction treatment in psychiatric populations. *Psychiatric Annals, 24*, 413–418.

Osher, F. C., & Kalofed, K. L. (1989). Treatment of patients with psychiatric and psychoactive substance abuse. *Hospital and Community Psychiatry, 40*, 1025–1030.

Reiger, D. A., Farmer, M. E., Rae, D. S., Locke, B. Z., Keith, S. J., Judd, L. L., & Goodwin, F. K. (1990). Co-morbidity of mental disorders with alcohol and other drug abuse. *Journal of the American Medical Association, 264*, 2511–2518.

Reis, R. (1994). *Assessment and Treatment of Patients with Coexisting Mental Illness and Alcohol and Other Drug Abuse.* Rockville, MD: USDA&HS Substance Abuse and Mental Health Services Administration.

Safer, D. J. (1987). Substance abuse by young adult chronic patients. *Hospital and Community Psychiatry, 38*, 511–514.

Wallen, D., & Weiner, H. D. (1989). The impediments to effective treatment of the dually diagnosed patient. *Journal of Psychiatric Drugs, 21*, 161–168.

Zahourek, R. P. (1995). Dual diagnosis: A challenge for mental health and substance abuse caregivers. In E. Sullivan (ed.), *Nursing Care of Clients with Substance Abuse* (pp. 345–373). St. Louis: Mosby Year Book.

BIBLIOGRAPHY

Alcoholics Anonymous (1993). *Dual Diagnosis Recovery Book.* New York: World Services.

Brown, V. B., Ridgely, M. S., Pepper, B., Levine, J. S., & Ryglewicz, H. (1989). The dual crisis: Mental illness and substance abuse. *American Psychologist, 44* (3), 565–569.

Clement, J. A., Williams, E. B., & Waters, C. (1993). The client with substance abuse/mental illness: Mandate for collaboration. *Archives of Psychiatric Nursing, 7* (4), 189–196.

Hospital and Community Psychiatry Service (1993). *Dual Diagnosis of Mental Illness and Substance Abuse: Collected Articles from Hospital and Community Psychiatry.* Washington, DC: American Psychiatric Association.

Janssen, E. (1994). A self psychological approach to treating the mentally ill, chemical abusing and addicted (MICAA) patient. *Archives of Psychiatric Nursing 8* (6), 381–389.

The Dual Disorders Recovery Book. A Twelve Step Program for Those of Us with Addiction and an Emotional or Psychiatric Problem (1993). Minnesota: Hazelden Foundation.

Salloum, I. M., Moss, H. B., & Daley, D.C. (1991). Substance abuse and schizophrenia: Impediments to optimal care. *American Journal of Drug and Alcohol Abuse, 17* (3), 321–336.

Sciacca, K. (1991). An integrated treatment approach for severely mentally ill individuals with substance abuse disorders. *New Directions for Mental Health Services, 50* (summer) 69–84.

Wilson, H. K. (1995). Their names are legion: Clients with substance-related and psychiatric comorbidities. *Capsules and Comments in Psychiatric Nursing, 2,* 7–10.

THIRTY THREE

The Client Who Has Dementia

Mary Beth Husseini*

OVERVIEW:

Description
Differential Diagnosis of Dementia
Clinical Manifestations
Assessment Tools
Client's Emotional Responses to
    Deficits

Prognosis
Nurses' Nonproductive Reactions
Nursing Interventions

DESCRIPTION

Dementia is an acquired cognitive impairment associated with temporary or permanent dysfunction of the brain. Persons with dementia have impairment of at least three of the following behavioral domains (Cummings & Benson, 1983):
1. Memory
2. Language
3. Visuospatial skills
4. Personality or mood
5. Cognition
Whereas mental retardation is present at birth, dementia is acquired. Delirium or acute confusional state is different from dementia (Cummings & Benson, 1983). Refer to Table 33-1 for the differences.

DIFFERENTIAL DIAGNOSIS OF DEMENTIA

Dementia syndromes are more prevalent among the elderly but are not confined to old age (Weiner, 1991). Dementia syndrome is a result of many conditions that impair brain function including (Weiner, Tintner, & Goodkin, 1991):
1. Thyroid and adrenal gland dysfunction
2. Hepatic encephalopathy
3. Schizophrenia
4. Korsakoff's syndrome

*The author would like to acknowledge Marie C. Smith for her chapter "The Client Who Is Organically Brain Damaged" in the first edition.

TABLE 33-1
Clinical Differences Between Delirium and Dementia

	DELIRIUM	DEMENTIA
Onset	Sudden	Insidious
Duration	Hours to days	Months to years
Memory	Temporary impairment	Increasing amnesia over time
Speech	Slurred	Normal but can progress to aphasia
Perception	Hallucinations and illusions	Hallucinations not prominent
Mood	Fear, anxiety, suspiciousness, and irritability	Labile moods, previous personality traits are exaggerated
EEG	Pronounced, diffuse slowing or fast cycles	Normal or mildly slow

Adapted from Cummings, J. L., & Benson, D. F. (1983). Dementia: Definition, prevalence, classification, and approach to diagnosis. In J. L. Cummings & D. F. Benson (eds.), *Dementia: A Clinical Approach* (pp. 1–14). Boston: Butterworths; and Cleary, B. L. & Varcarolis, E. M. (1990). Organic mental syndromes and disorders. In E. M. Varcarolis (ed.), *Foundations of Psychiatric Mental Health Nursing* (pp. 533–571). London: W. B. Saunders Company.

5. Neurosyphilis
6. Trauma, subdural hematoma, hypoxia
7. Brain neoplasm
8. Multiple sclerosis
9. Multi-infarct dementia
10. Huntington's disease
11. Parkinson's disease
12. AIDS dementia complex
13. Alzheimer's disease
14. Pick's disease

CLINICAL MANIFESTATIONS

Symptoms vary in dementia depending on the specific brain involvement. The following symptoms can be seen alone or in clusters (Stuart & Sundeen, 1991):

1. Disorientation—first affected is time, then place, and last is person
2. Memory loss—first affected is immediate recall, then remote memory deteriorates as the disease progresses
3. Confabulation
4. Labile affective behavior
5. Decreased inhibition
6. Impaired judgment
7. Decreased concentration
8. Apathy
9. Deterioration in social skills
10. Perceptual disturbances
11. Agitation
12. Restlessness
13. Sleep–wake disturbances (Weiner, 1991)
14. Suspiciousness

15. Delusional thinking
16. Loss of intellectual capacities
17. Impairment of abstract thinking
18. Aphasia
19. Apraxia
20. Agnosia
21. Hallucinations
22. Global cognitive impairment as the disease progresses to end stage

ASSESSMENT TOOLS

Several tools have been designed to assess for dementia. These include the:
1. Dementia questionnaire (Breitner & Folstein, 1984)
2. Global Deterioration Scale (Reisberg, Ferris, de Leon, & Crook, 1982)

CLIENT'S EMOTIONAL RESPONSES TO DEFICITS

Although psychiatric symptoms are seen in combination with dementia symptoms, it is important to note that many psychiatric symptoms represent the client's emotional response or defense against the acknowledgment of intellectual deficits. The emotional responses may become pronounced whenever the client notices self-deficits or the deficits of other clients. Frequently, these reactions gain much attention from nurses without a full understanding that they are defenses against anxiety and loss and are to be dealt with as such. Some of these defenses are (Weiner, 1991):
1. Reduced ego strength
2. Blaming of others for their own inadequacies
3. Hopelessness
4. Helplessness
5. Mild to profound depression
6. Denial
7. Delusional projection
8. Distortion
9. Displacement
10. Reaction formation
11. Regression
12. Anxiety
13. Hyperalert state
14. Focus on somatic symptoms
15. Suspiciousness
16. Exaggeration of previous personality behavior

PROGNOSIS

The clinical prognosis can be divided into three levels (Cummings, 1992):
1. Reversible (e.g., hypothyroid dementia)
2. Treatable but does not reverse the existing cognitive damage (e.g., prevention of further ischemic injury in vascular injury)
3. Progressive (e.g., Alzheimer's disease)

NURSES' NONPRODUCTIVE REACTIONS

Nurses who work with clients with dementia are frequently confronted with their own human limitations in effecting change in their clients, especially when deficits are irreversible and become progressively worse over time. Repeating oneself constantly, knowing that the client will soon forget, is inherently frustrating. Attempts to control the inevitable deterioration of some clients and the subsequent failure cause a number of emotional reactions in the nurse. The responses of nurses are viewed as psychological processes that must be examined and changed to restore the nurse's functioning to a more realistic potential. Some of these responses are:

1. Overprotectiveness
2. Chronic helpfulness
3. Emotional and physical withdrawal
4. Frustration
5. Disgust
6. Anger
7. Impatience
8. Avoidance of client
9. Coercive manipulation of client to behave
10. Impotence
11. Helplessness
12. Depression
13. Lack of caring, leading to mechanical, impersonal nursing care
14. Transfer to a different client care setting because of "burnout"

NURSING INTERVENTIONS

Interventions for clients with dementia are palliative and supportive. The core theme in all nursing interventions for the cognitively impaired is to facilitate their highest level of functioning in all aspects of life. See Table 33-2 for interventions and rationales.

TABLE 33-2
Problems, Interventions, and Rationales in the
Nursing Care of Clients with Dementia

INTERVENTION	RATIONALE
Problem: Altered Thought Processes	
1. Ask significant others about client's baseline behavior.	1. What may appear abnormal may in fact be part of the client's "normal." For example, the client may have always had fears and phobias or believed in the supernatural.
2. Approach client in a calm, slow manner.	2. A fast approach may be frightening, especially if people and the environment appear distorted.
3. Acknowledge client's feelings and reinforce reality.	3. Helps client feel understood. Helps with reorientation.
4. Avoid challenges to the client's delusions.	4. Challenging can enhance adherence to false beliefs, and may increase distress.
5. Talk about real people and events.	5. Increases the client's sense of reality, self-worth, and personal dignity.
6. Avoid forcing activities and communication.	6. Force can increase suspiciousness and delusions.
7. Encourage interaction on a one-to-one or group level.	7. Helps maintain a social interaction, improves self-esteem, and increases reality orientation.
8. Provide magazines, books, and newspapers.	8. Helps maintain intellectual stimulation.
9. If client becomes agitated, place in a quiet setting and offer firm limits.	9. Aids in defusing the situation and gives the client time to gain emotional and behavioral control.
10. Accept the client's fear.	10. Decreases aggression.
11. Avoid isolating the client.	11. Hallucinations often increase when the client is alone.

TABLE 33-2 *(continued)*

INTERVENTION	RATIONALE
Problem: Altered Perceptions	
1. Assess degree of sensory/perceptual impairment.	1. By determining a baseline, an individual plan of care can be developed.
2. Encourage use of glasses and hearing aids when needed.	2. Enhances sensory input. Helps reduce distortions.
3. Have easy-to-read clocks and calendars available.	3. Reorients client and reduces confusion.
4. Display personal items (Bible, pictures).	4. Aids in maintaining personal identity.
5. Prevent overstimulation by decreasing noise and objects in the environment.	5. Overstimulation may lead to suspiciousness.
6. Remove pictures and objects if the client perceives them in a way not intended.	6. Distorted perceptions may increase suspiciousness, fear, anxiety, and confusion.
7. Assess the client's interpretation of touch and offer it appropriately.	7. Touch can enhance perception of self/body boundaries, convey warmth and acceptance, or may be interpreted as an intrusion into personal space.
8. Use sensory games for individual or group interventions. Have clients discuss what memories are stirred up by smelling items from different seasons, or Vicks Vapor Rub, flowers, foods, and so forth.	8. Stimulates memories and interaction.
9. Encourage significant others to show affection.	9. Even with cognitive impairment, a client has basic needs for affection.
10. Use restraints as a last resort.	10. Lowers self-esteem, enhances sensory deprivation, and may increase anxiety.
Problem: Altered Verbal Communication	
1. Identify yourself and the client by name.	1. Frequent orientation is needed owing to short-term memory loss. Individual recognition and self-identity are reinforced by using the person's name.
2. Assess client's degree of comfort.	2. Clients may not be able to communicate when they are uncomfortable. Clients may not perceive correctly when clothes or shoes are too tight, or if they are incontinent.
3. Speak slowly, using short, simple sentences.	3. Prevents confusion and misinterpretation of complex statements or abstract ideas.
4. Talk face-to-face with the client.	4. Verbal and nonverbal cues help client understand.
5. Speak at the lowest pitch and volume needed.	5. Loud sounds distort the quality. High volume and pitch can convey stress and anger, increasing client's anxiety.
6. Ask one question at a time; repeat it exactly the same if needed.	6. The client can process one group of words at a time, avoiding confusion.
7. Interpret hidden meaning in client's statements or behaviors.	7. A client calling for mama may benefit from a hug. Anxiety over searching for children might be decreased by carrying a doll.
8. Use "I" instead of "we" when addressing the client.	8. Helps maintain client's individuality.
9. Be aware of statements of helplessness and hopelessness or desire to die.	9. Depression is common with dementia.

(Continued)

TABLE 33-2 *(continued)*

INTERVENTION	RATIONALE
Problem: Ineffective Family Coping	
1. Assess the family's current pattern of care and various persons and agencies used for support.	1. Establishes a baseline. Identifies flaws in care or support. An intervention plan can be adopted.
2. Include family members in discussions about home care.	2. Eases the transition back home. Lessens anxiety of caregivers.
3. Be realistic, honest, and try to focus on the present.	3. When families realize the client is not going to improve, they may adjust their goals to cope with current, less intense issues.
4. Encourage family members to vent their feelings.	4. Prevents buildup of anger and resentment.
5. Encourage participation in support groups.	5. Lessens feelings of isolation. Mortality rates are higher for the primary caregiver than for the client with Alzheimer's dementia.

Adapted from Doenges, M. E., Moorehouse, J. F., & Geissler, A. C. (1993). *Nursing Care Plans: Guidelines for Planning and Documenting Patient Care* (3rd ed.). Philadelphia: F. A. Davis Company; and Rawlins, R. P., & Heacock, P. E. (1993). *Clinical Manual of Psychiatric Nursing* (2nd ed.). St. Louis: Mosby–Year Book.

REFERENCES

Breitner, J. C. S., & Folstein, M. F. (1984). Alzheimer dementia: A prevalent disorder with specific clinical features. *Psychological Medicine, 14* (1), 63–80.

Cleary, B. L., & Varcarolis, E. M. (1990). Organic mental syndromes and disorders. In E. M. Varcarolis (ed.), *Foundations of Psychiatric Mental Health Nursing* (pp. 533–571). London: W. B. Saunders Company.

Cummings, J. L. (1992). Neuropsychiatric aspects of Alzheimer's disease and other dementing illnesses. In S. C. Yudofsky & R. E. Holis (eds.), *Textbook of Neuropsychiatry* (2nd ed., pp. 605–618). Washington, DC: American Psychiatric Press.

Cummings, J. L., & Benson, D. F. (1983). Dementia: Definition, prevalence, classification, and approach to diagnosis. In J. L. Cummings & D. F. Benson (eds.), *Dementia: A Clinical Approach* (pp. 1–14). Boston: Butterworths.

Doenges, M. E., Moorehouse, J. F. & Geissler, A. C. (1993). *Nursing Care Plans: Guidelines for Planning and Documenting Patient Care* (3rd ed.). Philadelphia: F. A. Davis Company.

Rawlins, R. P., & Heacock, P. E. (1993). *Clinical Manual of Psychiatric Nursing* (2nd ed.). St. Louis: Mosby–Year Book.

Reisberg, B., Ferris, S. H., de Leon, J. L., & Crook, T. (1982). The global deterioration scale for assessment of primary degenerative dementia. *American Journal of Psychiatry, 139* (9), 1136–1139.

Stuart, G. W., & Sundeen, S. J. (1991). Impaired cognition. In G. W. Stuart & S. J. Sundeen (eds.), *Principles and Practices of Psychiatric Nursing* (4th ed., pp. 566–593). St. Louis: C. V. Mosby Company.

Weiner, M. F. (1991). *The Dementias: Diagnosis and Management.* Washington, DC: American Psychiatric Press.

Weiner, M. F., Tintner, R. J., & Goodkin, K. (1991). Differential diagnosis. In M. F. Weiner (ed.), *The Dementias: Diagnosis and Management* (pp. 77–106). Washington, DC: American Psychiatric Press.

BIBLIOGRAPHY

Beck, C. K., Heacock, P., Rapp, C. G., & Shue, V. (1993). Cognitive impairment in the elderly. *Nursing Clinics of North America, 28* (2), 335–347.

Emery, V. O., & Oxmon, T. E. (1992). Update on the dementia spectrum of depression. *American Journal of Psychiatry, 149* (3), 305–317.

Hoffman, S. B., & Platt, C. A. (1991). *Comforting the Confused: Strategies for Managing Dementia.* New York: Springer Publishing Company.

Koss, E., & Barry, M. A. (1994). Neuropsychological testing of older persons with dementia. *American Journal of Alzheimer's Care and Related Disorders and Research, 9* (3), 22–27.

Kuhn, D. R. (1994). The changing face of sexual intimacy in Alzheimer's disease. *American Journal of Alzheimer's Care and Related Disorders and Research, 9,* 7–14.

Price, R. W., Sidtis, J. J., Navia, B. A., et al. (1989). The AIDS dementia complex. In M. L. Rosenblom, R. M. Levy, & D. E. Bredesen (eds.), *AIDS and the Nervous System* (pp. 203–219). New York: Raven Press.

Reifler, B. V. (1990). Depression with and without dementia. *Hospital Practice, 25* (4A), 47–66.

Winiarski, M. G. (1991). *AIDS-Related Psychotherapy.* New York: Pergamon Press.

Wolf-Klein, G. (1993). New Alzheimer's drug expands your options in symptom management. *Geriatrics, 48* (8), 26–36.

THIRTY FOUR

The Client Diagnosed as Schizophrenic

Hildegard E. Peplau

OVERVIEW:

Introduction
Common Dysfunctional Human Responses
Language–Thought Disorder
Hallucinations

INTRODUCTION

Schizophrenia is a cumulative, dysfunctional adaptation to experiences the client found disturbing during the formative years. While much contemporary research suggests that inborn biologic, genetic, or biochemical factors put certain individuals at risk for schizophrenia, as yet there is no hard evidence for this theory (Horgan, 1993). The dysfunctional patterns of behavior used by these clients are at least in part transmitted to them experientially and acquired incrementally in interpersonal situations. By the same token, the distressing human responses of these clients can be remediated by therapeutic interpersonal encounters with nurses.

COMMON DYSFUNCTIONAL HUMAN RESPONSES

The role of the nurse is to diagnose clients' dysfunctional human responses, recognize their theoretical meanings, and intervene based on theory. Table 34-1 lists common dysfunctional patterns of these clients, theoretical explanations, and nursing interventions.

LANGUAGE–THOUGHT DISORDER

As children move from infancy to childhood, language emerges. By the end of childhood, language influences thought, which influences action. Most often feelings are evoked by events and are a response to the language–thought–action sequence. We see in clients diagnosed as schizophrenic language that has been influenced by problems in the thought process. The nurse can help clients correct faulty thought processes by helping clients change their language. This requires nurses to listen for and note clients' problematic verbalizations and respond every time with a remedial verbal stimulus. Clients hear the remedial stimuli, take them in, and make them their own, which alters their thinking, and then the client acts upon the new thinking. Table 34-2 lists common language–thought patterns observable in clients diagnosed as schizophrenic, nursing interventions, and rationales for the nursing actions.

(Text continues on page 294)

TABLE 34-1
Dysfunctional Human Response Tendencies of
Clients Diagnosed as Schizophrenic

DYSFUNCTIONAL HUMAN RESPONSE TENDENCY	THEORETICAL EXPLANATION	NURSING INTERVENTION
1. Lack of a separate identity.	1. Significant others have incorporated clients into their identity, for example, the mother might say, "We don't get angry."	1. Asks to whom the plural pronoun refers, calls the client by name, and is careful to use separate pronouns to designate client and nurse.
2. Lack of boundaries (react negatively to any hint of intrusion or closeness).	2. Significant others have acted with intrusive and oversolicitous behavior.	2. Takes care to respect the client's personal space, for example, the nurse therapist does not perform physical exams or treatments on therapy clients, secretly search their rooms, or intrude in other ways.
3. Low self-esteem, self-derogation (call themselves "stupid," "no good," act beneath their potential, make themselves physically unattractive).	3. Significant others have derogated client or missed the opportunity to allow healthy development of self-worth.	3. Questions the origin and validity of the low self-view. "When did you get that idea about yourself?" Or "Who said that about you?"
4. Lack of self-worth.	4. Client has missed the opportunity for a close childhood relationship validating mutual self-worth with a chum.	4. Provides regard without overwhelming the client. Does not act as a "pseudochum."
5. Lack of trust.	5. Client has found significant others to be inconsistent, and expects others to be the same.	5. Fulfills all promises made to the client.
6. Role disorientation (feel obliged to put aside or fail to recognize their own needs, acting subservient to others).	6. Significant others expected clients to serve their narcissistic irrational needs rather than recognize the client's needs apart and separate from them.	6. Helps clients recognize what they themselves want and need, taking care to avoid any hint of exploitation of the client.
7. Inappropriate self-reference (believe the behavior of others refers to themselves or that they can control or influence others nonverbally).	7. Clients have not experienced a separate identity and clear boundaries in early years.	7. Takes care to keep clear separate identities and boundaries of client, nurse, and others. Addresses client by name.
8. Withdrawal (are mute, use private language, and other distancing behaviors).	8. Clients have learned to move out of situations to avoid anxiety-evoking events.	8. Spends specific times with the client, announcing arrival and departure, promising to return, and returning as promised. Encourages client to communicate in a public way that can be validated.
9. Overuse of autistic invention.	9. Withdrawal has led to autistic inferences as to the what and why of events. These inferences are not validated by others and are expanded upon by the client.	9. Validates reality, but inquires about inferences of client.
10. Loss of control over focal attention, failure to notice and correct errors of speech.	10. Private thought, neither confirmed nor validated by others, has led to an inability to distinguish between inner and outer reality; the subjective world has become more compelling than the objective world.	10. Provides communication and interaction that pulls the client into the outer reality, toward change.

TABLE 34-2
Common Language–Thought Patterns Observable in Clients Diagnosed as Schizophrenic, Nursing Interventions, and Rationales

PROBLEMATIC PATTERN REFLECTED IN LANGUAGE OF THE CLIENT	TYPICAL LANGUAGE INDICATING CLIENT'S PROBLEM	NURSING INTERVENTION: VERBAL STIMULI AND VARIATIONS OF NURSE INPUTS TO COUNTERACT PROBLEM	RATIONALE OF NURSING ACTION
1. Pronouns that signify incorporation of client with other persons.	1. "We" "Let's" "Our" "Us"	1. "To whom are you referring?" "You and who else?" "Who are us?" Nurse refers to client by name.	1. Helps clients to speak for themselves using the personal pronoun "I," and to name other persons being talked about. Promotes separate identity.
2. Pronouns that signify loss of identity of persons referred to.	2. "They" "The people" "Themselves" "The doctors"	2. "Who are they?" "Who are the people?" "Who, for instance?" "What are their names?"	2. Helps clients to progress toward naming people about whom they are speaking. Fosters autonomy and direct communication.
3. Depersonalized statements that indirectly imply separate identity.	3. "She wants to go out." "One never knows." "You sometimes think you are lost."	3. "Who is she?" "Who is the one?" "Who is the you that is lost?"	3. Helps clients speak for themselves using "I," "me," "mine," and to identify referents, separate from themselves.
4. "Should-type" injunctions.	4. "I should have known better." "I must do that." "I ought to."	4. "Who said so?" "When did you first think that?" "Where did you get that idea?" "What would happen if you didn't do that?"	4. Helps clients become aware of the source of the injunction, and later their incorporation of the source.
5. Automatic knowing: The client acts as if other persons know something without the client telling them.	5. "You know." "You see." "You understand." "You get what I mean."	5. "What is it I'm supposed to know?" "What is it you want me to see?" "What do you mean?" "No, I don't know. Tell me." Nurse does not use automatic knowing language.	5. Helps clients realize they cannot influence others in this autistic way. Encourages direct communication.
6. Neologisms: Highly private words often coined by juxtaposition of common terms, which can be decoded by the nurse.	6. "I was out-blued by my voices." Decoded: "The voices came out of the blue."	6. Decodes to understand the meaning. Asks the client: "Are you speaking in a private way?" If so, asks the client to "Put what you said into public words."	6. Shows clients the nurse's effort and ability to understand.
7. Delusions: In a situation of high anxiety or panic, in which observation is reduced, an inadequate conclusion is drawn, which provides the client with an explanation that produces relief. The client clings to the delusion to prevent recurring panic.	7. "My husband brought me to the hospital because he knows I am being hunted by the FBI. I'll be safe here."	7. Helps client name the anxiety. Develops client's competence in describing and analyzing the interpersonal situation. Eventually gets to the description of the panic–delusion-forming event.	7. This is a long psychotherapeutic process. When the client has gained self-control over anxiety, understands and works through the interpersonal problems, and finally the delusion-producing event, then the need for the delusion is gone.

HALLUCINATIONS

This phenomenon arises from human capacities common to all people, but is used by the client diagnosed as schizophrenic to mitigate loneliness. A need to interact with people leads to inner events being experienced and expressed as though they were external events. The phenomenon of hallucinating is amiable to remedial nursing intervention. When clients report that voices are talking to them, the nurse is careful to:

1. Avoid reinforcing the so-called voice as real.
2. Shed doubt.
3. Keep the identity of the nurse and patient separate. For example, the nurse says, "What are these *so-called* voices *you say you hear* saying to you?" or "Talk about these *so-called voices*." Table 34-3 describes the four phases of the development of auditory hallucinations and provides nursing interventions for each phase.

As the nurse–patient relationship develops over time, the client's loneliness abates, and the hallucinations are relinquished. As one client said, "Now that I talk to you, I don't hear the voices anymore."

TABLE 34-3
Phases in the Development of Auditory Hallucinations and Nursing Interventions

DESCRIPTION OF PHASES		NURSING INTERVENTIONS
Phase 1.	In a situation of great stress or need, a helping figure from past experience is recalled, or invented, and the reverie of the client interacting with the figure aids in problem-solving and produces immense relief.	None. Become aware of this as a personal experience.
Phase 2.	The client courts relief by repetition of Phase 1. Anxiety has led to withdrawal from people, possibly felt as loneliness. The client recalls or invents an experience similar to Phase 1. A "listening state" develops along with anticipatory anxiety: "Will I again feel relief as before?"	Observe and disrupt the withdrawal. Observe for the "listening state." Seek psychotherapy time for the client.
Phase 3.	Greater loss of focal attention occurs. The hallucinating becomes public; others notice; embarrassment and shame are felt; effort is made at concealment.	Observe "inappropriate" laughter (appropriate only to client's inner experience). Ask "What's going on now?" Provide psychotherapy.
Phase 4.	Concealment fails. Social agents diagnose illness. Hospitalization occurs. New stress is added and may evoke panic. Control of the client shifts to others. Greater shame is felt. The client now taps into negative components of the self-system, saying, "The voices terrorize me." With chronicity the client negotiates, bargains, and pleads with the so-called voices: "I won't talk to others about you if you don't leave me."	Provide psychotherapy to explore progressively interpersonal situations, gradually leading to investigation of withdrawal and loneliness.

Adapted from Peplau, H. E. (1989). Anxiety, self, and hallucinations. In A. O'Toole & S. Welt (eds.), *Interpersonal Theory in Nursing Practice: Selected Works of Hildegard E. Peplau* (pp. 312–316). New York: Springer.

REFERENCES

Horgan, J. (1993). Eugenics revisited. *Scientific American,* June, 123–131.

Peplau, H. E. (1989). Anxiety, self, and hallucinations. In A. O'Toole & S. Welt (eds.), *Interpersonal Theory in Nursing Practice: Selected Works of Hildegard E. Peplau* (pp. 312–316). New York: Springer.

BIBLIOGRAPHY

Bellak, L. (1994). Enabling conditions for the ambulatory psychotherapy of acute schizophrenics. In T. B. Karasu & L. Bellak (eds.), *Specialized Techniques for Specific Clinical Problems in Psychotherapy* (pp. 76–84). Northvale, NJ: Jason Aronson, Inc.

Giovacchini, P. (1993). Schizophrenia, the pervasive psychosis: Paradoxes and empathy. *Journal of the American Academy of Psychoanalysis, 21* (4) 549–565.

Gottesman, I. I. (1991) *Schizophrenic Genesis: The Origins of Madness.* New York: W. H. Freeman & Company.

Green, H. (1964). *I Never Promised You a Rose Garden* (novel). New York: Henry Holt.

Greenspan, S. I. (1986). The development of psychopathology: Perspectives from clinical work with infants, young children, and their families. In D. B. Feinsilver (ed.), *Towards a Comprehensive Model for Schizophrenic Disorders.* Hillsdale, NJ: Analytic Press.

Karon, B. P. (1989). Psychotherapy versus medication for schizophrenia: Empirical consideration. In S. Fisher & R. P. Greenberg (eds.), *The Limits of Biological Treatments for Psychological Distress* (pp. 105–150). Hillsdale, NJ: Lawrence Erlbaum Assoc.

Karon, B. P., & Vandenbos, G. R. (1994). *Psychotherapy of Schizophrenia. The Treatment of Choice.* Northvale, NJ: Jason Aronson.

Lotterman, A. (1995). *Specific Techniques for the Psychotherapy of Schizophrenic Patients.* Madison, CT: International Universities Press.

Peplau, H. E. (1989). An explanatory theory of the process of focal attention. In A. O'Toole & S. Welt (eds.). *Interpersonal Theory in Nursing Practice: Selected Works of Hildegard E. Peplau* (pp. 338–347). New York: Springer.

Peplau, H. E. (1989). Thought disorder in schizophrenia: Corrective influence of nursing behavior on language of patients. In A. O'Toole & S. Welt (eds.), *Interpersonal Theory in Nursing Practice: Selected Works of Hildegard E. Peplau* (pp. 327–337). New York: Springer.

Schiller, L., & Benett, A. (1994). *The Quiet Room. A Journey Out of the Torment of Madness.* New York: Warner Books.

Strauss, J. S., Bowers, M., Downey, W. T., Fleck, S., Jackson, S., & Levine, I. (eds.) (1993). *The Psychotherapy of Schizophrenia.* Northvale, NJ: Jason Aronson.

35
THIRTY FIVE

The Client Who Has Been Battered

Christine A. Grant

OVERVIEW:

Introduction
Myths and Misconceptions
Profile of the Battered Woman
Profile of the Batterer
Description of Battering
The Cycle of Violence
Identifying the Battered Woman
Assessment
    Physical Exam
    Psychosocial Interview

Nursing Interventions
Providing Information
Documentation
Individual Psychotherapy
Couples Therapy
Evaluation of Psychotherapy

INTRODUCTION

Violence against women* by their intimate partners is a major health problem in the United States. In 1995, 25–35% of the women presenting to emergency departments had complaints directly related to battering. The leading cause of injury to women in the United States is a violent partner (Browne, 1993; Kandel-Englander, 1992; Straus & Gelles, 1990). Battering does not stop when a woman is pregnant, and the effects on the outcome of pregnancy are being studied by nurse researchers (Bullock, McFarlane, Bateman, & Miller, 1989; Bullock & McFarlane, 1989; Helton, McFarlane, & Anderson, 1987; Stewart & Cecutti, 1993; Helton, 1987). Two other groups who are victims of domestic violence are the aged and persons with HIV/AIDS. Although researchers and clinicians agree that battering may affect 3–4 million women per year, it remains the most unreported crime in our country (Campbell, 1982; Cirillo & DiBlasio, 1992; Gelles & Cornell, 1990).

MYTHS AND MISCONCEPTIONS

Battering an intimate partner is a crime. Battering can occur at any time during a relationship and breaks all barriers of race, class, age, and sexual orientation. Myths and misconceptions are seen in Table 35-1 along with facts.

---

*Since 95% of those battered are women (Chez, 1988), the female pronoun will be used to designate the battered partner.

TABLE 35-1
Myths, Misperceptions, and Facts About Battering

MYTHS AND MISPERCEPTIONS	FACTS
1. "It is only happening to me. Everyone else has a perfect relationship."	1. Battering happens to many women.
2. "It will never happen again. He promised."	2. Battering is rarely an isolated occurrence; usually it escalates.
3. "That's not really battering, so I'm not a battered woman."	3. All forms of aggression toward a woman by an intimate partner, whether physical, emotional, or sexual, are acts of violence.
4. "It's my fault. I made him angry."	4. It is never the fault of the battered person. Physical, emotional, and sexual violence are unacceptable in any relationship.
5. "There's nowhere I can go for help."	5. There are many resources for the battered woman, and nurses can help locate them.

PROFILE OF THE BATTERED WOMAN

There is no consistent personality or background factor predictive that a woman will be abused. Battering is not a result of individual female deviance, but rather a product of the batterer's need for power and control over an intimate partner and his denial of those needs.

PROFILE OF THE BATTERER

The following risk factors have been found to characterize batterers (Hotaling & Sugarman, 1986; Tolman & Bennett, 1990; Dutton & Strachan, 1987; Jaffe, Wolfe, & Wilson, 1990; Barling & Rosenbaum, 1986):
1. Both witnessing and experiencing violence in childhood
2. Low socioeconomic status
3. Chronic use of alcohol
4. Inability to respond appropriately by communicating verbally about perceived rejections, challenges from an intimate partner, and feelings of jealousy
5. Anger, frustration, or stress at work

DESCRIPTION OF BATTERING

The following behaviors often escalate over time, and represent the most common forms of abuse:
1. *Physical battering:* throwing objects, pushing, shoving, grabbing, slapping, hitting, smacking, punching, kicking, biting, pulling hair, choking, hitting with objects, beatings, tying up and torturing with lethal objects and weapons
2. *Emotional/psychological battering:* making unreasonable demands, orders, and directions; calling names; yelling; screaming; belittling; humiliating; degrading; interrogating; intimidating; isolating from contacts; depriving of sleep, food, safety, economic resources; coercing; threatening with death, disfigurement, physical injury, harm to loved ones, physical violence
3. *Sexual battering:* forced oral or anal sex, rape, forced involvement with pornography

THE CYCLE OF VIOLENCE

A three-stage repetitive battering cycle explains why women remain in abusive relationships and includes the following:

1. Tension-building phase
   - Increased tension occurs in the relationship.
   - Unreasonable demands, humiliation, and degradation increase.
   - Small arguments and disagreements occur, leading to threats and interrogations.
   - The batterer slaps, pushes, and hits the woman.
   - Intimidation continues to escalate.
   - The woman withdraws from the relationship to avoid battering.
   - The woman behaves increasingly compliant to please the batterer.
   - Emotional distance between the couple increases.
   - Minor abusive incidents occur.
   - The batterer may increase drinking or drug use.

2. Acute battering phase
   Actual battering incident(s) and aggressiveness occur.

3. Contrition phase
   This phase is also known as the "honeymoon phase" or the "loving phase." The batterer retreats, may apologize or ask for forgiveness, express remorse, try to make amends, behave calmly, and commit acts of kindness. This phase is marked by an absence of violence. However, the battered person may experience:
   - Blackened eyes
   - Abdominal injuries or vague pain (especially in pregnancy)
   - Burns
   - Open wounds

   or less overt signs or complaints of battering:
   - Anxiety or panic reactions
   - Sleep disturbance
   - Eating disturbance
   - Generalized tenderness, pain, or aches such as backaches, dyspareunia, or headaches
   - Menstrual complaints
   - Generalized lethargy or malaise

   Other associated problems of battering include:
   - Depression
   - Suicidal ideations or gestures
   - Acute stress reactions
   - Alcohol dependence and abuse
   - Drug dependence and abuse
   - Complaints of rape
   - Spontaneous abortions

IDENTIFYING THE BATTERED WOMAN

Battered women often report to the emergency departments of hospitals, psychiatric emergency services, and obstetrical–gynecological clinics following battering. They often attribute the injury to causes other than battering as they experience humiliation, fear of retribution, and embarrassment about their battering. Women may feel the need to cover for their partners in the attempt to be viewed favorably by the batterer or by the care provider. The nurse needs to be aware of the immediate physical effects of battering. Overt signs of battering include:

1. Bruises, swelling, bites, at varying stages of healing
2. Lacerations
3. Dislocations or fractures
4. Hematomas

ASSESSMENT

PHYSICAL EXAM

The client is asked to disrobe and is given a complete history and physical examination. With her consent, colored photographs are taken of all injuries and a body map is used for documentation. Laboratory and diagnostic tests are ordered including imaging if needed.

PSYCHOSOCIAL INTERVIEW

1. After getting dressed the client is given the self-report questionnaire in Box 35-1 to fill out. It is used as a guide in the interview.

2. If possible, a female conducts the interview, as many abused women feel more comfortable talking to another woman.

3. The nurse interviews the client alone, without her partner or children present. An abused woman will not answer questions about being battered in front of her abuser or children. Doing so could put her or her children in danger of future abuse (Migrant Clinician's Network, 1994).

4. Using her own words, the nurse takes care to sound nonjudgmental and supportive. She asks:
   - What was your reason for coming to the emergency room today?
   - Have you had similar complaints or injuries in the past?
   - How did this happen?
   - Where were you injured?
   - What was happening just before you were injured?
   - How did you respond after you were injured?
   - How do you feel now?
   - How much time has passed since you were injured? If she delayed coming for help: What prevented you from coming here right away? If the client responds positively to any of the following four questions, further questions are warranted, and she is considered a candidate for crisis counseling:
   - Do you feel your partner controls your behavior too much?
   - Does your partner ever threaten you?
   - Does your partner ever push, shove, punch, or kick you? While pregnant?
   - Does your partner ever force you to have unwanted sex?

5. The client is also asked about her
   - Economic and financial situation
   - Resources and sources of support
   - Self-destructive behaviors such as suicidal gestures, thoughts, drug or alcohol dependence, and forced involvement in illicit activities

6. The nurse is alert to:
   - Explanations inconsistent with the nature of the injury
   - Delay in seeking medical care

BOX 35-1: Migrant Clinicians Network
Domestic Violence Assessment Form

Note to Provider: If the client chooses to talk about child abuse which occurs in her home, the law in your state may require you to report suspicions of child abuse to state authorities. If this occurs, you need to discuss the reporting process with the client. Other than suspected child abuse, all information recorded on this form should remain confidential.

Client Name: _____ Chart No.: _____ Date: _____

Provider: _____ Clinic: _____

1. Within the last year, have you been hit, slapped, kicked, or otherwise physically hurt by someone?   YES   NO

   If YES, by whom? (circle all that apply)   HUSBAND   BOYFRIEND   RELATIVE   STRANGER   OTHER

   Total number of times: _____

   Please mark the area of injury on the body map. Score each incident according to the following scale:
   - 1 = Threats of abuse including use of a weapon
   - 2 = Slapping, pushing, no injuries and/or lasting pain
   - 3 = Punching, kicking, bruises, cuts and/or continuing pain
   - 4 = Beating up, severe contusions, burns, broken bones
   - 5 = Head injury, internal injury, permanent injury
   - 6 = Use of weapon, wound from weapon

2. If pregnant, since the pregnancy began have you been hit, slapped, kicked, or otherwise physically hurt by someone?   YES   NO

   Total number of times: _____

   Please mark the area of injury on the body map. Score each incident according to the following scale:
   - 1 = Threats of abuse including use of a weapon
   - 2 = Slapping, pushing, no injuries and/or lasting pain
   - 3 = Punching, kicking, bruises, cuts and/or continuing pain
   - 4 = Beating up, severe contusions, burns, broken bones
   - 5 = Head injury, internal injury, permanent injury
   - 6 = Use of weapon, wound from weapon

3. Within the last year, has anyone forced you to have sexual activities?   YES   NO

   If YES, who? (circle all that apply)   HUSBAND   BOYFRIEND   RELATIVE   STRANGER   OTHER

   Total number of times: _____

4. Are you afraid of your partner or anyone you listed above?   YES   NO

This form was developed by Dr. Judith McFarlane, College of Nursing, Texas Women's University, Houston, TX. This form was adapted by the Migrant Clinicians Network for use in a migrant health center setting and used with permission. This form may be duplicated as needed. For more information, contact MCN at 1515 Capital of Texas Highway South, Suite 112, Austin, TX 78746, (512) 327-2017.

- Multiple sites of injury
- Repeated or chronic injuries
- Injuries to the head, neck, breasts, chest, or abdomen
- Partner's overly attentive or threatening behavior with the client or women staff members

NURSING INTERVENTIONS

1. The nurse tells the woman:
   - "You are safe."
   - "This is not your fault."
   - "No one deserves to be battered."
   - "Battering is common. This happens to many women."
   - "Battering seldom happens only once. Your risk for more severe injuries may increase each time you are battered."
2. The nurse treats the injuries.
3. The nurse provides crisis counseling. The emphasis in counseling the battered woman is to help her develop a realistic and rational perception of her battering situation and to provide her with the information needed to help her make decisions. Crisis intervention is most beneficial when the nurse maintains the client's privacy and ensures confidentiality. The nurse approaches the woman in a nonjudgmental manner and recognizes that battered women may be embarrassed and fearful of condemnation. The nurse avoids criticizing or deriding the batterer but rather focuses on the woman's need for safety. The nurse asks the woman to examine her present situation, encouraging her to verbalize her feelings and allowing for the expression of both anger and affection toward the batterer. The client is helped to outline the consequences of the battering and the level of dangerousness she has experienced as a result of the battering. The nurse correlates the woman's present functioning, injuries, and complaints to the battering experience, helping her develop a realistic perception of the battering situation. Past coping responses and adaptations to battering are discussed.

PROVIDING INFORMATION

To help the client determine her options, the nurse provides her with information about:
1. Reporting the battering to the police.
2. Getting legal assistance to obtain an Order of Protection (also known as a Protection Against Abuse Order). See Box 35-2.
3. Obtaining temporary custody of minor children.
4. Local women's organizations, advocacy services, and emergency women's shelters.
5. Counseling services.
6. Vocational counseling.
7. Legal aid services.

Immediate crisis counseling also involves very concrete steps toward developing a plan for safety including:
1. Helping the woman develop a plan of escape by identifying supportive individuals and identifying locations to get away from the batterer
2. Developing an emergency kit to take when forced to leave in an emergency situation, including money, clothing, car keys, marriage license, birth certificates, medical cards, important phone numbers, apartment lease or papers pertaining to joint ownership of property
3. Securing information about partner's place of employment, including name, address of company, and employer's name
4. If children are involved, encouraging the woman to have birth certificates, immunization and medical records available, reminding her that schools and day care centers must be notified of moves

> ## BOX 35-2: The Legal Response to Battering
>
> If a woman has been physically abused or threatened with abuse, her batterer can be arrested. Police will need the following information:
>
> 1. The woman's statement of abuse
> 2. Evidence of either a visible injury (bruise or cut), evidence of damage to her property, or the statement of another witness
>
> If weapons were used in the assault these can be removed by the police. After the batterer is arrested he will be taken before a court and charged. A woman may obtain a Protection from Abuse Order from the police.
>
> 1. Once this order is signed by a judge, the batterer will be served a copy of the order. The order is entered into the police computer system.
> 2. In many states, after the police serve the batterer with the order and it has been signed by the batterer, the signature page is returned to the woman to provide her with proof of the Protection from Abuse Order.
> 3. If the batterer fails to appear in court, he may be rearrested or the judge may automatically decide to issue a Final Protection from Abuse Order to the woman by default.
> 4. The batterer may be fined for failure to appear in court.
> 5. Modification to a Protection from Abuse Order must be accomplished by an attorney.

Crisis counseling is considered to have a positive outcome when the client:

1. Identifies herself as being battered
2. Is aware of the consequences of the battering to herself and her family
3. Is knowledgeable about available resources

DOCUMENTATION

Chart documentation is very important, as it may be used later in litigation. Documentation includes:

1. *History:* Preface woman's verbal statements with "Patient states . . . ." Describe the specific incident including:
   - Circumstances of the battering, using the client's own words
   - Length of battering event
   - Abuse experienced
   - Description of past battering
   - Duration and frequency of battering
   - Assessment of woman's present danger and potential for danger to children or other relatives
   - Complete medical history
   - Social history as relevant
   - Your opinion about whether injuries were adequately explained
2. *Physical:* Be as complete and thorough as possible. Use descriptive terminology. Include:
   - Color photographs taken with the woman's consent
   - Results of laboratory or diagnostic tests
   - Imaging results when applicable

3. *Diagnosis:* Use terminology consistent with the woman's presentation. If the woman states she has experienced abuse, then add "alleged abuse" to your description. If the woman denies abuse but you are suspicious, document "injuries suggestive of battering" or "suspected abuse." Be careful to record all nonbodily evidence of abuse such as "torn clothing," "ripped handbag."

4. *Referrals:* Include the following:
   - Description of referral information you gave to the client
   - Client's decision about the referral

INDIVIDUAL PSYCHOTHERAPY

The nurse who holds a master's degree and is certified by the ANA as a clinical specialist in adult psychiatric–mental health nursing may engage in psychotherapy with battered women. The goals of individual psychotherapy are to (Herman, 1992):

1. Mourn the old self the trauma has destroyed
2. Develop a new self

Over time, in the context of a safe therapeutic relationship, the client is able to:

1. Take care of her body, her immediate environment, her material needs, her children, and her other relationships
2. Discover her own ambitions
3. Increase her sense of power and control
4. Protect herself against future danger
5. Deepen her alliances with those whom she has learned to trust

COUPLES THERAPY

When the couple agrees that battering is an issue they both want to work on together to save their relationship, couples therapy may be used. The goal is to "decrease the frequency and intensity of the battering by interrupting the cyclic nature of their interactions" (Morton, 1984, p. 472). Methods used are to:

1. Gather a detailed history of how the battering occurred
   - What are the stressors in the family that increase tension?
   - What are the couple's individual coping mechanisms?
2. Encourage the couple to identify patterns in their interactions
3. Teach the phases of the battering cycle
4. Help the partners identify the phases of their own cycle
5. Help the couple learn new ways to decrease tension without battering
6. Teach assertiveness
7. Help the couple learn positive coping skills
8. Strengthen the support system for the couple and each individual

EVALUATION OF PSYCHOTHERAPY

Because work with battered clients is highly charged and can be demanding and frustrating, channels for ventilating concerns and obtaining support are recommended (Morton, 1984). These include case review with peers and supervision or consultation. The best objective evaluation of success in this work is cessation of the battering. Other signs of improvement are:

1. Increased self-esteem, power, and control over life
2. Decreased alcohol and drug abuse
3. Decreased physical symptoms
4. Increased satisfaction in relationships

REFERENCES

Barling, J., & Rosenbaum, A. (1986). Work stressors and wife abuse. *Journal of Applied Psychology, 71,* 346–348.

Browne, A. (1993). Violence against women by male partners. *American Psychologist, 48* (10), 1077–1087.

Bullock, L., & McFarlane, J. (1989). Higher prevalence of low birthweight infants born to battered women. *American Journal of Nursing, 89,* 1153–1155.

Bullock, L., McFarlane, J., Bateman, L., & Miller, V. (1989). Characteristics of battered women in a primary care setting. *Nurse Practitioner, 14,* 47–55.

Campbell, J. C. (1992). Violence against women. *Nursing and Health Care, 13* (9), 464–470.

Chez, R. A. (1988). Woman battering. *American Journal of Obstetrics and Gynecology, 158* (1), 1–4.

Cirillo, S., & DiBlasio, P. (1992). *Families That Abuse.* New York: Norton.

Dutton, D. G., & Strachan, C. E. (1987). Motivational needs for power and spouse-specific assertiveness in assaultive and nonassaultive men. *Violence and Victims, 2,* 145–156.

Gelles, R. T., & Cornell, C. P. (1990). *Intimate Violence in Families* (2nd ed.). Newbury Park, CA: Sage.

Helton, A. S. (1987). Prevention of battering during pregnancy: Focus on behavior change. *Public Health Nursing, 4,* 166–174.

Helton, A. S., McFarlane, J., & Anderson, E. T. (1987). Battered and pregnant: A prevalence study. *American Journal of Public Health, 77,* 1337–1339.

Herman, J. L. (1992). *Trauma and Recovery.* New York: Basic Books.

Hotaling, G. T., & Sugarman, D. B. (1986). An analysis of risk markers in husband to wife violence: The current state of knowledge. *Violence and Victims, 1,* 101–124.

Jaffe, P. G., Wolfe, D. A., & Wilson, S. K. (1990). *Children of Battered Women.* Newbury Park, CA: Sage.

Kandel-Englander, E. (1992). Wife battering and violence outside the family. *Journal of Interpersonal Violence, 7,* 462–470.

Migrant Clinician's Network (1994). Domestic violence tips for clinicians. *Migrant Health Newsletter,* Jan.–Feb. 1–3. Austin, TX: National Migrant Resource Program.

Morton, T. (1984). The client who has been battered. In S. Lego (ed.), *The American Handbook of Psychiatric Nursing.* Philadelphia: J. B. Lippincott.

Stewart, D. E., & Cecutti, A. (1993). Physical abuse in pregnancy. *Canadian Medical Association Journal, 149* (9), 1257–1263.

Straus, M. A., & Gelles, R. J. (1990). *Physical Violence in American Families.* New Brunswick, NJ: Transaction.

Tolman, R. M., & Bennett, L. W. (1990). A review of research on men who batter. *Journal of Interpersonal Violence, 5,* 87–118.

BIBLIOGRAPHY

Barnett, O. W., & LaViolette, A. D. (1993). *It Could Happen to Anyone: Why Battered Women Stay.* Newbury Park, CA: Sage.

Campbell, J. C., & Woods, S. J. (1993). Posttraumatic stress in battered women: Does the diagnosis fit? *Issues in Mental Health Nursing, 14* (2), 173–186.

Kerr, N. J. (1995). The degrading of America: Violence toward women. Editorial. *Perspectives in Psychiatric Care, 31* (4), 3–4.

Peled, E., Jaffe, P. G., & Edleson, J. L. (1994). *Ending the Cycle of Violence: Community Responses to Children of Battered Women.* Newbury Park, CA: Sage.

Walker, L. E. A. (1994). *Abused Women and Survivor Therapy.* Washington, DC: American Psychological Press.

36
THIRTY SIX

The Client Who Has Been Raped

Christine A. Grant

OVERVIEW:

Introduction
Categories of Rapists
Types of Rape
Myths and Facts
Rape Trauma Syndrome

Emergency Care
Posttraumatic Stress Disorder
Treatment
Future Role of the Nurse

INTRODUCTION

Rape is defined as carnal knowledge forcibly and against one's will, including sexual penetration of the victim's vagina, rectum, or mouth. One out of every three women will be raped or sexually assaulted in her lifetime* (Vachss, 1993). There is gross under-reporting of rape owing to:
1. Fear of retaliation
2. Fear of being further victimized
3. Lack of encouragement or support to report
4. Lack of information about how to report

CATEGORIES OF RAPISTS

Crime Classification Manual (Douglas, Burgess, Burgess, & Ressler, 1992) classifies rapists as follows:
1. The *power-reassurance rapist* uses rape to express his fantasies. The rapist has a history of sexual preoccupation, bizarre masturbation practices, voyeurism, exhibitionism, obscene telephone calls, cross-dressing, and fetishism. The rapist is compensating for his felt inadequacies as a male and fantasizes that his victim will enjoy the experience and may even date and fall in love with him. The motivation for rape stems from the offender's belief that he is so inadequate no woman would ever voluntarily have sex with him.
2. The *exploitative rapist's* motive is to force the victim to submit sexually. The rape is an expression of an impulsive, predatory act and has little psychological meaning to

---

*Though men are raped as well, the majority of rape victims are women, so the female pronoun will be used to designate the victim, and the male to designate the offender.

the offender. This is a rapist who is on the prowl for a woman and will act more on the opportunity to rape rather than a conscious fantasy. This rapist forces his victim to comply and is not concerned for her welfare.

3. The *anger rapist* is motivated by aggression. The victim represents the hated individual(s) in the rapist's life who have psychologically injured and insulted him either in reality or fantasy. This rapist is a misogynist whose aggression is excessive in relation to the force needed to subdue his victim.

4. The *sadistic rapist* is expressing sexual-aggressive fantasies that heighten his sexual arousal. There is no differentiation between sexual and aggressive feelings and the offender becomes increasingly angry as he becomes sexually aroused. The rape is characterized by bizarre and intense forms of sexual-aggressive violence. This violence is typically directed at body parts that have a sexual meaning to the rapist, including the breasts, anus, buttocks, genitals, and mouth.

TYPES OF RAPE

All rapes involve aspects of power, anger, and sexuality through an act of aggression. Rapes have been differentiated as follows:

5. *Situationally motivated sexual assaults* are committed to fulfill sexual and other needs. The rape is not simply for arousal or gratification, but is an expression of power and control. Situational rapes are impulsive acts, involving opportunistic and predatory behaviors. The rape occurs at the spur-of-the-moment, sometimes called "blitz rape," involving no premeditation.

6. *Preferentially motivated sexual assaults* are rapes involving patterned behaviors or rituals necessary for the offender to become sexually aroused. The ritualism can include specific characteristics or belongings of the victims, or specific use of words or phrases. These rapes are often well planned, with the victim sought out by the rapist.

MYTHS AND FACTS

Table 36-1 lists myths about rape as well as facts.

TABLE 36-1
Rape Myths and Rape Facts

RAPE MYTHS	RAPE FACTS
1. Rape is provoked by the victim, either consciously or by default.	1. Eighty percent of rapes are planned in advance by rapists, and the victim is threatened with death or injury if she resists. No person's dress or behavior is license for violence.
2. Only young, beautiful women are raped, particularly if they are "promiscuous" or have "bad" reputations.	2. Rapists choose victims without regard for beauty, age, race, or socioeconomic class. Victims range in age from 3 months to 93 years.
3. If women stay at home, they will not be raped.	3. Half of all rapes occur in a private residence; one third to one half of all rapes occur in the victim's home. Women are raped by their husbands, ex-husbands, boyfriends, lovers, friends, and neighbors.
4. Women who avoid strangers will avoid being raped	4. Over half of *reported* rapes are by strangers; the majority of adults report rape by strangers, whereas the majority of children and adolescents report rape by persons known to them. Victims who know the rapist often do not report for fear that others will not believe them.

TABLE 36-1 *(continued)*

RAPE MYTHS	RAPE FACTS
5. No woman can be raped against her will.	5. A majority of victims are threatened with death if they resist. Eighty percent of rapists carry a weapon or threaten death, 30% manhandle victims, 20% use verbal threats, and 15% use no force (usually with child victims); percentages reflect use of more than one mode of force.
6. Rape occurs only in large cities.	6. Rape occurs everywhere. Reported rapes in urban areas are increasing. People in rural communities often believe rape myths and do not report rapes.
7. Most rapes involve black men and white women.	7. Rape is predominantly *intraracial*. Three percent of rapes involve interracial assaults.
8. Rape is an impulsive act to achieve sexual gratification.	8. Rapists report a lack of sexual gratification from rape and describe their motives as power, anger, and sadism aimed at humiliating or degrading the victim.
9. Rapists are abnormal perverts or mentally deranged.	9. Rapists exhibit poor impulse control and a greater tendency toward expressing violence; otherwise they do not differ from the "normal" man.
10. It is easy to prosecute rapists, thus failure to prosecute implies that the victim is guilty.	10. Only 3% of *reported* rapes result in convictions; when multiplied by estimates of unreported rapes, the rate is 0.3%. Rapists report 13 offenses for every convicted offense.
11. Women frequently cry rape for revenge.	11. The false report rate for rape is the same as for other felonies (2%).
12. Rape is a minor crime affecting only a few women.	12. The U. S. Department of Justice statistics indicate 700,000 forcible rapes occur annually. For every rape reported, 3 to 10 go unreported. One out of every 8 American women has been the victim of rape.
13. Rape is predominantly a hot-weather crime.	13. Research reports a higher incidence of *reported* rape in summer months and warmer weather areas. Rape occurs year round.
14. Elderly women are not bothered by rape because they have already had sex.	14. Rape of elderly women is more brutal and violent than rape of younger victims.
15. Psychiatrically ill women are raped more often than women without prior psychiatric histories.	15. Victims with psychiatric histories are not raped more frequently but do have a more severe response to being raped.
16. Homosexual rapes differ from heterosexual rapes.	16. Motives for homosexual rape are the same as for heterosexual rape; only the available object (person) differs, and more brutality may occur as the offender subdues a resisting victim.
17. Gang rape is harmless activity by young boys "sowing wild oats."	17. Gang rapes occur for hours and are brutal as each offender attempts to outdo the "performance" of his predecessor in demonstrating masculinity and "adequacy." Alcohol and drug abuse, which lowers inhibitions toward violence, is frequently associated with gang rapes.
18. Victims of repeat rape are unlike first-time victims.	18. Repeat rape reflects greater victim vulnerability. Victims of repeat rape tend to be newly relocated or transient, have a higher incidence of seeking help for emotional problems, and come from lower socioeconomic classes; otherwise repeat rape victims are similar to first-time victims.

Adapted from Foley, T. (1984). The client who has been raped. In S. Lego (ed.), *The American Handbook of Psychiatric Nursing* (pp. 475–495). Philadelphia: J. B. Lippincott.

**RAPE TRAUMA
SYNDROME**

Victims of rape show a wide variety of responses ranging from extreme emotional distress to no visible reaction. The common phases of rape trauma syndrome include (Burgess & Holmstrom, 1986):

Immediate or Acute Phase   The period immediately after the assault, marked by disorganization

1. Physical responses
   - Physical trauma/injury to specific body parts involved in the assault
   - Headaches
   - Skeletal muscle tension
   - Fatigue
   - Gastrointestinal disturbances
   - Genitourinary disturbances, e.g., dysmenorrhea
   - Stiff muscles and joints
   - Generalized malaise and physical illness
   - Sleep pattern disturbance
   - Eating disturbance
   - Sexual disturbance

2. Emotional responses
   - Fear
   - Shock
   - Anger
   - Numbness
   - Guilt
   - Disbelief and denial
   - Self-blame
   - Irritability

3. Behavioral responses
   - Development of specific or generalized fears
   - Seeking out or refusing medical care and counseling
   - Seeking out or reporting rape to law enforcement
   - Refusal to tell family or friends about the rape

Reorganization Phase (Long-Term Process)

1. Physical responses
   - Gastrointestinal disturbances
   - Chronic, vague complaints such as musculoskeletal pain
   - Genitourinary difficulties
   - Gynecological and menstrual problems

2. Psychological responses
   - Dreams and nightmares
   - Specific fears and phobias, e.g., fears of being alone, of the outdoors, of sexual relations
   - Generalized anxiety or fears
   - Depression
   - Denial, suppression, or repression of feelings and thoughts about rape
   - Apathy
   - Sexual/intimacy dysfunction or disturbance

3. Social lifestyle responses
   - Disruption in daily routine
   - Change in school, employment, or residence

- Disruptions in relationships with family and friends
- Change in leisure activities
- Increased alcohol/drug use

Complications, or mediating factors that may influence the long-term reorganization process include the following:

1. Delayed reporting or failure to disclose
2. Development of posttraumatic stress disorder
3. Prior history of assault
4. Psychiatric history
5. Suicidal behavior
6. Sexual promiscuity
7. Alcohol or drug abuse

EMERGENCY CARE

Psychiatric nurses are most likely to come in contact with rape victims when they enter the emergency room for care. Immediate care consists of:

1. Introduction of the nurse and her role in the rape examination
2. Obtaining written consent to provide care and treatment
3. Providing privacy and any emergency care needed
4. Informing the client of her rights and ensuring confidentiality
5. Safeguarding the client's well-being through nonjudgmental care, psychological support, and the projection of a caring yet professional demeanor throughout the examination
6. Providing the client with the opportunity to meet with a rape crisis center advocate
7. Helping the client notify friends, family, and law enforcement personnel
8. Providing for aftercare and appropriate referrals

See Box 36-1 for the physical examination of the rape victim and Box 36-2 for an interview guide.

(Text continues on page 313)

BOX 36-1: Physical Examination of the Rape Victim

History

A history should be obtained and a statement taken about time and place of the event, relationship to the assailant, if any, nature of suspected physical and sexual acts, time lapse between assault and current examination, victim's physical state, and whether there have been any physical changes since the assault (e.g., if victim bathed, douched, showered, urinated or defecated, changed clothes, used or removed a tampon, treated wound, etc., prior to examination).

Examination, Treatment, and Follow-Up Care

Equipment Recommended for Evidentiary Material

1. Fresh-sealed package of microscopic slides with frosted ends
2. Eyedropper bottle with 0.9% saline
3. Six to 12 packages of sterile cotton swabs
4. Nine to 12 test tubes with stoppers
5. Urine container
6. Sterile, new comb
7. Sterile scissors
8. Nail scraper—plastic or orangewood
9. Envelopes
10. Package of gummed labels
11. Glass-cutting pencil
12. Sterile gauze and envelope for saliva sample

Complete Physical and Gynecologic Examination

1. Evaluate vital signs, general appearance, and mental status.
2. Identify and measure cuts, bruises, and scratches; record and photograph.
3. Take fingernail scrapings, particularly if nails are broken or victim scratched the assailant.
4. Examine for extragenital sexual trauma to mouth, breasts, neck, and other body parts. Take swabs and smears from mouth, throat, or anus in the case of sodomy to check for semen presence. *(Continued)*

BOX 36-1 *(continued)*

5. Do a baseline check for sexually transmitted diseases (STDs). Treatment regimens vary for each STD. If antibiotics are prescribed, the victim is reminded to take them as prescribed. STDs require follow-up examinations to ensure successful treatment.

6. Discuss with the victim her birth control practices, use of oral contraceptives and IUDs, and belief system surrounding abortion. A discussion of possible types of postcoital contraception with a full explanation of possible effects is indicated (diethylstilbestrol [DES] has been shown to cause nausea and vomiting, and cancer in daughters born to women who have taken it during pregnancy).

7. Discuss with the victim the sexual functioning of the rapist (impotence, retarded ejaculation, premature ejaculation, masturbation).

8. Provide pregnancy testing and information on abortion, location of free clinics, women's health services, and crisis counseling centers in the community.

9. Pelvic examination should include the following:
   a. Observation for matted or free hair
   b. Combings of pubic and head hair to find any traces of assailant's hair and collection of pubic and head hairs from victim for reference
   c. Description of vulvar trauma, redness, lacerations, and bruises and photography in black and white
   d. Examination of condition of hymen
   e. Determination of parity
   f. Determination of date of last menstrual period
   g. Determination of date and time of last voluntary coitus
   h. Determination of condition of anus and rectum
   i. Vaginal examination with lubricated, water-moistened speculum
   j. Specimen of victim's blood for matching
   k. Examination of adnexa for hematoma
   l. Swabs and smears from vagina, vulva, rectum, and thighs to check for presence of semen

10. Clothing should be checked for tears, blood, semen, and stains. Victim's clothing should be preserved, marked, photographed, and collected in a paper bag (never plastic).

11. Discuss with the victim HIV blood testing. An HIV screening test (ELISA) is repeated if positive results are reported. A Western Blot test is performed if the repeat ELISA is positive. Inform the victim that it may take as long as a year for HIV antibodies to develop. Link the victim to pretesting and posttesting counseling services in her area.

Evidentiary Material

Evidentiary material should be gathered and held for release to the police. It should not be released without consent of the patient or guardian, except by subpoena or court order. Specimens should be gathered and handled as follows:

1. Take swab from the vaginal pool and from any suspicious area about the vulva and protect in dry test tube. These can be examined by a hospital or police laboratory for the following:
   a. Acid phosphatase test
   b. Blood group antigen of semen test
   c. Precipitin test against sperm and blood

2. Examine wet sample from fornix immediately for motile sperm. This examination should be performed only by an experienced person who understands the limitations of examining sperm material.

3. Take separate smears from vulva.

4. Culture for *Neisseria* in appropriate medium such as Thayer-Martin.

5. Comb pubic and head hair for free hairs; pull (do not cut) a minimum of 25 of victim's pubic and head hairs.

6. Take fingernail scrapings.

7. Chain of evidence; laboratory specimens should be gathered by a physician in presence of a witness and personally handed to a technician or pathologist. Slides and containers should be clearly labeled with patient's name. Victim should be advised that turning bloody, torn, or stained clothing over to police may help their investigation and prosecution of case (if she chooses to prosecute). It is critical that a chain of evidence be established identifying all persons responsible for handling or keeping evidentiary material.

Follow-Up Care

Patient should be examined for lacerations, contusions, and other wounds. Retesting and examining for pregnancy, STDs, and HIV should be completed. Counseling to assess and prevent long-term psychological effects should be provided or made available.

Medical Records

Medical records should contain complete documentation of history, examination, and treatment provided. They should describe physician's findings and what was done. They should state what evidentiary materials were given and to whom. Only medical conclusions, opinions, and diagnosis should be in medical records. Above all, they must be legible, and preferably typed, to avert case dismissal in court proceedings. Medical personnel and records may be subpoenaed. Misinterpretations can be avoided if all data are exact and detailed. Negative findings are as important as positive ones and may assist in protection of all concerned parties.

From Foley, T. S. (1984). The client who has been raped. In S. Lego (ed.), *The American Handbook of Psychiatric Nursing* (pp. 484–485). Philadelphia: J. B. Lippincott.

BOX 36-2: Interviewing Guidelines with Rape Victims in Crisis

Date _____ Time _____

General Information

Introduction: Hello. This is _____

from _____.

   How can I help you?

Name of victim/caller_____

Phone number calling from _____

Address or general area _____

   Location/neighborhood of assault _____

   Why in the area_____

When did assault occur (date, time)?_____

Are you in a safe place? _____

Are you hurt?_____

How are you feeling now? _____

Time between assault and call to crisis line _____

Demographic Data

Age of victim _____

Race and sex of victim _____

Marital status _____

Description of assailant:

   Who did it? _____

   Age _____

   Race and sex _____

   Acquainted with victim _____

      Describe relationship:

Crisis Status

Perception of the event _____

Response to the event _____

Situational supports _____

Coping mechanisms_____

Type of Assault

_____ Rape

_____ Attempted rape

_____ Involuntary deviate sexual intercourse

_____ Indecent assault

_____ Sexual assault of a minor

_____ Other degrading acts

      Describe:

_____ Use of weapon

      Type:

_____ Struggle by victim

      Feelings now about that

_____ Threats (describe)

      Verbal _____

      Physical _____

Services Requested and Questions to Consider

1. Medical intervention (hospital): Has the victim had a medical examination? Encourage going to the emergency room for treatment of injuries and collection of evidence pending decision to prosecute.

   a. *If not examined:* If she does not want to go to the hospital, does she know about the importance of testing for HIV, STDs, and pregnancy now and later? Is she injured other than the sexual assault? What supportive network is available to her? Does she want/need an advocate to accompany her to a shelter/care facility? Give her information about the local hospital procedure and what to expect, her rights.

   b. *If examined:* How did she get to the hospital? What did she expect would be done for her at the hospital? Were tests for HIV, STDs, and pregnancy done? Did she change clothes or clean up before going to the hospital? Was medical evidence collected (what, where)? Was she treated for lacerations, abrasions, bruises? Is she on any medications or DES? Specify these. Does she know their side effects and risks involved? Is she having any medical problems? Was follow-up care discussed/planned? How does she feel she was treated by the health professionals? What is her reaction to the experience? Did she decide to obtain help or did someone else pressure her to seek help?

   c. *Abuse:* Is there evidence of physical abuse to a child or elderly person or battered wife syndrome? Describe the data. Has the evidence been reported to the police, hospital, and/or Child Welfare?

(Continued)

BOX 36-2 *(continued)*

2. Shelter and transportation intervention: Does she need emergency transportation?
   From _____ to _____ Date _____
   Time _____
   Does she need emergency shelter? _____
   Contributing factors _____
   Length of time requested _____
   Accompanied (children) or alone _____
   Economic/financial concerns (describe) _____
3. Police and legal intervention: Has she reported to the police?
   a. *If not reported:* Does she want to report? Does she want the report kept anonymous? Does she want to press charges? Does she want to talk about the pros and cons of not reporting/reporting? What feelings/factors are contributing to a no-report decision? Does she know about victim compensation-restitution (that she can be compensated for unpaid medical expenses if she reports the crime within 72 hours)?
   b. *If reported:* Does she understand the legal procedure and what to expect at the preliminary hearing, pretrial, trial? Is she aware of the possibility of a trial postponement and of a not-guilty verdict? To whom did she report (which police station and name of officer taking the report? Was a report taken? Was she encouraged or discouraged from prosecuting? What is happening with the police follow-up at this time? Is she aware of the procedures necessary to identify the assailant? Has the assailant been picked up by the police? Is the assailant in jail, out on bond? Is she being harassed or threatened by him or others? Describe. Does she have any intent to retaliate against the assailant? Name of officer arresting the assailant and police station(s) is assigned to? Who is the district attorney? How does she feel the police treated her? What is her reaction to the experience of reporting?
4. Psychological intervention
   a. *The victim:* How did she feel at the time of the assault? And now? Does she feel the rape was her fault? Does she believe in the myths? Which ones and their impact on her as noted by _____.
      Does she perceive anyone as able to assist her? Did she go or not go to the police/hospital as a result of outside pressure/advice? Is she ambivalent regarding what to do? Describe. Is she seeking others' opinions? (Whose? What content? What action taken?) Was she or the assailant affected by the use of alcohol and/or drugs? (What ingested? When? Amount? By which party?) Feel-

ings about this? Is she unable to verbalize her needs? Is she psychotic? Mentally retarded? History of social difficulties? History of physical difficulties? Hospitalized or under a physician's care now or previously? Mental status is (describe). What is the most painful part to recall/discuss? Has she been raped before? Is this her first sexual experience? What is her usual sexual style? What does this sexual assault mean to her? How did she react to sexual acts demanded (feelings, behaviors, e.g., compliance, resistance)?
   b. *Family and friends:* Who are her friends, relatives? Where do they live? Quality and frequency of contacts? Persons most and least in touch with? Does she have a therapist, minister? Does she attend any women's groups, any rap sessions? Does she want to talk with other victims of rape? Can she rely on her support systems if she wants to talk about the rape? Will they listen? How will she feel if they don't or reject her? How is her church community a support system for her? Has she decided to talk about the incident? (Discuss pros/cons of doing so and with whom—she is the best judge of her situation.) Who knows about the assault? Describe their response. Do family/friends want to talk with a counselor, or does she want a counselor to talk with them? Is the family responding with (1) caring for the victim's welfare, empathy, support, anger directed at the assailant, ability to give to the victim or (2) blaming the victim, caring for their own welfare (e.g., what others will think), recriminations, anger directed at the victim, blaming themselves?
5. Narrative summary
   Services requested _____ Medical
                        _____ Police/legal
                        _____ Shelter
                        _____ Transportation
                        _____ Counseling (specify type)
                        _____ Other
   Nursing diagnosis _____
   Plans _____
   Contacts made (e.g., police, hospital, name of person/agency)
   Referrals made or suggested _____
   Follow-up indicated and type _____
   Self-evaluation
   Describe feelings about the call, personal reactions, influence of biases/myths. List additional information/training that would help improve services. Delineate learning needs.

From Foley, T. S. (1984). The client who has been raped. In S. Lego (ed.), *The American Handbook of Psychiatric Nursing* (pp. 486–487). Philadelphia: J. B. Lippincott.

POSTTRAUMATIC STRESS DISORDER

Recovery from the traumatic experience of rape is varied owing to the individual characteristics of the victim and the level of intervention provided. Many individuals who have been raped meet the criteria for posttraumatic stress disorder as outlined in the DSM-IV (American Psychiatric Association, 1994). The essential feature of posttraumatic stress disorder is the development of characteristic symptoms following an extreme traumatic stressor with direct personal experience of an event involving actual or threatened death or serious injury, or other threats to physical integrity. Rape and sexual assault are traumatic events that are experienced directly and lead to the following symptoms:

1. Persistent reexperiencing of the trauma
   - Recurrent and intrusive recollections of the rape
   - Recurrent distressing dreams of the rape
   - Acting or feeling as if the rape were recurring
   - Intense psychological distress at symbolic events
   - Physiological reactivity to events resembling the rape

2. Persistent avoidance and numbing of rape associations
   - Avoidance of thoughts and feelings about rape
   - Avoidance of social activities
   - Inability to recall aspect(s) of the rape
   - Feelings of detachment from others
   - Restricted range of affect
   - Sense of a foreshortened future

3. Persistent symptoms of increased arousal
   - Difficulty falling or staying asleep
   - Irritability or outbursts of anger
   - Difficulty concentrating
   - Hypervigilance
   - Exaggerated startle response

TREATMENT

See Table 36-2 for three treatments employed by nurses to help clients recover from the trauma of rape.

FUTURE ROLE OF THE NURSE

Nurses are currently being trained as sexual assault nurse examiners (SANEs). These nurses are taught to:
1. Interview the client
2. Complete the physical examination
3. Collect evidence
4. Present the evidence in a court of law as an expert witness

TABLE 36-2
Systems of Treatment for Rape Victims

PRINCIPLE	METHOD/TECHNIQUE	SETTING	POSITIVE OUTCOME
Crisis intervention: brief, here-and-now intervention aimed at reestablishing equilibrium	Investigate precipitating event. Assess client's reaction, strengths, and coping mechanisms. Offer emotional support, guide client through decisions, and help her find adaptive solutions.	General hospitals, emergency departments, community agencies, psychiatric units, crisis units, telephone crisis lines	Client returns to precrisis functioning or higher.
Cognitive behavioral therapy: based on changing distorted views the client has of herself and her world	Offer cognitive restructuring and self-monitoring to change irrational thinking through exposure and response prevention. Through guided self-dialogue the client is taught to think certain thoughts before acting, to stop anxiety-producing thoughts, and to keep journals describing these memories, feelings, and thoughts. (See Chapter 13.)	General hospital, psychiatric hospitals or units, outpatient clinics, private practice	Client's view is restored to optimal level through identification and correction of faulty cognitions.
Systematic desensitization: designed to help client overcome anxiety related to the rape by exposing her to harmless but feared stimuli	Expose client to her own tape-recorded account of the rape while she practices relaxation techniques.	Same as above	Client depersonalizes the event and is desensitized to memory of the rape.

REFERENCES

American Psychiatric Association (1994). *Diagnostic and Statistical Manual of Mental Disorders* (4th ed.). Washington, DC: American Psychiatric Association.

Burgess, A. W., & Holmstrom, L. L. (1986). *Rape: Crisis and Recovery.* West Newton, MA: Awab.

Douglas, J. E., Burgess, A. W., Burgess, A. G., & Ressler, R. K. (1992). *Crime Classification Manual.* New York: Lexington Books.

Foley, T. S. (1984). The client who has been raped. In S. Lego (ed.), *The American Handbook of Psychiatric Nursing* (pp. 475–495). Philadelphia: J. B. Lippincott.

Sampselle, C. M. (1991). The role of nursing in preventing violence against women. *Journal of Obstetric, Gynocologic and Neonatal Nursing, 20* (6), 481.

Vachss, A. (1993). *Sex Crimes.* New York: Random House.

BIBLIOGRAPHY

Calhoun, K. S., & Atkeson, B. M. (1991). *Treatment of Rape Victims: Facilitating Psychosocial Adjustment.* New York: Pergamon Press.

Foa, E. B., Feske, U., Murdock, T. B., Kozak, M. J., & McCarthy, P. R. (1991). Processing of threat-related information in rape victims. *Journal of Abnormal Psychology, 100* (2), 156–162.

Foa, E. B., & Rothbaum, B. O. (1989). Behavioral psychotherapy for post-traumatic stress disorder. *International Review of Psychiatry, 1,* 219–226.

Frank, E. (1988). Efficacy of cognitive behavior therapy and systematic desensitization in the treatment of rape trauma. *Behavior Therapy, 19,* 403–420.

Gelles, R. T., & Cornell, C. P. (1990). *Intimate Violence in Families* (2nd ed.). Newbury Park, CA: Sage.

Groth, A. N. (1979). *Men Who Rape.* New York: Plenum.

Hazelwood, R. B. (1987). Analyzing the rape and profiling the offender. In R. R. Hazelwood and A. W. Burgess (eds.), *Practical Aspects of Rape Investigations.* New York: Elsevier.

Janssen, E. (1995). Understanding the rapist's mind. *Perspectives in Psychiatric Care, 31* (4), 9–13.

Knight, R. A., & Prentky, R. A. (1990). Classifying sexual offenders: The development and corroboration of taxonomic models. In W. L. Marshall, D. R. Laws, & H. E. Barbaree (eds.), *Handbook of Sexual Assault.* New York: Plenum.

Lanning, K. V. (1986). *Child Molesters: A Behavioral Analysis.* Washington, DC: National Center for Missing and Exploited Children.

Ledray, L. E. (1990). Counseling rape victims: The nursing challenge. *Perspectives in Psychiatric Care, 26* (2), 21–27.

Ledray, L. E. (1993). Sexual assault nurse clinician: An emerging area of nursing experience. *AWHONN's Clinical Issues, 4* (2), 180–190.

Ledray, L. E., & Arndt, S. (1994). Examining the sexual assault victim: A new model for nursing care. *Journal of Psychosocial Nursing, 32* (2), 7–12.

Lenehan, G. P. (1991). Sexual assault nurse examiners: A SANE way to care for rape victims. Letter to the editor. *Journal of Emergency Nursing, 17* (1), 1–2.

Minden, P. B. (1989). The victim care services: A program for victims of sexual assault. *Archives of Psychiatric Nursing, 31* (11), 7–14.

Prentky, R. A., Cohen, M. L., & Seghorn, T. K. (1985). Development of a rational taxonomy for the classification of sexual offenders: Rapists. *Bulletin of the American Academy of Psychiatry and the Law, 13,* 39–70.

Solomon, S. D., Gerrity, E. T., & Muff, A. M. (1992). Efficacy of treatments for posttraumatic stress disorder. *Journal of the American Medical Association, 268* (5), 633–638.

Stewart, D. E., & Cecutti, A. (1993). Physical abuse in pregnancy. *Canadian Medical Association Journal, 149* (9), 1257–1263.

THIRTY SEVEN

The Client Who Was Sexually Abused

Claire Burke Draucker

OVERVIEW:	Introduction	Group Therapy
	Long-Term Effects	Male Survivors
	Individual Therapy	

INTRODUCTION

Childhood sexual abuse is a significant issue for many adults who receive psychotherapy or other nursing services. It is estimated that between 20% and 40% of all American women and between 10% and 20% of all American men have experienced a sexual abuse incident before the age of 18 (Finkelhor, Hotaling, Lewis, & Smith, 1990; Urquiza & Keating, 1990). Reported rates of childhood sexual abuse in the histories of individuals who seek psychotherapeutic services range from 20% to 70% (Bolton, Morris, & MacEachron, 1989; Briere & Zaidi, 1989; Doob, 1992; Jacobson, 1989). Therefore, psychiatric nurses frequently work with individuals in therapy who have experienced sexual trauma in their childhoods.

In this chapter, childhood sexual abuse is considered any sexual activity perpetrated on a child to meet the sexual or emotional needs of a person who has power over the child by virtue of older age, authority or privileged position, physical strength, or relationship to the child, whether or not direct physical contact occurred (Draucker, 1992).

LONG-TERM EFFECTS

Whereas only a small portion of adults who were sexually abused as children manifest severe psychopathology (Browne & Finkelhor, 1986), there are several long-term psychological and behavioral effects that are believed to be related to childhood sexual abuse. Table 37-1 lists these effects with examples of related symptomatology.

INDIVIDUAL THERAPY

Several basic assumptions about the nature and the impact of childhood sexual abuse experiences underlie the basic principles of therapy aimed at resolving sexual abuse trauma. These assumptions and principles are outlined in Table 37-2.

The stages of therapy for adult survivors of childhood sexual abuse, the major therapeutic issues, and suggested therapeutic interventions for each stage are outlined in Table 37-3. Although stages are identified for the sake of description, the processes

(Text continues on page 322)

TABLE 37-1
Long-Term Effects of Childhood Sexual Abuse

LONG-TERM EFFECTS	EXAMPLES
1. Posttraumatic effects (Briere, 1992)	
a. Intrusive symptoms	a. Nightmares, flashbacks, repetitive thoughts or memories
b. Avoidant symptoms	b. Phobias, numbing
c. Arousal symptoms	c. Sleep disturbances, irritability
2. Dissociative effects (Loewenstein, 1993)	
a. Amnesia symptoms	a. Blackouts, fugues, fragmentary recall of life experiences
b. Autohypnotic symptoms	b. Trances, voluntary analgesia, depersonalization
c. Dissociative process symptoms	c. Presence of distinct personality states, pseudohallucinations, passive-influence experiences
3. Impaired sense of self	Low self-esteem, identity confusion, boundary disturbances
4. Chronic affective disturbances	Depression, anxiety
5. Disturbed interpersonal relationships	Continued victimization, sexual dysfunction, social isolation, intimacy disturbances, aggression
6. Tension-reducing or self-destructive behaviors (Briere, 1992)	Suicidality, self-mutilation, substance abuse, bingeing and purging, compulsive sexual behavior

TABLE 37-2
Assumptions Regarding Childhood Sexual Abuse and
Implications for Therapy

ASSUMPTIONS	PRINCIPLES OF THERAPY
1. Childhood sexual abuse can cause the various symptoms and emotional distress often exhibited by adult survivors seeking therapy.	1. Exploratory therapy focusing on the abuse, when conducted within the context of a supportive and empowering relationship, can facilitate trauma resolution and result in relief of symptoms, intrapersonal growth, and actualization of potential.
2. Childhood sexual abuse often involves the betrayal of a significant other, the abuse of power, and an invasion of the child's personal boundaries.	2. Therapy must not recapitulate any aspects of the abuse (Briere, 1992). The therapist must clearly articulate the ground rules and boundaries of therapy (e.g., limits of the therapist's availability, length of sessions, parameters of the therapeutic relationship); engage the client in mutual decision making and goal setting related to the therapy experience; avoid any exploitative or seductive behaviors; and seek ongoing supervision or personal therapy to address the therapist's own issues related to abuse and to identify possible countertransference (e.g., identification with the survivor or with the perpetrator).
3. Children who are victims of sexual abuse develop behavioral and psychological responses to the trauma that are necessary for their survival. These responses are often carried into adulthood.	3. Therapy is based on respect and acknowledgment of the client's survival. The client's presenting symptoms are viewed as coping mechanisms that were once needed to adapt to trauma, rather than as pathological processes. Survivors' inner strengths and resources are identified and the courage required to undertake therapy aimed at trauma resolution is acknowledged.
4. Childhood sexual abuse frequently occurs in the context of family dysfunction and always occurs in the context of a society that allows the victimization or oppression of groups of lesser power (Briere, 1992).	4. While resolution of sexual abuse trauma is the focus of treatment, issues related to the broader family and social forces that served as the context of the abuse are also addressed.

TABLE 37-3
Stages of Individual Therapy for Adult Survivors of
Childhood Sexual Abuse

GOALS	THERAPEUTIC ISSUES	THERAPEUTIC INTERVENTIONS

Stage One: Disclosing the Abuse

1. Providing an opportunity for client to disclose childhood sexual abuse experiences
2. Considering the possible relevance of these experiences to client's current concerns or distress

Trust: Often clients have had prior negative experiences (e.g., disbelief, rejection) when disclosing abuse to others and initially may choose not to share a history of abuse with the therapist.

Minimization: Clients may not consider exploitative sexual experiences as abusive and may not believe that their abuse is significant or relevant to their current concerns. This may be owing to a protective psychological process, such as denial of the abuse impact, or may reflect messages from family or prior therapists that the sexual experiences were not significant, influential, or harmful.

Repression: Survivors of abuse often have partial or total amnesia for the sexual abuse incidents, especially if the abuse occurred early, was severe, or was accompanied by physical violence. Clients may have no clear memories of the abuse but may believe "something" traumatic happened during their childhood (Dinsmore, 1991; Walker, 1994).

Assessment: A complete interview that addresses the overall quality of childhood experiences and family relationships, and includes direct, sensitive questions about sexual experiences that were hurtful, discomforting, embarrassing, or frightening, is the most effective way to facilitate disclosure.

Development of trust: Because survivors have typically experienced a major betrayal, disclosure often occurs only after the client and therapist have developed a trusting relationship.

Addressing minimization: When a client discloses a sexual abuse experience but minimizes its significance, the therapist may explore the possible impact of the abuse on the client's development and discuss any possible relationships between the abuse and the client's current concerns.

Addressing repression: If the client's presenting symptoms or family history are strongly suggestive of a sexually abusive or traumatic experience, and if the client suspects but does not remember being sexually abused, the therapist may explore with the client the possibility of repressed trauma. Therapists should consider the increasing concern related to therapy-induced "false memories," and explore the possibility of repression responsibly, while avoiding premature interpretations related to the etiology of the client's symptoms (Loftus & Ketcham, 1994; Yapko, 1994).

Responding to disclosure: Revealing a history of childhood sexual abuse can be a frightening or painful experience for survivors. Therapeutic responses to difficult disclosures of childhood sexual abuse include:

1. Responding calmly while exhibiting concern and interest
2. Acknowledging the difficulty of disclosure
3. Validating the significance of the disclosure
4. Providing support and reassuring the client of therapist availability
5. Inviting clients to discuss the abuse at their own pace
6. Evaluating the client's mental status
7. Determining the client's immediate safety needs

TABLE 37-3 *(continued)*

GOALS	THERAPEUTIC ISSUES	THERAPEUTIC INTERVENTIONS

Stage Two: Preparing for Exploratory Therapy

1. Determining if the sexual abuse, rather than symptom relief or the presenting concern, shall be the focus of therapy
2. Preparing for exploratory work related to the abuse trauma

Abuse-focused versus symptomatic treatment: Survivors have often been treated by many therapists for numerous and varied symptoms without having the relationship of their sexual abuse experience to their current distress addressed.

Power and control: Sexual abuse robs children of control over their own lives. Issues related to power, control, and choice are always important concerns in therapy with survivors.

Symptom exacerbation: When exploratory work begins, the client will likely experience an exacerbation of symptoms and increased emotional distress (e.g., anxiety, depression, anger). Clients who have a history of self-destructive behaviors (e.g., suicidality, substance abuse, eating disorders) or who have a tendency to neglect their self-care needs may be at risk during this time.

Therapy contract: Survivors are naturally fearful, and often initially resistant, to begin the painful work of trauma resolution. While these feelings can be addressed, the choice to focus on the sexual abuse in therapy must be mutually agreed upon by client and therapist (Draucker, 1992).

Self-care planning: The therapist explains that some exacerbation of symptoms and increase in affect is a normal part of trauma resolution and requires some preparation regarding self-care and safety. A self-care plan may be aimed at basic needs (e.g., an agreement to engage in some form of relaxation, such as a recreational activity, following a particularly difficult session) or may be more extensive and involved (e.g., a year's sobriety for a client actively abusing substances; a suicide contract and plan for a client with a history of suicide attempts) (Draucker, 1992).

Stage Three: Focusing on the Abuse Experience

1. Decreasing denial or minimization
2. Beginning the process of trauma resolution

Trauma response: Traumatic events threaten physical and psychological integrity and exceed normal capacities for coping. When an individual experiences a trauma such as childhood sexual abuse, from which escape is not possible, the victim typically "escapes" through some dissociative processes, which often extend into adulthood. Trauma that is unresolved and unassimilated results in continuing symptoms and psychic distress in the life of the survivor (Briere, 1992; Loewenstein, 1993).

Abuse work: In therapy, the individual becomes aware of and reexperiences the traumatic events in a safe and supportive environment while learning to tolerate previously dissociated affect. The availability, support, and reassurance of the therapist are important during this process. Abuse work results in the integration and resolution of the trauma and involves several interventions:

1. Exploration of the significant factors of the abuse experience that survivors remember or suspect. Such factors may include:
   a. The duration and frequency of the abuse
   b. The client's relationship to the offender
   c. Methods used to carry out the abuse
   d. The sexual activities involved
   e. The survivor's and the offender's ages at the time of the abuse
   f. Circumstances that altered or ended the abuse
   g. The role of family in the abuse
   h. Results of disclosure, if it occurred
2. Description of remembered abuse incidents and the experiencing of feelings associated with those memories (Briere, 1992). The client is asked to:
   a. Describe verbal memories (i.e., What is the first thing you remember happening? What happened next?)
   b. Describe sensory memories (i.e., What can you see, smell, feel?)

(Continued)

TABLE 37-3 *(continued)*

GOALS	THERAPEUTIC ISSUES	THERAPEUTIC INTERVENTIONS
Stage Three (continued)		

c. Identify, label, and discuss feelings that are associated with the memories. Guilt, shame, anger, and sadness may be experienced initially. Deeper feelings that arise as the abuse work continues may include terror, despair, and a sense of abandonment (Blake-White & Kline, 1985).

3. Retrieval of repressed memories. Repression is generally considered a protective defense and interventions for memory retrieval should be used cautiously at a pace dictated by the client's progress. Memories are often retrieved during the normal course of therapy while childhood experiences are being addressed. Interventions used to facilitate memory retrieval include:

   a. Viewing old family photographs, scrapbooks, or diaries from the period in which abuse is believed to have occurred
   b. Reading literature written by other survivors
   c. Attending group therapy
   d. Talking with family members (e.g., siblings)
   e. Hypnosis and guided imagery (These are more invasive procedures that should only be used judiciously by therapists with sufficient training and supervision.)

Consolidation work: The use of interventions to facilitate abuse exploration should be carefully paced and the client's symptoms, affect, and level of dissociation should be continuously monitored (Briere, 1992). Exacerbation of trauma effects is anticipated during the working through of the abuse experience, but too great an exacerbation may reflect problems with the timing or intensity of the therapeutic process. Consolidation interventions to pace the therapeutic process and to assure the client's safety include:

1. Normalizing symptom exacerbation. Clients are reassured that the exacerbation of symptoms and the increase in painful feelings that occur during abuse work, while distressing, are related to healing.
2. Focusing on the present. Discussion of the client's current concerns and reviewing progress made thus far can help the client maintain a sense of control and can modulate the intensity of therapy.
3. Grounding techniques. These techniques can cognitively remove the survivor from childhood memories and modulate the affect associated with those memories (Blake-White & Kline, 1985; Cole & Barney, 1987). During flashbacks clients may be taught to:
   a. Repeat their name, age, and current location
   b. Plant their feet firmly on the ground and grasp the arm of a chair
4. Hypnotic distancing techniques. Clients can be taught to control the intensity of their affect and to manage dissociative symptomatology. Techniques include (Loewenstein, 1993):
   a. Developing the image of a "safe" place to go to achieve inner peace
   b. Having a hypnotic "screen" on which to project and control disturbing visual imagery (e.g., "zoom in" and "zoom out")
   c. Imagining having one's own "rheostat" with which to turn down anxiety
5. Focusing on the self-care plan. Reviewing and reinforcing the self-care plan is indicated during times of symptom exacerbation.

TABLE 37-3 *(continued)*

GOALS	THERAPEUTIC ISSUES	THERAPEUTIC INTERVENTIONS

Stage Four: Reinterpreting the Sexual Abuse Experience from an Adult Perspective

1. Addressing the distorted beliefs and perceptions of self, others, and the world that developed in response to the abuse experience
2. Reinterpreting the sexual abuse experience from an adult perspective

Cognitive distortions: Common distorted perceptions and beliefs exhibited by survivors are as follows:
1. Blaming the self. Survivors often have received the message, either directly or indirectly, by "society" or family, that they were to blame for their victimization because they enjoyed the attention or affection associated with the abuse, found the experience sexually pleasurable, didn't tell anyone, or were inherently bad. These messages are internalized by survivors who come to believe the abuse was their fault.
2. Lack of self-efficacy. Because survivors experienced a traumatic event they were powerless to stop, they come to believe they have little control over the course of their lives and limited ability to influence their environment in ways they desire.
3. Equating love with sex. Survivors of abuse often believe they must provide sex to be loved.
4. Viewing all relationships from an abuse perspective. Survivors, especially those whose abuse occurred within the context of the nuclear family, assume that all relationships are based on power dynamics. Those with power are always seen as potential abusers and those without power are seen as potential victims.

Cognitive restructuring: This is a therapeutic technique used to address distorted thoughts related to the abuse by (Jehu, Klassen, & Gazan, 1986):
1. Discussing how beliefs, feelings, and behaviors can be related
2. Identifying distressing beliefs related to the abuse
3. Recognizing distortions in those beliefs
4. Exploring alternate beliefs

Experiential reinforcing of new beliefs: Techniques that reinforce survivors' "new" beliefs on a feeling level are helpful adjuncts to the cognitive approach (Draucker, 1992). Techniques include:
1. Viewing childhood photos to reinforce the client's "childlikeness" at the time of the abuse.
2. Using an empty chair technique in which the client asserts the offender's responsibility for the abuse.
3. Having the client write an unsent letter to an offender reaffirming the offender's responsibility for the abuse.
4. Having the client confront offenders or family members (Gelinas, 1993). These experiences can be powerful, but must follow careful planning. A survivor who confronts an offender with hopes of the offender showing remorse may feel revictimized if the offender does not respond in this manner.

Stage Five: Addressing the Context of the Sexual Abuse

Understanding the sociocultural and family context of the sexual abuse experience

The abuse context: To fully understand the sexual abuse experience and to integrate this aspect of one's childhood into ones's life history, an appreciation of other influential life experiences is necessary. The sexual abuse therefore does not remain "out of context."

The following childhood issues may be explored:
1. Family communication and interaction patterns
2. Concomitant physical and emotional abuse
3. Family alcoholism and mental illness
4. Perceived role of nonoffending family members in the abuse dynamics
5. Significant losses and illnesses
6. Positive experiences and relationships
7. The impact of societal forces (e.g., sex-role stereotyping, oppression, the historical denial of the sexual abuse of children) on one's childhood

Stage Six: Making Desired Life Changes

Making desired behavioral and lifestyle changes in areas that were previously influenced by abuse effects

Lifestyle changes: Many aspects of the client's lifestyle (e.g., relationships, sexuality, career) were likely to be influenced by the abuse experience. Once significant abuse work has been completed, many survivors seek to make changes in one or more aspects of their lives.

1. Family or couples treatment
2. Sex therapy (Bolen, 1993; Maltz & Holman, 1987)
3. Career counseling

(Continued)

TABLE 37-3 *(continued)*

GOALS	THERAPEUTIC ISSUES	THERAPEUTIC INTERVENTIONS

Stage Seven: Addressing Resolution Issues

Integrating the sexual abuse experience into one's identity so that the abuse no longer serves as the primary guiding force in one's life	*Resolution of philosophical and spiritual issues related to the abuse:* These issues include:
	1. Forgiveness. As survivors begin to heal, they often wrestle with the issue of forgiveness. Two "styles" of forgiveness have been identified (Maltz & Holman, 1987):
	  a. Releasing offenders from responsibility for the abuse by justifying their activities (e.g., "He was mentally ill," "He was drunk all the time"). This may represent an attempt at premature resolution by denial of anger and hurt.
	  b. Recognizing the offender's limitations, history, and weaknesses and no longer experiencing bitterness and need for revenge. Although forgiveness is always a choice, not a prerequisite for healing, this style of forgiveness can facilitate the resolution.
	2. Finding purpose. Determining the "greater meaning" of the abuse, as it relates to the overall purpose of one's life, is a poignant issue for survivors as they more fully resolve their traumatic childhood experiences. Survivors often ponder their relationship with God or reflect on their spiritual beliefs. While fully acknowledging the pain that the abuse itself caused, survivors often come to believe that healing from that abuse made them stronger, more compassionate, or more empowered individuals than they might have otherwise been.
	3. Identity issues. Establishing a clear sense of one's identity, including the integration of the abuse experience, often results in giving up the identity of "survivor." Clients accept the abuse as an important aspect of their childhoods but no longer define themselves solely in relationship to their abuse experiences. They grow to appreciate the many dimensions of their personality and the many aspects of their lives.
		Termination: Resolution issues discussed earlier, such as forgiveness, finding meaning, and identity, often arise as clients prepare to end therapy because termination represents closure on work related to trauma. Therefore, such issues are often discussed during this last phase of therapy.
		
		As termination inevitably represents a loss, the process also includes:
		1. Saying good-bye
		2. Reviewing progress
		3. Discussing future plans

they reflect are in actuality neither discrete nor linear. Healing is more accurately described as a spiral process in which a client may complete one task of recovery only to return to it later, often from a different perspective and with greater insight (Dinsmore, 1991).

GROUP THERAPY

Group therapy is an effective treatment modality for adult survivors of childhood sexual abuse and is often used in conjunction with, or following, individual therapy. Three basic types of therapy groups for sexual abuse survivors have been identified. Short-term, structured groups have a limited number of sessions, often between 6 and 12, and typically limit membership to those individuals who begin the group initially. Long-term, open-ended groups are ongoing and allow members to enter the group at various times. Time-limited, consecutive group programs include a series of group "cycles," each of which runs for a limited time period (e.g., for 12 sessions) and is followed by a hiatus before the next "cycle" begins. The goals, activities, advantages, and disadvantages of each type of group are outlined in Table 37-4. Specific issues to consider when planning group therapy for survivors of sexual abuse are described in Table 37-5.

MALE SURVIVORS

While men and women who were sexually abused as children exhibit many similar responses to their victimization, unique treatment issues for male survivors, related to the sociopolitical context of their abuse, have been identified (Bolton et al., 1989; Struve, 1990). Sex role expectations for males often result in gender-specific responses to childhood sexual abuse. These responses influence recovery and therefore should be considered when conducting therapy with male survivors (Struve, 1990). Table 37-6 outlines relevant sex role expectations, related gender-specific responses to victimization, and implications for therapy with male survivors.

TABLE 37-4
Types of Therapy Groups for Adult Survivors of Childhood Sexual Abuse

TYPE OF GROUP	GOALS	ACTIVITIES	ADVANTAGES	DISADVANTAGES
Long-term, open-ended groups (Briere, 1989; Hall & Lloyd, 1989)	Exploration of sexual abuse with others who have had similar experiences. Decreasing feelings of isolation, shame, stigma. Developing trust and interpersonal skills. Developing a social support network.	Typically, open forum for discussion of issues brought up by group members.	New members may be added throughout life of group. Members can achieve goals at their own pace. Members further along in the healing process can provide hope for newer members. Long-term relationships among group members can result in greater cohesion.	Potential for the development of sub-grouping. Interpersonal conflicts are likely to arise. This could provide opportunity for learning regarding the impact of abuse on relationships. However, such conflicts, if allowed to become the primary focus of the group, could interfere with other activities aimed at trauma resolution, such as processing memories of sexual abuse incidents.
Short-term, structured groups (Briere, 1989; Hall & Lloyd, 1989)	Focus on a specific abuse issue with others who have similar healing needs.	The agenda of each session is typically predetermined. Sessions may be planned around topics (e.g., self-esteem) or around activities (e.g., sharing childhood photos).	Structure encourages focus on a particular healing task. Some survivors feel more comfortable committing to a group with a limited number of sessions.	Limited number of sessions may interfere with the development of trust and group commitment. Issues may not be explored in depth and individual needs of members may not be addressed.
Time-limited, consecutive groups (Sgroi, 1989)	Combination of above.	A theme (e.g., dealing with fears) is determined for one group cycle. Following a hiatus, another cycle focusing on a different theme occurs.	Survivors may commit to a group experience with a finite number of sessions while still having the opportunity to continue group therapy when the next cycle begins.	Disadvantages of other approaches are lessened.

TABLE 37-5
Issues in Planning Groups for Adult Survivors of
Childhood Sexual Abuse

ISSUES	CONSIDERATIONS
Choice of Facilitators	
1. Qualifications	1. Group facilitators should have both group leadership skills and expertise in treating abuse survivors.
2. Number	2. Co-facilitators are recommended to share leadership tasks and to provide emotional support and peer supervision for one another.
3. Gender	3. For single-gender groups, leaders of the same gender as group members are typically recommended to engender trust earlier in the group process (Cole, 1985). However, mixed-gender co-facilitator teams have potential benefits. For example, a male facilitator in a women's survivor group would provide opportunities for members to experience a nonexploitative relationship with a man.
Composition of Groups	
1. Gender	1. While mixed gender groups have the advantage of allowing members to appreciate the universality of the victimization experience, male and female survivors may have difficulty trusting one another initially in group. Also, because men and women deal with their abuse recovery in unique ways, a single gender group may be preferable, especially for a survivor's initial group experience.
2. Other traits	2. Balancing other traits (e.g., sexual orientation, race) within a group is generally recommended. However, the potential for any one group member to feel different or isolated (e.g., having one lesbian or one woman of color) should be considered (Dinsmore, 1991).
3. Types of abuse	3. Some groups mix individuals who were physically, sexually, or emotionally abused based on the belief that survivors of all types of abuse share similar issues (Gil, 1990). However, groups limited to only sexual abuse survivors may be preferable to deal with issues related specifically to sexual abuse (e.g., shame, secrecy, sexuality).
Screening	
1. Screening meeting	1. A screening meeting with individuals prior to the beginning of the group is used to determine survivors' appropriateness for group membership and to give potential members an opportunity to meet the leaders and learn about the group.
2. Criteria for membership	2. Exclusionary criteria include psychosis or disorientation, active suicidality, current substance abuse, or an inability to discuss the abuse experience with the group leader at the screening session. Many groups require that members have an individual therapist to provide support in the event of a crisis or decompensation.
Ground Rule and Boundaries	
1. Confidentiality	1. Material discussed in group is to remain confidential. The leaders, however, cannot guarantee confidentiality and it should be stated that all group members share the responsibility of maintaining confidentiality. Limits of confidentiality include instances in which group members are of danger to themselves or others.
2. Safety	2. Physical safety needs are respected and no physical violence is tolerated. Group members' emotional safety is also of concern in the group. Whereas helpful confrontation is encouraged, verbal abuse is not accepted.
3. Group time	3. The times of the beginning and ending of the group should be specified and respected.
4. Attendance	4. While most support groups allow members to attend periodically, most therapy groups require regular attendance. Many group members experience anxiety and shame after disclosing their abuse in group and may experience the impulse to quit the group. Members should be encouraged to work through those feelings with the support of the group. Nonetheless, if any member chooses to leave the group, that choice should be respected.

TABLE 37-6
Male Survivors of Childhood Sexual Abuse

MALE SEX ROLE EXPECTATIONS	GENDER-RELATED RESPONSES TO VICTIMIZATION	THERAPY IMPLICATIONS
Men, as members of the dominant class in a patriarchal society, should not be seen as victims (Struve, 1990).	Male survivors often exhibit reluctance to seek treatment. Male survivors often resist viewing exploitative childhood sexual experiences as abusive.	The therapist must provide a supportive environment that facilitates disclosure. Avoiding labels "victim" or "abuse" is recommended until trust is developed (Bolton et al., 1989). A clear explanation of the therapeutic process is recommended. A goal of therapy is to disrupt the survivor's association between the concepts of "victimization" and "weakness," and to focus on the power differential between a child and the older offender, i.e., the abuse occurred because the offender had more knowledge, experience, and power; not because the survivor was "weak" (Bolton et al., 1989).
Power, strength, and control are defining male characteristics.	Male survivors often believe that as males, they should have protected themselves from victimization in childhood (Bolton et al., 1989; Struve, 1990). Exaggerated masculine behaviors, e.g., aggression, "macho" activities, exerting excessive control in interpersonal relationships, may be exhibited by the male survivor to reestablish a sense of control (Struve, 1990).	Therapy addresses irrational beliefs related to sex role socialization, e.g., "real men" are always in control, and explores how these beliefs may be related to the self-image, attempts to compensate for abuse experiences, and impaired interpersonal relationships (Bolton et al., 1989).
Men should not express "feminine" feelings, e.g., sadness, vulnerability, depression, but may externalize anger.	Male survivors may engage in victimizing or aggressive behaviors toward others. Substance abuse is often the male survivor's way of dealing with unacceptable feelings, i.e., "to deaden the pain."	Therapy may include assertive training, substance abuse treatment, and anger management. The cultural basis for the injunction against men expressing feelings can be addressed in therapy and cultural beliefs related to feelings, e.g., experiencing feelings equals loss of control, feelings necessitate action, can be challenged (Bolton et al., 1989).
Men are valued according to their productivity (Struve, 1990).	Male survivors may engage compulsively in activities-related achievement, e.g., work, sex, sports.	Specific techniques related to such behaviors, e.g. treatment for sexual dysfunction, may be integrated into the therapy plan (Bolton et al., 1989).

REFERENCES

Blake-White, J., & Kline, C. M. (1985). Treating the dissociative process in adult survivors of childhood incest. *Social Casework: The Journal of Contemporary Social Work, 66,* 394–402.

Bolen, J. D. (1993). Sexuality-focused treatment with survivors and their partners. In P. Paddison (ed.), *Treatment of Adult Survivors of Incest* (pp. 55–76). Washington, DC: American Psychiatric Press.

Bolton, F. G., Morris, L. A., & MacEachron, A. E. (1989). *Males at Risk: The Other Side of Child Sexual Abuse.* Newbury Park, CA: Sage.

Briere, J. (1989). *Therapy for Adults Molested as Children.* New York: Springer.

Briere, J. (1992). *Child Abuse Trauma: Theory and Treatment of Lasting Effects.* Newbury Park, CA: Sage.

Briere, J., & Zaidi, L. Y. (1989). Sexual abuse histories and sequelae in female psychiatric emergency room patients. *American Journal of Psychiatry, 144,* 1426–1430.

Browne, A., & Finkelhor, D. (1986). Initial and long-term effects: A review of the research. In D. Finkelhor (ed.), *A Source Book on Child Sexual Abuse* (pp. 143–179). Newbury Park, CA: Sage.

Cole, C. H., & Barney, E. E. (1987). Safeguards and the therapeutic window: A group treatment strategy for adult incest survivors. *American Journal of Orthopsychiatry, 57,* 668–670.

Cole, C. L. (1985). A group design for adult female survivors of childhood incest. *Women and Therapy, 4* (3), 71–82.

Dinsmore, C. (1991). *From Surviving to Thriving: Incest, Feminism, and Recovery.* Albany, NY: State University of New York Press.

Doob, D. (1992). Female sexual abuse survivors as patients: Avoiding retraumatization. *Archives of Psychiatric Nursing, 6* (4), 245–251.

Draucker, C. B. (1992). *Counseling Adult Survivors of Childhood Sexual Abuse.* London: Sage.

Finkelhor, D., Hotaling, G., Lewis, I. A., & Smith, C. (1990). Sexual abuse in a national survey of adult men and women: Prevalence, characteristics, and risk factors. *Child Abuse & Neglect, 14,* 19–28.

Gelinas, D. J. (1993). Relational patterns in incestuous families, malevolent variations, and specific interventions with the adult survivor. In P. Paddison (ed.), *Treatment of Adult Survivors of Incest* (pp. 1–34). Washington, DC: American Psychiatric Press.

Gil, E. (1990). *Treatment of Adult Survivors of Childhood Abuse.* Walnut Creek, CA: Launch Press.

Hall, L., & Lloyd, S. (1989). *Surviving Childhood Sexual Abuse.* New York: Falmer Press.

Jacobson, A. (1989). Physical and sexual assault histories among psychiatric outpatients. *American Journal of Psychiatry, 146,* 755–758.

Jehu, D., Klassen, C., & Gazan, M. (1986). Cognitive restructuring of distorted beliefs associated with childhood sexual abuse. *Journal of Social Work and Human Sexuality, 4,* 49–69.

Loewenstein, R. J. (1993). Aspects of the treatment of dissociative disorders in survivors of incest. In P. Paddison (ed.), *Treatment of Adult Survivors of Incest* (pp. 77–100). Washington, DC: American Psychiatric Press.

Loftus, E., & Ketcham, K. (1994). *The Myth of Repressed Memory: False Memories and Allegations of Sexual Abuse.* New York: St. Martin's Press.

Maltz, W., & Holman, B. (1987). *Incest and Sexuality: A Guide to Understanding and Healing.* Lexington, MA.: D. C. Heath and Company.

Sgroi, S. M. (1989). Healing together: Peer group therapy for adult survivors of child sexual abuse. In S. Sgroi (ed.), *Vulnerable Populations: Vol 2. Sexual Abuse Treatment for Children, Adult Survivors, and Persons with Mental Retardation* (pp. 131–166). Lexington, MA: Lexington Books.

Struve, J. (1990). Dancing with the patriarchy: The politics of sexual abuse. In M. Hunter (ed.), *The Sexually Abused Male: Vol 1. Prevalence, Impact, and Treatment* (pp. 3–46). Lexington, MA: D. C. Heath and Company.

Urquiza, A. J., & Keating, L. M. (1990). The prevalence of the sexual victimization of males. In M. Hunter (ed.), *The Sexually Abused Male: Vol 1. Prevalence, Impact, and Treatment* (pp. 89–104). Lexington, MA: D. C. Heath and Company.

Walker, L. E. A. (1994). *Abused Women and Survivor Therapy.* Washington, DC: American Psychological Press.

Yapko, M. (1994). *Suggestions of Abuse: True and False Memories of Childhood Sexual Abuse Trauma.* New York: Simon & Schuster.

BIBLIOGRAPHY

Blume, E. S. (1990). *Secret Survivors: Uncovering Incest and Its Aftereffects in Women.* New York: Wiley.

Courtois, C. A. (1988). *Healing the Incest Wound.* New York: W. W. Norton & Company.

Gonsiorek, J. C., Bera, W. H., & LeTourneau, D. (1994). *Male Sexual Abuse. A Trilogy of Intervention Strategies.* Newbury Park, CA: Sage.

Herman, J. L. (1992). *Trauma and Recovery.* New York: Basic Books.

Hunter, M. (1990). *Abused Boys: The Neglected Victims of Sexual Abuse.* New York: Fawcett Columbine.

Hunter, M. (1995). *Adult Survivors of Sexual Abuse.* Newbury Park, CA: Sage.

Kluft, R. P. (ed.) (1990). *Incest Related Syndromes of Adult Psychopathology.* Washington, DC: American Psychiatric Association Press.

Lee, S. A. (1995). *A Survivor's Guide: For Teenage Girls Surviving Sexual Abuse.* Newbury Park, CA: Sage.

Mendel, M. P. (1994). *The Male Survivor: The Impact of Sexual Abuse.* Newbury Park, CA: Sage.

Russell, D. E. H. (1986). *The Secret Trauma: Incest in the Lives of Girls and Women.* New York: Basic Books.

Salter, A. (1995). *Transforming Trauma: A Guide to Understanding and Treating Adult Survivors of Childhood Sexual Abuse.* Newbury Park, CA: Sage.

Smith, M. (1993). *Ritual Abuse: What It Is, Why It Happens, How to Help.* New York: HarperCollins.

Terr, L. (1994). *Unchained Memories: True Stories of Traumatic Memories, Lost and Found.* New York: Basic Books.

Wiehe, V. R. (1990). *Sibling Abuse: Hidden Physical, Emotional, and Sexual Trauma.* Lexington, MA: Lexington Books.

Wilson, M. (1994). *Crossing the Boundary: Black Women Survive Incest.* Seattle: Seal Press.

Wingerson, N. (1992). Psychic loss in adult survivors of father–daughter incest. *Archives of Psychiatric Nursing, 6* (4), 239–244.

The Client Who Is an Incest Perpetrator

Suzanne Lego

OVERVIEW:

DEFINITION

The incest perpetrator is one who has sexual contact with a person who is biologically related or a stepchild.*

MYTHS AND FACTS

Many people believe that incest perpetrators act out only in their own families. A study showed that 49% of subjects also abused female children outside the family at the same time they abused children at home (Abel, Becker, Cunningham-Rathner, Mittleman, & Rouleau, 1988). Other myths and facts are shown in Box 38-1.

---

*While males are sometimes victims of incest, this chapter will focus mainly on father–daughter incest.

BOX 38-1: Myths and Facts About Incest Perpetrators

Myths	Facts
Many believe incest perpetrators to be:	Rather they are often:
1. Dirty old men	1. Churchgoing
2. Strangers to their victims	2. Respected
3. Retarded	3. Hardworking
4. Alcoholic or drug addicted	4. Competent
5. Sexually frustrated	5. Successful
6. Insane	
7. Increasingly violent over time	

From Ballard, D. T., et al. (1990). A comparative profile of the incest perpetrator: Background characteristics, abuse history and use of social skills. In A. Horton, B. L. Johnson, L. M. Roundy, & D. Williams (eds.), *The Incest Perpetrator: A Family Member No One Wants to Treat* (pp. 43–64). Newbury Park, CA: Sage.

PROFILE OF THE OFFENDER

In a study of 383 offenders in prisons, mental health agencies, Parents United (a self-help group), and private practice, the following demographics were found (Ballard, Blair, Devereaux, Valentine, Horton, & Johnson, 1990):

1. Gender: 97.9% male
2. Age: mean age 38.8 years
3. Ethnicity: 84.6% white
4. Education: 12.1 years
5. Employment: 65.1% employed full-time
6. Religion: 47.1% Protestant
7. Current use of alcohol: 79% never/seldom
8. Current use of drugs: 45.6% never/seldom
9. History of psychiatric problems: 15.4%
10. Hospitalization for psychiatric problems: 18.9%
11. Current marital status: 56% married
12. Previous marital status: 79.8% married
13. Number of marriages: 56.4% had one; 30.1% had two
14. Previous marital satisfaction on a scale from 1–10: sexual 4.5; emotional 3.6; overall 4.0
15. History of abuse: 52% were physically abused; 53% were sexually abused. Pelto (1981) found 10 times more abuse, and Langevin (1983) found 5 times more abuse in offenders' histories than control groups.
16. Incest perpetrators demonstrated strong confirmation of poor social skills (Ballard et al., 1990).
17. Isolation: Offenders were isolated in their families of origin, relationships with peers, and marriages (Gilgun & Connor, 1990).

DYNAMICS IN INTACT FAMILIES

CLASSIC PICTURE

Both the family and the father prefer that he remain in the family to have his sexual needs met, rather than leave. The mother plays a vital role by overtly or covertly condoning the behavior. Frequently the marriage is conflictual and the mother does not want sex with the father. The mother may be phobic about sex, having been abused herself, may fear pregnancy, or may be overwhelmed and fatigued. Often she has abdicated the role of housekeeper and the oldest daughter has taken over. She then takes her mother's sexual role as well.

MORE RECENT FINDINGS

There is great variety in these findings. Mothers often do not desire or benefit from the incest, more than one child is abused, and many fathers abuse outside the home. The most constant family dynamic is male dominance over dependent wives.

DYNAMICS IN STEPFATHER INCEST

1. Absence of the incest taboo exists along with role confusion. He enters as a boyfriend and becomes a father.
2. In a study of 63 cases, frequently the stepfather was younger than the mother and became "another child" in the family.
3. In the same study, one-third of the children had been sexually maltreated by their biological fathers. This may have increased their vulnerability as they had been socialized to expect sexual behavior from adult males, and may have acted in ways perceived as seductive by their stepfathers. Also, the stepfather may have been titillated by this knowledge, and may have used this knowledge to rationalize his own behavior (Faller, 1990).

DYNAMICS IN ABUSE BY NONCUSTODIAL FATHERS

1. There is a lack of structure and monitoring of interaction between father and daughter.
2. Frequently the mother initiated the breakup. The father is angry, bewildered, and desolate, and transfers these feelings to the child.
3. The father may seek comfort from the child and this interaction becomes sexualized.
4. The father may regress under the stress of the marital demise and may feel more comfortable with an immature sex object (Faller, 1990).

THE GROOMING PROCESS

Christianson and Blake (1990) outlined six steps in the process of grooming daughters for incest:

1. *Developing trust:* 90% of perpetrators revealed to Warner-Kearney (1987) that they deliberately built trust with their daughters first, before beginning any sexual activity. This reduces the risk of exposure. They did this by (Christianson & Blake, 1990):
   - Giving them presents of candy, food, money, clothing
   - Spending time with them
   - Assuring them of the "rightness" of what they were doing
   - Telling them the sexual acts would not hurt them

   Interviews by Passey (1987) confirmed that the fathers had indeed convinced their daughters to trust them, and this had led to the incest.
2. *Favoritism:* The daughter is often given gifts, candy, and clothes with the idea she will have to "be nice" in return. Role blurring leads to the idea she is a special friend to her father and more valued than her mother or siblings. Her father may disclose his loneliness to her, encouraging her to want to fill this loneliness, and thus increasing her self-esteem.
3. *Alienation:* These girls are alienated from their mothers because they have taken over the role of confidante, intimate friend, and sex partner. They are alienated

from their siblings, owing to their special status with their father, and from their friends because their fathers come to dominate their lives. The incest serves to make them feel different from their peers.

4. *Secrecy:* Fathers may use persuasive, subtle, and confusing rationalizations to develop secrecy as a part of their "special" relationship, for example, "Mom wouldn't understand how special we are together. Ours is a special love that others wouldn't understand" (Christianson & Blake, 1990, p. 91).

5. *Boundary violations:* These begin as early as infancy:
   Bathing: Fathers may insist on bathing their daughters, washing them all over, and may bathe with them, asking them to reciprocate.
   Dressing: Fathers may dress their daughters, dress together, or watch them dress.
   Bathroom behaviors: Fathers watch and participate with their daughters in bathroom behavior, which lends itself to conversations about bodily and sexual functions.
   Sexually explicit and vulgar conversation: Fathers use sexually explicit language to refer to daily experiences, thus eroticizing the child, and providing easy movement from talk to action.

6. *Evaluation of the grooming phase:* The father attempts to evaluate whether the grooming has prepared the girl to move into the overtly sexual stage.

ONGOING PHASE

This phase involves planning, scheming, and execution of strategies (Christianson & Blake, 1990):

1. *Stepwise progression of sexual acts:* Touching, kissing, hugging, fondling, breast stimulation, reciprocal fondling, masturbation, oral stimulation of breast and genitals, reciprocal masturbation, oral sex and, finally, coitus. If the daughter is pubescent there is less intercourse, owing to a fear of pregnancy.

2. *Repeated checking of risks:* Fathers watch their daughters carefully to be sure it is safe to proceed.

3. *Selecting a place:* The most frequently used place is the daughter's bedroom; the second is the living room. This serves to eliminate a place that is "safe" for the child.

4. *Selecting a time:* Rather than choosing a time when others are out of the house, most perpetrators fit the sex act into late evening, relaxing routines such as bathing, showering, preparing for bed, watching television.

5. *Bribes, threats, and punishments:* Fathers offer gifts and may act more kindly to the daughters than to other siblings. If the girls are reluctant to continue, they may be physically threatened. If disclosure is threatened, the fathers may threaten the girls by saying if anyone found out, they would lose their jobs, their mothers would divorce the fathers, and the children would be put in foster homes. Alcohol is sometimes used by both father and daughter.

AMELIORATION PHASE

The incest ends and the father shifts the blame to the daughter, saying she was seductive. Any negative outcomes are seen by the girl as her fault. Edmonds and Christianson (1988) found that obtaining a confession from the father with a full apology to the daughter tends to reduce the daughter's guilt in both the short term and long term.

ONGOING INCEST CUES

Christianson and Blake (1990) describe the following cues that a girl is involved in incest:

1. Girls display low self-esteem, antisocial behavior, withdrawal, sexual acting out, sudden lack of interest or motivation in school, and mood changes.

2. Fathers place unusual demands on the girl's time and do not welcome her peers.
3. Fathers spend much time with the girls in their rooms or the living room late at night, or attending them while they bathe or dress.
4. Girls display apprehension, owing to threats and intimidation, or they have physical evidence of actual assaults.
5. Fathers and daughters use alcohol and drugs.

STAGES IN THE SYSTEM OF SERVICE

1. *Allegation stage:* Child, wife, or victim comes forth.
2. *Crisis intervention stage:* Perpetrator is separated from family. The arrangements in order of preference are:
   - The father leaves the home.
   - The mother and children leave the home.
   - The child moves to another relative's home.
   - The child is placed in foster care.
3. *Investigation stage:* A child protective agency is notified and investigates.
4. *Judicial process stage:* If charges are filed, a trial may be held.
5. *Treatment stage:* Treatment may be by self-referral or court mandated.
6. *Reintegration stage:* Gradual move from individual and group to family therapy, increasing contact with the family, referral to Parents United and other self-help groups, etc. (See Box 38-2.)
7. *Maintenance stage:* Lifelong treatment and monitoring to offender, victim, and family (Ingersoll & Patton, 1990).

LEGAL ISSUES

Duty to Report   In most states clinicians have a duty to report child abuse or suspected abuse to a child protection agency. In some states past abuse disclosed by an adult must be reported. In others there is a statute of limitations. Once the therapist files the initial

---

▌BOX 38-2: Organizations Helping Incest Perpetrators and Victims

AlexAndria Associates, 911 W.W. 3rd Street, Ontario, OR 97914.

Center for the Prevention of Sexual and Domestic Violence, N. 34th Street, Suite 105, Seattle, WA 98103.

Channing L. Bete Co., Inc., 200 State Road, South Deerfield, MA 01373-0200, (800) 628-7733.

Child Sexual Abuse Curriculum for Social Workers, 9725 East Hampden Avenue, Denver, CO 80231-4919, (303) 695-0811.

Child Help USA, 6463 Independence Avenue, Woodland Hills, CA 91367, (818) 347-7280.

Effectiveness Training, Inc., 531 Stevens Avenue, Solana Beach, CA 92075.

Ending Men's Violence National Referral Directory, To RAVEN, P.O. Box 24159, St. Louis, MO 63130, (314) 725-6137.

Family Resources, 429 Forbes Avenue, Pittsburgh, PA 15261, (412) 562-9440.

National Adolescent Perpetrator Network, Denver, CO 80231, (303) 321-3963.

National Self-Help Clearing House, Graduate School, City University of New York, 33 West 42nd Street, Rm. 1222, New York, NY 10036, (212) 840-1259.

Parents Anonymous (P.A.). To locate a P.A. group in your area, call toll free outside California (800) 421-0353. Inside California call (800) 352-0386.

Parents United treatment and self-help. Call to locate a P.U. group in your area. (409) 280-5055.

Society's League Against Molestation, 524 S. 1st Avenue, Arcadia, CA 91006, (818) 445-0802.

report, client disclosures in therapy are considered privileged and confidential (*People v. Stritzinger,* California, 1983).

Duty to Warn or Duty to Protect If the therapist has "a reasonable suspicion that a client may endanger another person, the therapist must use 'reasonable care' in protecting the other person" (Kelly, 1990, p. 241).

BASIC ASSUMPTIONS OF TREATMENT

Basic assumptions exist in psychotherapy. However, in therapy with the incest perpetrator, these assumptions cannot be taken for granted. Table 38-1 shows the usual assumptions in psychotherapy versus the reality of therapy with the incest perpetrator.

BIASES IN THE TREATMENT OF INCEST PERPETRATORS

Refer to Roundy and Horton (1990) for a more detailed account of biases.

CULTURAL/SOCIAL BIASES

1. Some are reluctant to acknowledge what the high pressure of incest suggests about our society.
2. Therapists who want to treat rather than incarcerate perpetrators are seen as perpetuating the problem.
3. Many lack faith in the value of psychotherapy for this population.
4. Upper-class perpetrators are less likely to be incarcerated, and their children are less likely to be placed in foster care, than are those in lower socioeconomic groups.

RELIGIOUS VALUE BIASES

1. Clergy may be unwilling to acknowledge the presence of incest perpetrators in their congregations.
2. Conflict exists over what constitutes adequate and sufficient intervention, the clergy believing that confession and repentance is sufficient, while clinicians believe more is necessary.
3. Perpetrators may believe they have been forgiven by God and have no need for clergy *or* clinicians.

PROFESSIONAL BIASES

1. Therapists may be unable to give "unconditional positive regard" or empathy.
2. Therapists may feel unable to trust these clients.
3. Therapists may be maligned by colleagues for treating this population.
4. Pedophiles, often including incest perpetrators, are considered by many in the field to be incurable.
5. Turf battles may ensue between therapists and agencies.

PERSONAL BIASES

1. Therapists with unresolved sexual conflicts may "side with" the perpetrator, seeing the child as seductive and blameworthy.
2. Gender biases may exist in either direction. Female therapists see this as evidence that men are bad; male therapists see this as evidence that girls are seductive.
3. Biases may excuse the offender if his wife did not perform her "wifely duties."
4. Biases related to Oedipal theory may lead psychoanalysts to disregard accounts of incest by children, believing them to be Oedipal wishes, and other therapists to accept any incestuous account as fact.

TABLE 38-1: Differences in Basic Assumptions in Psychotherapy with Psychotherapy of the Incest Perpetrator

BASIC ASSUMPTIONS OF THERAPY	THERAPY WITH THE INCEST PERPETRATOR
Therapy requires:	
1. An identified client with a problem	1. Incest perpetrators see themselves as the victims; they do not recognize they have a problem.
2. An identified strategy to ameliorate the problem	2. Research has not identified one strategy, though a team approach involving all of the family seems to work best.
3. A commitment to change	3. Often treatment is court ordered. However, once therapy begins, the offender often values it.
4. A willingness to treat on the therapist's part	4. Often this is lacking in those who have not had experience treating offenders.
5. An awareness of countertransference	5. This nearly always exists and bears careful and ongoing evaluation.
6. A belief that therapy is an appropriate response to the problem	6. If the therapist believes the offender should be incarcerated, the therapy is doomed to fail. Therapists who do not believe therapy is the answer should refer the client to another therapist.

Roundy, L. M., & Horton, A. L. (1990). Professional and treatment issues for clinicians who intervene with incest perpetrators. In A. Horton, B. L. Johnson, L. M. Roundy, & D. Williams (eds.), *The Incest Perpetrator: A Family Member No One Wants to Treat.* Newbury Park, CA: Sage.

TRANSFERENCE

Incest perpetrators may (Roundy & Horton, 1990):
1. Seek to seduce, imitate, intimidate, or invalidate the therapist
2. Become passive and overcompliant, seeing the therapist as a powerful parent
3. Fear being controlled by the therapist, and employ strong resistance
4. Be acutely sensitive to abandonment or what they see as betrayal

COUNTER-TRANSFERENCE

Therapists of incest perpetrators may (Roundy & Horton, 1990):
1. Fear discomfort as it is painful to hear about the incest and its aftermath
2. Feel discomfort with the emotional intensity
3. Feel discomfort with the specifics of the abusive behavior
4. Be manipulated by claims of improvement and terminate prematurely, or may become frustrated or discouraged
5. Have trouble confronting dysfunctional behaviors of clients
6. Be unable to persist in confronting clients' resistance
7. Identify with the client's despair over loss of home and family and his stigma in the community (Conte, 1990)

GENERAL PRACTICAL GUIDELINES FOR THERAPISTS

It is recommended that therapists who work with incest perpetrators (Roundy & Horton, 1990):
1. Identify and resolve personal biases.
2. Accept the obligation to build and maintain clinical competence.
3. Anticipate and work to reduce burnout.
4. Establish a network of fellow clinicians to gain support and process cases.
5. Be open to observation and feedback from fellow clinicians or supervisors.
6. Be alert for the "quick cure" play.

7. Establish realistic clinical expectations regarding success with this population.

8. Measure success in small increments. The average length of treatment is 2 years but treatment may last longer.

9. Develop and implement a general response strategy to perpetrators' anticipated behaviors and defenses.

10. Do not bargain away court involvement in the treatment process. The "legal ax" is a powerful motivation.

11. Do not make promises of favorable legal outcomes if the offender discloses all. Therapists have no real control over court process. Clients who tell all will feel betrayed, angry, resentful, and resistive to therapists and therapy in general if these promises are not kept.

12. Deal directly with difficult issues rather than avoid them.

CLINICAL PHENOMENA AND INTERVENTIONS

Table 38-2 shows clinical phenomena that arise in work with incest perpetrators, and interventions.

TABLE 38-2: Clinical Phenomena and Interventions in Therapy with Incest Perpetrators

PHENOMENON	INTERVENTION
1. Clients often use denial as a defense against the anxiety of realizing and disclosing the incest (Mayer, 1983; Sanford, 1982).	1. Build trust so that the client can begin to face what he has done.
2. Clients use rationalization to explain their behavior and decrease anxiety. "She asked me to do it."	2. Point out to the client he is the father and she is the child.
3. Clients use self-deception to justify their actions, convincing themselves the daughter wanted them to do this (de Young, 1982; Sanford, 1982).	3. Point out the client is feeling guilty and is attempting to deflect the guilt.
4. Clients minimize the abuse behavior (Mayer, 1983; Sanford, 1982).	4. Be perfectly realistic in pointing out what the offender did and how it affected others, though not in a hostile, confrontational, or "abusive" way.
5. Clients appear manipulative and "slick," perhaps to appear in control (Mayer, 1983).	5. Explore the need for this facade, and the impulses underlying it.
6. Clients may use dissociation in regard to the incest or in the session (Justice & Justice, 1979).	6. Help client to stay with the anxiety of the past or of the moment. If the client seems to be "fading out" in the session, point this out.
7. Clients often act egocentric and narcissistic, unaware of the suffering they have caused their victims and family (Crewdson, 1988; de Young, 1982).	7. Help clients to begin to take the role of the other. Narcissism takes a long time to overcome.
8. Clients experience jealousy of daughter's association with boys, often projecting their own sexual desires onto the boys (Justice & Justice, 1979).	8. Explore these jealous feelings, helping clients to gain insight, to shift their feelings to other endeavors, and to understand how this affects the daughter.
9. Clients feel isolated from others (Gilgun & Connor, 1990).	9. Help client realize he is not alone, his behavior can be understood, and worked through. Group therapy is very helpful, as are couple and family therapy.
10. Clients confuse sex and love (Mayer, 1983).	10. Help client see that these are not necessarily the same.

TABLE 38-2 *(continued)*

PHENOMENON	INTERVENTION
11. Clients experience a need to be traditionally "masculine" (Mayer, 1983; Williams & Finkelhor, 1984).	11. Help clients over time to see the useless energy tied up in this.
12. Clients often fear adult females (Finkelhor, 1984) owing to early exposure to hostile females who acted superior to the men in their lives. They may appear as "mama's boys" (Mayer, 1983; Williams & Finkelhor, 1988).	12. Explore early relationships with females and their effect on the transference.
13. Clients may tend to sexualize all behavior and to be overly preoccupied with sex (Carnes, 1983).	13. Explore the origins of this behavior and other ways to express feelings.
14. Clients often are very stressed and have poor stress management skills (Justice & Justice, 1979; Mayer, 1983; Williams & Finklehor, 1988).	14. Reduce anxiety by exploring and working through conflicts. Recommend relaxation techniques. (See Chapter 16.)
15. Clients often engage in other forms of abuse as well, i.e., emotional abuse, physical child abuse, or spouse abuse (de Young, 1982; Williams & Finklehor, 1988).	15. Explore this and attempt to explore each situation, helping clients to observe and analyze their behavior by asking: Who? What? When? Where? As clients begin to understand the meaning of this behavior, it decreases.
16. Clients may abuse alcohol and drugs, using their influence to explain the incest (Williams & Finklehor, 1988).	16. Explore this and recommend a 12-step program.
17. Clients often believe sex is their "right," and if they don't get it in marriage, they have the prerogative to go elsewhere (Mayer, 1983).	17. Explore how this idea began. Group members often help dispel this kind of irrationality.
18. Clients display authoritarian parenting in the home but are submissive to authority themselves (de Young, 1982; Herman, 1981).	18. Discuss these episodes of authoritarian behavior with a view toward understanding it is a need to control one's own impulses by controlling others.
19. Clients display low impulse control at home but are controlled elsewhere (de Young, 1982).	19. Help client understand and explore the impulses driving this behavior and to develop more constructive ways of behaving.
20. Clients have frequently experienced childhood sexual abuse themselves (Williams & Finklehor, 1988; Groth, 1979; de Young, 1982; Mayer, 1983; Pelto, 1981).	20. Explore early abusive experiences and their impact.
21. Clients describe a poor relationship with parents (de Young, 1982). Themes include abandonment, power-lessness, maternal seduction, and paternal rejection (Williams & Finklehor, 1982).	21. Explore the feelings the client had as a child and their impact on the incest experience.
22. Clients believe their children are possessions and they therefore have a right to do whatever they wish with them (de Young, 1982).	22. Explore the roots of this idea, e.g., the role of their own parents toward them.
23. Clients blur generational boundaries, acting like suitors of their daughters, especially when the daughter looks like his wife did when they first met (Justice & Justice, 1979).	23. Discuss the first meeting, what attracted him to his wife, the history of the marriage.
24. Clients exhibit low self-esteem and depression (Mayer, 1983; Williams & Finklehor, 1988).	24. Explore feelings including early losses and current losses.
25. Clients exhibit paranoia, owing to the virtually universal stigma of incest (Williams & Finklehor, 1988).	25. Help clients separate out what is genuine hostility toward them and what is a reflection of their own guilt and projected anger.
26. Clients may expect complete forgiveness in response to simplistic apologies, and be angry when their wives or victims remain angry and unforgiving (Williams & Finklehor, 1988).	26. Help clients see how devastated others feel, and that forgiveness may take a long time or may never come.

INDICATORS FOR TERMINATION OF THERAPY

Termination is appropriate when clients are (Ingersoll & Patton, 1990, p. 78):

1. Able to recognize their own shortcomings and problem areas
2. Spontaneous with their interactions with the therapist
3. Able to express a full range of emotions
4. Able to reach out to and help others
5. Noticeably less egocentric than when they began treatment
6. Motivated in most areas of their lives
7. Fully responsible for their crime and concerned with their family's healing
8. Ready to assume financial responsibility for their own counseling and that of their victims
9. Considering some practical and concrete means of making amends for their behavior
10. Working on making new or restoring previous social connections
11. Exhibiting new and functional coping behaviors
12. Developing a plan for continuing counseling
13. Exhibiting a restored sense of humor consistent with their own style

REFERENCES

Abel, G., Becker, J., Cunningham-Rathner, J., Mittleman, M., & Rouleau, J. L. (1988). Multiple paraphiliac diagnoses among sex offenders. *Bulletin of the American Academy of Psychiatry and the Law, 16* (2), 153–168.

Ballard, D. T., Blair, G. D., Devereaux, S., Valentine, L. K., Horton, A., & Johnson, B. L. (1990). A comparative profile of the incest perpetrator: Background characteristics, abuse history, and use of social skills. In A. Horton, B. L. Johnson, L. M. Roundy, & D. Williams (eds.), *The Incest Perpetrator: A Family Member No One Wants to Treat* (pp. 43–64). Newbury Park, CA: Sage.

Carnes, P. (1983). *The Sexual Addiction.* Minneapolis, MN: Compcare.

Christianson, J. R., & Blake, R. H. (1990). The grooming process in father–daughter incest. In A. Horton, B. L. Johnson, L. M. Roundy, & D. Williams (eds.), *The Incest Perpetrator: A Family Member No One Wants to Treat* (p. 88–98). Newbury Park, CA: Sage.

Conte, J. R. (1990). The incest offender: An overview and introduction. In A. Horton, B. L. Johnson, L. M. Roundy, & D. Williams (eds.), *The Incest Perpetrator: A Family Member No One Wants to Treat* (pp. 19–28). Newbury Park, CA: Sage.

Crewdson, J. (1988). *By Silence Betrayed: Sexual Abuse of Children in America.* Boston: Little, Brown.

de Young, M. (1982). *The Sexual Victimization of Children.* Jefferson, NC: McFarland.

Edmonds, B., & Christianson, J. R. (1988). Father's apologies in father–daughter incest. Paper presented at the Western Social Sciences Association, Denver, CO.

Faller, K. C. (1990). Sexual abuse by paternal caretakers: A comparison of abusers who are biological fathers in intact families, stepfathers, and non-custodial fathers. In A. Horton, B. L. Johnson, L. M. Roundy, & D. Williams (eds.), *The Incest Perpetrator: A Family Member No One Wants to Treat* (pp. 65–93). Newbury Park, CA: Sage.

Finkelhor, D. (1984). *Child Sexual Abuse: New Theory and Research.* New York: Free Press.

Gilgun, J. F., & Connor, T. M. (1990). Isolation and the adult male perpetrator of child sexual abuse. In A. Horton, B. L. Johnson, L. M. Roundy, & D. Williams (eds.), *The Incest Perpetrator: A Family Member No One Wants to Treat.* Newbury Park, CA: Sage.

Groth, A. N. (1979). Sexual trauma in the life histories of rapists and child molesters. *Victimology: An International Journal 8* (1), 10–16.

Herman, J. L. (1981). *Father–Daughter Incest.* Cambridge, MA: Harvard University Press.

Ingersoll, S. L., & Patton, S. O. (1990). *Treating Perpetrators of Sexual Abuse.* Lexington, MA: Lexington Books.

Justice, B., & Justice, R. (1979). *The Broken Taboo: Sex in the Family.* New York: Human Sciences Press.

Kelly, R. J. (1990). Confidentiality issues with incest perpetrators: Duty to report, duty to protect, duty to treat. In A. Horton, B. L. Johnson, L. M. Roundy, & D. Williams (eds.), *The Incest Perpetrator: A Family Member No One Wants to Treat* (pp. 238–245). Newbury Park, CA: Sage.

Langevin, R. (1983). *Sexual Strands: Understanding and Treating Sexual Anomalies in Men.* Hillsdale, NJ: Lawrence Erlbaum.

Mayer, A. (1983). *Incest: A Treatment Manual for Therapy with Victims, Spouses, and Offenders.* Holms Beach, FL: Learning Publications.

Passey, L. S. (1987). Behaviors leading to father–daughter incest: A further test of the Warner–Kearney hypothesis. Paper presented at the Western Social Science Association, El Paso, TX.

Pelto, V. L. (1981). Male incest offenders and non-offenders: A comparison of early sexual history. *Dissertation Abstracts International, 42* (3), 1154.

People v. Stritzinger, 2.34 Ca.L.3d 437 (1983).

Roundy, L. M., & Horton, A. L. (1990). Professional and treatment issues for clinicians who intervene with incest perpetrators. In A. Horton, B. L. Johnson, L. M. Roundy, & D. Williams (eds.), *The Incest Perpetrator: A Family Member No One Wants to Treat.* Newbury Park, CA: Sage.

Sanford, L. T. (1982). *The Silent Children.* New York: McGraw-Hill.

Warner-Kearney, D. (1987). The nature of grooming behavior used by sexual offenders in father–daughter incest. Paper presented at the Western Criminology Association, Las Vegas, NV.

Williams, L. M., & Finkelhor, D. (1988). The characteristics of incestuous fathers: A review of recent studies. In W. L. Marshall, D. R. Laws, & H. E. Barbaree (eds.), *The Handbook of Sexual Assault: Issues, Theories and Treatment of the Offender.* New York: Plenum.

BIBLIOGRAPHY

Parker, H., & Parker, S. (1986). Father–daughter sexual abuse: An emerging perspective. *American Journal of Orthopsychiatry, 56,* 531–549.

Salter, A. C. (1988). *Treating Child Sex Offenders and Victims: A Practical Guide.* Newbury Park, CA: Sage.

Trepper, T. S., & Barrett, M. J. (1989). *Systemic Treatment of Incest: A Therapeutic Handbook.* New York: Brunner/Mazel.

39

THIRTY NINE

The Client with HIV Infection

Suzanne Lego

OVERVIEW:

Introduction
Early Phase
Middle Phase
Group Therapy
  Assessment
  Coleadership
  Group Composition

Setting
Group Process
Leadership
Confidentiality
Late Phase

INTRODUCTION

HIV/AIDS has become one of the major mental health problems of the 1990s (Knox, 1989). Psychiatric diagnoses linked to AIDS include organic mental syndromes, adjustment disorder with depressed or anxious mood, panic disorder, major depression, psychoactive substance abuse, and sleep disorders. The major thrust in counseling clients who are HIV infected is to help them improve their daily well-being and maintain a sense of control over as many aspects of their lives as possible. While some clients may be treated in individual psychotherapy, the majority are treated in groups.

EARLY PHASE

During the initial early phase of HIV/AIDS the client experiences a myriad of feelings and clinical phenomena. These are listed in Table 39-1 along with nursing interventions.

MIDDLE PHASE

The middle phase of HIV/AIDS is often the longest phase and may last years. Table 39-2 lists clinical phenomena and nursing interventions in this stage. Table 39-3 lists special concerns arising in this stage, nursing interventions, and theoretical rationales.

TABLE 39-1
Clinical Phenomena and Nursing Interventions in the Early Phase of HIV/AIDS

CLINICAL PHENOMENON	NURSING INTERVENTION
1. Shock, anger, panic	1. Provides quiet, emotional connectedness.
2. Disappointment, loss, sadness	2. Offers quiet reassurance, mobilization of a supportive network.
3. Fear of incapacitation, physical and mental deterioration, deformity, pain	3. Encourages client to express all thoughts and feelings. Reassures client that professional help will be available.
4. Shame, both internal and external	4. Examines personal values. Explores internal conflicts.
5. Denial	5. Helps the client gently to accept the diagnosis.
6. Suicidal thoughts	6. Evaluates a possible plan, its lethality, time frame. Intervenes to avert the suicide.
7. The "ego chill, a shudder that comes from the sudden awareness that our nonexistence is entirely possible" (Erikson, 1958)	7. Helps the person explore thoughts and feelings about death.

This table is adapted from Lego, S. (1994). *Fear and AIDS/HIV: Empathy and Communication.* Albany, NY: Delmar Publications.

TABLE 39-2
Clinical Phenomena and Nursing Interventions in the Middle Phase of HIV/AIDS

CLINICAL PHENOMENON	NURSING INTERVENTION
1. Loss of control	1. Helps clients find ways to gain control of life, for example, seeking treatment for infections, leading a healthy lifestyle through good nutrition, exercise, meditation, and communion with others.
2. Helplessness and vulnerability	2. Empowers clients by encouragement to reach out to others through cultural, political, or altruistic endeavors that give purpose to life.
3. Passivity and victimization	3. Replaces negative thinking with positive attitudes by encouraging clients to live life to its fullest and to be proactive.
4. Severe reduction in self-esteem	4. Encourages clients to continue work even if it must be scaled down, and to spend time with supportive family and friends, helping others, attending a support group or individual psychotherapy.
5. Changes in physical appearance	5. Helps clients reorder priorities, pointing out that relationships, work, connections with the world at large may supersede personal appearance.
6. Sense of isolation	6. Helps clients decide who can be of the most support and who should be present at death. A support group and individual psychotherapy help overcome loneliness and stigmatization.
7. Guilt over lifestyle when the client is gay, bisexual, an intravenous drug abuser, or a female partner who has been victimized	7. Helps clients explore the roots of this guilt, that is, who has caused them to feel bad or wrong. Explores ways to expiate guilt, for example, by repaying money stolen for drugs.
8. Anger and acting out	8. Helps clients express rage verbally rather than act it out, validating the reasons for realistic anger such as problems with health care delivery or victimization by discrimination. Helps clients identify displaced anger as well.
9. Depression	9. Helps clients realize they are turning the anger they feel toward themselves rather than expressing it openly. Encourages open expression of anger.
10. Paranoia	10. Helps clients sort out behaviors that reflect actual anger at others, and paranoia that represents their own anger that is projected onto others.
11. Fear of violence	11. Explores sources of violence at home and in the community, helping clients avoid these. May refer family and friends to support groups or involve social agencies.
12. Sense of betrayal by partners, family, or friends who may have deceived or deserted the client	12. Helps clients grieve the loss of belief in the other, at the same time helping them acquire new sources of comfort including the nurse, a support group, or a higher being. *(Continued)*

TABLE 39-2 *(continued)*

CLINICAL PHENOMENON	NURSING INTERVENTION
13. Escape into alcohol or other drugs	13. Helps clients talk about their thoughts and feelings, rather than escape them. Helps clients get access to prescribed pain medication when needed.
14. Somatic preoccupation	14. Provides health information to allay unrealistic worries.
15. Projective identification	15. When clients unconsciously infuse the nurse with their own feelings of panic, anger, helplessness, and so forth, the nurse steps back, notices what is happening, and attempts to react with empathy and understanding.

This table is adapted from Lego, S. (1994). *Fear and AIDS/HIV: Empathy and Communication.* Albany, NY: Delmar Publications.

TABLE 39-3
Special Concerns of the Middle Phase of HIV/AIDS, Nursing Interventions, and Rationale

SPECIAL CONCERNS	NURSING INTERVENTIONS	RATIONALE
1. How to tell parents or children	1. Each case must be individually assessed and evaluated. The nurse helps clients look at all the dimensions and ramifications.	1. Some factors such as health status of elderly parents or life phase of the children have a bearing on how the information is accepted. On the other hand, thinly veiled family secrets can be destructive.
2. Questions about sexuality	2. Helps clients explore safer sex methods and nonsexual physical contact. May encourage discussion of feelings about this with partners.	2. Most human beings need physical contact. Partners may withdraw, owing to fear of contagion or anticipatory grief.
3. Reconciliation with estranged family members	3. Helps clients decide if reconciliation is desired even if they seem strongly defended. Agrees to be present at the reconciliation if desired, and to meet with the client afterward.	3. A tough exterior may cover a fear of rejection. The reconciliation is likely to arouse strong feelings that require expression and acceptance.
4. A "limbo" phase	4. When opportunistic infections are in check, encourages an "enjoy the moment" philosophy, but is alert to underlying depression.	4. Clients can fall into a state of denial when they feel physically healthy but suffer intense depression when an infection returns.
5. Unfinished business	5. Moves at the client's pace but may offer encouragement to put legal and personal affairs in order. This may include helping to plan the funeral or memorial service, or to leave letters or tapes behind.	5. Clients may fear that to do this planning hastens the end. Owing to low self-esteem, they may not realize the importance letters or tapes may have for others after they are gone, for example, to children.
6. Resurrection fantasies as others recover from an infection	6. Helps clients explore thoughts, feelings, wishes, dreams, keeping reality in mind, e.g., "It's good to see John feeling better. I guess we all wish it could last forever."	6. As with all forms of denial the client is vulnerable to "crashing" when reality sets in. Resurrection fantasies represent the wish to reverse the dying process.
7. Talk about death	7. Remains alert to signs the patient is ready, for example, "How come your books about HIV/AIDS are on the same shelf as books on death and dying?" Asks clients if they have been thinking about death.	7. Thoughts and feelings about dying are always present, though often kept in abeyance. The nurse may be the only person with whom the client can openly discuss death.
8. Rational suicide (see also Chapters 20 and 71)	8. Depending on ethical and moral beliefs, may allow clients to discuss and explore a rational suicide plan.	8. Many clients are reassured by knowing they have a means of controlling their own death with dignity. If nurses are in accord, they can help the client accept this without guilt. If nurses believe death is "in the hands of God," they will be unwilling and unable to enter into this discussion.

This table is adapted from Lego, S. (1994). *Fear and AIDS/HIV: Empathy and Communication.* Albany, NY: Delmar Publications.

GROUP THERAPY* Though many HIV-infected persons choose to be in individual psychotherapy, most clients are treated in support groups. These groups have special qualities that make them conducive to the treatment of HIV-infected persons. Rosenberg (1984) listed the following properties of support groups:

1. Homogeneity
2. Victimization by a system, as opposed to psychopathology
3. Public confession of qualification for membership
4. A common language
5. Horizontal structure
6. Educational and information exchanges
7. Reality testing
8. Development of coping skills

The goals of group therapy in this case are that the HIV-infected persons be able to (Lego, 1994):

1. Accept the illness
2. Express otherwise unacceptable feelings of rage, sadness, jealousy, shame, and guilt
3. Decrease anxiety
4. Regain the ability to manage their lives
5. Reach out to others for practical and emotional support
6. Face the fear of loss and death
7. Increase self-esteem
8. Reduce high-risk behaviors
9. Deal with substance abuse if it is present
10. Find new meaning in life
11. Reconcile with estranged family members
12. Find ways to show concern for significant others who may be overwhelmed by the member's illness
13. Examine the ways they may leave a legacy unique to their own lives (Lego, 1993)

The technique of group psychotherapy with HIV-infected persons is modified to meet the unique needs of the members.

ASSESSMENT

HIV-infected persons are likely to enter a group after the shock of diagnosis has subsided and they are ready to consider how to best live their lives with HIV. An intake interview is done to explore the person's reasons for entering a group, prior group experiences, acceptance of the diagnosis and initial adjustment, available social supports, current physical capacity, mental status and apparent coping capacity, and anticipated or actual reservations about being in a group with other HIV-infected persons who are ill and may die (Gambe & Getzel, 1989).

COLEADERSHIP

Group coleadership is recommended as a way to share responsibilities. For example, coleadership can make it easier for nurses to make follow-up phone calls when members are absent and to visit hospitalized or homebound members. Coleadership also provides mutual support and emotional outlets for the group leaders as they identify with the members' tragedy and pain (Gambe & Getzel, 1989).

*This section is reproduced by permission from *Fear and AIDS/HIV* by Suzanne Lego, Delmar Publishers, Inc. Albany, NY, 1994.

GROUP COMPOSITION

As with many other groups, a membership of seven is ideal. The group should not contain more than 10 members, as groups of this size tend to break into subgroups. The group should not have less than seven members since there may be frequent absences because of illness. If the group is composed of IV drug abusers, the members should also be receiving separate, ongoing individual treatment, if possible (Gambe & Getzel, 1989).

SETTING

Sessions should be held in a warm room since HIV-infected persons are often thin and vulnerable to the cold. Smoking is not usually permitted and ventilation should be good so that those recovering from pneumonia have clean air. The setting must allow for access by wheelchairs and intravenous equipment. If sessions are held in a hospital they should be held off the AIDS unit so that patients are not further stigmatized.

GROUP PROCESS

The first session of a group is the time for the nurses to introduce themselves, describe their professional backgrounds, tell why they want to work with HIV-infected persons, and reassure members that their stories will be understood. In this session it is important to discuss and agree to confidentiality. Members are introduced and tell the group how and when they were diagnosed (Gambe & Getzel, 1989).

Nurses should be supportive, point out underlying themes, and avoid elaborate interpretations. Care is taken to leave control of the group in the hands of the members, as they may feel out of control in other areas of their lives.

As the group progresses, the members focus on the current crises and developing plans for remaining as healthy as possible. As members become comfortable with one another they may begin to discuss their personal lives, looking for common bonds. Often unconscious competition and testing of the nurses occur. Eventually, conflict among the members and transference to the nurses emerge. Group interaction often reveals ambivalence about being cared for and caring for others (Gambe & Getzel, 1989).

The concept of universality is important in groups of HIV-infected persons because members often feel isolated and alone. In the group they discover that their thoughts, feelings, and actions are similar to those of others. Thoughts or feelings they may have considered unacceptable, such as rivalry for group attention, a greed for life itself, even resentment toward healthy nurses or a secret wish to infect them, may be felt to some extent by every group member. Those "bad" or "odd" thoughts come to be seen as a normal part of living with a fatal disease.

Discussions often center on experimental drugs and medical procedures. Subgrouping may divide the group into those who want to return to prediagnosis functioning, and those who view AIDS as an experience from which they will never recover and who are able to talk openly about their own death and the deaths of others (Gambe & Getzel, 1989). The nurses encourage the open expression of feelings, helping to make overt what has been covert (Lego, 1984).

LEADERSHIP

Before assuming the leadership of a group of HIV-infected persons, nurses must carefully examine their own personal values and possible bias toward homosexuality or drug use. Also, they must be able to discuss death and dying and be comfortable working with persons whose death may be imminent.

Nurses must be able to avoid dominating the group and let natural leaders emerge as the group moves forward. They must be able to accept and be comfortable discussing sex (Spector & Concklin, 1987). They must also be aware of and honest about their own concerns, for example, about being at risk themselves.

Nurses should be highly knowledgeable about AIDS. Knowledge will allow them to clear up any misconceptions the group members may have, to recommend community resources, to monitor the mental states of group members, and to recognize the early signs of central nervous system complications.

One role of the nurse is to encourage problem solving and self-care so that members can begin to feel they have some control over their lives (Child & Getzel, 1990). In addition, the leader encourages the members to help one another and to reach out to others for help. Unlike some conventional therapy groups in which meetings outside the group are discouraged (Lego, 1984), HIV-infected persons do meet outside the group, since their social isolation is severe (Beckett & Rutan, 1990).

The nurse should report the death of a member to all the other members by telephone as soon as possible. This alleviates members' anxiety about arriving at a session only to learn that a group member died a few days earlier (Beckett & Rutan, 1990). Members are urged to grieve for members who die by talking about them in the group (Tunnell, 1991).

CONFIDENTIALITY

Confidentiality is of major concern to HIV-infected persons, as the knowledge of the HIV status could lead to the loss of their families, friends, jobs, health insurance, housing, and civil liberties. The nurse is sometimes faced with the "duty to warn" dilemma, such as when HIV-infected persons are having sex with persons who are unaware of their partner's HIV status. Nurses encourage discussion of these confidentiality concerns in the group.

In the case of destructive behavior, an advantage of group therapy is that the members provide not only understanding but peer pressure to encourage the destructive member to act in a responsible way (Posey, 1988). The nurse and the other group members can help members explore their reluctance to inform their partners and others at risk. Beckett and Rutan (1990) found that many times the group helped other members exercise self-restraint and altruism.

Other than when a group member's behavior can cause harm to others, confidentiality is carefully guarded by nurses. Group members must also be able to rely on each other to maintain confidentiality. Issues of confidentiality arise when group members accidentally meet in public, when they must leave telephone messages for one another, and when they meet the families and friends of group members (Posey, 1988). The nurse helps group members explore these issues in the context of support and trust.

LATE PHASE

In the late stage of HIV/AIDS, death is relatively near. In a high percentage of cases, dementia appears. Other personality changes such as acute psychosis may be caused by high anxiety and are therefore treatable with psychopharmacology and psychotherapy. Others may be caused by HIV invading brain tissue. CT scans, MRIs, or spinal taps may help with differential diagnosis. For more information about dementia, see Chapter 33.

As in all clients close to death, those with HIV/AIDS experience phenomena related to withdrawal of energy from this world and placement in the next. Table 39-4 shows some of these phenomena and nursing interventions. See Chapter 20 for more information about the dying process.

TABLE 39-4
Phenomena Observed in Late Phase of
HIV/AIDS and Nursing Interventions

CLINICAL PHENOMENON	NURSING INTERVENTION
1. Disinterest	1. Realizing the client's need to disengage, the nurse remains emotionally available but avoids unnecessary demands.
2. Ambivalence	2. Recognizing clients' simultaneous feelings of anger and neediness, the nurse realizes clients may need to be with loved ones, or may need to die alone. "I'm here for you. Don't be afraid to ask for anything."
3. Life review	3. Realizing clients may want to review happier times or talk about regrets, the nurse is emotionally available. Any and all feelings are encouraged and accepted. The nurse may ask if there are friends or relatives to call or messages to be sent.
4. Resolution	4. Recognizing death is near, the nurse helps clients to accept death.

This table is adapted from Lego, S. (1994). *Fear and AIDS/HIV: Empathy and Communication.* Albany, NY: Delmar Publications.

REFERENCES

Beckett, A., & Rutan, J. S. (1990). Treating people with ARC and AIDS in group psychotherapy. *International Journal of Group Psychotherapy, 40,* 19–28.

Child, R., & Getzel, G. S. (1990). Group work with inner city persons with AIDS. *Social Work with Groups, 12,* 65–80.

Erikson, E. H. (1958). *Young Man Luther: A Study in Psychoanalysis and History.* New York: W. W. Norton.

Gambe, R., & Getzel, G. S. (1989). Group work with gay men with AIDS. *Social Casework, 70,* 172–179.

Knox, M. D. (1989). Community mental health's role in the AIDS crisis. *Community Mental Health Journal, 25,* 185.

Lego S. (1984). Group therapy. In S. Lego (ed.), *The American Handbook of Psychiatric Nursing.* Philadelphia: J. B. Lippincott.

Lego, S. (1993). Group psychotherapy with HIV-infected persons and their care-givers. In H. Kaplan & B. Sadock (eds.), *Comprehensive Group Psychotherapy* (3rd ed.). Baltimore: Williams & Wilkins.

Lego, S. (1994). *Fear and AIDS/HIV: Empathy and Communication.* Albany, NY: Delmar.

Posey, E. C. (1988). Confidentiality in an AIDS support group. *Journal of Counseling and Development. 66,* 226–227.

Rosenberg, P. R. (1984). Support groups: A special therapeutic entity. *Small Group Behavior, 15,* 173–186.

Spector, I. C., & Conklin, R. (1987). Brief reports: AIDS group psychotherapy. *International Journal of Group Psychotherapy, 37* (3), 433–439.

Tunnell, G. (1991). Complications in group psychotherapy with AIDS patients. *International Journal of Group Psychotherapy, 41,* 481–497.

BIBLIOGRAPHY

Bor, R., Miller, R., & Goldman, E. (1993). *Theory and Practice of HIV Counseling: A Systematic Approach.* New York: Brunner/Mazel.

Flaskerud, J. H. (1992). Psychological aspects. In J. H. Flaskerud & P. J. Ungvarski (eds.), *HIV/AIDS: A Guide to Nursing Care.* Philadelphia: W. B. Saunders.

Landau-Stanton, J., & Clements, C. D. (1993). *AIDS, Health and Mental Health: A Primary Sourcebook.* New York: Brunner/Mazel.

Lego, S. (1996). Individual psychotherapy with the HIV-infected patient. In K. M. Casey, F. Cohen, & A. Hughes (eds.), *ANAC's Core Curriculum for HIV/AIDS Nursing.* Philadelphia: Nursecom, Inc. At press.

Lego, S. (1996). Support groups with HIV-infected patients. In K. M. Casey, F. Cohen, & A. Hughes (eds.), *ANAC's Core Curriculum for HIV/AIDS Nursing.* Philadelphia: Nursecom, Inc. At press.

Tasker, M. (1992). *How Can I Tell You? Secrecy and Disclosure with Children When a Family Member Has AIDS.* Bethesda, MD: Association for the Care of Children's Health.

40
FORTY

The Client with Obsessive-Compulsive Disorder or Phobias

Suzanne Lego

OVERVIEW:

Obsessive-Compulsive Disorder
   Description
   Incidence
   Comorbidity
   Biological Factors
   Genetic Factors
   Psychodynamic Factors
   Symbolic Meaning of the Obsession or
      Compulsion
   Psychopharmacology
   Somatic Therapies
   Psychotherapy

Phobias
   Description
   Incidence
   Genetic Factors
   Psychodynamic Factors
   Psychopharmacology
   Psychotherapy

OBSESSIVE-
COMPULSIVE
DISORDER

DESCRIPTION

Clients with obsessive-compulsive disorder (OCD) are often plagued by intrusive thoughts, called obsessions, and pressures to commit repetitive acts, called compulsions. These acts may include checking, counting, cleaning, repeating a phrase, or avoiding certain objects or situations. The diagnostic criteria for OCD are shown in Box 40-1. These clients usually realize the irrationality of these thoughts and acts but feel powerless to stop.

INCIDENCE

OCD is reported in varying studies to include 2–3% of the U.S. population. In adults OCD is distributed evenly in men and women, but in teens, it is more prevalent in boys. OCD is a disorder of young people, and it can start in childhood (Kaplan, Sadock, & Grebb, 1994).

BOX 40-1: DSM-IV (300.3) Criteria for Obsessive-Compulsive Disorder

A. Either obsessions or compulsions:

Obsessions as defined by (1), (2), (3), and (4):

(1) Recurrent and persistent thoughts, impulses, or images that are experienced, at some time during the disturbance, as intrusive and inappropriate and that cause marked anxiety or distress.

(2) The thoughts, impulses, or images are not simply excessive worries about real-life problems.

(3) The person attempts to ignore or suppress such thoughts, impulses, or images, or to neutralize them with some other thought or action.

(4) The person recognizes that the obsessional thoughts, impulses, or images are a product of his or her own mind (not imposed from without as in thought insertion).

Compulsions as defined by (1) and (2):

(1) Repetitive behaviors (e.g., hand-washing, ordering, checking) or mental acts (e.g., praying, counting, repeating words silently) that the person feels driven to perform in response to an obsession, or according to rules that must be applied rigidly.

(2) The behaviors or mental acts are aimed at preventing or reducing distress or preventing some dreaded event or situation; however, these behaviors or mental acts either are not connected in a realistic way with what they are designed to neutralize or prevent or are clearly excessive.

B. At some point during the course of the disorder, the person has recognized that the obsessions or compulsions are excessive or unreasonable. *Note:* This does not apply to children.

C. The obsessions or compulsions cause marked distress, are time-consuming (take more than 1 hour a day), or significantly interfere with the person's normal routine, occupational (or academic) functioning, or usual social activities or relationships.

D. If another Axis I disorder is present, the content of the obsessions or compulsions is not restricted to it (e.g., preoccupation with food in the presence of an Eating Disorder; hair pulling in the presence of Trichotillomania; concern with appearance in the presence of Body Dysmorphic Disorder; preoccupation with drugs in the presence of a Substance Use Disorder; preoccupation with having a serious illness in the presence of Hypochondriasis; preoccupation with sexual urges or fantasies in the presence of Paraphilia; or guilty ruminations in the presence of Major Depressive Disorder).

E. The disturbance is not due to the direct physiological effects of a substance (e.g., a drug of abuse, a medication) or general medical condition.

Specify if:

With Poor Insight: If, for most of the time during the current episode, the person does not recognize that the obsessions and compulsions are excessive or unreasonable.

From American Psychiatric Association (1994). *Diagnostic and Statistical Manual of Mental Disorders* (4th ed.). Washington, DC: American Psychiatric Association.

COMORBIDITY

Clients with OCD often have other disorders including major depressive disorder, social phobia, alcohol use disorders, specific phobia, panic disorder, and eating disorders.

BIOLOGICAL FACTORS

A dysregulation of serotonin and a decrease in size of caudates bilaterally have been noted in clients with OCD. However, it is not certain whether these changes cause the disorder, or are a result of the disorder.

GENETIC FACTORS

Though some data support the hypothesis that OCD has a genetic component, these data "do not yet distinguish the influence of cultural and behavioral effects on the transmission of the disorder" (Kaplan, Sadock, & Grebb, 1994, p. 600).

PSYCHODYNAMIC FACTORS

The client who develops OCD frequently undergoes the following process:

1. The client experiences disturbances in growth and development related to the anal-sadistic phase, for example, growing up in a household where strict arbitrary control is maintained over the child's behavior.
2. The child feels anger at this constant overcontrol.
3. The child uses reaction formation to keep the anger in check, becoming a pleasant, "perfect" child.
4. The client experiences some stimulation in the environment, or reaches a developmental stage touching off extreme anxiety. This stimulation may be sexual or aggressive, or both.
5. The client unconsciously regresses to the earlier anal-sadistic phase of development.
6. The anal-sadistic impulses are reinforced, augmented, and strengthened.
7. The pressure of reactivated anal and aggressive impulses arouse new anxiety and new conflicts.
8. Reaction formation no longer works, and isolation, undoing, and displacement come into play.
9. The client experiences an idea or impulse that:
   - Intrudes persistently
   - Is ego alien
   - Produces anxiety and dread
   - Leads to taking countermeasures
   - Is seen by the client as absurd and irrational

SYMBOLIC MEANING OF THE OBSESSION OR COMPULSION

The obsessions and compulsions are often patently symbolic when the client's life experiences are explored. Table 40-1 shows the mechanisms described above with examples. In the case of Diane referred to in the table, she grew up in a rigid Italian Catholic home. Her parents fought and often left one another. They would ask her to keep confident the complaints each had about the other. She learned to keep these secrets, and acted like a "perfect" daughter. In adulthood when a stressful event occurred she developed the impulse to shout out hostile secrets in public.

PSYCHOPHARMACOLOGY

The standard treatment is to start with a serotonin-specific drug such as clomipramine (Anafranil) or a serotonin-specific reuptake inhibitor (SSRI) such as fluoxetine (Prozac) and then move to another drug if the SSRIs are not effective (Kaplan, Sadock, & Grebb, 1994). (See Chapter 67.)

SOMATIC THERAPIES

Both electroconvulsive therapy (ECT) and psychosurgery are being used to treat clients who have proven treatment-resistant.

PSYCHOTHERAPY

Neither psychopharmacology nor somatic therapies address the underlying interpersonal situation that has produced the client's aggression or that keeps it going. Nurse psychotherapists and others report success in the use of insight-oriented psychotherapy with these clients (Gabbard, 1992). Therapy is directed at:

TABLE 40-1
Defense Mechanisms Used by Clients with OCD and Clinical Examples

MECHANISM	DEFINITION	CLINICAL EXAMPLE
Isolation	An unacceptable idea or image is isolated from the affect or feeling.	Diane has impulses to yell out in church hostile comments about the priests. Yet she feels no conscious anger.
Undoing	An unacceptable idea is nullified by opposite acts.	John fears he will bump people in the street and hurt them, so he must check over and over to be sure he hasn't.
Reaction formation	The unacceptable ideas are hidden over time by character traits that are the opposite.	Diane is oversolicitous of the priests.
Ambivalence	Love and hate are experienced simultaneously. The impulse to destroy is converted into an impulse to control or win over the other.	John is very angry with his mother and refuses to abide by "house rules." Yet he won't move out on his own. His rituals are very disruptive to the house.
Magical thinking	The idea that thoughts or acts can control events.	John turns around to check every person for signs he has harmed them. This ritual is designed to control his aggression.

1. Uncovering the underlying aggression
2. Exploring the defense mechanisms used to keep the anger in check
3. Allowing the aggression to appear and be worked through in the transference

PHOBIAS

DESCRIPTION

A phobia is an irrational fear resulting in a conscious avoidance of the feared object, activity, or situation. Either the presence or the anticipation of the phobic entity elicits severe distress in the affected person, who recognizes that the reaction is excessive. Nevertheless, the phobic reaction results in a disruption of the person's ability to function in life. (Kaplan, Sadock, & Grebb, 1994, p. 592)

See Box 40-2 for the diagnostic criteria for specific phobia.

INCIDENCE

Phobias are the most common mental disorder in the United States, occurring twice as often in women as men. An estimated 5–10% of the population is affected.

GENETIC FACTORS

First-degree relatives of persons with social phobia are about three times more likely to have social phobias than are people without relatives who are phobic. It is clear that this need not mean the client has inherited a tendency to be phobic. Instead, we must wonder how much is transmitted interpersonally or culturally. It has also been speculated that phobic clients were born with a predisposition to fearfulness. Again it is nearly impossible to isolate these variables from the interpersonal or cultural environment.

BOX 40-2: DSM-IV (300.29) Criteria for Specific Phobia
(formerly Simple Phobia)

A. Marked and persistent fear that is excessive or un-reasonable, cued by the presence or anticipation of a specific object or situation (e.g., flying, heights, animals, receiving an injection, seeing blood).

B. Exposure to the phobic stimulus almost invariably provokes an immediate anxiety response, which may take the form of a situationally bound or situationally predisposed Panic Attack. *Note:* In children, the anxiety may be expressed by crying, tantrums, freezing, or clinging.

C. The person recognizes that the fear is excessive or unreasonable. *Note:* In children, this feature may be absent.

D. The phobic situation(s) is avoided or else is endured with intense anxiety or distress.

E. The avoidance, anxious anticipation, or distress in the feared situation(s) interferes significantly with the person's normal routine, occupational (or academic) functioning, or social activities or relationships, or there is marked distress about having the phobia.

F. In individuals under age 18 years, the duration is at least 6 months.

G. The anxiety, Panic Attacks, or phobic avoidance associated with the specific object or situation is not better accounted for by another mental disorder, such as Obsessive-Compulsive Disorder (e.g., fear of dirt in someone with an obsession about contamination), Posttraumatic Stress Disorder (e.g., avoidance of stimuli associated with a severe stressor), Separation Anxiety Disorder (e.g., avoidance of school), Social Phobia (e.g., avoidance of social situations because of fear of embarrassment), Panic Disorder With Agoraphobia, or Agoraphobia Without History of Panic Disorder.

Specify type:

Animal Type: If the fear is cued by animals or insects. This subtype generally has a childhood onset.

Natural Environment Type: If the fear is cued by objects in the natural environment, such as storms, heights, or water. This subtype generally has a childhood onset.

Blood-Injection-Injury Type: If the fear is cued by seeing blood or an injury or by receiving an injection or other invasive medical procedure. This subtype is highly familial and is often characterized by a strong vasovagal response.

Situational Type: If the fear is cued by a specific situation such as public transportation, tunnels, bridges, elevators, flying, driving, or enclosed places. This subtype has a bimodal age-at-onset distribution, with one peak in childhood and another peak in the mid-20s. This subtype appears to be similar to Panic Disorder With Agoraphobia in its characteristic sex ratios, familial aggregation pattern, and age at onset.

Other Type: If the fear is cued by other stimuli. These stimuli might include the fear or avoidance of situations that might lead to choking, vomiting, or contracting an illness; "space" phobia (i.e., the individual is afraid of falling down if away from walls or other means of physical support); and children's fears of loud sounds or costumed characters.

From American Psychiatric Association (1994). *Diagnostic and Statistical Manual of Mental Disorders* (4th ed.). Washington, DC: American Psychiatric Association.

PSYCHODYNAMIC FACTORS

Table 40-2 lists the steps in the process of phobia development, examples of a classic case of phobia, and examples from a modern case.

PSYCHOPHARMACOLOGY

The drugs used most frequently are (Kaplan, Sadock, & Grebb, 1994):
1. Phenelzine (Nardil)
2. Alprazolam (Xanax)
3. Clonazepam (Klonopin)

TABLE 40-2
The Development of a Phobia with Examples

STEPS	EXAMPLE OF "LITTLE HANS"	CURRENT EXAMPLE
1. The client has "unacceptable" drives, e.g., anger, aggression, separation.	1. Little Hans had reached the Oedipal stage and had unconscious sexual feelings toward his mother.	1. Jim felt aggression and anger toward his mother, but at the same time was very dependent on her. She was helping him find an office for his dental practice.
2. These are kept unconscious.		
3. The unacceptable drive is projected onto a specific object.	3. Hans unconsciously projected his sexual/aggressive feelings onto his father.	3. Jim developed a fear of elevators.
4. The object is then seen as aggressive toward the client.		
5. The person finds relief by avoiding the object *or* The anxiety attached to the object is displaced further to another object that is symbolically linked to the first.	5. Hans could not avoid his father, so he developed a fear of horses. The horse was a symbol of his father.	5. Jim avoided elevators, making his life in New York City difficult. In therapy he described a fear that he would be shut up in the elevator and his mother would not be able to get to him. The fear then was a wish that 1. He could escape her smothering control. 2. He could control his aggression toward her.

PSYCHOTHERAPY

A number of psychotherapies are used:
1. Behavior therapy (see Chapter 12)
2. Cognitive therapy (see Chapter 13)
3. Psychodynamic therapy aimed at uncovering the meaning of the symptom through an examination of underlying aggression

REFERENCES

American Psychiatric Association (1994). *Diagnostic and Statistical Manual of Mental Disorders* (4th ed.). Washington, DC: American Psychiatric Association.

Gabbard, G. O. (1992). Psychodynamic psychiatry in the "decade of the brain." *American Journal of Psychiatry, 149,* 991–1000.

Kaplan, H. I., Sadock, B. J., & Grebb, J. A. (1994). *Kaplan and Sadock's Synopsis of Psychiatry* (7th ed.). Baltimore: Williams and Wilkins.

PART FOUR

Designing Programs

41

Designing a Crisis Center

Wendy Lewandowski*

OVERVIEW:

Introduction
Process for Developing a Crisis Center
    Determining Need
    Gaining Support
    Specifying Mission
    Getting Approval
    Marketing
    Program Evaluation

Guidelines for Establishing and
    Maintaining an Effective
    Crisis Center
Affiliation
Crisis Delivery Systems
Accountability Through Record Keeping

INTRODUCTION

Deinstitutionalization and the movement of psychiatric care into the community since the 1950s has led to community-based crisis intervention services. Such services provide aid to people in crisis at primary, secondary, and tertiary levels of care. Designing, implementing, and evaluating a center for crisis intervention requires that the nurse be familiar with concepts and principles of community mental health, community action, and program development.

PROCESS FOR DEVELOPING A CRISIS CENTER

DETERMINING NEED

During the planning phase of the crisis intervention center, data are gathered to document and justify the need for this service in a specific community. What are the primary sources of crisis intervention in the community? Are these adequate? Is there a need for additional or alternative crisis services? Results of the needs assessment can be included in a proposal for federal, state, or local funding.

GAINING SUPPORT

Certain groups will have vital interest in the project, whereas others will not. Interest cannot be assumed where there is none; similarly, allies must not be overlooked. History is useful. Learning what mistakes were made in the past can prevent repetition of them. Issues of territoriality may be avoided by involving key members of service agencies already in existence. Supporters already recognized as credible in the community should be enlisted (Kobberger & Tousley, 1984, p. 46).

*Appreciation is extended to Kathleen O'Brien Kobberger and Martha Merritt Tousley, who wrote this chapter in the first edition.

SPECIFYING MISSION

A mission is identified for the crisis intervention center; for example, to intervene with severely mentally disabled adults at a community level, thereby offering an alternative to hospitalization. Specific goals and objectives are set, along with outcome indicators. Initial planning is kept flexible.

GETTING APPROVAL

The project is legitimized by obtaining funding (federal, state, or local) and public approval (sponsorship) from influential community members (Kobberger & Tousley, 1984).

MARKETING

The crisis center advertises its services to the public. Other service agencies are informed so they can make referrals. The following methods can be used to inform the public of services: broadcast media, print media, posters in public places, and speakers' bureaus (Kobberger & Tousley, 1984).

PROGRAM EVALUATION

An ongoing method of quality assurance and program evaluation should be developed to ascertain its effectiveness in reaching stated objectives and goals.

GUIDELINES IN ESTABLISHING AND MAINTAINING AN EFFECTIVE CRISIS CENTER

1. The extent of need in the community is determined by considering the following:
   a. Who decided such a need exists here?
   b. How was that need determined?
   c. Has the need been documented adequately?
   d. Are anyone's personal motives at work?
2. The length of time devoted to program planning is less important than the quality of time spent.
3. Having one or two key persons manage the planning process proves more efficient than doing so by committee.
4. Planning continues indefinitely throughout the life of the program.
5. An attitude that values and permits change should be nourished as the program develops.
6. Knowledge of the local power structure keeps the program's goals congruent with changes in the local social, economic, and political climate.
7. Although professional consultations and collaboration are necessary, power and control rightfully belong to the program.
8. The impact of this new crisis service on the operation of existing agencies is kept in mind.
9. Representatives from those outside the mental health field are valuable resources and collaborators, for example, police or paramedics.
10. Turnover rate is kept to a minimum by selecting key personnel carefully.
11. Needs of the center's staff members are recognized and addressed.
12. Alternative plans for permanent funding are included in the earliest planning.
13. Key persons, that is, those from industry, banking, and business, are invited to sit on the center's board of directors.
14. Public funding carries a price. It may require surrendering some control or compromising some program goals.
15. The agency acts as though it deserves recognition in the community; it must take up an identifiable space and assume responsibility for a particular type of service.

AFFILIATION

A crisis center can stand alone or can be affiliated with the local community mental health center (CMHC). There are advantages and disadvantages to either approach (Kobberger & Tousley, 1984).

Advantages of CMHC Affiliation
1. *Funding:* Access to local, state, and federal monies.
2. *Acceptance:* Entry into an established community power structure.
3. *Quality assurance:* Quality of mental health service is already being assessed by CMHC.

Disadvantages of CMHC Affiliation
1. *Funding:* When local funding is no longer "matched" by federal or state dollars, certain crisis services may become expendable.
2. *Control:* Philosophy, purpose, and methods of the crisis center may be inconsistent with those of the CMHC, jeopardizing the crisis center's autonomy.

Alternatives to Affiliation
1. Operation by an independent corporation contracting with a number of different agencies to provide service
2. Conceptualization of the crisis intervention service as a non–mental health program providing its own unique service

CRISIS DELIVERY SYSTEMS

A crisis service provides short-term assistance to distressed individuals, families, significant others, or groups. People in crisis can seek such help directly, or they can be referred by others (Kobberger & Tousley, 1984, p. 48). Efforts are directed at early intevention, eliminating, or defusing a stressful event before decompensation occurs. Comprehensive crisis services can be delivered in the following ways.

Twenty-Four-Hour Telephone Counseling   This service is operated by predominantly lay volunteers. It is their responsibility to help with the presenting crisis situation itself, and to provide linkages to the other essential crisis services in the community. Crisis center developers should plan ahead for an adequate telephone system because it is difficult to change telephone systems once they have begun operation. Guidelines for installing a telephone system include the following (Kobberger & Tousley, 1984, p. 48):
1. Install a separate business line in addition to the crisis line.
2. Install rotary connections on the crisis line so that when one crisis line is busy, another will ring automatically.
3. Install a separate telephone instrument for each emergency line. This permits emergency calls during the time that the original incoming call is still on the line, thereby eliminating the need to put a caller on hold.
4. Install an automatic dial telephone with an unlisted number so that outgoing emergency calls can be made.
5. List the center's telephone numbers in all local telephone directories and in adjacent area directories as well.
6. Index both the business and emergency numbers in the white pages section.
7. Index both the business and emergency numbers in the classified section under several eye-catching categories, for example, Crisis Center, Suicide Prevention.
8. Include the center's emergency numbers in the emergency listings section located in the front of the telephone directory.

9. Receive calls on a full-time basis in the crisis center. Commercial answering services carry with them a number of disadvantages:
   a. *Control*—When total responsibility for telephone counseling is not provided by a trained crisis worker, the center's control over the service is diminished considerably.
   b. *Ethics*—When a 24-hour service is advertised and something less than that is provided, an ethical question arises as to whether the center is, in fact, providing what it has promised to deliver to the public.
   c. *Contact*—When the client's initial contact is not with the crisis worker, the fragile connection with the caller may be broken. Delays in rendering service can result. Callers who want anonymity are prevented from having any access to the crisis worker (Kobberger & Tousley, 1984, pp. 48–49).

Face-to-Face Counseling—Walk-In Service   A crisis center must have an independent, identifiable base from which its operations are directed and conducted. The walk-in service is located in the crisis center itself. Consider these questions in planning a base of operations (Kobberger & Tousley, 1984, p. 48):

1. *Location:* Is the proposed center
   - Accessible to the community in need?
   - On a main street?
   - Served by public transportation?
   - Housed in an easily recognized building?
   - Identifiable with a sign?
   - Near adequate parking facilities?
2. *Physical setting:* Has adequate space been allotted so that
   - Records can be stored?
   - Business can be conducted?
   - Telephone counseling can be provided?
   - Walk-in counseling can be done in separate, private quarters?
   - Seclusion areas are available for psychiatric emergencies?

Mobile or Outreach Service   The goal of outreach services is to resolve the crisis and maintain the individual, family, or group in the community with appropriate referrals and follow-up (Kobberger & Tousley, 1984). If a psychiatric emergency exists, as when someone is threatening suicide or homicide, the person(s) cannot be forcibly removed from the home. Probate procedures or police intervention must be instituted.

1. *Criteria:* A mobile service may be indicated when
   - A crisis cannot be assessed adequately over the telephone and the person(s) cannot come to the center.
   - Police or rescue squad intervention seems inappropriate, is unavailable, or is refused by the person(s) in crisis.
   - The person is a threat to self and cannot or will not come for help, but is agreeable to outreach services.
   - The person is a threat to others. In such cases collaboration with police is carefully considered. Crisis workers do not place themselves in dangerous situations.
   - Transportation to community resources is urgently needed and no other means of transportation is available. The mobile crisis service is not merely a transportation service for people in crisis.
   - A disruption in a family requires resolution.

2. *Staff:* Usually two crisis workers go to the crisis scene together (additional workers may actually increase anxiety and confusion in the crisis situation).
3. *Equipment:* Certain items prove useful in the operation of a mobile unit:
   - Automobile with safety locks and a screen to separate the back and front seats.
   - Two-way radio system enables the crisis worker to get to the crisis scene as quickly as possible and facilitates involvement of other community services (e.g., police, rescue squad).
   - Maps of the community.
   - First aid kit.
   - Flashlights.
4. *Crisis setting:* Wherever crisis service is rendered, the rapport between crisis worker and the person(s) in crisis is enhanced when certain conditions exist:
   a. *Quiet*—Counseling is conducted in an area that is as quiet, calm, private, and as conducive to concentration as possible (e.g., in an automobile, office, home, or outdoor place away from noise or activity).
   b. *Comfort*—The comfort of the person(s) in crisis should be addressed. The client is provided warmth, food, and water.
   c. *Safety*—A safe environment is essential not only for the person in crisis but for the crisis worker as well. When a person is potentially dangerous, it is essential that
      - Potential weapons are removed, such as glasses, plates, and heavy bookends
      - Access to help has been anticipated
   (Kobberger & Tousley, 1984, p. 50)
5. Potential dangers of operating a mobile crisis team must be considered in developing policies and procedures (Zealberg, Santos, & Fisher, 1993):
   a. Dealing with violent patients or family members on their own home turf.
   b. Neighborhoods that may be dangerous to enter in the daytime and life-threatening at night.
   For this reason, the crisis worker collaborates with law enforcement agencies, for example, requesting a police escort when working with a person who is homicidal, requesting police intervention for a person who is actively suicidal but not willing to come to the crisis center for evaluation.

Crisis Residential Service   A crisis-oriented residential service is geared to the severely mentally disabled (SMD) adult in crisis. The goals are to remove the person from an unsafe crisis situation, and provide an accessible, effective alternative to state hospitalization. This is not a substitute for needed inpatient hospitalization; rather, evaluation, early intervention, and linkage with interagency and intraagency services will help the SMD person remain in the community.

1. Criteria for admission to a crisis residential service are:
   a. The client is in crisis and can be evaluated and maintained in a setting with low restrictions. The person voluntarily consents to stay at the crisis residential center.
   b. Families of SMD clients require a temporary "time-out" when psychotic symptoms become too difficult to manage, or when the family is experiencing a specific stressful event that the SMD person finds overwhelming.
2. Exclusion criteria are (Britton & Mattson-Melcher, 1985):
   a. Clients who require medical treatment

   b. Clients who require a closed unit
   c. Clients who are actively threatening suicide, homicide, or assault
   d. Clients with a history of arson
   e. Clients who are acutely intoxicated on alcohol or other drugs
   f. Clients requiring more medications than can safely be administered in the crisis unit
   g. Clients merely needing a place to stay
3. Operating expenses include:
   a. Equipment—furnishings, kitchen, laundry
   b. Full-time and part-time staff
   c. Occupancy expenses—telephones, utilities, housekeeping, maintenance
   d. Operating supplies—kitchen, linen, activity, food

Referral Service Whenever crisis resolution requires services beyond the scope of the center, referral is made to other appropriate community resources and follow-up is provided. When a referral is needed, the crisis worker considers the following:

1. *Who* is to initiate the referral? (Will the client make the contact, or is the helper to do it?)
2. *What* is the appropriate resource (contact person's name, telephone number)?
3. *Where* is the resource located (address and client's means of transportation)?
4. *When* can referral arrangements be made (date, time of appointment)?
5. *Why* is this particular resource chosen (purpose; anticipated outcome)?
6. Was the contact made?
7. What were the results?
8. Is further intervention needed?

(Kobberger & Tousley, 1984, p. 50)

A center's referral service is more effective and efficient when it has:

1. Access to a *directory* of community resources
2. Knowledge of the *admission criteria* for each
3. Formal written *referral procedures* and agreements with all agencies involved in crisis work, including a review process
4. Initial and continuing *personal contact* with other agencies so that communication is maintained

(Kobberger & Tousley, 1984, p. 50)

ACCOUNTABILITY THROUGH RECORD KEEPING

Accountability to the community is indicated by the emphasis placed on documentation and record keeping. A crisis center's systematic collection, recording, and filing of information about itself and its clients can be useful for a number of reasons:

1. *Continuity of service:* Clients who have made prior contact are better served when their records at the center indicate what was tried and found to be effective in the past.
2. *Quality of service:* The effects of crisis intervention can be documented. Individual workers and the center as a whole can profit from this knowledge and be held accountable for their actions.
3. *Assessment of needs:* Recorded data can reveal characteristics and patterns of the population of clients served by the crisis center, the agency services most in demand, the adequacy of funding, and the justification of further funding.

4. *Accreditation:* Meticulous record keeping prepares the center for external evalua-
tion. Beyond protecting the public from substandard care, accreditation brings
- Stimulation toward self-improvement
- Public recognition
- Eligibility for government funding
- Protection from external pressures, which enables the program to keep legiti-
mate control over its own growth and development

(Kobberger & Tousley, 1984, p. 52)

REFERENCES

Britton, J. G., & Mattson-Melcher, D. M. (1985). The crisis home: Sheltering patients in emotional crisis. *Journal of Psychosocial Nursing, 23* (12), 18–23.

Kobberger, K. O., & Tousley, M. M. (1984). Designing a crisis center. In S. Lego (ed.), *The American Handbook of Psychiatric Nursing* (pp. 45–54). Philadelphia: J. B. Lipppincott.

Zealberg, J. J., Santos, A. B., & Fisher, R. K. (1993). Benefits of mobile crisis programs. *Hospital and Community Psychiatry, 44* (1), 16–17.

BIBLIOGRAPHY

Caplan, G. (1993). Organization of preventive psychiatry programs. *Community Mental Health Journal, 29,* 367–395.

Chiu, T. L., & Primeau, C. (1991). A psychiatric mobile crisis unit in New York City: Description and assessment, with implications for mental health care in the 1990's. *International Journal of Social Psychiatry, 37,* 251–258.

Dubin, S. E., Ananth, J, Bajwa, B. G., & Stuller, S. (1990). Three day crisis resolution unit. *Indian Journal of Psychiatry, 27,* 287–291.

Piersma, H. L., & VanWingen, S. (1988). A hospital-based crisis service for adolescents: A program description. *Adolescence, 23,* 491–500.

Putnam, J. F., Cohen, N. L., & Sullivan, A. M. (1985–86). Innovative outreach services for the homeless
mentally ill. *International Journal of Mental Health, 14* (4), 112–124.

Reynolds, I., Jones, J. E., Berry, D. W., & Hoult, J. E. (1990). A crisis team for the mentally ill: The effect on
patients, relatives and admissions. *Medical Journal of Australia, 152,* 646–652.

Silver, T., & Goldstein, H. (1992). A collaborative model of a county crisis intervention team: The Lake
County experience. *Community Mental Health Journal, 28,* 249–256.

Taylor, J. R., & Dees, J. P. (1993). How to design a mental health system to optimize mental health. *AAOHN Journal, 41,* 330–336.

Woodward, H. L. (1993). One community's response to the multi-system service needs of individuals with
mental illness and developmental disabilities. *Community Mental Health Journal, 29,* 347–359.

FORTY TWO

Designing a Debriefing Program

Karen Evanczuk

OVERVIEW:

Introduction
Victims of Critical Incidents
Stress Responses
Stress Syndromes
Interventions

Types of Debriefing Teams
Establishing a Team
Team Composition
Training
Evaluation

INTRODUCTION

Persons who experience a stressful event out of the range of ordinary human experience can suffer cognitive, affective, behavioral, and physical reactions. These events, called *critical incidents* (Mitchell & Everly, 1993), can affect occupational and social functioning and cause people to become vulnerable to "burnout" and posttraumatic stress disorder. Interventions, called *critical incident stress debriefings* (CISD), provide victims an opportunity to ventilate, share experiences, and discover they are not unique in their responses. The educational component of CISD informs participants about the normalcy of their responses and teaches them coping responses. Debriefing teams can be set up specifically for emergency services personnel (paramedics, firefighters, police, and emergency department staff) as well as for nonemergency community members.

VICTIMS OF CRITICAL INCIDENTS

Victims of critical incidents are categorized according to degree of exposure:
1. *Primary victims* are those with direct exposure to the incident, e.g., survivors of a plane crash.
2. *Secondary victims* are those who have seen the effects of the trauma on the primary victims, e.g., rescue workers or emergency technicians.
3. *Tertiary victims* are those who have seen the effects of the trauma on primary or secondary victims or who have been exposed to the scene of the tragedy, e.g., families of the victims or of the rescue workers. It is clear that natural and man-made disasters produce a ripple effect involving persons, families, and communities (Erikson, 1994).

STRESS RESPONSES   Responses to the overpowering stress of critical incidents occur in the following realms.

Cognitive   Blaming; confusion; poor attention; difficulty with decision making; heightened or lowered alertness; poor concentration; memory difficulties; hypervigilance; difficulty identifying familiar people or objects; increased or decreased awareness of surroundings; poor problem solving; poor abstract thinking; disorientation to time, place, or person; nightmares; intrusive images.

Affective   Anxiety; guilt; grief; denial; panic; shock; fear; uncertainty; loss of emotional control; depression; anger; irritability; agitation; helplessness; frustration.

Physical   Fatigue; headaches; visual difficulties; nausea and vomiting; weakness; dizziness; lightheadedness; sweating; chills; tachycardia; muscle tremors or twitches; chest tightness; gastrointestinal problems; shortness of breath; dry mouth.

Behavioral   Withdrawal; emotional outbursts; suspiciousness; change in activity level; change in speech patterns; change in usual communications; appetite increase or decrease; use of alcohol or drugs; pacing; change in sexual functioning.

Spiritual   Inability to integrate the incident with spiritual beliefs; anger at God; refusal to pray or attend church services; resentment toward religion.

STRESS SYNDROMES   Responses to stress have been categorized on a temporal basis as follows.

Acute Stress Syndrome   This response occurs during or just following the incident and includes fatigue, nausea, muscle tremors, twitches, profuse sweating, chills, dizziness, gastrointestinal upset, and other shock symptoms.

Delayed Stress Response Syndrome   This response occurs after the acute phase has passed and may continue for years if not treated. Symptoms include intrusive images, fear of repetition, physical symptoms, and the emotional symptoms associated with posttraumatic stress disorder.

Cumulative Stress (Burnout)   This response occurs when people are exposed to stress daily over time, resulting in physical and emotional exhaustion, apathy, and deterioration in performance.

INTERVENTIONS   *Defusing*   This intervention uses small group process instituted as soon as possible after the incident in hopes of:
1. Reducing the stress response
2. Defining the person's response as "normal"
3. Returning people to their jobs as soon as possible
4. Reestablishing a social network
5. Giving all the information available about the incident to everyone involved
6. Teaching stress survival
7. Determining if a debriefing is necessary

Debriefing   Debriefing uses small group process for crisis intervention and education 24–72 hours after the incident to:
1. Lessen the impact of the event on the victims
2. Speed up the healing process

3. Teach survival skills
4. Allow emotional ventilation
5. Reassure victims they will recover
6. Foster group cohesiveness
7. Prevent mental illness
8. Refer for mental health services if needed

Demobilization Demobilization is a primary prevention technique used for personnel who participate in a large-scale disaster rescue effort. It is used immediately after they return from the scene and before they leave to resume their usual duties with the goals of:
1. Forming a transition from the disaster to normal life
2. Reducing the intensity of stress reactions
3. Assessing needs for supplementary services
4. Forewarning workers about possible future responses
5. Providing information about the disaster
6. Teaching stress management
7. Fostering a positive attitude about recovery

TYPES OF DEBRIEFING TEAMS

Critical incident stress debriefing is carried out in teams, organized and led by psychiatric–mental health nurses or other mental health professionals. Critical incident stress management services can be developed in the following settings:
1. Emergency workers, such as police, EMS personnel, firefighters, and staff of emergency departments of hospitals. These teams can be organized and funded in a variety of ways, e.g., by city or county governments, hospitals, corporations, or a combination of these.
2. Employee assistance programs (EAPs), organized and funded by the agency using the program.
3. Private practitioners who contract with agencies to provide debriefing services when needed.

ESTABLISHING A TEAM

The first step in establishing a CISD team is to develop a needs assessment. The crucial questions in assessment are:
1. How many critical incidents occur that require intervention?
2. Is there support for a team from the people who will be using it?

Once a need has been established, the next steps are to:
1. Obtain approval
2. Convene a steering committee
3. Develop the structure of the team
4. Develop a membership application process
5. Provide training
6. Write policy guidelines
7. Begin team operations
8. Evaluate operations

TEAM COMPOSITION

The CISD team consists of:
1. Steering committee/board of directors.
2. Clinical director.

3. Administrative director.
4. Team coordinator(s).
5. Mental health professionals who serve as team leaders during debriefings.
6. Peer support personnel from emergency agencies, hospital, school, or other agencies in which the team will be located. The peers participate in defusings, debriefings, and demobilizations for emergency workers or any interventions for their professional counterparts.

TRAINING

It is recommended that basic training be provided by the International Critical Incident Stress Foundation located in Ellicott City, Maryland (telephone 410/730-4311). Because of possible future certification processes, contacting this agency or persons approved by them to teach basic training is suggested. Sixteen hours of basic training will provide the following content:
1. Stress: causes, sources, effects, and management
2. Types of critical incidents
3. The emergency worker personality
4. Team development
5. Interventions
6. Resources, disposition, and referrals
7. The family of the emergency worker
8. Mock debriefing
9. Crisis intervention
10. Communication

EVALUATION

A CISD team is considered successful if:
1. It is known and used by those it is designed to serve
2. It responds within the designated time periods with appropriate interventions
3. It is "driven" by emergency services peers in interventions provided for them
4. It provides follow-up for participants within a week to 10 days
5. It provides mental health referral services as needed
6. It provides services for families of those it serves

REFERENCES

Erikson, K. (1994). *A New Species of Trouble: Explorations in Disaster, Trauma, and Community.* New York: W. W. Norton.

Mitchell, J. T., & Everly, G. S. (1993). *Critical Incident Stress Debriefing (CISD): An Operations Manual for the Prevention of Traumatic Stress Among Emergency Services and Disaster Workers.* Ellicott City, MD: Chevron.

BIBLIOGRAPHY

Biley, F. C. (1989). Stress in high-dependency units. *Intensive Care Nursing, 5,* 134–141.

Clark, K. M. (1992). Pulling together: Building a community debriefing team. *Journal of Psychosocial Nursing, 30* (7), 27–32.

Freehill, K. M. (1992). Critical incident stress debriefing in health care. *Critical Care Clinics, 8* (3), 491–500.

Harris, R. B. (1989). Reviewing nursing stress according to a proposed coping-adaptation framework. *Advances in Nursing Science, 11,* 12–28.

Jimmerson, C. (1988). Critical incident stress debriefings. *Journal of Emergency Nursing, 14,* 43a–45a.

Lane, P. S. (1993–94). Critical incident stress debriefing for health care workers. *Omega, 28* (4), 301–315.

Linton, J. C., Kommor, M. J., & Webb, C. H. (1993). Helping the helpers: The development of a critical incident stress management team through university/community cooperation. *Annals of Emergency Medicine, 22* (4), 34–39.

Mitchell, J. T. (1982). Recovery from rescue. *Response, The Magazine of Emergency Management,* Fall, 7–10.

Mitchell, J. T. (1983). When disaster strikes . . . the critical incident debriefing process. *Journal of Emergency Medicine Service, 8* (1), 36–39.

Mitchell, J. T. (1984). The 600-run limit. *Journal of Emergency Medicine Service, 9,* 52–54.

Mitchell, J. T. (1984). High tension: Keeping stress under control. *Firehouse, 9,* 86–88.

Mitchell, J. T. (1984). Special report: No time for goodbyes. *Journal of Emergency Medicine Service, 9,* 28.

Mitchell, J. T. (1986). Teaming up against critical incident stress. *Chief Fire Executive, 1* (1), 24, 36, 84.

Mitchell, J. T. (1988). Stress: The history, status, and future of critical incident stress debriefings. *Journal of Emergency Medicine Service, 11,* 47–52.

Mitchell, J. T. (1988). Stress: Development and functions of a critical incident stress debriefing team. *Journal of Emergency Medicine Service, 13,* 43–46.

Rubin, J. G. (1990). Critical incident stress debriefing: Helping the helpers. *Journal of Emergency Nursing, 16* (4), 255–258.

Schaefer, K. M., & Peterson, K. (1992). Effectiveness of coping strategies among critical care nurses. *Applied Research, 11* (1), 28–34.

Shannon, P. A. (1991). The crisis of the caregivers. *Critical Care Nursing Clinics of North America, 3* (2), 353–359.

Troiani, T. A., & Boland, R. T. (1992). Critical incident stress debriefing: Keeping your flight crew healthy. *Journal of Air Medical Transport, 10,* 21–24.

FORTY THREE

Designing a Psychiatric Consultation–Liaison Nurse Program

Mary Grace Fitzgerald

OVERVIEW:

INTRODUCTION

Psychiatric consultation–liaison nursing (PCLN), a subspecialty of psychiatric–mental health nursing, focuses on the emotional, spiritual, developmental, cognitive, and behavioral responses of clients admitted to a health care facility, and of their significant others. These clients are usually admitted for a physical health care problem, and their significant others become known to the PCLN as visitors. The PCLN may be a part of the nursing service department or the department of psychiatry.

SETTINGS

Psychiatric consultation–liaison nursing may take place in:
1. General hospitals
2. Clients' homes
3. Rehabilitation facilities
4. Long-term care facilities
5. Home health nursing agencies
6. Primary and specialty care clinics
7. Health maintenance organizations
8. Hospices

COLLABORATION

To provide the most comprehensive delivery of service, the PCLN regularly exchanges ideas with, gathers information from, and shares treatment plans with team members, including:

1. Staff nurses
2. Primary care physicians, consulting physicians, physician assistants, and nurse practitioners
3. Nursing assistants and care partners
4. Administrators
5. Consultation–liaison psychiatrists
6. Psychologists
7. Social workers
8. Chaplains
9. Translators or international liaisons
10. Volunteers
11. Other staff including dietitians, physical therapists, occupational therapists, child life specialists, respiratory therapists, phlebotomists

PROFESSIONAL QUALIFICATIONS

The PCLN holds a master's degree in psychiatric nursing; demonstrates depth of knowledge, skill, and competence in the practice of psychiatric–mental health nursing; and is certified as a specialist in psychiatric–mental health nursing by the American Nurses Association. It is also recommended that the nurse have experience working on a medical-surgical unit.

PERSONAL QUALIFICATIONS

Because PCLNs work in such a wide range of situations, they are required to (Stokoloff, 1993):

1. Communicate easily with individuals with a wide range of educational and cultural backgrounds
2. Work well with others, put other people at ease
3. Work autonomously and flexibly, while continuously updating their own knowledge
4. Interact comfortably across disciplines
5. Teach in a creative way, using a variety of educational resources

FACTORS THAT PROMOTE OPTIMAL FUNCTIONING

The PCLN is able to function best when the following factors exist:

1. Administrative support
2. Acceptance and respect by members of the health care team
3. Identification of sources of frustration and pursuit of personal support systems
4. Peer group meetings to reduce isolation
5. Conferences to provide continuing education
6. Psychotherapy supervision

THE THERAPIST'S ROLE

The PCLN helps clients or their significant others to:

1. Gain insight into the nature and source of their problem
2. Identify and acknowledge their feelings related to the problem
3. Mobilize both internal strengths and environmental resources for effective coping
4. Eliminate or change the problem
5. Learn new and adaptive methods of coping

6. Formulate plans for prevention of future maladaptations
7. Reduce anxiety by participating in support groups

THE CONSULTANT'S ROLE

The PCLN helps staff members to:
1. Gain insight into the nature and source of their problem
2. Interpret their observations
3. Establish realistic goals
4. Formulate a plan to manage the problem
5. Identify resources for resolving or changing the problem
6. Identify the components of job stress and separate these from the delivery of client care
7. Build upon internal strengths and maximize coping skills
8. Evaluate the outcome of their actions

THE EDUCATOR'S ROLE

The PCLN helps staff to learn by:
1. Providing informal teaching during client care rounds
2. Organizing intradisciplinary client care conferences when a client's care is complex
3. Assessing for learning needs and developing inservice programs
4. Developing and presenting formal workshops on psychosocial topics that are relevant to the staff
5. Modeling therapeutic communication and behaviors

THE RESEARCHER'S ROLE

The PCLN helps staff members appreciate the value of research and use research in their practice by:
1. Encouraging a review of literature for solutions to client care problems
2. Approaching client care problems using the results of previous nursing research
3. Defining the problem in concrete and measurable terms
4. Using the scientific method in data collection
5. Analyzing the data as they apply to the research question
6. Providing a format for communicating the findings to colleagues

STEPS IN THE PROCESS

Upon receiving a request for consultation, usually from a nurse or physician, the PCLN takes the following steps:
1. Interviews the consultee to elicit the reason for the referral
2. Interviews the client or family
3. Conducts behavioral observations
4. Collects data from collaborative sources such as friends, families, caregivers, past and current medical records, community agencies
5. Records assessment data (see Box 43-1 for an assessment guide)
6. Formulates a psychiatric diagnosis, if appropriate, using the DSM-IV (see Chapters 1 and 2)
7. Formulates a nursing diagnosis, identifying human responses to actual or potential health problems, such as:
   - Impaired functioning or self-care limitations for which the etiology is mental or emotional distress, physical illness, or family dysfunction
   - Stress or crisis components of illness, pain, self-concept changes, and developmental changes

---

BOX 43-1: Assessment Guide for the Liaison Nurse

1. History of present illness and reason for referral with emphasis on the client or client's family's responses to illness, treatment regimes, and the caregiving environment
2. History of psychiatric disorders that would place the individual at increased risk when stressed with physical disability
3. Social history including significant life events that influence the coping ability of the client/family with identification of supportive individuals
4. Family history including family integrity, structure, and members' experience with illness as well as their coping strategies
5. Developmental history including patterns of coping and adaptation
6. Medical history and current medical status including drug and alcohol use, current medications, laboratory and test findings, and health beliefs and practices including cultural factors
7. Mental status examination (see Chapter 1)

  - Emotional problems related to illness experiences, such as guilt, anxiety, anger, loss, helplessness, loneliness, and grief
  - Alterations in cognition, perceiving, symbolizing, communicating, decision-making abilities
  - Sources of conflict, stress, or dysfunction in health care systems
8. Revises diagnoses as needed with subsequent data
9. Develops and initiates a plan of treatment or helps the staff in the development and implementation of a care plan that is:
  - Based on realistic goals
  - Built on the strengths of the client/family
  - Adaptable to the immediate circumstances and needs of the client/family
  - Reflective of collaborative resources in the milieu
  - Communicated to the staff through chart notes and verbal discussions
10. Evaluates the effectiveness of treatment through:
  - Ongoing communication with nurse consultee
  - Periodic reassessment of the client/family for adaptive coping skills

AIDS

Staff members often require help from the PCLN in caring for clients who have AIDS. Problems raised by nursing staff and suggested interventions are found in Table 43-1. See Chapter 39 for problems experienced by clients who are HIV-positive.

ORGAN TRANSPLANTATION

PROBLEMS OF THE NURSES

Problems experienced by staff nurses and operating room nurses in the care of clients who are transplant candidates, recipients, or donors and their families include:

1. Emotional fatigue and discouragement at seeing patients return repeatedly because of rejection and infection
2. Ethical aspects related to transplantation and organ allocation
3. Conflict over the glorification of transplant procedures by the media versus the realities

TABLE 43-1
Problems of Nursing Staff Caring for Persons with AIDS and Suggested Nursing Interventions of the PCLN

PROBLEMS	NURSING INTERVENTIONS
1. Fear of contagion and transmission to themselves, other patients, colleagues, family, and friends	1. Help staff members separate the emotional, behavioral, and physical needs of the client and significant others from their own emotional and personal conflicts.
2. Discomfort with clients' lifestyles when they differ from the nurses'	2. Provide individual support for the nurse's own responses through values clarification exercises.
3. Fatigue from the burden of intense emotional and physical needs of hospitalized persons with AIDS; identification with clients who may be dying and who are close to their own age	3. Provide a support group; teach stress management.
4. Difficulty responding to the neuropsychiatric sequelae of AIDS including organic brain disorders, major depression, psychosis, and personality disorders	4. Provide educational programs, clarification of emotional needs of clients and significant others; act as a role model in caring for clients and helping significant others.
5. Ethical conflicts regarding quality of life, prolongation of life, and rational suicide	5. Encourage discussion of these conflicts in informal contacts or support groups, helping staff members to explore all the dimensions of these conflicts. (See Chapter 71.)

4. Observation of healthy-looking, life-sustaining organs being removed from a cadaver donor who does not appear dead
5. Reality of death as life supports to the donor are discontinued, the rest of the surgical team leaves, and the body is prepared for the morgue
6. Physical, emotional, and intellectual demands of an 8–24-hour surgical procedure

HELPING THE NURSES

The PCLN:
1. Recognizes practice areas that are high emotional risk areas: the transplant operating room, intensive care units, and pretransplantation and posttransplantation wards and outpatient clinics
2. Plans for emotional and teaching support through allocation of time on these units
3. Teaches stress reduction and crisis intervention techniques to staff members
4. Encourages staff members to express their feelings and discuss the conflicting ethical issues in a support group

PROBLEMS OF THE ORGAN TRANSPLANT CLIENT OR FAMILY

Clients or families experience:
1. Conflict resulting from their anticipated quality of life and less satisfying reality.
2. Emotional and physical side effects of medications including emotional lability, delirium, depression, anxiety, tremor, nausea, hirsutism, weight gain, cushingoid features.
3. Frustration over frequent returns to the physician or hospital.

4. Need to take medications daily on a structured schedule.
5. Conflict between hope and guilt because the availability of a suitable donor necessitates the death of another.
6. A long and uncertain wait for a donor organ. As it gets longer, anger and hopelessness increase.
7. Fear of not being considered a suitable candidate and fear of being removed from the candidate list.
8. Trading a diseased organ for a new, unknown "disease" called organ transplantation.
9. Fear of rejection of the new organ.
10. Fear of infection and subsequent isolation.
11. Discomfort with shifts from the illness to the wellness role and vice versa.
12. Guilt feelings in family members who may feel responsible for the consequences of their decision if they believe they have coerced the patient.
13. Triggering or exaggeration of preexisting family problems owing to stress.
14. Role strain and role reversal.
15. Severe financial burden of medical expenses and travel and housing expenses.
16. Anxiety over lifestyle changes or decisions, e.g., about pregnancy, employability, insurability.
17. Altered developmental courses for children, adolescents, and young adults.
18. Social isolation or the belief that it is impossible for others to understand what the experience of the transplantation process is like.
19. Body image changes in physical appearance: flushing, tremor, rounding of face, increased body hair, thinning hair, weight gain/loss, aggravated acne, large surgical scar, and muscle wasting.

INTERVENTIONS FOR CLIENTS AND FAMILIES

1. Assess family stress and coping resources before and after transplantation.
   - Pretransplant evaluation includes identification of the demands on the family unit and the resources or strengths, coping behaviors, and types of support available to family members to manage these demands.
   - Posttransplant evaluation determines how families are adapting and whether they need further help and intervention to enhance coping and improve family life.
2. Provide anticipatory guidance regarding care and socioemotional needs.
3. Organize support groups for clients and families to communicate their thoughts, feelings, and concerns.
4. Review financial concerns and help families identify sources of financial support.
5. Support and counsel families in letting go and avoiding overprotection of the client after transplantation.
6. Support the client to develop independence.
7. Discuss with families their children's developmental needs.
8. Assess clients' level of functioning after they have arrived home.
9. Provide psychotherapy to support self-concept and social competence.

ESTABLISHING PCLN SERVICES

Table 43-2 shows two models for PCLN organization: one within a department of nursing, the other in a department of psychiatry.

TABLE 43-2
A Comparison of PCLN Organizational Models

PCLN IN A NURSING DEPARTMENT	PCLN IN A PSYCHIATRY DEPARTMENT
1. Functions as a clinical nurse specialist.	1. Functions as a clinical nurse specialist.
2. Referrals are encouraged from the nursing staff.	2. Referrals are more likely to come from physicians.
3. A physician's order is not required for consultation.	3. Consultation is often made through a physician's order.
4. Encourages nurse-to-nurse consultation, built on a nursing model, with benefits for the entire nursing department.	4. Encourages nurse–physician consultation, built on the medical model. Consultation involves only the PCLN, the physician, and the client.
5. Psychotherapy supervision is often provided outside the nursing department.	5. Psychotherapy supervision is provided within the department of psychiatry.
6. May have administrative authority over staff members who request the consultation.	6. Has no administrative authority over staff members who request the consultation.
7. Communicates with nursing administration, helping to plan organizational changes in the nursing department.	7. Has no responsibility for the nursing department.
8. Is evaluated by the nursing department using case logs, written evaluations of workshops, and reports from staff, clients, and families.	8. Is evaluated by the psychiatry department.

REFERENCE

Stokoloff, S. (1993). Psychiatric nurse consultant. *Canadian Nurse, 79* (4), 42–45.

BIBLIOGRAPHY

Chisolm, M. (1991). The psychiatric consultation–liaison nurse and the challenge of AIDS: Caring for nurses. *Clinical Nurse Specialist, 5* (2), 123.

Council of Psychiatric and Mental Health Nursing (1990). *Standards of Psychiatric Consultation–Liaison Nursing Practice.* Washington, DC: American Nurses Association.

Hart, C. A. (1990). The role of psychiatric consultation liaison nurses in ethical decisions to remove life-sustaining treatments. *Archives of Psychiatric Nursing, 4* (6), 370–378.

Kurlowicz, L. H. (1991). Psychiatric consultation–liaison nursing interventions with nurses of hospitalized AIDS patients. *Clinical Nurse Specialist, 5* (2), 124–129.

Mallory, G. A., Lyons, J. S., Scherubel, J. C., & Reichelt, P. A. (1993). Nursing care hours of patients receiving varying amounts and types of consultation/liaison services. *Archives of Psychiatric Nursing, 7* (6), 353–360.

Newton, L., & Wilson, K. G. (1990). Consultee satisfaction with a psychiatric consultation–liaison nursing service. *Archives of Psychiatric Nursing, 4* (4), 264–270.

Robinson, L. (1987). Psychiatric consultation liaison nursing and psychiatric consultation doctoring: Similarities and differences. *Archives of Psychiatric Nursing, 1* (2), 73–80.

Schaal, P. G., & Slemenda, M. B. (1984). Nurses' response to transplants: A systems view. *AORN Journal, 39* (1), 42–45.

Talley, S., & Caverly, S. (1994). Advanced-practice psychiatric nursing and health care reform. *Hospital and Community Psychiatry, 45* (6), 545–547.

Talley, S., Davis, D. S., Goicoechea, N., Brown, L., & Barber, L. L. (1990). Effects of psychiatric liaison nurse specialist consultation on the care of medical-surgical patients with sitters. *Archives of Psychiatric Nursing, 4* (2), 114–123.

Tommasini, N. R. (1992). The impact of a staff support group on the work environment of a specialty unit. *Archives of Psychiatric Nursing, 6* (1), 40–47.

Uzark, K. (1992). Caring for families of pediatric transplant recipients: Psychosocial implications. *Critical Care Nursing Clinics of North America, 4* (2), 255–261.

Weiner, M. F., & Caldwell, T. (1983–84). The process and impact of an ICU nurse support group. *International Journal of Psychiatry in Medicine, 13* (1), 47–55.

Designing a Forensic Program

Anne Barker Dunn
Joyce A. Selzer
Patricia M. Tomcho

OVERVIEW:

Introduction
Definition of Terms
Settings
Diagnostic Categories

Ethical and Legal Issues
Components of a Forensic Program
Nursing Interventions
Future Directions

INTRODUCTION

Forensic psychiatric nurses provide mental health services to clients who are involved in some way with the criminal justice system and show evidence of mental or emotional illness. An alarming increase in crime, violence, and substance abuse along with the return to a punitive approach toward criminals with psychiatric problems makes it imperative that psychiatric mental health nurses respond with holistic and comprehensive services in forensic settings. The forensic nurse in psychiatric–mental health nursing possesses the knowledge and skills to ensure balance in the treatment of offenders and to create bridges between three systems sometimes at odds: the criminal justice system, the mental health system, and community agencies.

DEFINITION OF TERMS

1. *Forensic services* provide mental health care to inmates in correctional facilities, parolees in community mental health centers, and patients in forensic psychiatric units.
2. *Forensic nurses* are generalist registered nurses who provide holistic care to clients in clinical forensic psychiatric settings.
3. *Forensic clinical nurse specialists* hold a master's degree in nursing and function as expert clinicians, educators, researchers, consultants, and administrators in forensic psychiatric settings.
4. *Correctional facility* is a federal, state, or local institution providing confinement for those convicted of a crime or those awaiting trial. Jails are generally used for those awaiting trial and prisons for those serving sentences.
5. *Community mental health center* is an agency providing psychiatric services to clients in a particular catchment area.
6. *Forensic psychiatric units* offer specialized services for the evaluation or treatment of persons who are mentally ill and involved with the criminal justice system. This

specialized care includes assessment of competency to stand trial, care of persons found not guilty by reason of insanity, and treatment of clients who exhibit psychiatric symptomatology while in a correctional setting.

7. *Population* to be served includes clients who show mental illness or emotional problems and are involved in some way with the criminal justice system.

SETTINGS

Forensic psychiatric nurses practice in:
1. Correctional facilities: juvenile detention facilities, jails, and prisons
2. Forensic psychiatric units
3. Community mental health centers with parolees, clients of a conditional release program, and ex-offenders

DIAGNOSTIC CATEGORIES

Patients in forensic settings exhibit a wide variety of psychiatric diagnoses. The following DSM IV categories are represented in the forensic population: Substance-Related Disorders, Schizophrenia and Other Psychotic Disorders, Mood Disorders, Anxiety Disorders, Somatoform Disorders, Factitious Disorders, Dissociative Disorders, Sexual and Gender Identity Disorders, Eating Disorders, Sleep Disorders, and Personality Disorders.

In addition to the above categories, a number of individuals may be dually diagnosed or carry a diagnosis from childhood or adolescence. The forensic psychiatric nurse must exercise caution when assessing and providing care based on the DSM IV diagnoses, because "there are significant risks that diagnostic information can be misused or misunderstood" (American Psychiatric Association, 1994, p. xxi).

ETHICAL AND LEGAL ISSUES

An understanding of ethical and legal issues and guidelines is essential to forensic psychiatric nursing. Some of these are (see also Chapters 70 and 71):
1. Confidentiality and the right to privilege
2. Informed consent
3. Types of admissions—voluntary versus involuntary, indefinite commitment (state and institutional rules/regulations)
4. Patients' rights
5. Competency issues, criminal responsibilities, nonguilt by reason of insanity
6. Voluntary versus involuntary use of medication or other techniques for behavioral change
7. Seclusion and restraint policy and procedures

COMPONENTS OF A FORENSIC PROGRAM

Essential components of a forensic program include:
1. A mission statement and philosophy
2. A clear protocol of rules, regulations, and policies
3. A clear protocol for assessing competency
4. Written standards of care
5. Guidelines for confidentiality
6. A cost-effective plan
7. Attainable goals and objectives mutually defined by client and nurse
8. A system for nursing intervention
9. Documentation
10. Evaluation of all of the above

NURSING INTERVENTIONS

Nursing interventions and their rationales are shown in Table 44-1.

TABLE 44-1
Tasks of the Forensic Psychiatric Nurse with Rationales

TASK	RATIONALE
Assess for:	
1. Physical/Problems • communicable diseases such as TB, STDs, HIV • side effects of medications • health education and health promotion needs • ability to engage in self-care behaviors	1. A comprehensive assessment ascertains a clear database and identifies physical problems that can affect psychological functioning Communicable diseases must be identified, treated, contained
2. Psychological Issues • depression/hopelessness/powerlessness • homicidal or suicidal ideation • history of violence as victim or perpetrator • potential for violence • history of sexual, physical, or emotional abuse • level of current stress • psychotic symptoms • ability to participate in individual or group therapy • sexual history • gender orientation • current sexual relationships • family and support system • addiction history • side effects of psychotropic medications and potential drug interaction	2. A comprehensive psychological assessment gives an accurate picture of the client's past and current level of psychological functioning. Assessment of risk of harm to self and others ensures safety and maintains the therapeutic milieu
3. Ethical/Legal Issues • competency • abuse of client from within the system (staff or patients) • perceived infringement of legal rights	3. A comprehensive assessment of ethical/legal issues ensures that appropriate services are rendered to the client
4. Other Issues • literacy and comprehension • spiritual orientation • vocational/employment history	4. A comprehensive assessment of diverse issues ensures the provision of holistic care
Intervene by:	
1. Providing individual psychotherapy	1. Helps clients to alleviate symptoms, develop self-esteem, and plan for the future
2. Providing group therapy	2. Helps clients to see themselves as others see them, alleviate symptoms, develop self-esteem, and plan for the future
3. Providing family therapy	3. Helps clients resolve family conflicts
4. Providing sexual abuse counseling	4. Helps clients work through reactions to victim or perpetrator roles
5. Providing HIV/AIDS counseling	5. Helps clients confront psychological changes, grief, and relationship changes. Encourages safe sex to prevent further infection.
6. Providing relaxation and stress-management training	6. Helps clients manage anxiety and increases coping skills
7. Providing assertiveness training	7. Helps clients learn appropriate personal advocacy

TABLE 44-1 *(continued)*

TASK	RATIONALE
8. Providing a safe milieu via medication, or other techniques for behavioral change	8. Helps clients feel safe in the least restrictive environment
9. Providing health education and medication teaching	9. Helps clients increase knowledge base, empowers decision making
10. Providing addiction counseling	10. Helps client to begin recovery
11. Providing referral to appropriate psychiatric resources or facilities	11. Helps clients to gain access to appropriate services

Evaluate for:

1. Symptom reduction

2. Improvement in physical/psychological functioning

3. Integration of health teaching

4. Access to appropriate resources

5. Verbalization of future goals

FUTURE DIRECTIONS   Opportunities in forensic psychiatric nursing will continue to proliferate. The following list illustrates areas for potential role development and expansion in the future:

1. Sexual assault nurse examiner (see Chapter 36)
2. Forensic nurse investigator
3. Forensic nurse educator, researcher, consultant
4. Clinical forensic nurse specialist
5. Nurse coroner/death investigator
6. Legal nurse consultant
7. Nurse attorney
8. Correctional nurse
9. Forensic pediatric nurse
10. Forensic geriatric nurse
11. Forensic psychiatric nurse
12. Emergency/trauma or critical care forensic nurse
13. Nurse specializing in the application of clinical or community-based nursing practice involving victims of intentional or nonintentional injuries (International Association of Forensic Nurses, 1994)
14. Hostage negotiator
15. Battered women specialist

REFERENCES   American Psychiatric Association (1994). *Diagnostic and Statistical Manual of Mental Disorders* (4th ed.). Washington, DC: American Psychiatric Association.

International Association of Forensic Nurses (IAFN) (1994). *Forensic Nursing in Leadership in the Health Care Response to Violence* (available from Slack Inc., 6900 Grove Road, Thorofare, NJ 08086).

BIBLIOGRAPHY   Alexander-Rodriguez, T. (1983). Prison health—A role for professional nursing. *Nursing Outlook, 31* (2), 115–118.

Baier, M. (1982). Group therapy with parolees in a Community Mental Health Center. *Journal of Psychosocial Nursing and Mental Health Services, 20* (2), 26–40.

Bernier, S. L. (1986). Corrections and mental health. *Journal of Psychosocial Nursing and Mental Health Services, 24* (6), 20–26.

Birk, S. (1992). Emerging specialties expand opportunities. *American Nurse, 24* (9), 7, 9, 24.

Caplan, C. A. (1993). Nursing staff and patient perceptions in a maximum security forensic hospital. *Archives of Psychiatric Nursing, 7* (1), 23–29.

Halleck, S. L. (1986). *The Mentally Disordered Offender.* Maryland: U.S. Department of Health and Human Services. Public Health Services.

Hufft, A. G., & Fawkes, L. S. (1994). Federal inmates, a unique psychiatric nursing challenge. *Nursing Clinics of North America, 29* (1), 35–42.

Laben, J. K., Dodd, D., & Snead, L. (1991). King's theory of goal attainment applied in group therapy for inpatient juvenile sexual offenders, etc. *Issues in Mental Health Nursing, 12* (1), 51–64.

Laben, J. K., & MacLean, C. P. (1989). *Legal Issues and Guidelines for Nurses Who Care for the Mentally Ill* (2nd ed.). Maryland: National Health Publishing.

Lynch, V. (ed.) (1993). Forensic nursing (special issue). *Journal of Psychosocial Nursing and Mental Health Services, 31* (11).

Lynch, V. (1993). Forensic aspects of health care: New roles, new responsibilities. *Journal of Psychosocial Nursing and Mental Health Services, 31* (11), 5–6.

Masters, R. E. (1994). *Counseling Criminal Justice Offenders.* Newbury Park, CA: Sage.

Niskala, H. (1986). Competencies and skills required by nurses working in forensic areas. *Western Journal of Nursing Research, 8* (4), 400–413.

Osborne, M. (1991). The many faces of mental health nursing. *Alberta Association Registered Nurses Newsletter, 47* (5), 5–6.

Pepper, J. (1982). Psychiatric assessment on a forensic unit. *Canadian Nurse, 78,* 50–51.

Phillips, M. S. (1983). Forensic psychiatry: Nurses' attitudes revealed. *Dimensions in Health Services, 60* (9), 41–43.

FORTY FIVE

Designing a Mental Health Home Care Program

Edith Brogan de la Fuente
Lou Ann Fulmer

OVERVIEW:

Introduction
Definition of Mental Health Home Care
Client Population
Needs Assessment
Reimbursement
Staffing

Method of Service Delivery
Productivity Standard
Referrals
Assessment of Clients
Marketing
Evaluation

INTRODUCTION

The 20th century has seen a movement in the care of those diagnosed mentally ill from asylums to long-term public and private hospitals, to short-term psychiatric units in general hospitals, and recently to their own homes. The mentally ill are hospitalized only when they are a threat to themselves or others, and then only for brief stays. As life expectancy has increased, more elderly are living at home, many with depression or dementia. Owing to shortened stays in hospitals, many people are coping with acute, chronic, and life-threatening illnesses at home. Caretakers of the mentally ill, elderly, and physically ill are stressed and need the help of psychiatric home care nurses to reduce this stress.

**DEFINITION OF
MENTAL HEALTH
HOME CARE**

Traditionally mental health home care (MHHC) was designed for persons with mental illness who could not use outpatient mental health services, because of the nature of their mental illness or an accompanying physical disability. Buckwalter (1991) writes that "psychiatric nursing home care is designed to smooth the transition from hospital to community, to promote the highest level of functioning possible in the community setting, and to reduce recidivism—all in a cost-effective manner" (p. 897). However, today MHHC involves far more than treatment of psychiatric patients.

CLIENT POPULATION

Clients receiving MHHC include:
1. Clients with a psychiatric diagnosis who are homebound
2. The elderly with psychiatric or physical problems who are homebound

3. Clients with emotional problems related to physical problems who are home-bound
4. Caretakers of the homebound

Table 45-1 lists examples of clients treated by psychiatric nurses at home, and the interventions offered.

TABLE 45-1
Examples of Clients Cared for in an MHHC Program and Nursing Interventions

EXAMPLES OF CLIENTS	NURSING INTERVENTIONS
Clients with acute anxiety	1. Provide psychotherapy. Help client to recognize anxiety, and identify feelings and events that precede anxious feelings or behavior. (See Chapter 22.) 2. Teach techniques for reducing anxiety, including guided imagery. 3. Prescribe antianxiety medication, or refer to one who can evaluate and prescribe. (See Chapter 69.)
Clients with depression	1. Explore the source of the mood change, for example, dementia, structural changes in the brain following cerebral vascular accidents, reactions to chemotherapy or reactions to losses. 2. Help client understand and work through the cause, using psychotherapy. 3. Prescribe antidepression medications or refer to one who can evaluate and prescribe.
Clients who need blood levels drawn for clozapine, lithium, and so forth	Explain procedures necessary to prepare for drawing, for example, that patient should not take lithium in the morning of the day blood is drawn for lithium levels.
Clients with cancer who are experiencing side effects of treatment as well as interpersonal problems	1. Help patient understand or expect fatigue, possible depression, and anxiety. 2. Evaluate for akathisia, neuropsychiatric problems, such as hallucinations, changes in cognition, frank psychosis from steroids, and depression with suicide ideation seen with interferon at certain doses. 3. Provide psychotherapy, relaxation, and guided imagery. 4. Recommend community resources such as support groups and cancer hotlines for information of the disease and the latest treatment modalities. 5. Provide assertiveness training when needed.
Clients with acute or chronic disabilities from cardiovascular or other disorders	1. Provide psychotherapy as needed. 2. Use creative ideas to help client deal with maintaining sexuality, such as colostomy intimacy pouches or crotchless underwear for clients with foley catheters, and so forth. 3. Recommend support groups and educational groups.
Clients with chronic pain	1. Provide psychotherapy as needed. 2. Teach relaxation and guided imagery techniques. 3. Recommend support and educational groups.
Clients with HIV/AIDS	1. Provide psychotherapy as needed. (See Chapter 39.) 2. Recommend HIV/AIDS support groups. 3. Assess periodically for any changes in cognition.
Clients who are dying	See Chapter 20 for in-depth information.
Caretakers experiencing stress and exhaustion	1. Educate about the illness, symptom management, respite care available, the use of volunteers from groups such as Time Out or churches. 2. Recommend support groups. 3. Provide psychotherapy as needed.

NEEDS ASSESSMENT
The first step in establishing an MHHC is to perform a needs assessment. Before starting an MHHC program there must be:

1. Agency ability to support the service
   - Financial
   - Human resources
2. Community support for such a service
   - Physician (psychiatry and general medicine)
   - Hospital (psychiatric and general)
   - Community mental health centers
   - Assisted living centers
   - Community-based senior services

REIMBURSEMENT
Agencies wishing to start an MHHC program must become familiar with basic guidelines developed by third-party payers, such as Medicare, Medicaid, private insurance, and managed care providers. Because a majority of home care patients are 65 and over, knowledge of Medicare guidelines is essential. Federal guidelines for reimbursing Medicare home health care stipulate that:

1. Patient must be homebound and in need of skilled nursing care
2. Care is provided by a home health agency that does not primarily provide care and treatment in mental illness, such as a community mental health center
3. Services must be provided by a psychiatrically trained nurse either 2 years post-baccalaureate or master's level
4. The plan of care is established and reviewed by a psychiatrist (1989 Health Care Financing Administration: Home Health Regulations and Guidelines HIM-11)

STAFFING
Table 45-2 lists the team members who may be involved with the psychiatric home care patient, and the role of each.

METHOD OF SERVICE DELIVERY
When designing the MHHC program, decisions must be made initially regarding the method of service delivery. The team may be composed of hourly employees or contract nurses who are paid per visit.

PRODUCTIVITY STANDARD
A productivity standard must be established, for example, that the nurse will see four to five patients per day.

REFERRALS
Patients are referred to MHHC agencies by:

1. Hospital coordinators
2. Advanced practice nurses
3. Physicians
4. Social workers
5. Psychologists
6. Community mental health centers
7. Other nurses in the agency

Referrals are either done by phone through the intake nurse or program coordinator, or through a written referral. The case is then assigned to a nurse by the coordinator.

TABLE 45-2
Psychiatric Home Care Team

TEAM MEMBER—CREDENTIALS	ROLE
Program Coordinator—master's degree in geriatric or adult psychiatric nursing	1. Directs program 2. Checks appropriateness of referrals 3. Assigns cases 4. Oversees quality assurance activities 5. Directs marketing 6. Oversees program evaluation 7. Hires and evaluates employees
Psychiatric Clinical Nurse Specialist— master's degree in psychiatric nursing, ANA certified in adult psychiatric nursing	1. Provides psychiatric assessment 2. Provides psychotherapy 3. Provides clinical supervision to nurses managing client's psychiatric problems, when third-party reimbursement is denied for psychiatric services or client refuses services 4. Provides intradepartmental coordination when client with limited cognitive or coping abilities is in need of multiple services, such as diabetic educator, social services, physical therapy, skilled nursing, and so forth 5. Provides consultation, for example, to hospice nurses 6. Presents community workshops, for example, on living with or providing support to people with a life-threatening illness 7. Presents professional workshops, for example, on managing difficult emotions such as depression or anger
Psychiatric Staff Nurse—registered nurse with 2 years of experience in inpatient, outpatient, or community mental health	1. Provides counseling 2. Provides case management including blood draws and skilled nursing care 3. Monitors and evaluates clients' response to medication 4. Refers clients to community resources
Nursing Staff Educator—master's degree in nursing or education	1. Orients new nurses to agency 2. Coordinates inservice education
Skilled Nurse—registered nurse with at least 2 years of medical-surgical nursing	1. Provides ongoing skilled nursing care 2. Processes doctor's orders
Medical Social Worker—bachelor's degree in social work with 1 year of health care experience and licensure	Assesses need for, educates about, and refers client to community resources
Physical, Occupational, and Speech Therapist—bachelor's degree in specialty, and 1 year of experience in acute care setting or rehabilitation center	Provides specialized services

ASSESSMENT OF CLIENTS

Once a referral is received, the psychiatric nurse does a full mental health assessment that includes a mini–mental health assessment to identify any cognitive deficits. (See Chapter 1.) This assessment, along with a plan of care, is placed in the patient's record to guide care, and as a resource for other professionals involved in the care of the patient.

MARKETING

A well-developed MHHC program has to support itself. This can be accomplished by a sound creative internal and external marketing plan. Marketing requires the administrator to:

1. Analyze the community needs assessment survey
2. Develop a brochure describing mental health home care services (see Box 45-1)
3. Develop a checklist of appropriate patients for referring agencies, practitioners both generalist and psychiatric, managed care providers, and discharge planners to use or have as a guideline when ordering services (Thobaben, 1989)
4. Contact all referring agencies by letter and with a follow-up visit using a brochure listing services (see Box 45-1)
5. Provide inservice programs on mental health problems to staff in referring agencies
6. Provide speakers for community and professional programs, to explain the program
7. Advertise the program in various media formats, offering free information upon request

---

BOX 45-1: Example of Marketing of MHHC

Psychiatric Nursing Program

The Psychiatric Clinical Nurse Specialist (PCNS) provides psychotherapeutic counseling to homebound patients who are diagnosed as experiencing a psychiatric disorder. The services are provided by registered nurses, with masters degrees in nursing and clinical specialization in psychiatric mental health nursing.

Patients Who Benefit

Patients who benefit from the program include individuals experiencing difficulty adjusting to physical disabilities which are associated with acute or chronic illness. Individuals with psychiatric diagnoses are also referred to this program.

Benefits of Using VNS Psychiatric Program

- Home visits by the psychiatric clinical nurse specialist enhance existing community programs.

- Services are made available to homebound patients who are unable to obtain services on an outpatient basis.

- The PCNS provides a comprehensive mental health assessment of the patient and involves the patient and family in developing a plan for therapy.

- The therapy focuses on promoting day-to-day functioning, including reality orientation and structural activities to improve or maintain mental health.

- The PCNS interacts in consultation and collaboration with the patient's psychiatrist and/or attending physician to implement a treatment plan. The nurse provides periodic written progress reports of the patient's status to the physician.

- Arrangements can be made for a psychiatrist to make a home visit and evaluate those patients who do not have a private psychiatrist.

- When the patient is no longer homebound, but still in need of therapy, the patient is referred to the physician, appropriate community agency or outpatient facility for ongoing intervention.

Visiting Nurse Service, Akron, OH. Reprinted with permission.

EVALUATION

An MHHC program is considered a success if:

1. Early intervention prevents exacerbation of mental health problems into full-blown incapacitating illness
2. Patients are able to avoid hospitalization
3. Unsafe situations are resolved by methods such as providing mobile meals, a home health aide to help with bathing, community service agencies like Passport providing caregivers for 4 hours a day in lieu of a nursing home, connecting clients to Adult Protective Service, and so forth
4. The program meets the need of the community as measured by increase in referrals

REFERENCES

Buckwalter, K. C. (1991). Community mental health and home care. In G. K. McFarland & M. D. Thomas (eds.), *Psychiatric Mental Health Nursing* (pp. 893–902). Philadelphia: J. B. Lippincott.

Health Care Financing Administration (1989). *Medicare Home Health Agency Manual* (HIM-11). HCFA-Pub. 11, 205.1.

Thobaben, M. (1989). Developing a psychiatric home health service. *Caring, 8* (6), 10–14.

BIBLIOGRAPHY

Blazek, L. E. (1993). Development of a psychiatric home care program and the role of the CNS in the delivery of care. *Clinical Nurse Specialist, 7* (4), 164–168.

Dittbrenner, H. (1994). Psychiatric home care: An overview. *Caring, 13* (6), 26–28, 30.

Harper, M. S. (1989). Providing mental health services in the homes of the elderly: A public policy perspective. *Caring, 8* (6), 4–6, 8–9, 52–53.

Hellwig, K. (1993). Psychiatric home care nursing: Managing patients in the community setting. *Journal of Psychosocial Nursing and Mental Health Services, 31* (12), 21–24.

Kozlak, J., & Thobaben, M. (1992). Treating the elderly mentally ill at home. *Perspectives in Psychiatric Care, 28* (2), 31–35.

Miller, M. P., & Duffey, J. (1993). Planning and program development for psychiatric home care. *Journal of Nursing Administration, 23* (11), 35–41.

Richie, F., & Lusky, K. (1987). Psychiatric home health nursing: A new role in community mental health. *Community Mental Health Journal, 23* (3), 229–234.

Thobaben, M., & Kozlak, J. (1990). Home health care's unique role in serving the elderly mentally ill. *Home Health Care Nurse, 8* (4), 37–39.

46

Designing an Inpatient Psychiatric Unit

Peggy A. Sawyer

OVERVIEW:

INTRODUCTION

Inpatient hospitalization can be a stressful event for the most emotionally healthy among us. The provision of a safe, structured, clinically sound environment is of paramount importance in helping clients weather the acute phase of psychiatric illness and return to the community.

RECENT DEVELOPMENTS IN HEALTH CARE

Changes in reimbursement for psychiatric care have produced changes in the structure of inpatient psychiatric units. Lengths of stay are shorter than they used to be, averaging about 1 week. Only the most acute portion of an individual's illness is treated in the hospital and only the most acutely ill are admitted. In the modern psychiatric inpatient unit:

1. *Crisis intervention and relief of acute symptoms* is the purpose of hospitalization.
2. *Multidisciplinary critical care paths* provide a clear, concise care plan for the clinical team to follow. Programs are 7 days per week, 24 hours per day, with no slack time. All scheduled activity leads to achievement of short-term measurable goals. Critical paths are monitored manually or with specialized software.
3. *Information systems* are programmed to prompt required care, monitor variances from critical paths, assure that variances occur only when patients change unexpectedly, and detect inefficiencies in the hospital's systems or clinicians.
4. *Patient outcome tracking tools,* both manual and automated, assist in continuously monitoring patient clinical outcomes and progress toward goals.

5. *Communication* among multiple practitioners in various geographic locations uses advanced communication methods, including information systems. Such systems include patient clinical and financial data from prior and current inpatient and out-patient episodes. All members of the team as well as insurers can regularly access and add to the data using security codes to ensure confidentiality.

6. *Continuous quality improvement* efforts actively involve all clinical staff members as their ongoing feedback is sought to address clinical issues and efficiencies and to implement solutions.

7. *Skill mix* of the staff members is designed for maximum patient benefit and efficiency. Cross-trained staff is the norm. Highly skilled staff are held accountable for designing care plans and monitoring patient progress toward goals. Nursing staff, including nurse practitioners and clinical nurse specialists, are part of the clinical team along with multiskilled care partners. Expert staff members are available 7 days a week, 24 hours a day, with no downtime on weekends.

8. *Therapeutic milieu and psychopharmacology* are both important aspects of the patient's care, with quality-of-life research outcomes and patients' needs balanced with medication dosages.

ADVANTAGES OF INPATIENT HOSPITALIZATION

Hospitalization of psychiatric patients:
1. Provides patients who may be suicidal or potentially violent with a safe, nurturing, nontoxic environment to begin treatment
2. Provides families with safety and respite from patients who may be suicidal or potentially violent
3. Provides communities with safety from patients who may be suicidal or potentially violent

DISADVANTAGES OF INPATIENT HOSPITALIZATION

Hospitalization of psychiatric patients:
1. May lead patients and families to believe treatment is only needed for the acute episode
2. May lead family and friends to hold patients in less regard once they have been labeled "mental patients"
3. May lead to community stigma
4. May have concrete consequences when patients apply for jobs or other positions after hospitalization

PHYSICAL DESIGN OF INPATIENT UNITS

General The unit should be pleasant and soothing in color. Pictures on the walls are covered with shatterproof glass or Plexiglas and secured with tamperproof screws. Maximum attention is paid to patient safety including use of shatterproof glass throughout the unit, locked windows, double-hinged doors, absence of hooks in patient areas, and other patient safety measures. The physical plant must meet state and federal building codes as well as requirements of accrediting bodies.

Maximum Size Capacity should not exceed 40–50 patients.

Nursing Stations One main station and two or three smaller pods dispersed around the unit discourage the concentration of staff in one station and allow for maximum interaction between staff and patients and maximum staff observation of patients. Pods should have computer terminals, allowing for ease of data input and access.

Medication Room   Stock medications, emergency medications, and unit doses are stored in the medication room. This room may be adjacent to the main nurses' station and should be in staff view.

Locked Area   Contraband and unsafe objects brought onto the unit by patients or visitors are stored in the locked area.

Staff Lounge   This space allows for break time of two or three staff members at one time, near the main nursing station.

Dictation Room   Data are dictated in this room. The dictation system is preferably one designed to automatically turn the spoken word into type as dictation is occurring.

Treatment Room   Physical exams and medical treatments are carried out in the treatment room, where medical supplies and a crash cart are stored.

Conference Room   Daily patient team conferences, patient/family education meetings, group therapy, and staff meetings can be held in the conference room.

Private Offices   These offices are generic rooms for meeting privately with patients, families, and significant others.

Seclusion/Restraint Section   This section is a five- or six-room area for quiet time, seclusion, or restraint. It should be blocked off and soundproofed from the rest of the unit to provide for patient privacy and to prevent disturbance of the rest of the milieu.

Patient Rooms   Private and semiprivate rooms with bathrooms are designed for safety and must not present opportunities for suicidal threats to be carried out.

One-to-One Section   This section is a patient room alcove where five or six patients on close or constant observation can be observed by one or two caregivers without disrupting the rest of the unit.

Lounges/Dining Rooms   Two or three dining rooms/lounges are provided for patients' free time, community meetings, dining, and visitors. Lounges should be pleasant and comfortable with enough chairs, couches, and tables for patients and visitors.

Activity Rooms   Two to three rooms should allow for patient groups of up to 15 for games, crafts, meetings, and recreation.

Linen Room   This area is for storing clean linen.

STAFFING PATTERNS

TRADITIONAL MODEL

Box 46-1 shows a traditional staffing pattern for 23–25 patients over 7 days/week. This model can absorb one patient on a one-to-one level of observation, but adjustments can occur if more patients need close observation. According to the Joint Commission on Accreditation of Healthcare Organizations (JCAHO), every psychiatric unit must have a staffing plan for minimum staffing that includes provisions to increase staff if patient acuity increases. Software is available to calculate staffing plans based on patient acuity. Inpatient units often employ homegrown plans that are developed with sound judgment and are easily understood and implemented. Either plan will satisfy accrediting bodies. In addition to the JCAHO, the National Council for Quality Assurance (NCQA) has been formed to monitor managed care organizations.

BOX 46-1: Nursing Staffing Pattern for a 25-Bed Inpatient Psychiatric Unit Using a Traditional Model

Staff	Day Shift	Evening Shift	Night Shift
Clinical coordinator	1–5 days/week (Can manage two such units)		
RN	3	2	1
Mental health workers	2	2	2
Unit clerk	1		
Social worker	1		
Therapist (art/occupational)	1 / 2	1 / 2	
Psychologist	1		
Clinical nurse specialist	1 (swing shift: days & eves)		
Psychiatrist	1		

PATIENT-FOCUSED MODEL

This model employs fewer nurses and more staff members called *care partners*. Care partners are highly skilled paraprofessionals who preferably have a bachelor's degree in a behavioral science and who replace the traditional nursing assistants. Nurses supervise care partners and perform only those tasks that paraprofessionals are prohibited by law from performing. This model is more cost-effective and has been shown to be as effective at reaching patient goals as traditional staffing patterns. Box 46-2 shows the nursing

BOX 46-2: Nursing Staffing Pattern for a 25-Bed Inpatient Psychiatric Unit Using a Patient-Focused Model

Staff	Day Shift	Evening Shift	Night Shift
Clinical coordinator	1–5 days/week (Can manage two such units)		
RN	2	1	1
Care partners	3	3	3
Unit clerk	1		
Social worker	1		
Therapist (art/occupational)	1 / 2	1 / 2	
Psychologist	1		
Clinical nurse specialist	1 (swing shift: days & eves)		
Psychiatrist	1		

staffing pattern for the same 23- to 25-bed unit with one patient on one-to-one observation using the patient-focused model. Because patients are in the hospital for such a short period, nurses ensure that the best possible use is made of the time. While each patient will be on an individual schedule or critical pathway, the general goals of the nursing staff are to:

1. Provide safety
2. Set short-term and long-term goals
3. Structure therapeutic interpersonal interactions
4. Meet with the interdisciplinary team daily to evaluate patients' movements toward goals

DAILY SCHEDULE

Box 46-3 shows a sample daily activity schedule for a psychiatric unit.

BOX 46-3: Sample Daily Activity Schedule for a Psychiatric Inpatient Unit

TIME	MONDAY	TUESDAY	WEDNESDAY	THURSDAY	FRIDAY	SATURDAY	SUNDAY
7:00 – 8:00 A.M.	A.M. Care	A.M. Care	A.M. Care	A.M. Care	A.M. Care	A.M. Care	A.M. Care
8:00 – 8:30	Breakfast/Meds	Breakfast/Meds	Breakfast/Meds	Breakfast/Meds	Breakfast/Meds		
8:30 – 9:00						Breakfast	Breakfast
9:00 – 9:30	Community Meeting	Community Meeting	Community Meeting	Community Meeting	Community Meeting	Community Meeting	Community Meeting
9:30 – 10:00	Rec/Walk	Rec/Walk	Rec/Walk	Rec/Walk	Rec/Walk	Meds	Meds
10:00 – 11:00	Education/Art Therapy	Education/Art Therapy	Education/Art Therapy	Education/Art Therapy	Education/Art Therapy	Group Therapy	Group Therapy
11:00 – 12:00						Walk/Recreation Activity	Walk/Recreation Activity
12:00 – 12:15 P.M.	Vital Signs	Vital Signs	Vital Signs	Vital Signs	Vital Signs	Vital Signs	Vital Signs
12:15 – 1:00	Lunch	Lunch	Lunch	Lunch	Lunch	Lunch	Lunch
1:00 – 2:00	Meds/Activities	Meds/Activities	Meds/Activities	Meds/Activities	Meds/Activities	Meds	Meds
2:00 – 3:00	Group Therapy	Group Therapy	Group Therapy	Group Therapy	Group Therapy	Visiting/Recreation Activity	Visiting/Recreation Activity
3:00 – 4:00	OT	OT	OT	OT	OT		
4:00 – 5:00	Vital Signs	Vital Signs	Vital Signs	Vital Signs	Vital Signs	Vital Signs	Vital Signs
	Walk/Personal Time	Walk/Personal Time	Walk/Personal Time	Walk/Personal Time	Walk/Personal Time	Walk/Personal Time	Walk/Personal Time
5:00 – 6:30	Meds/Dinner	Meds/Dinner	Meds/Dinner	Meds/Dinner	Meds/Dinner	Meds/Dinner	Meds/Dinner
6:30 – 8:30	On/Off Unit Activities/Visiting	On/Off Unit Activities/Visiting	On/Off Unit Activities/Visiting	On/Off Unit Activities/Visiting*	On/Off Unit Activities/Visiting	On/Off Unit Activities/Visiting	On/Off Unit Activities/Visiting
8:30 – 9:00	Day End Group	Day End Group	Day End Group	Day End Group	Day End Group	Day End Group	Day End Group
9:00 – 11:00	Meds/Personal Time	Meds/Personal Time	Meds/Personal Time	Meds/Personal Time	Meds/Personal Time	Meds/Personal Time	Meds/Personal Time

*Family Education Meeting, 8:00 P.M.

With permission: Pocono Medical Center, East Stroudsburg, PA.

CRITICAL PATHS

A critical path is a multidisciplinary care plan mapped out on a daily basis for each patient. Critical paths came into existence to provide organized, measurable, multidisciplinary treatment to patients with common diagnoses or symptom(s). Once care delivery is somewhat standardized, patient outcome data can be predicted and measured. Critical paths are usually developed by a multidisciplinary team of clinicians who will be using them. Critical paths can be purchased and then customized to suit the unit. Companies selling critical paths and published works relating to critical paths include but are not limited to the following:

1. Center for Case Management (The center is comprised of consultants on and vendors of critical paths. The center's paths are largely related to nursing care versus the care provided by the entire team, although there is a multidisciplinary component for documentation. The center is in the process of streamlining its pathways, which have tended to be long.)

   6 Pleasant Street
   South Natick, MA 01760
   (508) 651-2600

2. Wallace, Carol (1994). *Monitoring with Indicators. Evaluating the Quality of Patient Care.* Gaithersburg, MD: Aspen Publishers. (This publication is an annually supplemented manual. The information contained is not in pathway format, although it can be formatted as such.)

3. American Health Consultants (Atlanta, GA) publishes *The Hospital's Critical Path Manual,* a good reference book on critical pathways. It does not, however, contain psychiatric/mental health pathways. Trial copies are available by calling 1-800-688-2421.

Box 46-4 shows an example of a draft critical path, using a patient who is depressed. The boxes are filled in by a multidisciplinary team member as consensus is reached regarding specific care delivery for the particular diagnosis or symptom(s) being addressed. Usually a manager is designated to monitor the patient's daily adherence to the path. Daily, the case manager notes variations and intervenes immediately to achieve expected delivery. Variation data are summarized and analyzed regularly and a method to address commonly occurring variances is developed. This information is reviewed regularly by a multidisciplinary committee, and should be shared with all other clinicians. Table 46-1 shows examples of pathway variances and interventions to correct them.

EFFECTIVE LEADERSHIP

Employee productivity has never been more in the forefront of health care than it is today. Managers at every level are testing and adopting effective behaviors for enhancing employee satisfaction, job commitment, and concurrently, productivity. Table 46-2 shows management actions, anticipated results, and examples.

INFORMATION SYSTEM IMPLICATIONS AND REQUIREMENTS

Table 46-3 shows the information system needs on a psychiatric unit and the rationale for each.

Patients' records include:
1. Multidisciplinary charting
2. Multidisciplinary treatment notes and care plans
3. Automated group and individual treatment notes, some of which may be standardized based on diagnoses, symptoms, and courses of treatment
4. Centralized documentation rather than decentralized documentation from each treatment area

BOX 46-4: Draft of a Critical Pathway for a Patient with Major Depression with Suicidal Features

Date/Time: _____ Exp. LOS: _____ Reviewed by MD: _____

PROCESS	DAY 0	DAY 1	DAY 2	DAY 3	DAY 4	DAY 5	DAY 6
Assessment	Suicide Evaluation Nursing Assessment	Physical Exam Psych. Work-Up → O.T. Assess. Social Assess.	Ortho. BPs → →	Comm. Disease Clearance → →	→ →	→ →	→
Lab		CBC, UA, SMA 18 Thyroid Function If Indicated: Preg. Test Urine TDX Ther. Drug Level					
Care Plan	Initiated by Nursing	Update	Multidisciplinary Care Plan in Place	Multidisciplinary Care Plan in Place		Care Plan Review	
Meds	Antianxiety Drugs PRN	→ Antidepressant Initiated	→ Eval. Side Effects Eval. Effects	→ → → Adjust Dose	→ → →	→ → →	→ → →
Therapeutic Activities		50% Record Observation	75% →	100% →	→	→	→
Therapy and Observations	Psychiatrist Nursing	→ → Psychologist Social Worker	→ → → →	→ → → →	→ → → →	→ → → →	→ → → →
Discharge Planning	Data Collection	Interview	Tentative Plan	→	→	Review Plan with Patient	Finalized Plan
Patient and Family Education	Orientation to Unit and Patient Rights	Med. Ed. Informed Consent for Meds. Obtained by M.D.	Med. Education	→	→	→	→ O.P. Instruction in Meds.

Admission Criteria
DSM-IV Axis I Diagnosis
Cannot be safely therapeutically treated in less restrictive setting

Discharge Criteria
Patient no longer actively suicidal
Patient can be safely and therapeutically discharged to less restrictive level of care

Outcome Criteria
Patient will not be readmitted within 30 days
Patient will not leave AMA
GAF score?

With permission: Dept. of Psychiatry, St. Joseph's Hospital of Orange County, CA.

TABLE 46-1
Examples of Critical Pathway Variance Data and Case Manager Interventions

VARIANCE	CAUSE	INTERVENTION
Discharge planning not begun the day of admission. Discharge may be delayed.	Responsible individual out ill. No one scheduled to cover her.	Coverage immediately scheduled. System put in place to cover all patients daily regardless of staff "sick calls."
Patient not discharged when acute psychiatric admission symptoms resolved.	Medical illness developed requiring IV antibiotics.	Patient to be discharged with home infusion therapy in 2 days when medical symptoms are expected to be under control.
Patient not begun on discharge medication dosage today.	Necessary blood levels not available on the system. No record of blood having been drawn.	Blood level redrawn stat. Patient to have new dosage started as soon as results are available. No expected delay in treatment.

TABLE 46-2
Effective Leadership Behaviors, Anticipated Outcomes, and Examples

NURSE MANAGER	ANTICIPATED RESULTS	EXAMPLES
Acts as role model to challenge processes, empower staff, and question the status quo, allowing for mistakes along the way.	Invites entrepreneurship and new and improved methods for accomplishing goals. Promotes trust.	Consistent problems getting lab results in 24 hours. Nurse manager to empower staff to examine lab results, reporting processes and test solutions.
Encourages and supports staff members to inspire common goals and vision. Enthusiastically enlists others in implementing new ideas.	Promotes unity, cohesion, and team pride.	Nurse manager invites staff as a group to set goals for the unit. She or he then encourages them to set up working groups to examine and identify the best methods and work plans for achieving these goals.
Fosters collaboration and cooperation.	Allows for development of the sharing of knowledge, building of confidence, and group cohesiveness.	Clinical specialists with specialty in group therapy are hired on one unit. Nurse manager invites clinical specialists to participate in Ph.D.-led family sessions in return for staff nurses attending the new clinical specialist–led group sessions. This will lead to collaborative therapy sessions for the patients in the institution based on clinicians' expertise and interest. It also allows for the sharing of new knowledge and expertise among staff.

TABLE 46-3
Information System Needs and Rationales for a Psychiatric Unit

NEED	RATIONALE
Point-of-care technology (bedside/pod terminals)	Automates all clinical information. Updates care plans. Automates flow sheets.
Clinical protocol development	Standardizes those aspects of care related to diagnostic categories, symptoms, interventions, and expected outcomes.
Longitudinal patient record	Serves as repository of all clinical and financial data collected during each patient encounter.
Computer-based record of current and historical clinical and financial data	Serves as repository of documentation, clinical results, and images to help with clinical decision making.

PROGRAM EVALUATION

Today's environment requires continuous improvement in all processes, both administrative and clinical. A formal or homegrown evaluative tool and process may be employed. Some suggested sources for seeking out processes for improvement are:

1. Quality improvement reports that include both quality and quantity indicators
2. Patient/family satisfaction surveys
3. Patient complaint/reports
4. Risk management reports
5. Case manager reports including summarized variance reports from critical path data
6. Payer satisfaction information usually available from the finance department

Mail-in surveys to patients and families postdischarge, in-person questionnaires, and information system management reports can all lead to collection, summarization, and ultimate analysis of data. Management should employ a standardized process of summarizing and analyzing data to allow for an objective, systematic, and scientific review. Reviews should be regularly completed by a multidisciplinary team with results regularly shared with all caregivers. The outcome is positive if the patient's acute episode is stabilized in a cost-effective way with which patients, families, friends, and caregivers are satisfied.

BIBLIOGRAPHY

Bigbee, J. L., Collins, J., & Deeds, K. (1992). Patient classification systems: A new approach to computing reliability. *Applied Nursing Research, 5* (1), 32–38.

Finnigan, S. A., Abel, M., Dobler, T., Hudon, L., & Terry, B. (1993). Automated patient acuity. Linking nursing systems and quality measurement with patient outcomes. *Journal of Nursing Administration, 23* (5), 62–71.

Health care reform for Americans with severe mental illnesses: Report of the National Advisory Mental Health Council (1993). *American Journal of Psychiatry, 150* (10), 1447–1465.

Johns, V. (1993). Capturing the activity factor. *Nursing Management, 24* (12), 26–29.

Joint Commission for Accreditation of Healthcare Organizations (1995). *The 1996 Comprehensive Accreditation Manual of Hospitals.* Oakbrook, IL: JCAHO.

Jung, F. D., Pearcey, L. G., & Phillips, J. L. (1994). Evaluation of a program to improve nursing assistant use. *Journal of Nursing Administration, 24* (3), 42–47.

LeCuyer, E. A. (1992). Milieu therapy for short stay units: A transformed practice theory. *Archives of Psychiatric Nursing, 6* (2), 108–116.

McCue, M. J., & Clement, J. P. (1993). Relative performance of for-profit psychiatric hospitals in investor-owned systems and nonprofit psychiatric hospitals. *American Journal of Psychiatry, 150* (1), 77–82.

McKeown, M. (1994). Skill-mix reviews: The need to be aware. *Nursing Standard, 8* (32), 37–39.

McNeese-Smith, D. (1993). Leadership behavior and employee effectiveness. *Nursing Management, 24* (5), 38–39.

Nygaard, L., & Hansen, J. (1991). Making computerized PCS (patient classification system) work for psychiatric care. *Nursing Management, 22* (1), 40–42, 44.

O'Leary, C. (1991). A psychiatric patient classification system. *Nursing Management, 22* (9), 66.

Phillips, C. Y., Castorr, A., Prescott, P. A., & Soeken, K. (1992). Nursing intensity. Going beyond patient classification. *Journal of Nursing Administration, 22* (4), 46–52.

Trimpey, M., & Davidson, S. (1994). Chaos, perfectionism, and sabotage: Personality disorders in the workplace. *Issues in Mental Health Nursing, 15* (1), 27–36.

Tuck, I., & Keels, M. C. (1992). Milieu therapy: A review of development of this concept and its implications for psychiatric nursing. *Issues in Mental Health Nursing, 13* (1), 51–58.

Warner, S. (1993). The milieu enhancement model: A nursing practice model, part I. *Archives of Psychiatric Nursing, 7* (2), 53–60.

47

FORTY SEVEN

Designing a Partial Hospitalization Program

Christine A. Heifner

OVERVIEW:

Introduction
Reasons for Admission
Advantages of Partial Hospitalization
Facility
Types of Programs
Staff
Assessment

Programming
Reimbursement
Documentation
Quality Assurance
Linkage
Discharge

INTRODUCTION

Partial hospitalization is "a time-limited, ambulatory, outpatient treatment program that offers intensive, coordinated, clinical services within a stable therapeutic milieu" (Block & Lefkovitz, 1990, p. 1). Programming employs "an integrated, comprehensive and complementary schedule of acknowledged treatment approaches" and is designed "to serve individuals with significant impairment resulting from psychiatric, emotional, or behavioral disorders" (Block & Lefkovitz, 1990, p. 2).

REASONS FOR ADMISSION

Clients are admitted for partial hospitalization (P.H.) when (Block & Lefkovitz, 1990):
1. They exhibit symptoms that impair social, vocational, or emotional functioning
2. They are not a threat to themselves or others, but need external support to gain control of their behavior
3. They are ready for discharge from an inpatient unit but not yet ready for outpatient treatment only, as they still need crisis stabilization, daily monitoring, support, and ongoing therapeutic intervention
4. They have the capacity to participate actively in the program

ADVANTAGES OF PARTIAL HOSPITALIZATION

Advantages are that clients:
1. Maintain their usual psychosocial roles
2. Avoid the stigma of inpatient hospitalization
3. Spend about one-half the cost of inpatient hospitalization
4. Gradually taper off their participation and move into the community

FACILITY

The facility should be seen as an independent unit separate from the hospital but physically close enough that clients can use hospital facilities. There must be access to public transportation or parking (Block & Lefkovitz, 1990; Rosato, 1984). Table 47-1 lists rooms needed and their uses.

TABLE 47-1
Rooms and Their Uses in a Partial Hospitalization Program

PROGRAM ROOMS	USES
Large meeting room	Morning meeting area for daily goal setting and day end groups
Psychotherapy group rooms	Group psychotherapy, aftercare support groups, relaxation training, staff inservices
Conference rooms	Psychoeducation, expressive therapies, nutrition classes, stress management, assertiveness training, problem-solving conferences
Library	Journal writing, bibliotherapy groups, special projects
Activity room	Emotive-expressive therapy sessions, support groups, work skills, role-playing, psychodrama, family support groups, team/staff meetings, special presentations
Staff offices	Individual, couple, and family sessions, case management work, program work
Dining area	Lunch, snacks, socialization

C. McGowan, personal communication, 1993.

TYPES OF PROGRAMS

P.H. programs were originally designed for the chronic mentally ill who had been deinstitutionalized but still needed the structure of a daily program. These are called intermediate programs. Today P.H. programs are also used for brief crisis stabilization. Table 47-2 compares these two programs.

STAFF

Table 47-3 lists the titles, preparation, and duties of staff members in a P.H. program.

ASSESSMENT

Formal, comprehensive assessment is completed at the time of admission. Documented assessment should address medical, emotional, behavioral, social, recreational, vocational, legal, and nutritional needs and resources and include psychiatric history, presenting symptoms, mental health status exam, and diagnostic impression (Block & Lefkovitz, 1990). See Chapter 1 for assessment tools.

PROGRAMMING

Box 47-1 shows a typical weekly program schedule.

REIMBURSEMENT

Coverage for partial hospitalization, especially crisis stabilization programs, is improving, though standard third-party benefits have not yet emerged. Establishing communication lines with (1) designated persons in the P.H. program patient accounts and accounting offices, (2) administrative staff in other partial hospitalization programs, and (3) administrative staff in the private and public insurance industry contributes to the constant updating of reimbursement information needed to successfully obtain or negotiate coverage for treatment. To secure third-party payment (Cuyler & Galbraith, 1988; Leibenluft & Leibenluft, 1988; Lefkovitz, 1991):

TABLE 47-2
Comparison of Crisis Stabilization and
Intermediate Partial Hospitalization Programs

	CRISIS STABILIZATION PROGRAM	INTERMEDIATE PROGRAM
Purpose	To provide short-term help to resolve a crisis	To provide intermediate-term care
Target population	Individuals experiencing acute psychiatric symptoms or decompensating clinical conditions that might require inpatient hospital care, but are tried in P.H. first	Individuals with chronic illness who are not likely to respond to short-term intervention or treatment
Length of stay	3–6 weeks, with 50% of clients remaining longer than 30 treatment days per episode of care	Less than 9 months, with no more than 50% of clients remaining longer than 180 treatment days per episode of care
Staff–patient ratio	1:4	1:6
Programming	At least 65% of program hours specifically addressing the presenting problems	At least 50% of program hours specifically addressing the presenting problems
Treatment planning	Initial treatment plan: within 5 treatment days after admission	Initial treatment plan: within 5 treatment days after admission
	Formalized treatment plan: within 10 treatment days after admission	Formalized treatment plan: within 20 treatment days after admission
Plan revision	Every 5 treatment days	Every 20 treatment days

Block, R., & Lefkovitz, P. (1990). *American Association for Partial Hospitalization (AAPH) Standards and Guidelines for Partial Hospitalization.* (Available from the American Association for Partial Hospitalization, Alexandria, VA.)

1. Contact the third-party payer or health maintenance organization to determine benefits for partial hospitalization prior to admission.
2. Identify availability of reimbursement and requirements.
3. Precertify admission to partial hospitalization.
4. Identify the health insurer's case manager for ongoing reviews and treatment planning.
5. Document information exchanged during contacts with third-party payers or health maintenance organizations, noting next scheduled case management review. Use documented information as reference for future contacts with third-party payers and health maintenance organizations.
6. Keep client updated on status of coverage. Provide the client with payment plan options when health care coverage does not cover all P.H. costs. When coverage for partial hospitalization is not a benefit, negotiating extracontractual or "out of contract" coverage becomes an option (Cuyler & Galbraith, 1988; Leibenluft & Leibenluft, 1988; Lefkovitz, 1991).
   a. If partial hospitalization coverage is not a benefit, talk to the insurer about going "out of contract" to provide coverage for partial hospitalization services.
   b. Identify the cost for inpatient and outpatient services. Negotiate for equivalent inpatient benefits for coverage of partial hospitalization services.
   c. Identify the health insurer's case manager, claims supervisor, or manager with authority to negotiate out-of-contract agreement.
   d. Present clinical rationale for extracontractual arrangements. Describe clinical picture, especially noting risk factors, history of previous inpatient admissions,

TABLE 47-3
Staff Titles, Preparation, and Duties in a Partial Hospitalization Program

TITLE	PREPARATION	DUTIES
Administrative director (full-time)	Master's or doctorate degree in relevant clinical area with functional major in business administration	Oversees administration, marketing, and public relations activities; participates in ongoing assessment of program effectiveness and development; negotiates with health insurance companies and health maintenance organizations; provides individual, group, and family therapy; provides clinical supervision.
Clinical nurse specialist (full-time)	Master's degree in psychiatric nursing and ANA certification as a clinical specialist in adult psychiatric nursing	Provides clinical supervision; individual, group, and family therapy; psychoeducation. Manages quality assurance review, communicates with third-party payers, participates in program development and public relations, prescribes and dispenses medication.
Medical director (part-time)	Psychiatrist	Prescribes medication; participates in program development and public relations; provides psychoeducation.
Social worker (full-time)	Master's degree in social work	Provides individual, group, and family therapy and supervision; participates in program development and public relations; serves as liaison with community agencies.
Caseworker (full-time)	Bachelor's degree in social work, nursing, or psychology	Helps client with discharge planning, facilitates client contact with community agencies, participates in program activities. Communicates with insurers regarding client's progress.
Occupational therapist, art therapist, music therapist, or mental health rehabilitation counselor	Bachelor's degree or higher in mental health specialty field	Coordinates, develops, and leads groups focused on art, music, crafts, or recreation.

Block, R., & Lefkovitz, P. (1990). *American Association for Partial Hospitalization (AAPH) Standards and Guidelines for Partial Hospitalization.* (Available from the American Association for Partial Hospitalization, Alexandria, VA.); Rosato, J. (1984). Designing a day hospital program. In S. Lego (ed.), *The American Handbook of Psychiatric Nursing* (pp. 103–111). Philadelphia: Lippincott.

and proposed treatment plan. Provide specific information to establish "medical necessity."

e. Present financial rationale for extracontractual agreement (aversion/shortening of inpatient stay, cost savings, results of program outcome studies).

f. Request written verification of negotiated agreement.

g. Document events of negotiations to use as future references.

h. Keep client updated on status of coverage. Provide the client with payment plan options when health care coverage does not cover all P.H. costs.

DOCUMENTATION

Clinical records are maintained for each client with daily documentation noting group attendance, participation, mental status, and progress made toward attainment of treatment objectives (Block & Lefkovitz, 1990).

QUALITY ASSURANCE

Quality assurance reflects the guidelines identified by accrediting and regulatory agencies, and should address "peer review, negative incident reporting, and goal attainment of programmatic, clinical, and administration quality indicators" (Block & Lefkovitz, 1990, p. 10).

BOX 47-1: Partial Hospitalization Weekly Schedule

	Monday	Tuesday	Wednesday	Thursday	Friday
9:00–9:45	Morning goal-setting group				
10:00–11:00	Wellness education	Work skills	Assertiveness training	Work skills	Expressive therapy
11:00–12:15	Group psychotherapy				
12:15–1:00	Lunch				
1:00–2:00	Stress management	Role-playing	Loss and grieving	Symptoms recognition	Journal to wellness
2:00–3:00	Expressive therapy	Care planning	Expressive therapy	Medication education	Social skills
3:00–3:30	Afternoon closure group				
6:00–7:15		Family support group		Aftercare support group	

Adapted from Block, B., & Lefkovitz, P. (1990). *American Association for Partial Hospitalization (AAPH) Standards and Guidelines for Partial Hospitalization.* (Available from the American Association for Partial Hospitalization, Washington, DC.); Cuyler, R., & Galbraith, J. (1988). *Insurance and Partial Hospitalization.* (Available from the American Association for Partial Hospitalization, Alexandria, VA.); C. McGowan (personal communication, 1993).

Courtesy of Akron General Medical Center, Akron, Ohio.

LINKAGE

Programs must maintain liaison relationships with psychiatric and human service providers, inpatient psychiatric programs, outpatient services, private industry through personnel departments and employee assistance programs, program accounting and patient accounts, and public and private health insurance providers (Cuyler & Galbraith, 1988; Block & Lefkovitz, 1990).

DISCHARGE

The client is discharged when (Block & Lefkovitz, 1990, pp. 7–8):
1. The client's clinical condition has improved as reflected in symptom relief and reduced interference with social, vocational, or educational goals to such a degree as to warrant a treatment regimen of less intensity
2. Treatment goals have been accomplished as established in the client's individualized treatment plan
3. The client is able to return to increased levels of independence in daily activities and is judged no longer to require the intensity of supervision, support, and therapeutic intervention provided by the partial hospitalization program
   – OR –
4. The client's clinical condition has deteriorated to the extent that the safety and security of inpatient care is necessary

REFERENCES

Block, B., & Lefkovitz, P. (1990). *American Association for Partial Hospitalization (AAPH) Standards and Guidelines for Partial Hospitalization.* (Available from the American Association for Partial Hospitalization, 301 North Fairfax Street, Suite 109, Alexandria, VA 22314.)

Cuyler, R., & Galbraith, J. (1988). *Insurance and Partial Hospitalization.* (Available from the American Association for Partial Hospitalization, Alexandria, VA.)

Leibenluft, E., & Leibenluft, R. (1988). Reimbursement for partial hospitalization: A survey and policy implications. *American Journal of Psychiatry, 145* (12), 1514–1520.

Lefkovitz, P. M. (1991). *Enhancing Third Party Coverage of Partial Hospitalization Services.* (Available from the American Association for Partial Hospitalization, Alexandria, VA.)

Rosato, J. (1984). Designing a day hospital program. In S. Lego (ed.), *The American Handbook of Psychiatric Nursing* (pp. 103–111). Philadelphia: J. B. Lippincott.

BIBLIOGRAPHY

Hoge, M., Davidson, L., Hill, W. L., Turner, V., & Ameli, R. (1992). The promise of partial hospitalization: A reassessment. *Hospital and Community Psychiatry, 43* (4), 345–354.

Parker, S., & Knoll, J. (1990). Partial hospitalization: An update. *American Journal of Psychiatry, 147* (2), 156–160.

48
FORTY EIGHT

Designing Residential Aftercare and Outreach Programs

Mary Beth Husseini

OVERVIEW:

INTRODUCTION

A large part of aftercare is focused on community residential care of the mentally ill. Since deinstitutionalization, an attempt has been made to maintain mentally ill clients in the community. Placement can be a real challenge, owing to the wide variety of clients, negative responses from the community, and limited resources. Sometimes the mentally ill seek out housing on their own, but through outreach programs nurses can help them through the hurdles they must face. Often community mental health centers are responsible for setting up and maintaining housing.

TYPES OF CLIENTS

The following conditions are often seen in individuals requiring residential aftercare:
    1. Chronic schizophrenia

2. Severe affective disorders
3. Borderline personality disorder
4. Mental retardation

GOALS OF RESIDENTIAL CARE

The goals of residential care include (Budson, 1983):
1. Improving self-esteem
2. Living at an independent level as much as possible
3. Preventing isolation
4. Improving social skills
5. Decreasing dependence on family caregivers
6. Decreasing hospitalizations

TYPES OF HOUSING

Owing to the variety of client needs and levels of independence, various types of residential care are needed. The most common forms of housing and characteristics of each are shown in Table 48-1 (Budson, 1983).

ESTABLISHING A COMMUNITY RESIDENTIAL PROGRAM

Establishing community residential programs entails much preparation. Guidelines are (Budson, 1983):
1. Perform a needs assessment of the community.
2. Determine the scope and size of the facility.
3. Contact a legal expert to facilitate compliance with zoning and other legal issues.
4. Make sure the building meets safety codes.
5. Have an affiliation with the county mental health center.
6. Formulate a network of services available to residents.
7. Define staff requirements.
8. Educate the staff about the program components such as specifics for a behavior modification program.
9. Plan strategies to introduce the new residence to the community.

SUGGESTIONS TO GAIN COMMUNITY SUPPORT

Residential housing for the mentally ill is almost certain to spark community opposition (Winerip, 1994). The following suggestions may help to prevent conflict or lessen it when it occurs (Rizzo, Zipple, Pisciotta, & Bycoff, 1992):
1. Anticipate and plan for problems.
2. Increase contact between residents and neighbors.
3. Offer community education.
4. Establish forums for ongoing meetings.
5. Encourage informal contact with the residents in the community.
6. Be persistent and patient.

CLINICAL CONSIDERATIONS

Placement into a residential setting requires planning to facilitate the least stressful transition. Specific considerations are (Budson, 1983):
1. Prior to placement, a detailed assessment is made. This should include all available sources to give the best all-round picture of the client including social skills, work potential, and the current family situation. Suggest family counseling if needed.
2. Discuss with the client and residential staff stressors that precipitated a relapse in the past. Discuss with the client and residential staff behaviors that might indicate an exacerbation.

TABLE 48-1
Types and Characteristics of Housing in Aftercare of the Mentally Ill

TYPE OF HOUSING	PURPOSE	STAFFING ON SITE	PROVISIONS	AVERAGE LENGTH OF STAY	NUMBER OF RESIDENTS	COUNSELING AVAILABLE	RESPONSIBILITIES OF RESIDENTS
Transitional halfway house	Transition from the hospital to the community	Available 24 hours a day	Room, board, and help with activities of daily living	6–8 months	10–20, varies with available space and staff	Yes	Cooking and cleaning the house
Long-term group home	Transition from the hospital to the community; sometimes residency	Available 24 hours a day	Room, board, and help with activities of daily living	Years to a lifetime	10–20, varies with available space and staff	Yes, as residents are often dependent and symptomatic	Cooking and cleaning the house
Single-room occupancy hotels	Residency	Dependent on availability of an outreach program	Room	Years to a lifetime	Up to hundreds	If a PMH CNS is available for outreach	Independent living
Cooperative apartments	Residency	None	Room	Years to a lifetime	2–4 clients per apartment	If a PMH CNS is available	Independent living
Foster care	Residency	None, but family is often supervised by case manager	Room and board	Years to a lifetime	Usually one	No	As required by foster family
Nursing home	To provide physical care as well as shelter	Nursing staff and sometimes PMH CNS or geriatric CNS	Room and board, custodial care by nursing staff	Dependent on physical care needed	Varies	If a PMH CNS is available	None
Crisis center	To prevent admission to a psychiatric unit, if client has begun to deteriorate	Available 24 hours a day. At least one staff member is a nurse	Close observation, support, medication, counseling	1–2 weeks	Varies	Yes	Participation in the program

Adapted from Budson, R. D. (1983). Residential care for the chronically mentally ill. In I. Barofsky & R. D. Budson (eds.), *The Chronic Psychiatric Patient in the Community: Principles of Treatment* (pp. 281–308). New York: SP Medical & Scientific Books.

3. Avoid more than one change in the client's life at a time. For example, if clients are moving into a new residence, try to keep everything else in their lives as stable as possible.
4. Encourage visits or participation in residence activities before the client moves in.

OUTREACH

Some mentally ill individuals live independent of mental health programs. This portion of the population may be unable or unwilling to use services offered in traditional medical and mental health settings. Psychiatric nurses work in outreach programs designed to provide therapeutic intervention to those who are at risk or who have been diagnosed mentally ill. Often these clients live in SROs (single room occupancies) in urban areas or in boarding homes.

CHARACTERISTICS*

Outreach

1. Is geared to the needs of the population, rather than to the needs and norms of the hospital
2. Implies intervention within the client's own territory rather than agency territory
3. May be initiated by telephone, mail, or a visit to the person's home
4. May include psychiatric clients, their relatives, neighbors, landlords, or other community agencies

THE POPULATION

The population in need of mental health outreach tends to possess one or more of the following characteristics:

1. A tendency to be passive in using health services
2. A lack of adequate support systems, such as families or friends
3. A lack of skills or resources to deal with predators
4. A minimal or unclear understanding of services that are available to them
5. An inability to use traditional systems

Outreach services cover the entire span of acute and chronic care, from crisis intervention to ongoing treatment.

Outreach programs can potentially encompass all aspects of community life. However, to be manageable, a program must set a narrow focus and reasonable limits. The SRO hotel program is one type of outreach program, which is examined here in detail.

THE MENTAL HEALTH OUTREACH TEAM IN THE SRO HOTEL

GENERAL DESCRIPTION

The mental health outreach team is a multidisciplinary team of mental health professionals and paraprofessionals, affiliated with a larger health care institution. The team is based on site in the SRO, 5 days a week, to provide a variety of services to the hotel population.

ORIGIN OF CONCEPT

The outreach concept developed in response to increasing awareness of the high concentration of people living in the SRO who were in need of community mental health services, while having difficulty obtaining them.

OVERALL GOAL

The overall goal is to help the SRO tenant gain or sustain maximum functioning within the community. Emphasis is on the individual becoming as autonomous as possible, and developing a working social support network. See Table 48-2 for specific program objectives.

---

*Material from this point is taken from Winter, J. S. (1984). Designing an outreach program in an SRO hotel. In S. Lego (ed.), *The American Handbook of Psychiatric Nursing*. Philadelphia: J. B. Lippincott.

TABLE 48-2
SRO Program Objectives and Rationales

OBJECTIVE	RATIONALE
1. Identify those tenants who are in need of health care; formulate a treatment plan (with tenant cooperation); implement and evaluate it	1. Tenants may not identify themselves as having problems, or may be unable to solve problems without assistance. Successful treatment may help them avoid hospitalization and promote their autonomous strengths.
2. Intervene in situations of acute mental or physical distress and, whenever possible, help the tenant remain in the community while obtaining treatment	2. Tenants' sense of self-control and self-esteem may be enhanced by the team's response to their distress and the team's willingness to coordinate treatment in the community.
3. When necessary, facilitate psychiatric or medical hospitalization, collaborate with the inpatient treatment team, and help with discharge planning for follow-up care	3. The many systems obstacles to hospitalization for the SRO tenant may be more effectively surmounted by an "inside" health worker–tenant advocate, who has knowledge of the system.
4. Help tenants use other outpatient and social agencies in the community	4. Tenants' dependence on the team and others decreases as tenants' knowledge of available resources and how to use them increases.
5. Help tenants take a more active and autonomous role in their dealings with hotel management, each other, and on-site health workers	5. This helps tenants learn to manage their own affairs, increasing self-esteem and satisfaction.
6. Help to build a "sense of community" among hotel tenants	6. This provides stability and durability in tenant interpersonal relationships.
7. Help tenants expand their "community" to include other area residents, local planning boards, and block associations, through responsible representation of tenants at these association meetings	7. Effective communication and understanding between area residents, politicians, and SRO tenants makes for a stronger, more integrated community.

Winter, J. S. (1984). Designing an outreach program in an SRO hotel. In S. Lego (ed.), *The American Handbook of Psychiatric Nursing* (pp. 156–166). Philadelphia: Lippincott.

CONTRACT WITH SRO HOTEL

It is necessary to have a contractual agreement between the SRO landlord and the sponsoring health agency. This contract:
1. Allows the agency to rent or use work space within the SRO
2. Allows outreach workers access to tenant areas of building
3. Indicates a degree of cooperation between the landlord (including hotel workers) and the health agency (the on-site health workers)
4. Ideally allows health workers to screen prospective tenants

TEAM STRUCTURE

TYPICAL COMPOSITION
1. Psychiatric/mental health clinical nurse specialists
2. Psychiatric social workers
3. Alcoholism counselor
4. Community mental health aide
5. Psychiatrist (part-time)

ADDITIONAL MEMBERS, AS PROGRAM FUNDS PERMIT
1. Recreational therapist
2. Clinical psychologist
3. Night counselor

Part-time staff for minimedical clinic in SRO consists of a nurse practitioner or primary care physician and a community health nurse.

NONSALARIED OTHERS

Students of nursing, social work, psychology, and psychiatry are generally a welcome, if temporary, addition to team strength. Their participation tends to revitalize mental health workers as well as tenants. Their fresh outlook on chronic problems tends to enhance others' investment in problem resolution.

Volunteers from the community may be successfully used, provided confidentiality concerning client information is not breached.

TEAM FUNCTION

The functions of team members tend to be role-blended as well as role-specific, depending on the members' areas of expertise and the identified needs of tenants. Thus, while any professional team member may assess a tenant's mental status, the nurse may be consulted to further assess physical complaints in relation to mental status.

The types of services offered by the teams cover a range of traditional therapeutic activities, as well as innovative approaches that are consonant with mental health principles. Basically, services can be categorized as:
1. Individual, group, and family therapy or counseling
2. Crisis intervention
3. Psychiatric evaluation
4. Medication
5. Education and treatment about drug and alcohol abuse
6. Advocacy services concerning basic needs
7. Socialization and facilitation of social support systems
8. Assistance in developing a sense of community

PROBLEMS OF MENTAL HEALTH WORKERS IN THE SRO

Because outreach reverses the traditional flow in which the consumer seeks out the professional, it poses unique problems for the workers "in the field." Table 48-3 offers problems, examples, and interventions.

TABLE 48-3
Potential Problems for Nurses in the SRO, Examples, and Interventions

AREA OF POTENTIAL PROBLEMS	EXAMPLES	INTERVENTIONS
1. *Territoriality*—is not under health workers' control, but is the "home turf" of hotel management and tenants.	a. Management suddenly denies team and tenants access to kitchen area, where a lunch program has been established.	a. The nurse tries to find out informally (from porters and tenants) why this is happening. May approach management diplomatically with a tenants' committee representative.
	b. Tenant asks the nurse not to knock on his door again.	b. The nurse must respect tenant's territorial rights. May try leaving a note in his mailbox, or phoning his room, if further outreach is indicated.

(Continued)

TABLE 48-3 *(continued)*

AREA OF POTENTIAL PROBLEMS	EXAMPLES	INTERVENTIONS
2. *Resistance of tenants*—may be related to tenant's fear of exposure, authority figures, the (traditional) health care system.	a. Tenant is ill or broke, but refuses to accept help. The nurse may become concerned, but feels helpless and inadequate.	a. The nurse confers with the team for support and to develop problem-solving strategies. Constructive manipulation of systems can be effective. If the tenant's friends and hotel management become concerned, they may exert pressure on the tenant to accept help.
	b. Tenant is "crisis-oriented"; he accepts help when in crisis, but refuses help designed to prevent crises.	b. The nurse relies on her own skill and ingenuity to form a relationship with the tenant, and then uses any possible opportunity for health teaching.
3. *Negotiations with hotel management*—is an ongoing necessity for health workers, for space and for improvement of services.	a. Management views the nurse alternately as intruder, troublemaker, or peer and is inconsistent in dealings with tenants.	a. The nurse tries to determine the motivation behind actions of management, then deal accordingly. While management may make the final decision, they can be influenced, especially if the nurse's desired outcome is presented as meeting the manager's needs as well. Health teaching with management may mean a positive change in the treatment of workers and tenants!
4. *Unique nature of the setting*—lack of external work structures and the broad range of needs presented may be disorienting to the health worker who is trying to define a professional role.	a. Tenant feels helpless and distraught when management removes her cat to the pound. Tenant has been a responsible pet owner, but management has decided that all pets must go. Nurse questions his "professional role" in this case.	a. The nurse confers with the team using a systems reference for assessing the problem. He recognizes the meaning of the pet, and the many negative consequences to the tenant when a beloved pet is removed.
5. *Multidisciplinary nature of the team*—each member comes from a discipline with certain preconceived notions or role functions; conflicts may arise regarding role definitions.	a. A solitary nurse is without discipline peers on the health team. Every physical complaint of tenants is referred to the nurse. Often, tenants already know the cause of the symptom, and the recommended treatment for the probem.	a. The nurse addresses this issue in the team meeting, clarifying her role, her strengths, and her limitations. Discussion may reveal that non-nurse members feel fearful or inadequate when confronted with tenants' dramatic complaints. Review of assessment skills may help these members shift more responsibility to themselves, and to the tenant.
6. *Supervision*—lack of on-site supervisor may increase the nurse's feelings of helplessness.	a. Situations involving all of the above examples may lead the nurse to doubt his own professional judgment.	a. A supervisor is always available by telephone. Conferring on the phone, requesting a site visit, or arranging supervision at the sponsoring agency is helpful. Peer/team supervision is of the utmost importance for the on-site health worker; this process generally serves to increase team cohesiveness and mutual support.

Source: Winter, J. S. (1984). Designing an outreach program in an SRO hotel. In S. Lego (ed.), *The American Handbook of Psychiatric Nursing* (pp. 156–166). Philadelphia: Lippincott.

CHARACTERISTICS OF THE NURSE ON THE SRO TEAM

To work in this unusual setting, the clinical nurse specialist must possess a variety of professional and personal attributes. The nurse (Rosamilia, 1977):

1. Is a skilled clinician, capable of independent judgment
2. Is willing to accept considerable responsibility
3. Possesses leadership skills to coordinate conflicting systems
4. Has a high degree of flexibility in working with other disciplines and defining a role
5. Is able to give and receive support, confront conflicts, share, teach, and learn with others on the team
6. Is able to achieve satisfaction with achievement of limited goals
7. Maintains expectations that tenants have the ability to change
8. Is available to clients, reacts to them openly and spontaneously, and deals with them in a variety of settings
9. Has a high tolerance for ambiguity and for deviant behavior
10. Is capable of self-direction, and actively seeks challenges

EVALUATION

The criteria used to determine whether or not program objectives have been met are varied; most frequently they are determined by the nurse's ongoing assessment of the client's response to program treatment. Evaluation is related to previously stated program objectives: Tenants identified as being in need of treatment have successfully been engaged in treatment, and are attempting to collaborate and cooperate in the implementation of their treatment plans. Specifically, there is:

1. A decrease in the recidivism rate for a significant number of chronic clients and an increase in tenant acceptance of home care and health teaching about physical illness
2. Increased acceptance of brief inpatient treatment, and more follow-up care
3. A decrease in the chronic use and abuse of the emergency room and, instead, use of other community services
4. Growing mutual responsibility among clients, that is, more awareness of neighbors who need help and willingness to "get involved" and help them
5. Increased self-advocacy and cooperation among clients in planning for shared goals and positive response of management to tenant requests
6. A more positive and less fearful regard of the client by the community so that local groups ask for tenants' opinions and cooperation in local matters

REFERENCES

Budson, R. D. (1983). Residential care for the chronically mentally ill. In I. Barofsky & R. D. Budson (eds.), *The Chronic Psychiatric Patient in the Community: Principles of Treatment* (pp. 281–308). New York: SP Medical & Scientific Books.

Rizzo, A. M., Zipple, A. M., Pisciotta, J., & Bycoff, S. (1992). Strategies for responding to community opposition in an existing group home. *Psychosocial Rehabilitation Journal, 15* (3), 85–95.

Rosamilia, J. D. (1977). Community mental health nursing in an urban setting. Paper presented at the Psychiatric–Mental Health Nursing Practice Conference Group Program at the New York State Nurses Association Convention.

Winter, J. S. (1984). Designing an outreach program in an SRO hotel. In S. Lego (ed.), *The American Handbook of Psychiatric Nursing* (pp. 156–166). Philadelphia: Lippincott.

BIBLIOGRAPHY

Esser, A. H., & Lacey S. D. (1989). *Mental Illness: A Homecare Guide.* New York: John Wiley & Sons.

Jacobson, J. W., Burchard, S. N., & Carling, P. J. (1992). *Community Living for People with Developmental and Psychiatric Disabilities.* Baltimore: The Johns Hopkins University Press.

Maluccio, A. N. (1980). *Alternatives to Institutionalization: A Selective Review of the Literature.* Saratoga, CA: Century Twenty One Publishing.

Segal, S. P., & Aviram, U. (1978). *The Mentally Ill in Community-Based Sheltered Care.* New York: John Wiley & Sons.

Winerip, M. (1994). *9 Highland Road.* New York: Pantheon Books.

49
FORTY NINE

Designing a Family Education Program

Catherine Kane

OVERVIEW:

Purpose
Conceptual Considerations
Structure

Organization
Program Topics

PURPOSE

Educational programs for families are a necessary adjunct to the treatment of severe mental disorders. The goals of family educational programs are to:

1. Provide family members with current and accurate information about the symptoms, course, and treatment of the illness
2. Enable family members to maintain a positive relationship with the ill relative and to interact in a supportive and constructive way
3. Teach family members effective strategies for encouraging treatment participation, monitoring their relative's functioning, intervening to avert relapse and rehospitalization
4. Enable family members to maintain a positive family environment
5. Encourage family members to effectively use the treatment system and community resources to receive the services they and their ill relative require
6. Enable family members to cope effectively with their feelings, reactions, and the stress of their relative's illness
7. Enable family members to maintain personal productivity and self-esteem

CONCEPTUAL CONSIDERATIONS

Psychiatric–mental health nurses are aware that families coping with mental illness of a relative need support, encouragement, and relevant skills. Conceptual models of mental illness that frame the family as the causative agent can contribute to the stigmatizing of these families and inhibit the development of constructive working relationships between the family and professional service system. Blaming attitudes on the part of professionals are inappropriate to the development and implementation of family educational programs. Family educational programs are best conceptualized within a stress and coping paradigm that appreciates the burdens faced by family members and supports the use and development of coping strategies (Hatfield & Lefley, 1987). Mastery of effective coping strategies will encourage families' competent management of the critical situations that occur with mental illness.

STRUCTURE

The family education program may be structured as follows:

1. *Length of program:* short-term (e.g., 1 full day or weekly evenings for 1 month) or long-term (e.g., regular meetings for a year or more)
2. *Format:* individual family education sessions or multifamily group sessions
3. *Group composition:* family members only; consumers and family members; special groups such as siblings, spouses, parents
4. *Setting:* office, conference room, community or church facility, family home
5. *Leaders/facilitators:* psychiatric–mental health nurses, psychiatrists, psychologists, social workers, family members or clients who are successfully coping, community service providers (police, lawyers, community program staff)
6. *Scheduling and length of sessions:* weekends or evenings; one or two weekend days, series of 1½- to 3-hour evening sessions
7. *Recruitment:* clinician referral, written invitations, posters, phone calls to client's home, hospital referral
8. *Confidentiality:* may need administrative policy to handle the problem of the client's objection to family education

ORGANIZATION

Educational sessions are organized to enable family members to be as comfortable as possible and to promote interactive discussion. Family members confronting the early stages of an illness are primarily interested in learning the meaning of psychiatric terms used in reference to the relative, as well as causes of the illness, prognosis, and treatments. Those families who have been coping with a chronic course are more likely to focus on managing problematic behaviors and planning for the future. Depending on the membership mix of the group, content may be tailored to meet the needs of the families. Meetings with individual families can enhance and reinforce the content provided in the group context. A format for a multifamily group educational session includes:

1. *Welcome:* Express appreciation for those participating; acknowledge that families have other demands on their time that compete with their attendance at the session; set the tone for learning and supportive interactions.
2. *Information sharing:* Lecture/discussion with appropriate audiovisuals; provide opportunities for participants to give examples from their own experience; provide handouts, information sheets, reference lists. Box 49-1 lists audiovisual resources. Box 49-2 lists publications for family members.
3. *Skill building:* Instruct and guide families in observing behavior, making accurate assessments, practicing problem-solving methods, implementing and evaluating new strategies.
4. *Review and homework:* Review the goals and objectives for the session and relevant homework assignments for family members to practice skills at home.
5. *Evaluation:* May be conducted session by session or at the conclusion of the program. Request written evaluations by participants to assess program impact, provide direction for improving the program, and assess the quality of the program.

PROGRAM TOPICS

The selection and arrangement of program topics is based on an assessment of the client population, the characteristics of the family members, and the treatment program. An ideal family educational program is integrated with the client's treatment pro-

---

BOX 49-1: Audiovisual Resources for Families of the Mentally Ill

The Brain, 8-part video series, produced by the Annenberg CPB Project. Introduction to basic brain function in everyday activities, one episode on mental illness. Available from the Annenberg CPB project (1-800-LEARNER or 202-879-9600).

The Mind, 9-part video series produced by PBS. Includes episodes on depression, pain, aging, violence. Available from PBS Films (1-800-328-PBS1).

Schizophrenia, video, specially adapted Phil Donahue program. Dr. E. Fuller Torrey reviews suspected causes, symptoms, prognosis, and strategies for family members, available from Films for the Humanities and Sciences (1-800-257-5126).

Living with Schizophrenia: A Video Manual for Families, video, available from David Katz, Washington University, One Brookings Drive, St. Louis, MO 63116 (314-935-6683).

When Mental Illness Invades a Marriage, video, available from AMI of Alabama, 6900 6th Avenue, South, Suite B, Birmingham, AL 35212 (205-833-8336).

Understanding and Communicating with a Person Who Is Hallucinating, video available from NurSeminars, Inc., W. 13523 Shore Road, Nine Mile Falls, WA 99206 (509-468-9673).

Shattered Dreams, video available from AMI of Pennsylvania, 2149 North 2nd Street, Harrisburg, PA 17110 (717-238-1514).

Coping With Depression, video, assists sufferers in implementing self-help strategies, available from New Harbinger Publications (1-800-748-6273).

Depression: Back from the Bottom, video, explains symptoms of depression and range of treatment options, available from Films for the Humanities and Sciences (1-800-257-5126).

Depression: Biology of the Blues, video, focuses on the biological causes of depression, current treatments and research, available from Films for the Humanities and Sciences (1-800-257-5126).

When the Music Stops: The Reality of Mental Illness, video, available from NAMI, 2101 Wilson Blvd., Suite 302, Arlington, VA 22201 (703-524-7600).

On the Road to Recovery, video, available from California AMI, 111 Howe Avenue, Suite 475, Sacramento, CA 95825 (916-567-0163).

Note: This list provides examples of videos useful for family education programs. Most sources have other related titles available.

---

gram, supporting and reinforcing content in client psychoeducational programs. Some topics include:

1. *Illness overview:* Definition, prevalence, common myths, stress-vulnerability model of mental illness. Typical categories are schizophrenia, depression, and bipolar disorder.
2. *Diagnosis and symptoms:* Diagnostic process, symptoms of the illness, distinguishing the illness from personality traits, alcohol and drug abuse.
3. *Treatment:* Medications, side effects, controlling side effects; psychosocial therapies, rehabilitation programs, importance of encouraging treatment participation.
4. *Stress reduction and behavior management:* Communication, problem solving, establishing reasonable expectations, limit setting, negotiating behavioral consequences, stress management, establishing and maintaining a balanced emotional home environment, signs of relapse, illness monitoring, relapse prevention strategies, healthful lifestyle, preventing and responding to crises, educating and including

---

BOX 49-2: Publications for Families of the Mentally Ill

Understanding Schizophrenia: A Guide to the New Research on Causes and Treatment, 1994, by Richard Keefe and Philip Harvey. Basic introduction for individuals interested in understanding schizophrenia.

Surviving Schizophrenia: A Family Manual, 1995 (revised), by E. Fuller Torrey, MD. Schizophrenia in understandable terms with practical suggestions for families.

Coping with Schizophrenia: A Guide for Families, 1994, by Kim Mueser and Susan Gingerich. Practical and readable book gives step-by-step strategies for coping with everyday issues of mental illness.

The Family Face of Schizophrenia, 1994, by Patricia Backlar. A family member's story on how to cope with schizophrenia. Includes comments, insights, and advice of mental health and legal professionals.

Tell Me I'm Here, 1991, by Anne Deveson. Poignant personal account of coping with son's schizophrenic illness.

The Depression Workbook, 1992, by Mary Ellen Copeland. Self-help workbook for those suffering from or wanting to understand more about depression.

Understanding Depression, 1993, by Donald Klein, MD, and Paul Wender, MD. A forthright definition of clinical depression as a biological illness, covering symptoms, causes, diagnosis, and treatment.

Living Without Depression and Manic Depression, 1994, by Mary Ellen Copeland. Self-help workbook for those suffering from or wanting to understand more about depression or manic depression.

We Heard the Angels of Madness: One Family's Struggle with Manic Depression, 1991, by Diane and Lisa Berger. Personal account of coping with the first few years of a relative's manic depressive illness.

What You Need to Know About Psychiatric Medications, 1991, by Stuart C. Yudofsky, MD, and Tom Ferguson, MD. Easy-to-read consumer guide to current psychiatric medications.

Note: These books and other resources can be purchased through the National Alliance for the Mentally Ill (703-524-7600, ext. 7992).

---

other family members, maintaining a social support system, interacting with the treatment system, participation in self-help groups such as local chapters of the National Alliance for the Mentally Ill.

5. *Planning for the future:* Encouraging social relationships and activities, reinforcing personal hygiene and social skill building, encouraging independence, finding and comparing community programs, comprehending the social service system, negotiating living arrangements, assessing the client's needs, making financial arrangements, considering the implications for a will, involving other family members in the planning process.

REFERENCE

Hatfield, A. B., & Lefley, H. P. (eds.) (1987). *Families of the Mentally Ill: Coping and Adaptation.* New York: Guilford Press.

BIBLIOGRAPHY

Abramowitz, I. A., & Coursey, R. D. (1989). Impact of an educational support group on family participants who take care of their schizophrenic relatives. *Journal of Consulting and Clinical Psychology, 57,* 232–236.

Anderson, C. M., Reiss, D. J., & Hogarty, G. E. (1986). *Schizophrenia and the Family: A Practitioner's Guide to Psychoeducation and Management.* New York: Guilford Press.

Ascher-Svanum, H., & Krause, A. A. (1991). *Psychoeducational Groups for Patients with Schizophrenia: A Guide for Practitioners.* Gaithersburg, MD: Aspen Publishers.

Berkowitz, R., Eberlein-Fries, E., Kuipers, L., & Leff, J. (1984). Educating relatives about schizophrenia. *Schizophrenia Bulletin, 10* (3), 418–429.

Bernheim, K. F., & Lehman, A. F. (1985). *Working with Families of the Mentally Ill.* New York: W. W. Norton.

Bisbee, C. C. (1991). *Educating Patients and Families About Mental Illness: A Practical Guide.* Gaithersburg, MD: Aspen Publishers.

Cole, R. E., & Reiss, D. (eds.) (1992). *How Do Families Cope with Chronic Illness?* Hillsdale, NJ: Lawrence Erlbaum.

Falloon, I. R. H. (ed.). (1985). *Family Management of Schizophrenia: A Study of Clinical, Social, Family, and Economic Benefits.* Baltimore: Johns Hopkins University Press.

Falloon, I. R. H., Boyd, R. L., & McGill, C. W. (1984). *Family Care of Schizophrenia: A Problem-Solving Treatment for Mental Illness.* New York: Guilford Press.

Hatfield, A. B. (1990). *Family Education in Mental Illness.* New York: Guilford Press.

Hatfield, A. B., & Lefley, H. P. (eds.). (1987). *Families of the Mentally Ill: Coping and Adaptation.* New York: Guilford Press.

Hill, D., & Balk, D. (1987). The effect of an education program for families of the chronically mentally ill on stress and anxiety. *Psychosocial Rehabilitation Journal, 10* (4), 25–40.

Kahana, E., Biegel, D. E., & Wykle, M. (eds.) (1994). *Family Caregiving Across the Lifespan.* Beverly Hills: Sage.

Kane, C. F., DiMartino, E., & Jimenez, M. (1990). A comparison of short-term psychoeducation and support groups for relatives coping with chronic schizophrenia. *Archives of Psychiatric Nursing, 4* (6), 343–353.

Kuipers, L., MacCarthy, B., Hurry, J., & Harper, R. (1989). Counselling the relatives of the long-term adult mentally ill: II. A low cost supportive model. *British Journal of Psychiatry, 154,* 768–775.

Lefley, H. P., & Johnson, D. L. (eds.) (1990). *Families as Allies in Treatment of the Mentally Ill: New Directions for Mental Health Professionals.* Washington, DC: American Psychiatric Press.

Malone, J. (ed.) (1992). *Schizophrenia: Handbook for Clinical Care.* Thorofare, NJ: Slack Inc.

Marsh, D. T. (1992). *Families and Mental Illness: New Directions in Professional Practice.* New York: Praeger.

Maurin, J. T. (ed.) (1989). *Chronic Mental Illness: Coping Strategies.* Thorofare, NJ: Slack Inc.

Mueser, K. T., & Gingerich, S. (1994). *Coping with Schizophrenia: A Guide for Families.* Oakland, CA: New Harbinger Publications.

Nguyen, T. D., Attkisson, C. C., & Stegner, B. L. (1983). Assessment of patient satisfaction: Development and refinement of a service evaluation questionnaire. *Evaluation and Program Planning, 6,* 299–314.

Smith, J. V., & Birchwood, J. (1987). Specific and nonspecific effects of educational intervention with families living with a schizophrenic relative. *British Journal of Psychiatry, 150,* 645–652.

The National Alliance of the Mentally Ill's (NAMI) Curriculum and Training Network is an exceptional resource for professionals developing family education programs. NAMI also operates a publication service, which is a source of relevant publications for educational programs. Obtain information about the network and publications through:

The National Alliance for the Mentally Ill (NAMI)
200 North Glebe Road, Suite 1015
Arlington, VA 22203-3754
(703) 524-7600

Designing a Private Practice

Suzanne Lego

OVERVIEW:

INTRODUCTION

Thousands of psychiatric–mental health advanced practice nurses are now offering psychotherapy in private practice. Most of these nurses hold full-time or part-time jobs as well, but some support themselves in full-time private practices. A number of factors may account for this, including the following:

1. A general dissatisfaction among nurses with institutionalized settings
2. Advanced nurse practice acts that recognize specialization in psychiatric–mental health (PMH) nursing
3. Insurance laws and regulations favorable to PMH nursing

4. Reimbursement practices favorable to PMH nursing
5. A trend in the United States toward home-based work
6. Satisfaction on the part of clients with advanced practice nurses, compared to physicians (Congress of the United States, Office of Technology Assessment, 1986)

ADVANTAGES

Private practice of psychiatric–mental health nursing provides the following advantages:

1. *Control of the scope of practice:* Nurses can select the kind of clients with whom they like to work, and their modality and theoretical framework. They can determine how many hours per week to devote to direct care, and how many to lecturing, consultation, writing, community work, and so forth. They can choose their own supervisors.
2. *Flexibility of hours:* Nurses can schedule office hours according to their own preferences, and can arrange days off and vacations as they see fit.
3. *Financial remuneration:* Nurses are generally paid more per hour for private practice than for institutional practice.

DISADVANTAGES

Some nurses shun the idea of private practice or become anxious upon entering private practice because private practice may generate fear about autonomy, independence, separation, individuation, and aggression. These internal feelings, which nurses experience consciously or unconsciously, are based on the following reality factors about private practice. The nurse:

1. Is fully responsible and accountable
2. Must have the ability to make decisions that have lasting consequences
3. Is involved in a 24-hour/day contractual arrangement
4. Often does not have daily contact with colleagues

QUALIFICATIONS

CERTIFICATION*

It is generally agreed that nurses who practice psychotherapy privately should be certified or in the process of becoming certified as a clinical specialist in adult psychiatric and mental health nursing or a clinical specialist in child and adolescent psychiatric and mental health nursing. Not only does this move the profession forward, but also third-party payers rely on certification as an important criterion for reimbursement. To apply for certification, nurses must (ANA, 1995):

1. Currently hold an active RN license in the United States or its territories; *and*
2. Be currently involved in direct patient contact in psychiatric and mental health nursing an *average* of 4 hours per week. Administrators, educators, researchers, and consultants can meet this requirement if they are involved in direct patient contact; *and*
3. Be currently involved in clinical consultation or clinical supervision; *and*
4. Have experience in at least two different treatment modalities; *and*
5. Hold a master's or higher degree in psychiatric and mental health nursing.†
   †If you do not meet requirement #5, your application will be reviewed if your educational preparation meets the following criteria:

*Eligibility requirements are subject to change from year to year. Please contact the American Nurses Credentialing Center for up-to-date information at 600 Maryland Avenue, Suite 100, Washington, DC 20024, or call (202) 651-7000.

a. A master's or higher degree in nursing outside the psychiatric and mental health nursing field with a *minimum* of 24 graduate- or postgraduate-level academic credits in courses that have a significant focus in psychiatric and mental health theory and supervised clinical training in two psychotherapeutic treatment modalities; *and*

6. Have at least 800 hours of direct patient/client contact in advanced clinical practice of psychiatric and mental health nursing; up to 400 of these hours may be earned through the clinical practicum in a master's program of study; at least 400 of these hours must be earned following completion of the educational preparation listed in #5 or #5a above; *and*

7. Document 100 hours of individual or group clinical consultation/supervision and submit endorsement(s) from the consultant/supervisor(s). Form A must be submitted for all supervision including practicum supervision and posteducation supervision. At least 50% of these hours must be earned following completion of the educational preparation listed in #5 or #5a above. These hours may be earned in the following manner:

   a. Up to 50% of the 100 hours may be earned within the master's-degree program.*

   b. A *minimum* of 65% (up to 100%) of the consultation/supervision must be provided by a nurse who is ANCC certified or eligible for ANCC certification as a clinical specialist in psychiatric and mental health nursing.*

   c. Up to 35% of the consultation/supervision may be provided by a non-nurse who meets one of the criteria listed below. (For those nurses who expect to hold prescriptive privileges, these hours might be applied toward supervision of the prescription of medications.) The non-nurse(s) may be:

      • A master's-prepared licensed/certified mental health social worker
      • A psychiatrist
      • A psychologist prepared at the doctoral level and listed in the National Register of Health Service Providers in Psychology
      • A psychologist prepared at the doctoral level in an APA accredited program in one of the following clinical areas: clinical psychology, counseling psychology, or school psychology

      *If the nurse consultant/supervisor is not ANCC certified as a clinical specialist in psychiatric and mental health nursing, documentation must be provided that she/he meets all ANCC eligibility requirements in education, practice, and supervision as outlined in the catalog.

CONTINUING EDUCATION

Although the private practitioner may be licensed and certified and hold advanced degrees, professional education does not end there. Because knowledge in the field of mental health is constantly expanding, the professional must keep abreast of current knowledge. A number of states now require continuing education for relicensure, and the ANA requires that certified specialists earn a specified number of continuing education units (CEUs) over each 5-year period of recertification. Ways to earn CEUs include:

1. Attendance at approved conferences sponsored by universities or private companies. Annual psychiatric nursing conferences are sponsored by:

Contemporary Forums
11400 Silvergate Drive, Suite A
Dublin, CA 94568-2257
(510) 828-7100

Medical College of Pennsylvania and Hahnemann University
Continuing Nursing Education
Box 12608
Philadelphia, PA 19129-9964
(215) 841-4345

2. Presentation at approved conferences.
3. Completing self-study exercises. These appear in the *Journal of Psychosocial Nursing and Mental Health Services*, the *Journal of the American Psychiatric Nurses Association*, and *Perspectives in Psychiatric Care.* Some states, e.g., Ohio, also offer self-study for CEUs.
4. Publications of books, chapters, articles, or participation in research. (For more information contact the American Nurses Credentialing Center at (202) 651-7000.)

PERSONAL PSYCHOTHERAPY

The clinical specialist who conducts psychotherapy as a private practitioner functions best when personal psychotherapy is a part of the professional preparation. This is because the practice of psychotherapy requires a close, intimate relationship over time with the client, who will present a wide range of irrational behaviors, which often touches off in the nurse an equally wide range of irrational thoughts and feelings. Through personal psychotherapy, nurses are helped to understand their own irrationalities so they can avoid acting out and can increase their useful, growth-promoting responses to clients.

FINANCIAL CONSIDERATIONS IN STARTING THE PRACTICE

START-UP COSTS

If an office is set up apart from home, start-up costs include:
1. Rent, including a security deposit
2. Furnishings and rugs for the waiting room and consultation room
3. Phone installation
4. Stationery, including:
   - Announcements of practice (see Box 50-1)
   - Letters and envelopes with letterhead
   - Business cards
   - Bills (see Box 50-2 for a sample bill and Box 50-3 for commonly used CPT codes)
   - An answering machine (if answering service is not used)
   - Legal fees for incorporation

ONGOING OPERATING COSTS

1. Office rent
2. Phone, electricity, heat
3. Answering service (if answering machine is not used)
4. Insurance
5. Supervision
6. Accountant fees for filing taxes and financial planning
7. Magazine subscriptions for office magazines

BOX 50-1: Sample Announcement of Practice

Suzanne Lego RN,PhD,CS,FAAN

Announces the relocation of her New York practice

to

Sewickley, PA and Kent, Ohio

for the practice of psychotherapy, psychoanalysis, and clinical supervision

Sewickley, PA   (412) 741-7930
Kent, Ohio   (216) 672-2044

BOX 50-2: Sample Bill

Dr. SUZANNE LEGO
334 Sycamore Road
Edgeworth
Sewickley, PA 15143

S.S. # XXX-XX-XXXX
ANA Cert. # XXXXX
Provider #

DIAGNOSIS	DATE	PROFESSIONAL SERVICE	CHARGE	PAYMENT	BALANCE
Axis I _____					
Axis II _____					
Axis III_____					
Axis IV_____					
Axis Va_____					
Axis Vb_____					

> **BOX 50-3: Commonly Used CPT Codes**
>
> | | |
> |---|---|
> | Diagnostic Interview | 90801 |
> | Individual Psychotherapy, 20–30 minutes | 90843 |
> | Individual Psychotherapy, 45–50 minutes | 90844 |
> | Family/Conjoint Therapy | 90847 |
> | Multiple Family Therapy | 90849 |
> | Group Psychotherapy | 90853 |
> | Telephone Consultation | 98920 |

These costs are reduced when nurses rent space in established offices, either by the day or hour. Disadvantages to this method are:

1. Lack of flexibility in scheduling clients
2. Office decor may not reflect the personality of the renter

HOME OFFICES

Many nurse psychotherapists practice at home. The advantages are:

1. Convenience
2. Economy

The disadvantages are:

1. Lack of privacy for the therapist and family
2. Some risk of danger if clients are unknown

THE SETTING

Whether the nurse's office is in the home or in another location, the following provisions are made:

PRIVATE WAITING ROOM

The waiting room should have a comfortable temperature, pleasant decor, quiet surroundings, a bathroom, a coat rack, and reading materials. If it adjoins the consultation room, privacy is maintained through soundproofing or a white noise machine.

PRIVATE CONSULTATION ROOM

The consultation room should be comfortable, pleasant, and quiet. Distractions such as phone calls, deliveries, pets, and other interruptions are avoided.

LOCATION

The office should be close to public transportation or have adequate parking facilities and should be in a quiet, safe neighborhood, if possible.

PERSONAL IMAGE

Personal image is very important in determining which therapists clients choose. Clients respond best when:

1. Therapists show interest, warmth, support, intelligence, and respect.
2. The office is comfortable, quiet, and nondistracting. Male clients may be uncomfortable if the therapist's office is too "feminine" and female clients may be turned off by a very traditional "cold"-looking office.

PRACTICE PROMOTION STRATEGIES

Ways to promote the practice include:

1. Becoming providers for preferred provider organizations (PPOs), health maintenance organizations (HMOs), and employee assistance programs (EAPs) who send clients directly
2. Providing services convenient to the work schedule or lifestyle of clients, e.g., in the evenings and on weekends, or telephone therapy (see Chapter 18)
3. Meeting individually with other nurses, ministers, priests, rabbis, physicians, school counselors, law enforcement agents, and court/juvenile authorities to explain the practice and ask for referrals
4. Reciprocal referral of clients to those who refer clients
5. Providing classes or lectures directed toward consumer needs in the community
6. Providing professional lectures or seminars and publishing in professional journals
7. Appearing as an expert guest on radio/television programs
8. Appearing in local newspapers
9. Voluntary consultation to nonprofit, community-based health agencies
10. Distributing professional business cards
11. Mailing announcements of a new practice to physicians, other health professionals, etc.
12. Actively participating in professional organizations
13. Becoming actively involved politically in issues affecting nursing and mental health
14. Advertising in the yellow pages. The nurse must take care to follow local, state, and professional advertising restrictions, including:
    - What titles may be used
    - What services may be offered

PRESCRIBING MEDICATION

In all but four states, at the time of this writing, nurses may apply for prescriptive practice. What this means varies widely from state to state. Some PMH advanced practice nurses do not want to prescribe medication, preferring instead to refer clients to another health care provider, probably a psychiatrist or nurse practitioner. When this happens, it is helpful if there is a good working relationship and similar philosophies of care between the professionals, for example, if both agree that a minimal amount of medication should be given to help the client function so that psychotherapy can proceed, or that hospitalization should be avoided if possible.

TAXES AND RETIREMENT PLANS

Since taxes are not withheld by an employing agency, it is up to the nurse to pay quarterly estimated taxes. An accountant determines what the quarterly payments should be, based on the previous year's earnings. If the nurse is not incorporated, these taxes are paid January 15, April 15, June 15, and September 15. When the nurse's income reaches a certain point, incorporation can provide advantages, such as a medical plan, retirement plan, automobile expenses, and much higher limits on nontaxable retirement contributions. Incorporation laws vary from state to state. Private practitioners must also plan their own retirement benefits using individual retirement accounts (IRAs) in which $2000 per year may be invested tax-free, or Keogh plans in which 15% of annual earned income may be invested. These retirement funds can be invested in bank accounts, insurance plans, investment trust funds, and so forth. An accountant is valuable for filing taxes and for providing information about deductions and financial plans.

INSURANCE

For the private practitioner, a number of kinds of insurance are necessary.

HEALTH AND LIFE INSURANCE

The nurse must contract independently for health and life insurance. Life insurance is available through the ANA at group rates (call 202-651-7000).

DISABILITY INSURANCE

Disability insurance provides monthly payments should the nurse become disabled through sickness or accidents. This kind of policy is available from private companies or at group rates through the ANA and other professional groups such as the American Orthopsychiatric Association.

MALPRACTICE INSURANCE

Malpractice insurance provides coverage for damages or court costs should the nurse be sued. It is available through private companies or the ANA.

PROPERTY AND CASUALTY INSURANCE

Property and casualty insurance provides coverage for damages or court costs should someone sue for damages as the result of an accident on the nurse's property (for example, in the waiting room or consultation room). If the office is in the home, "home owners" insurance can cover this if endorsed for professional use.

FIRE, THEFT, AND MALICIOUS MISCHIEF

If the nurse rents an office outside the home, fire, theft, and malicious mischief insurance may be desirable, and is fairly inexpensive in most locations. If the office is in the home, "home owners" insurance can cover this if endorsed for professional use.

LEGAL CONSIDERATIONS

It is generally accepted that the nurse practice acts in most states cover the practice of psychotherapy by the certified clinical nurse specialist. In addition, most states are in the midst of or have already added advanced nurse practice acts referring to the practice of nurse practitioners, nurse midwives, nurse anesthetists, and clinical nurse specialists. Some states require that advanced practice nurses practice with "supervision" by a physician, though the definition of supervision may be very loose. Other states require "collaboration" with a physician, and some allow for legally independent practice. Clinical nurse specialists have by and large been free of these restrictions if they were certified by the ANA. However, new advanced practice legislation and regulations may add new restrictions. It is important for nurse psychotherapists to be politically active in formulating these laws and regulations, and vital that they know them in their own states. To this end, nurse psychotherapists will want to hold membership in:
1. Their state nurses associations, many of which have advanced practice groups
2. The American Psychiatric Nurses Association, which has both an advanced practice committee and a national legislative network, (202) 857-1133.

RECORD KEEPING

Records of client visits are kept for the following reasons:
1. *Assessment and continuing evaluation:* Nurses keep records of early sessions and notes as sessions progress to record the client's progress.
2. *Supervision or peer review:* For supervision or peer review, a nurse will probably tape-record sessions or take notes during sessions or afterward. If tape recordings

are made, it is a good idea to have the client sign a simple release form stating that the nurse has the client's permission to tape-record for professional use.

3. *Billing:* A record of sessions is kept for billing the client each month.
4. *Taxes:* The nurse keeps a record of all income and expenses for tax purposes. A bound ledger is required for this purpose. Records must be retained for at least 3 years to be used in the event of a tax audit.

BECOMING A MANAGED CARE PROVIDER

PMH advanced practice nurses are eligible providers for many PPOs, EAPs, and HMOs. To become a provider nurses can:

1. Contact large companies in the area and talk to the person who coordinates health services for the company's employees (Gold, 1994).
2. Look for job openings in managed care companies in the newspaper. Contacting the managed care company can provide a contact person who can help you become a provider (Todd, 1994).
3. Contact the provider relations departments of the major managed care companies and request an application. Filling it out will be an arduous task, as most are very lengthy and require a lot of documentation.
4. Join the APA Employee Assistance Professional Association (EAPA). This is a way to meet with other EAP providers.
5. Network with providers already in current networks. They can provide names, addresses, and phone numbers of key people in the managed care systems (Todd, 1994).
6. Form a group of providers who are geographically diverse and can meet annually at the state nurses association meetings to share information. Geographic diversity reduces competition or conflict of interest (Todd, 1994).
7. Provide inservice training to clinicians in the system.
8. Maintain a good relationship with the system when you are a provider.

APPLYING TO A MANAGED CARE SYSTEM

Issues to emphasize in applying to a managed care system include (Todd, 1994):

1. Performance-based practice
   - Average number of sessions per diagnosis
   - Client satisfaction ratings
   - Range of problems dealt with
   - Percentage of cases with no administrative errors during a calendar year, e.g., concurrent reviews submitted on time
2. Specialties—Be specific. While family therapy is a specialty, you may say, "Families who have undergone trauma." While this limits the population, it may ensure you get every referral in that population.
3. Gender issues—If you specialize in women who were raped, or men whose wives were incest victims, say so.
4. Religiosity—If you are a "Christian counselor" or a counselor of some other religious group, say so.
5. Publications and presentations—Be sure to mention these as they establish you as an expert in certain clinical areas.
6. Specialization—Do not represent yourself as an expert in every area.
7. License and degree—Be specific, e.g., Ph.D. in nursing. Often there are quotas for each discipline.
8. Credentials—List any certifications you have, e.g.,

- Certified Employee Assistance Professional
- Certified Alcohol Counselor (list levels if pertinent)
- Certified Hypnotherapist
- Clinical member of the American Association for Marriage and Family Therapy
- Fluency in a foreign language
- American Sign Language
9. Geographic location—list all offices you have.
10. Group therapy is cost-effective and popular with managed care companies. If you have an ongoing group, say so.
11. Your clinical expertise.
12. Your understanding of the principles of managed care.

REVIEWS BY MANAGED CARE SYSTEMS

The prospective review "is a process whereby the managed care system reviews documentation by a provider prior to service delivery in nonemergency situations. The treatment plan is reviewed by either a person in charge of authorizing care or a panel of individuals. The outcome of the review process is that the provider is given a set number of authorized sessions (outpatient) or days (inpatient) before another review is needed" (Todd, 1994, p. 8).

Concurrent reviews "are conducted during the course of treatment. The provider supplies the managed care system with documentation justifying why further treatment should be authorized. The concurrent review process is the most common process used in managed care. It is generally through this process that managed care systems learn which providers in their network warrant future inclusion and which do not" (Todd, 1994, pp. 8–9). Suggestions regarding concurrent reviews are (Todd, 1994):

1. Use a primary diagnosis and all five axes.
2. Assessment—use verifiable facts rather than theory. Show a therapeutic direction. Assessment sets the stage for a reasonable treatment plan.
3. Treatment plan and goals—use specific behavioral goals, not theoretical goals.
4. Response to treatment—be specific, using goals.
5. Termination criteria—be specific, using Global Assessment Functioning (GAF). (See Chapter 2.)
6. Additional sessions—don't just put the allowable number. Typical coverage is 20 visits or $1000.

Provider profiling "is an activity that managed care companies engage in to monitor a therapist's performance. This process can be as informal as making notes in a provider's file, or it can be as complex as a computer database system in which many variables are measured and recorded. Typically, the variables that a managed care system will be examining are costs per treatment episode, client satisfaction, client complaints, the results of a records review, administrative performance, clinical effectiveness, and cooperativeness with the managed care system. These variables help the managed care system make decisions about referral patterns and, potentially, which contracts, if any, may not be renegotiated after they expire" (Todd, 1994, p. 8).

LEGAL CONCERNS IN MANAGED CARE SYSTEMS

The PMH advanced practice nurse must bear in mind the legal issues that may come up as a provider:

1. The nurse may be asked to sign a "no compete clause," meaning the nurse may not act as a consultant to other systems. Therapists may be providers for multiple systems (Todd, 1994).

2. The nurse may also be asked to sign a "hold harmless clause." This means the managed care system is held harmless for any act on the nurse's part. Nurses must be sure this works both ways, and they are held harmless for any adverse consequences resulting from a wrongful act by the managed care company. For example, providers can be held legally responsible when managed care systems deny services and the client goes without, even when the provider appealed the decision (Todd, 1994).

3. Treatment must be provided in accordance with community standards of care. Nurses must be sure their practice coincides with the manner in which most providers in their specialty would perform (Giles, 1993).

4. Individual providers also incur liability when they refuse a referral and instead recommend another provider within the panel (Giles, 1993).

5. Liability may result when there is a closed panel, a patient needs a specialist, and there is none on the panel, so a substitute "in house" is used. Informed refusal applies here (Giles, 1993).

6. Some managed care organizations withhold a part of clinicians' fees against the possibility of excess medical costs. If there are none, some of the withheld is returned. This is a disincentive to treat and has led to lawsuits (Giles, 1993).

7. Clients have a legal right to effective psychotherapeutic care. "Negligent failure to diagnose and properly treat a psychiatric condition may constitute cause-in-fact of harm to the patient and third parties if it in fact can be established that with proper care, the patient's condition and behavior could have been corrected or controlled" (Giles, 1993, p. 125). For example, a client was treated for depression using psychoanalytic treatment on an inpatient unit. Dissatisfied with his treatment, he went to a psychiatrist and was successfully treated with antidepressants. He sued the first providers for treating him with a method of unproven efficacy in place of one with proven efficacy (Giles, 1993).

8. It is considered legally fraudulent to charge patients different fees and waive copayments so that the therapist always gets the same fee but clients pay no copayments. For example, a therapist might charge patients with insurance $80, those with 20% copayments $100, and those with 50% copayments $160. This is unacceptable because the therapist misrepresented the fee to the insurance company, which has only agreed to pay 50% or 80% of the therapist's *actual* fee (Small, 1993). "Routine forgiveness of copayments is unacceptable. Whether it is actually illegal depends on state laws, specific insurance contracts, and federal regulations" (Small, 1993, pp. 36–37).

9. Therapists are taxed by the Internal Revenue Service (IRS) according to the amount *billed,* rather than the amount collected. For example, if the therapist bills an insurance company $80 for a session and the insurance company pays $40, the therapist must collect the other $40 from the client. If audited, the therapist must have record of a small claims judgment against the client. Otherwise the IRS assumes the money was collected and not reported (Gold, 1994).

ETHICAL CONCERNS IN MANAGED CARE SYSTEMS

The PMH advanced practice nurse must bear in mind the ethical issues that may come up as a provider:

1. To avoid patient abandonment therapists must treat patients until presenting problems are satisfactorily cleared, a referral is made, or care is terminated. This is often handled by reserving slots for low-fee patients (Giles, 1993).

2. In a capitated system "the fiscal incentive associates a decrease in delivered services with an increase in profit." Providers must be sure quality of care is not compromised (Giles, 1993, p. 120).
3. Therapists must be careful to provide services only in the areas in which they are trained. They may want to receive training and certification in brief therapy (Giles, 1993).
4. Conflicts arise over the need to give good care and the need to keep costs down (Giles, 1993).
5. Clients are entitled to "informed consent about benefits and expectations for care. This includes adequate disclosure about goal-driven therapy with concomitant time and economic constraints" (Giles, 1993, p. 122).
6. The ethical principle of fidelity dictates that therapists who do not feel loyal to managed care philosophy should refrain from provider membership (Giles, 1993, p. 122).
7. Therapists should communicate first with each other about known or suspected ethical violations or other examples of inappropriate clinical behavior before contacting employers, grievance boards, insurance commissioners, and attorneys (Giles, 1993).
8. Confidentiality issues arise when patient records can be accessed by nonclinical people and used inappropriately. There seem to be no laws or regulations requiring third-party payers to keep the information confidential (Small, 1993).

SIGNING OFF ON INSURANCE FORMS

"Perhaps the most scandalous and widespread unethical billing practice among mental health professionals is 'signing off' unlicensed therapists. Some practitioners will charge a flat amount, others a per-patient 'kickback' fee, while some 'sign off' with no remuneration as a favor for a friend. In any case, for practitioners to sign insurance forms for services that they did not perform or truly supervise is unethical and fraudulent practice. In fact, both the therapist and supervisor could find themselves liable. *Psychotherapy Finances* ('Legal Briefing,' 1987) reports that a licensed clinical social worker in Kentucky received a referral from a psychiatrist who continued to sign the bills that went to the insurance company. Blue Cross and Blue Shield of Kentucky pressed felony charges of theft by deception against only the social worker, who agreed to plead guilty to a misdemeanor. She was sentenced to a weekend in jail, 720 hours of community services, and 5 years of probation, and had to reimburse $37,000 to Blue Cross and Blue Shield. The psychiatrist was not charged by the state's attorney, but the Board of Medical Licensing charged him with dishonorable, unethical, or unprofessional conduct" (Small, 1993, p. 38)

Nurse psychotherapists must bear in mind that:
1. Supervisors or employees may perform services if it is clearly indicated on the form that this person and not the physician performed the services.
2. In some cases (e.g., Medicare and CHAMPUS) the supervisor signs the form, not the provider, and the services are rendered in this way:

> The physician must first render a covered personal professional service for which the services of the nonphysician can be considered incidental, although an integral part. [This indicates that the psychotherapeutic service must be eligible for Medicare reimbursement and would exclude such services as those for personal growth.] (Small, 1993, p. 39)

3. Some argue that while it is *legal* to have only the supervisor sign the Medicare and CHAMPUS form, it is not *ethical,* as it misrepresents services. Before adopting this procedure, one should carefully review the nursing code of ethics.
4. If the nurse works with a physician who signs forms, indicating the nurse provided the therapy, this is probably legal, but it is unethical, because the fee has been doubled, e.g., the patient or insurance company pays $150/session rather than the $75–$80 that would be paid if the nurse billed individually.

ACCEPTING ASSIGNMENT AS A PARTICIPATING PROVIDER

In this case the therapist accepts the insurer's "reasonable fee" as payment in full. The therapist is paid directly, e.g., by Medicare, Blue Shield, CHAMPUS, and a few private companies. If a private insurance company has no such arrangement, the patient must pay a copayment. Accepting assignment as a participating provider has these advantages (Small, 1993):

1. The therapist may receive increased referrals because patients may be required to see participating providers to receive reimbursement, or may be encouraged to through differential reimbursement.
2. Dealing directly with a single insurance company for numerous patients may also be convenient.

Disadvantages are (Small, 1993):
1. Delayed payment
2. Increased paperwork
3. Reduced fee

FEDERAL REIMBURSEMENT

The following federal programs reimburse PMH advanced practice nurses:
1. Medicare, Part B
   - CNSs in rural areas only, according to individual state regulations
   - NPs in rural areas and nursing facilities, according to state regulations

As this book goes to press, bills have been introduced in both the Senate and House of Representatives that will allow for direct reimbursement to advanced practice nurses.
2. Medicaid—Up to individual states
3. CHAMPUS—ANA-certified clinical nurse specialists
4. Federal Employee Health Benefit Program—ANA-certified clinical nurse specialists

ACCOUNTABILITY

Nurses in private practice are accountable to clients and to themselves in the following ways:
1. Nurses provide services as contracted with the client, keeping in mind the elements of the ANA Statement on Psychiatric and Mental Health Nursing (see Appendix A) (American Nurses Association, 1994).
2. Nurses are students of the problems that arise in the psychiatric–mental health field, checking and rechecking their assumptions and preconceptions, keeping an open and active mind, and laying aside their own needs so as to recognize and help resolve the needs of clients (Peplau, 1980).

EVALUATION

The success of a private practice for the nurse therapist may be measured in three ways:
1. The reduction of symptoms and emotional disturbance in the majority of clients
2. The satisfaction and growth of the nurse psychotherapist
3. Financial success

REFERENCES

American Nurses Association (1994). *A Statement on Psychiatric–Mental Health Clinical Nursing Practice and Standards of Psychiatric–Mental Health Nursing Practice*. Washington, DC: American Nurses Association.

American Nurses Association (1995). *1995 Certification Catalogue, American Nurses Credentialing Center*. Washington, DC: American Nurses Association.

Congress of the United States Office of Technology Assessment (Dec. 1986). *Nurse Practitioners, Physician Assistants and Certified Nurse–Midwives: A Policy Analysis, HCS 37*. Washington, DC: Office of Technology Assessment.

Giles, T. R. (1993). *Managed Mental Health Care: A Guide for Practitioners, Employers, and Hospital Administrators*. Boston: Allyn and Bacon.

Gold, M. I. (1994). *The Foundations of Your Private Practice. Vol 1*. Alameda, CA: Hunter House.

Peplau, H. E. (1980). The psychiatric nurse—accountable? To whom for what? *Perspectives in Psychiatric Care, 18,* 128–132.

Small, R. F. (1993). *Maximizing Third-Party Reimbursement in Your Mental Health Practice* (2nd ed.). Sarasota, FL: Professional Resource Press.

Todd, T. (1994). *Surviving and Prospering in the Managed Mental Health Care Marketplace* (2nd ed.). Sarasota, FL: Professional Resource Press.

51

Designing a Course in Psychiatric–Mental Health Nursing for Baccalaureate Students

Catherine Adams

OVERVIEW:

INTRODUCTION

In most undergraduate nursing programs a course in psychiatric–mental health nursing is taught by faculty members holding a master's degree in the specialty. These programs do not depend on the "integration" of psychiatric–mental health concepts throughout other courses to teach psychiatric nursing. However, threads relevant to the specialty run throughout the program. Some of these threads are:

1. Communication
2. Leadership
3. Clinical judgment
4. Critical thinking
5. Caring

In the psychiatric–mental health (PMH) course these concepts are refined for application with clients who are mentally ill or are experiencing other difficulties in living. Theory pertains to the various disorders or difficulties in living. The theory is applied to students' individual relationships with clients who range in age from adolescent to elderly and represent varying sociocultural backgrounds. Besides establishing a therapeutic relationship, students learn to:

1. Collaborate with other health care providers
2. Provide leadership in planning and implementing care
3. Assume accountability
4. Use clinical judgment

PLACEMENT OF THE COURSE

Because considerable maturity is required in the therapeutic use of the self with psychiatric clients, the PMH nursing course is usually taught in the senior year. In programs where students tend to be nontraditional (older) it may be offered in the later part of the junior year.

COURSE OBJECTIVES

Course objectives are written in behavioral terms and reflect the program's overall objectives, conceptual framework, and mission statement. These objectives describe the behavior the student is expected to exhibit as a result of one or more learning experiences (Reilly, 1975). The objectives are then used to evaluate students. Sample objectives are shown in Box 51-1.

BOX 51-1: Sample Objectives for a PMH Undergraduate Course

Upon completion of the course, the student will be able to:

1. Demonstrate competency in using the nursing process in mental health promotion, maintenance, and restoration.

2. Demonstrate clinical judgment in applying the nursing process to clients with potential or actual mental/emotional problems.

3. Develop an awareness of legal/ethical issues in the mental health system and demonstrate the ability to respond to them appropriately.

4. Apply communication skills in collaboration with other health care providers.

5. Use research findings in the practice of psychiatric–mental health nursing.

6. Take into account sociocultural factors in interventions with clients.

7. Recognize the need to collaborate with health care organizations.

CONTENT

The major topics covered in the course include an overview of theories of and intervention in mental and emotional disorders, an overview of the nurse's role in the psychiatric–mental health system, and psychopharmacology, including nursing implications.

ORGANIZATION OF COURSE CONTENT

Exposure to the major disorders such as schizophrenia precedes exposure to the less severe disorders such as obsessions, and the discussion of the underlying phenomena of stress, coping, anxiety, and grief for the following reasons:

1. Students are exposed to severely ill clients early in their clinical placement and need theory to match their observations.

2. By the time they begin the PMH course they have had considerable background content in the supporting courses of general psychology, sociology, and growth and development.

3. Psychotic and bizarre behavior provides students with the chance to learn in a dramatic way that all behavior has meaning. The skills they acquire in translating or decoding psychotic communication can be transferred to other less disturbed clients. Box 51-2 provides a sample lecture schedule.

BOX 51-2: Sample Lecture Schedule for an Undergraduate Course in Psychiatric–Mental Health Nursing

Week 1	Course Overview: Goals and Expectations Review of Therapeutic Communication and Crisis Orientation to Psychiatric–Mental Health Nursing
Week 2	Introduction to the DSM-IV
Week 3	Thought Disorders: Description, Theory, and Interventions Including Psychopharmacology
Week 4	Mood Disorders: Mania, Theory, and Interventions Including Psychopharmacology
Week 5	Mood Disorders: Depression, Theory, and Interventions Including Psychopharmacology
Week 6	Concepts of Mental Health and Illness: Historical, Ethical, Legal, and Cultural Implications
Week 7	The Concept of Anxiety: Theory and Intervention
Week 8	Models and Frameworks of Mental Health and Mental Illness: Stress and Coping
Week 9	Panic Disorders, Phobias, and Obsessions
Week 10	Substance Abuse and Dual Diagnosis
Week 11	Eating Disorders, Posttraumatic Stress Disorder, and Dissociative Identity Disorder
Week 12	Borderline Personality Disorder and Antisocial Personality Disorder
Week 13	Grief, Death, and Dying

TEACHING STRATEGIES

While some lectures are useful in the beginning of the course, critical thinking is enhanced by active participation in learning (Rubenfeld & Scheffer, 1994). Therefore, the teacher acts as a facilitator of group discussion using the techniques of:

1. Presenting controversial positions and asking for student opinions
2. Proposing clinical problems for group solution
3. Inviting or proposing questions from weekly reading assignments (McKeachie, 1978)

Owing to the knowledge explosion, information provided to students today is likely to be out of date by the time they are in positions of responsibility. Therefore, students are taught basic information, and more importantly to develop habits of critical thinking and inquiry (Rubenfeld & Scheffer, 1994). In addition to the lecture–discussion, students:

1. View videotapes
2. Read assigned material
3. Complete writing assignments
4. Attend field trips

ASSIGNMENTS

Learning and evaluation is enhanced by:

1. Quizzes and tests
2. Logs or journals
3. Process recordings
4. Case presentations

Box 51-3 presents an example of a creative writing assignment requiring the student to consider how it might feel to be mentally ill, as well as to think through the usefulness of nursing interventions.

BOX 51-3: Sample Assignment for Students in a Baccalaureate PMH Course

From the perspective of an outpatient schizophrenic client, answer the following two questions:

1. What about your illness has given you the greatest difficulty? What would you most like help with and what form should that help take?

2. What insight, learning, intervention, "trick", etc. has been the most helpful to you in dealing with your illness?

You may write this as though a journal entry, a letter of advice to another client or client's caretaker, mother, or nurse, or any other form you would like (poem, prose, etc.). This is a *creative* assignment and requires neither documentation nor designated length.

CLINICAL PLACEMENT

Clinical experience is important to students (Burnard, 1992) and affects their attitudes toward the specialty (Biordi & Oermann, 1993). Students approach clinical placements in psychiatric nursing with considerable fear and anxiety (Adams, 1993) owing to the ambiguity of their roles. The instructor's sensitivity to students' anxiety can make a difference in the students' overall opinion of the specialty. Settings used for clinical placement or observation are:

1. Psychiatric hospitals
2. Inpatient psychiatric units in general hospitals
3. Group homes
4. Homeless shelters
5. Substance abuse programs or agencies

If the course emphasis is on helping students see the impact of the nurse–patient relationship over time, students are placed in an agency where they can meet with the same client once a week for the whole semester, for example, in a group home. Field trips are then made to other settings, 12-step programs, and so forth.

CLINICAL SUPERVISION	Often the classroom teacher doubles as clinical instructor. This works well when the teacher is clinically active. When this is not the case, or when the instructor must supervise more than eight students, some students may be assigned to work with an experienced, master's-prepared clinical nurse specialist who is employed in the placement setting (Adams, 1993).
RECOMMENDED STUDENT ACTIVITIES	Student activities during the course of a clinical day vary from agency to agency. The following provide some suggested alternatives, and sites can be evaluated for their potential for supplying these experiences:

1. Treatment review meetings with interdisciplinary team
2. Nursing shift reports
3. 1:1 client interaction
4. Client/group interaction; community meetings
5. Activity group
6. Therapy group
7. Client assessments
8. Medication administration
9. Client teaching
10. Home visits
11. Charting
12. Case presentations
13. 1:1 clinical supervision
14. Group clinical supervision

CLINICAL CONFERENCES

PROCESS

The purpose of clinical conference is to provide a forum for discussion of clinical material so that theory and practice are integrated. Emphasis is placed on the process of intervention, focusing particularly on students' behaviors, feelings, and thoughts relative to the clinical situation.

Students come to preconference and postconference prepared to discuss their clinical experiences. This usually includes a brief description of a client and an account of an interaction with that client. Students are prepared with an idea, a question, or a problem they would like to discuss. The clinical supervisor might also present issues to discuss as they are relevant (e.g., confidentiality, self-disclosure, truth-telling, etc).

GOALS

Some goals of clinical conferences include:

1. To identify and succinctly define a particular clinical issue, problem, or theme (to carve away "fat" and get at the "crux")
2. To explore alternative and related clinical issues, problems, or themes, to expand the clinical possibilities
3. To determine and define a specific goal or direction of clinical intervention
4. To explore alternative and related clinical goals or directions of clinical intervention
5. To receive from peers critical and evaluative feedback with regard to clinical issues
6. To receive from preceptors critical and evaluative feedback with regard to clinical issues
7. To "practice" clinical experience through role-playing, example, and other facets of the group process

8. To work on personal issues relevant to clinical skill or judgment
9. To experience the emotional support of the group

STUDENT EVALUATIONS

TESTS AND QUIZZES

Tests and quizzes are given periodically to:
1. Encourage students to keep up with the reading
2. Help students identify problem areas
3. Provide students with the experience of taking examinations similar to the board examinations

Test and quiz items are continually reevaluated for (McKeachie, 1978):
1. Relevance to objectives
2. Ability of items to discriminate among learners
3. Appropriate level of difficulty

CLINICAL EVALUATION

Clinical practice should be evaluated on a pass/fail basis. It is appropriate for the classroom teacher to periodically check with the supervising preceptor to inquire about problems that may have arisen in the course of the clinical experience. Evaluation conferences between the preceptor or supervising instructor and the individual student should also occur on an ongoing basis. These conferences address two major questions from the point of view of both student and advisor:
1. What are the student's major strengths in working with psychiatric clients?
2. What are the areas in which the student needs to grow to increase/facilitate expertise?

In addition, students may be evaluated and evaluate themselves along a continuum of "excellent," "competent," or "needs work" in the following areas:
1. Commitment
2. Responsibility
3. Maturity
4. Energy
5. Motivation
6. Attitude
7. Comfort/anxiety level
8. Interpersonal skills
   - with clients
   - with staff

COURSE EVALUATION

Course evaluation should be ongoing and multifaceted. Methods include:
1. Faculty discussions.
2. Standardized tests, such as the National League for Nursing Achievement Test.
3. Student feedback sessions at the end of the course and at the end of the program.
4. Student evaluation forms. A particularly useful form is one that asks students to comment on any of the following areas they believe would be helpful in planning future courses:
   a. Overall course organization
   b. Specific content included in course
   c. Course materials

d. Course requirements
e. Class presentations
f. Faculty ability
g. Stimulation from course
h. Overall contribution from course
i. Additional comments about course or teaching approach

THE TEACHER AS A PERSON

Perhaps more crucial than any advice about the specifics of designing undergraduate experience is the observation that a teacher's enthusiasm and love of the work may be the single most important quality teachers have to offer. As McKeachie (1978) has noted, the full range of human needs is very much a part of the classroom. One function of the teacher as a person is to convey that the intellectual matters under discussion are not irrelevant to the conduct of a life. To be self-revealing, trustworthy, and warm not only encourages student openness, but increases the extent to which the teacher is revealed to be an ordinary mortal in pursuit of a recognizable and manageable set of goals. Students are affected by hearing how their teachers found their way into the field, and this can be as inspiring as course content or format.

REFERENCES

Adams, C. (1993). An evaluation of four student placements in psychiatric nursing. *Journal of the New York State Nurses Association, 24* (4), 19–22.
Biordi, B., & Oermann, M. H. (1993). The effect of prior experience on nursing students' attitude toward the disabled. *Rehabilitation Nursing, 18* (2), 95–98.
Burnard, P. (1992). Student nurses' perceptions of experiential learning. *Nurse Education Today, 12* (3), 163–173.
McKeachie, W. J. (1978). *Teaching Tips: A Guidebook for the Beginning College Teacher* (7th ed.). Lexington, MA/Toronto: D. C. Heath & Company.
Reilly, D. (1975). *Behavioral Objectives in Nursing: Evaluation of Learner Attainment.* New York: Appleton–Century–Crofts.
Rubenfeld, M. G., & Scheffer, B. K. (1994). *Critical Thinking in Nursing: An Interactive Approach.* Philadelphia: J. B. Lippincott.

BIBLIOGRAPHY

Kleehammer, K., Hart, A. L., & Keck, J. F. (1990). Nursing students' perceptions of anxiety producing situations in the clinical setting. *Journal of Nursing Education, 29* (4), 183–187.
Miller, L. (1991). Predicting relapse and recovery in alcoholism and addiction: Neuropsychology, personality, and cognitive style. *Journal of Substance Abuse Treatment, 8* (4), 227–291.
Pederson, C. (1993). Promoting nursing students' positive attitudes toward providing care for suicidal patients. *Issues in Mental Health Nursing, 14* (1), 67–84.

52
FIFTY TWO

Designing a Graduate Program in Psychiatric– Mental Health Nursing

Anita Werner O'Toole

OVERVIEW:

Description
Major Processes
Values
Core Courses
Cognates and Electives
Clinical Supervision
Personal Psychotherapy
Comparison of Supervision and
    Psychotherapy

Clinical Placement
    Settings
    Designing the Experience
    Evaluating the Agency
Evaluation of Student Clinical
    Performance
The PMH Nurse Practitioner

DESCRIPTION

Graduate education in psychiatric–mental health (PMH) nursing prepares nurses for advanced practice as clinical nurse specialists (CNS) or nurse practitioners. Specialization at the master's level helps nurses acquire expertise in the knowledge and practice of psychiatric–mental health nursing. Graduate education provides students with the opportunity to use an investigative approach as they develop breadth and depth in their understanding of theory and increased competence in nursing practice and research (Peplau, 1989). Curiosity and critical thinking are nurtured as students examine issues and question current nursing beliefs. Learning experiences increase in complexity as students move from learning to work with individuals, groups, and families to communities.

Students entering graduate programs in psychiatric–mental health nursing are heterogeneous; they bring with them a variety of experiences, attitudes, and interests. Recognition of what students bring with them and exploration of their needs are essential for the formulation of meaningful learning experiences.

A collaborative teacher–student relationship is essential, since a primary function of the teacher is the facilitation of students' learning and development. The teacher is responsible for developing an environment in which students have freedom and responsibility for self-direction and self-evaluation of their learning experiences in the program.

MAJOR PROCESSES

Experiences emphasize process as well as content. Content of knowledge and the nature of roles change; therefore, it is impossible to learn in any given program all one might need to know in the future. However, many educational processes have enduring characteristics. These processes are:

1. *Inductive:* The process of theorizing from clinical and empirical data, whereby concepts and categories arise from the data instead of being superimposed upon the data.
2. *Deductive:* The process of theory development whereby theories are applied to empirical data and revised accordingly.
3. *Experiential:* The process whereby one learns as one does. Like the inductive process of conceptualizing, experiential learning is based on the examination of the data of one's experience. In psychotherapy, clients learn new forms of behavior by examining current and past behavior and its antecedents and consequences. Likewise, in learning therapeutic skills, students are encouraged to apply theory and examine its usefulness in bringing about the desired outcome.
4. *Supervisory:* The process whereby students examine their clinical work over time with supervisors and peers to guide the learning process.
5. *Therapeutic:* The process whereby students learn to be therapists, which includes values inherent in the professional role of psychotherapist, either in formal, structured psychotherapy or in encounters on an inpatient unit, the client's home, or the community.
6. *Research:* The process of investigating phenomena in a logical, systematic way.

VALUES

Perhaps the most enduring outcome of an education experience is the acquisition of new values. Graduate students in psychiatric–mental health nursing should learn to value:

1. Their own intellectual and interpersonal competence and the importance of self-awareness
2. Nursing as a major profession in the mental health field
3. Professional development throughout one's career, including ongoing clinical practice with appropriate supervision, clinical research, and publication.

CORE COURSES

These courses are required of all students in the PMH program, and usually of students in the other advanced practice nursing programs. The courses usually include:

1. *Nursing theory:* Discusses kinds of theories, analyzes and critiques theories in nursing and in fields relevant to nursing
2. *Nursing research:* Includes statistics, research methodology, both quantitative and qualitative
3. *Advanced professional role development:* Discusses the role of advanced practice nurses and relevant topics such as certification, professional organizations, regulation, and legislation relative to advanced practice, etc.
4. *Social and health policy:* Includes social issues that influence the delivery of health care such as racism, poverty, homelessness, gender bias, etc.

COGNATES AND ELECTIVES

These courses support the clinical major and may include:

1. Measurement and evaluation of psychiatric illness
2. Psychopathology
3. Individual psychotherapy, with a practicum

4. Group psychotherapy, with a practicum
5. Family therapy, with a practicum
6. Community study, with a practicum
7. Psychopharmacology
8. Physiology
9. Consultation/liaison PMH nursing
10. PMH nurse management (elective)

Box 52-1 shows a sample master's curriculum in PMH nursing.

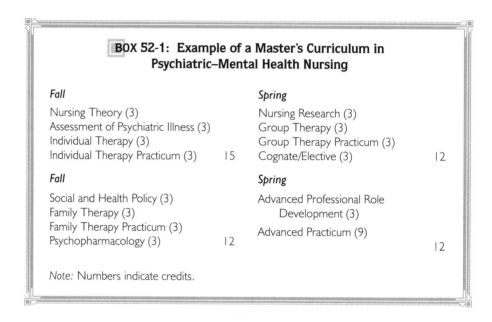

BOX 52-1: Example of a Master's Curriculum in Psychiatric–Mental Health Nursing

Fall		Spring	
Nursing Theory (3)		Nursing Research (3)	
Assessment of Psychiatric Illness (3)		Group Therapy (3)	
Individual Therapy (3)		Group Therapy Practicum (3)	
Individual Therapy Practicum (3)	15	Cognate/Elective (3)	12
Fall		**Spring**	
Social and Health Policy (3)		Advanced Professional Role Development (3)	
Family Therapy (3)			
Family Therapy Practicum (3)		Advanced Practicum (9)	
Psychopharmacology (3)	12		12

Note: Numbers indicate credits.

CLINICAL SUPERVISION

Supervision may be done by a faculty member or by a preceptor designated as adjunct faculty. Students may meet with the supervisor on a one-to-one basis or in small groups. During supervision seminars the student may:
1. Talk informally about the interactions with client(s)
2. Play an audiotape of the interaction
3. Show a videotape of the interaction

In some cases the supervisor sits in with the student as in group therapy, or may observe through a one-way mirror. It is important for supervisors to be ANA-certified clinical specialists, as students may later use a portion of their clinical supervision hours obtained in graduate school toward application for certification.
The purpose of supervision is:
1. To evaluate the use of self as a therapeutic variable
2. To assess intrapsychic and interpersonal processes that promote and impede communication
3. To develop psychotherapeutic skills with individuals, groups, and families
4. To demonstrate knowledge of and skills in the client–therapist relationship.

See Box 52-2 for guidelines in supervision sessions.

BOX 52-2: Supervision Guidelines

1. If first session, include presenting problem from the intake session.
2. State theme(s) of session.
3. State problem(s) presented.
4. Identify functional and dysfunctional behaviors.
5. State medicines prescribed, briefly identify actions, and evaluate effects on client(s).
6. Analyze and evaluate interventions that impeded or facilitated progress. Include one or more nontherapeutic interventions and one or more therapeutic interventions.
7. Provide theoretical rationale for interventions.
8. Comment on transference as it occurred.
9. Comment on countertransference as it occurred.
10. Plan modifications in interventions and rationale (that is, What will you do next time?).
11. If session is tape-recorded, identify sections of tape you want supervisor to focus on with specific questions/comments.

PERSONAL PSYCHOTHERAPY

Personal psychotherapy is desirable for all graduate students to:

1. Experience the client's side of the therapeutic alliance
2. Become aware of unresolved conflicts and resistances
3. Broaden students' range of self-awareness
4. Investigate factors underlying inappropriate responses to self, clients, and others

COMPARISON OF SUPERVISION AND PSYCHOTHERAPY

Similarities exist between psychotherapy and clinical supervision in that both are learning experiences. A comparison of supervision and psychotherapy is shown in Table 52-1.

TABLE 52-1: Comparison of Supervision and Psychotherapy

	SUPERVISION	PSYCHOTHERAPY
Objectives	1. Enhance quality of educational experience in relation to course objectives and learning needs. 2. Learn therapy skills and dynamics of behavior. 3. Become a psychotherapist.	1. Achieve resolution of personal problems over time. 2. Achieve self-awareness and self-knowledge over time.
Focus	Assess, intervene, and evaluate work with clients.	Explore personal experiences and resolve personal problems
Responses	Identify self-responses (thoughts, feelings, and behavior) that affect client positively and negatively.	Identify self-responses (thoughts, feelings, and behavior) that affect self positively and negatively.
Change	Identify and change behaviors that interfere with the therapeutic alliance.	Explore and resolve personal problems.
Evaluation	Assess work with client(s); expect a minimum learning level for the course.	Assess degree of change in self and in response to others; progress occurs over time with no time limit.

CLINICAL PLACEMENT

SETTINGS

Since graduate students have different past experiences and future goals, they choose the settings that meet their needs. Settings may include (Lego, 1992):

1. Inpatient psychiatric unit in a general hospital
2. Inpatient psychiatric hospital
3. Community mental health center
4. Family service center
5. Child guidance and counseling center
6. Home health care agency
7. Independent or group practice
8. Geriatric care setting
9. Group home
10. Single-room-occupancy hotels or boarding homes
11. Private practice

DESIGNING THE EXPERIENCE

1. Students are given a list of settings that faculty have previously contacted or that have been used in the past.
2. Students select a setting from the list or choose another agency on the basis of current professional interests, future goals, and geographic proximity.
3. Students contact agency staff and discuss clinical experiences in relation to the course objectives, performance expectations, and clinical hours (ideally 12–16 hours per week).
4. As needed, the clinical supervisor meets with agency staff to verify the student's status in the program, discuss the graduate program, and discuss the student's performance at the agency.

EVALUATING THE AGENCY

It is wise for future planning to have students complete a brief evaluation form in terms of the setting's ability to help meet course objectives.

EVALUATION OF STUDENT CLINICAL PERFORMANCE

The student and supervisor evaluate the student's progress together in relation to the course objectives and student's goals. The student's ability to perform the following activities is evaluated:

1. Identify themes and problems within the client–student interaction.
2. Identify functional and dysfunctional behaviors.
3. Provide therapeutic interventions.
4. Provide theoretical rationale for interventions.
5. Analyze and evaluate the effectiveness of interventions.
6. Plan modifications, as needed, in interventions and goals for treatment.
7. Assess effects of medications on clients.
8. Participate with agency staff by communicating activities with clients and sharing knowledge at staff meetings.

THE PMH NURSE PRACTITIONER

PMH nurse practitioners are prepared at the master's level to provide primary care to psychiatric patients, particularly the underserved in public mental hospitals, homeless shelters, inner-city clinics, and remote rural areas. In most states nurse practitioners have prescriptive practice. The CNS program described here can be adapted to prepare the PMH nurse practitioner by adding courses and clinical experiences in:

1. Advanced physical health assessment of psychiatric clients
2. Management of primary health delivery to psychiatric clients
3. Advanced pathophysiology
4. Pharmacology

REFERENCES

Lego, S. (1992). A practicum in private practice for graduate students in psychiatric nursing. *Archives of Psychiatric Nursing, 6,* 211–214.

Peplau, H. E. (1989). Investigative counseling. In A. W. O'Toole & S. R. Welt (eds.), *Interpersonal Theory in Nursing Practice: Selected Works of Hildegard E. Peplau* (pp. 205–229). New York: Springer.

BIBLIOGRAPHY

Greben, S. E. (1991). Interpersonal aspects of the supervision of individual psychotherapy. *American Journal of Psychotherapy, 45,* 306–316.

McNeill, B. W., & Worthen, V. (1989). The parallel process in psychotherapy supervision. *Professional Psychology: Research and Practice, 20,* 329–333.

Watkins, C. E. (1990). The separation–individuation process in psychotherapy supervision. *Psychotherapy, 27,* 202–209.

V
PART FIVE

Psychiatric Nursing Procedures

FIFTY THREE

Admission to the Hospital*

Fatima Ramos

OVERVIEW:

Standard of Care
Patient Care Outcome
Standard of Practice
Intake
Nursing Assessment Prior to Admission

Types of Admission
Nursing Intervention Prior to
    Admission
Admission Procedure
Continuous Quality Improvement

STANDARD OF CARE

Prior to accepting patients for admission, the hospital must have established mechanisms to ensure that patients are assessed and "to respect the patient's rights to care subject to the hospital's capability, mission, and applicable law and regulation" (Joint Commission on Accreditation of Health Care Organizations, 1994, p. 3)

PATIENT CARE OUTCOME

Patients will be admitted in a safe and efficient manner.

STANDARD OF PRACTICE

Qualified clinical professionals, determined by organizational and legal standards, such as advanced practice psychiatric nurses and physicians, gather and analyze assessment data to identify the best approaches to meeting the patients' needs.

INTAKE

Patients arrive at the hospital in the following ways:
1. Walk in unescorted
2. Walk in accompanied by family or friends
3. Brought by ambulance
4. Brought by police

They may arrive for an intake appointment, having been referred by an advanced practice nurse or physician, another professional, or they may be self-referred, and have no appointment. Patients may come to the hospital because of a psychiatric problem or may come for a medical problem, and be found to need psychiatric care. Generally they are seen either:
1. In an area designated for psychiatric admissions during business hours
2. In a psychiatric emergency room (ER)
3. In a general emergency room (ER)

*Laws and regulations in this chapter apply in New York. They may vary from state to state.

When patients arrive with a psychiatric emergency, they are seen immediately for intake and disposition. The disposition is determined, keeping in mind the hospital's policies and procedures, and may involve:
1. Admission to the hospital
2. Holding in the emergency room
3. Transfer to another hospital
4. Referral to outpatient treatment

NURSING ASSESSMENT PRIOR TO ADMISSION

The advanced practice psychiatric nurse conducting the intake asks for:
1. Patient's name, address, age, and the name of the person supplying the data if it is not the patient
2. Chief complaint or reason for coming to the hospital
3. Physical data including allergies, medical problems, physical injuries, sexual trauma, and current medications
4. Psychological data including description of current condition or illness, past psychiatric history, past psychiatric hospitalizations, current psychiatric medications, suicidal ideation, homicidal ideation, past suicidal or homicidal behavior, and family history of mental illness
5. Social data including living arrangements, employment, and communication barriers
6. Name and phone number of professional who recommended patient come to the hospital

Following the brief, initial assessment interview the nurse identifies a provisional diagnosis using the DSM-IV (see Chapters 1 and 2) and a decision is made in collaboration with the physician regarding the disposition. If admission is not required, the patient and significant others are informed about alternative care. If the patient is to be admitted, the nurse helps the patient and significant others through the admission process.

TYPES OF ADMISSION

Informal Admission   Patients request to be admitted to a psychiatric unit and agree to treatment at the time of admission. However, if at any time patients request to be discharged, the hospital has to freely discharge them. Informal admissions are much the same as admission to a medical/surgical unit. See Table 53-1 for nursing interventions and rationale in an informal admission.

Voluntary Admission   Patients request to be admitted to a psychiatric unit and agree to treatment at the time of admission. At any time during hospitalization, patients may submit a sign-out letter to leave the hospital. From the time the letter is received and acknowledged by staff, there is a 72-hour period to decide to either discharge the patient or convert the patient to involuntary status after examination by two physicians who sign certificates (known as 2PC). Those patients in need of hospitalization are usually encouraged to stay on a voluntary status and talk about why they want to leave the hospital. See Table 53-2 for nursing interventions and rationale in a voluntary admission.

Involuntary or Two-Physicians Consent   Two physicians, usually psychiatrists, examine the patient and both certify there are grounds to admit the patient involuntarily or to convert the patient from a voluntary to an involuntary status. For this to be done patients must present a danger to themselves or others. Patients may request a court hearing on this admission status.

TABLE 53-1
Nursing Interventions and Rationales in Informal Admissions

INTERVENTION	RATIONALE
1. Status and rights notice is provided to patients with the name and telephone number of Mental Hygiene Legal Service written on the form.	1. Patients have the right to know their legal admission status. They also have the right to know how to access legal services, advice, and representation independently of the hospital with regard to hospitalization.
2. Patients and the admitting physician discuss and then sign the informal admission form.	2. The form documents the patient's understanding of informal admission and treatment suitability.
3. Consent for treatment form is discussed and then signed.	3. It is required that written consent be attained from patients or their families for diagnostic tests, medical procedures, and so forth.
4. Consent for release of information is discussed and signed.	4. Patients must provide written consent for release of information before the treatment team can communicate with their family members, visitors, other treating health care professionals, and others.
5. A booklet with information on advance directives, health care proxy, and other insurance or legal materials is discussed with patients, who receive a copy. Patients may be asked to sign an acknowledgment form.	5. Patients, their families, and significant others must be informed about advanced directives as per the JCAHO standards, the State Department of Health, and the Office of Mental Health Law.

TABLE 53-2
Nursing Interventions and Rationales in Voluntary Admissions

INTERVENTION	RATIONALE
1. Status and rights notice is provided to patients on admission or conversion and every 120 days thereafter. This form must have the name and telephone number of Mental Hygiene Legal Service written on it. A copy of this document is placed in the medical record. New York State Office of Mental Health supplies legal documents in English and Spanish.	1. Patients have the right to know their legal admission status. They also have the right to know how to access legal services, advice, and representation with regard to hospitalization independently of the hospital.
2. Patients, their families, and the admitting physician discuss the Voluntary Request for Hospitalization.	2. The discussion helps the physician assess suitability and increases understanding about voluntary admission. It initiates a therapeutic relationship with patients, their families, and significant others.
3. Adult patients fill out the appropriate section of the form with their name, the name of the facility, reasons for request of admission, and then sign the form. For admission of minors, their parents or guardian must complete the appropriate section in the same format as for adults.	3. This procedure complies with Mental Hygiene Law.
4. Consent for Treatment is discussed and then signed.	4. It is required that written consent be attained from patients or their families for diagnostic tests, medical procedures, and so forth.
5. Consent for release of information is discussed and signed.	5. Patients must provide written consent for release of information before the treatment team can communicate with their family members, visitors, other treating health care professionals, and others.
6. A booklet with information on advance directives, health care proxy, and other insurance or legal materials is discussed with patients. Patients may be asked to sign an aknowledgment form.	6. Patients, their families, and significant others must be informed about advanced directives as per the JCAHO standards, the State Department of Health, and the Office of Mental Health Law.

Requesting a Court Hearing   This process must be followed on a timely basis. The steps include:

1. The patient requests in writing to leave the hospital.
2. The psychiatrist writes to the judge requesting a hearing for the patient.
3. The psychiatrist makes an application for order of retention.
4. The psychiatrist notifies by letter or phone call mental health legal services to obtain an attorney for the patient, if the patient does not already have an attorney.
5. The psychiatrist notifies the attorney representing the hospital.

Emergency Admission   There are specific requirements that must be met for patients to be accepted for this type of admission. In New York State, hospitals must be granted permission to admit on an emergency basis by the commissioner of mental health. Patients are examined by one physician who decides patients have met criteria for a mental illness and present a severe danger to self or others if admission does not occur immediately. Many psychiatric emergency rooms now have a holding area or crisis intervention units for these patients who remain for 48 hours and then are either released or admitted to a psychiatric hospital unit. The following steps are taken:

1. A physician, usually a licensed psychiatrist, must complete a second examination to confirm the need for extension of emergency admission beyond 48 hours.
2. The patient is admitted on emergency status for 15 days.
3. Next of kin is notified of the admission.
4. Before the 15 days are up, patients in need of continued hospitalization are encouraged to convert to a voluntary status.
5. If they refuse and ask to leave the hospital, arrangements for a court hearing must be made.

NURSING INTERVENTION PRIOR TO ADMISSION

See Table 53-3 for nursing interventions before the patient goes to the unit.

TABLE 53-3
Nursing Interventions and Rationales Prior to Admission

INTERVENTION	RATIONALE
1. Admission procedure and tentative plan of care is explained to the patient and significant others.	1. Increases collaboration and cooperation.
2. Clothing and belongings are examined. Potentially harmful articles are either: • Sent home with significant others • Locked up for use under supervision • Held until discharge	2. Provides a safe environment.
3. Weapons, drugs, or alcohol are confiscated and given to security staff.	3. Provides a safe environment.
4. The inpatient unit is informed the patient is coming. The nurse may accompany the patient to the unit, or a nurse from the unit comes for the patient. A comprehensive verbal report is given to the nurse in charge. The admission form is also given to the charge nurse when the patient arrives on the unit.	4. Provides a smooth transition and communication of information about the patient.

ADMISSION PROCEDURE

See Table 53-4 for nursing interventions and rationales once the patient has reached the inpatient unit.

TABLE 53-4
Nursing Interventions and Rationales During Admission on an Inpatient Unit

INTERVENTION	RATIONALE
The nurse	
1. Greets patient using last name, and introduces self to patient.	1. Conveys respect.
2. Shows patient to room.	2. Begins to build rapport.
3. Provides patient with a patient handbook (see Box 53-1).	3. Decreases anxiety, promotes cooperation, informs of legal rights.
4. Checks patient's clothing and belongings and confiscates any contraband that may have been missed earlier in the admission process.	4. Provides a safe environment.
5. Shows patient around the unit, introducing other patients and staff.	5. Decreases anxiety.
6. Provides patient with food or rest if hungry or tired. If not, nurse assesses: • Mental status • Reason for admission • Vital signs	6. Promotes a therapeutic relationship, begins assessment process.
7. Initiates a multidisciplinary treatment plan including: • Diagnosis • Patient's strengths and limitations • Goals (Later shared with patients and significant others) OR	7. Provides a guide for treatment.
8. Writes a nursing care plan including: • Nursing diagnosis • Goals • Nursing interventions	8. Provides a guide for nursing care.
9. Implements admission orders.	9. Assures effective and efficient inpatient care.

Note: A complete nursing assessment is performed within 24 hours. (See Chapters 1 and 2.)

CONTINUOUS QUALITY IMPROVEMENT

The clinical nurse manager or designee leads the team to systematically assess and improve the admission procedure of psychiatric patients.

BOX 53-1: Sample Patient Handbook

St. Barnabas Hospital
Third Avenue and 183rd Street
Bronx, New York 10457

Orientation Information
Kane 3

Patient Handbook
GENERAL INFORMATION & RULES AND REGULATIONS

1. LOCATION

The psychiatric unit at St. Barnabas Hospital is located in the main building on the 3rd floor. The floor is called Kane 3.

2. THE TREATMENT TEAM

Your treatment team consists of a psychiatrist, a psychologist, a social worker, nurses, activity therapists, and nursing attendants. Additionally, medical residents, medical students, nursing students and occupational therapy students are on the unit working with the team members. It is the aim of the treatment team to provide comprehensive care to help patients toward the highest level of health and to help them return to their families and communities.

3. ADMISSION

Upon your admission to Kane 3 a member of the nursing staff will help you get settled. A physical examination is routinely done on all patients. This will include certain laboratory tests, x-rays, and other special examinations which may be helpful in planning your treatment. Patients are asked to change into hospital pajamas or gown prior to a physical examination. Patients' belongings are checked to assure a safe environment.

4. TREATMENT PROGRAM

The treatment program for each patient may be quite different. Many types of activities may be planned, such as group therapy, individual psychotherapy, family therapy, activity groups, and others. Patients are strongly encouraged to participate in the activities scheduled for them by team members.

5. MEDICATION

Ordinarily, medication is given at 9:00 A.M., 1:00 P.M., 5:00 P.M., and 9:00 P.M. If you receive medication, kindly go to the medication room at the appropriate times or ask your nurse when you are to receive your medication. You should find out from your primary nurse what medication/s you are on, the reason/s and the side effects.

6. SECLUSION AND RESTRAINTS

Unfortunately, at times patients may need to be secluded or restrained to protect them from hurting themselves or others. When this happens staff will make every effort to make the experience brief and safe. Patients are encouraged to tell staff about what helps them calm down when they feel like hurting themselves or others.

7. MEALS

Meals are served in the day room as follows:

Breakfast	8:00 A.M.
Lunch	12:00 P.M.
Dinner	5:00 P.M.

Menus are distributed every morning so that you may choose your food preferences for the following day. These should be filled out and returned to the nurses station by 10:00 A.M. Food and drink must be confined to the dining room. No food or drinks are allowed in rooms. The only exception to the rule is in the case of candy that is wrapped.

8. DAILY ROUTINE

Unless a patient is physically ill it is common to be dressed before breakfast at 8:00 A.M. on weekdays and 9:00 A.M. on weekends and holidays. Patients are encouraged to make their own beds every day and to keep their rooms in order. Clean linen is available daily. Patients are also encouraged to shower daily. If patients need assistance with their hygiene, staff is available to help them.

9. LAUNDRY

Laundry is done from 9:00 A.M. to 5:00 P.M. on Tuesday, Thursday and Saturday in the laundry room located on the first door to the right as you enter Kane 3. There is a sign-up sheet on the door of the laundry room. No laundry is done during visiting hours.

10. SUPPLIES

Supplies, including towels, linens, refills on toiletry items, etc., will be given out by nursing staff in the morning between 9:00 A.M. and 11:00 A.M.

11. SHAVING

All shaving must be supervised by the nursing staff. Shaving is done after Community Meeting from 10:00 A.M. to 11:00 A.M. Patients will not keep shavers. Disposable razors are used and must be disposed of in the appropriate container designated by staff.

12. SMOKING

St. Barnabas Hospital is a NO SMOKING hospital. If anyone is found with cigarettes, matches or smoking

BOX 53-1 *(continued)*

implements, *visiting privileges will be restricted for three days.*

13. SOCIALIZING

Appropriate socializing is encouraged on Kane 3. All socializing should occur in the day room or TV room and not in individual rooms. Patients are discouraged from physical or sexual contact with others.

14. TELEPHONE

The telephones in the room are for the use of patients until 11:00 P.M. The telephone numbers are (XXX) XXX-XXXX and (XXX) XXX-XXXX. Please give these numbers to your relatives and friends. Out of consideration for other patients it is requested that calls be limited to 15 minutes.

15. CHECKING OF BELONGINGS

Upon admission patients will have belongings checked to ensure that forbidden items are confiscated or placed in a safe place to be returned back to patients at discharge. Staff will, on a daily basis, conduct random room searches. Patients are encouraged to be in their rooms at the time of the search.

To maintain safety the following items are not allowed to remain with patients in the unit:

1. Cigarettes/matches
2. Alcohol
3. Glass containers
4. Mirrors
5. Weapons
6. Shoelaces
7. Plastic bags
8. Belts
9. Electrical equipment
10. Lighters
11. Sharp objects

16. ADDITIONAL RULES AND REGULATIONS
   1. NO fighting (physical or verbal)
   2. NO physical contact of a sexual nature
   3. NO horseplay
   4. NO stealing

17. VITAL SIGNS

Your vital signs, which include blood pressure, pulse, respirations and temperature, will be taken upon admission and daily for the next five days. Blood pressure and pulse will be taken both on a lying-down and standing position to check for side effects of your medication. Vital signs are taken in the day room, unless patients have a condition that prevents them from coming out of their rooms.

St. Barnabas Hospital
Bronx, New York

DEPARTMENT OF PSYCHIATRY

VISITING RULES FOR KANE 3

1. Visiting Days and Hours:
   Monday, Wednesday, Friday   6:30 P.M. to 8:00 P.M.
   Saturday, Sunday, & Holidays   1:30 P.M. to 3:00 P.M. and
      6:30 P.M. to 8:00 P.M.

2. Only two visitors per patient are allowed in the unit.

3. Visiting time is limited to $1/2$ hour per visit.

4. There will be only 10 visitors at a time in the unit.

5. All visitors must check in with Security on the first floor before coming up to the unit.

6. Food and beverages from the outside are not allowed in the unit. Exceptions include food in cellophane bags and canned soft drinks. Staff will provide cups for soft drinks and will collect cans at the door.

7. Visitors will be issued a locker with a key outside of the unit and will be asked to place their belongings in the locker while they visit.

8. Patients and their visitors must stay in the dining room during the visit.

9. Visitors are not allowed to bring cigarettes, alcohol, drugs, weapons, matches, or lighters into the unit.

10. Visitors may be asked to show the contents of their pockets. A metal detector may be used at the door. Weapons and drugs will be confiscated and given to the Security Office.

St. Barnabas Hospital
Bronx, New York

DEPARTMENT OF PSYCHIATRY

NAME: _____

THE TREATMENT TEAM

The treatment team is a multidisciplinary group of health care professionals who work together with you to help you meet your health care needs. You are a member of the team and should share in all plans regarding your treatment. In addition to yourself, the team consists of

PRIMARY NURSE _____
ATTENDING PSYCHIATRIST_____

PSYCHOLOGIST _____
SOCIAL WORKER _____
ACTIVITY THERAPISTS _____
_____
OTHER (specify title) _____
_____

(Continued)

BOX 53-1 *(continued)*

Patient's Bill of Rights

As a patient in a hospital in New York State, you have the right, consistent with law, to:

1) Understand and use these rights. If for any reason you do not understand or you need help, the hospital must provide assistance, including an interpreter.

2) Receive treatment without discrimination as to race, color, religion, sex, national origin, disability, sexual orientation, or source of payment.

3) Receive considerate and respectful care in a clean and safe environment free of unnecessary restraints.

4) Receive emergency care if you need it.

5) Be informed of the name and position of the doctor who will be in charge of your care in the hospital.

6) Know the names, positions, and functions of any hospital staff involved in your care and refuse their treatment, examination or observation.

7) A no smoking room.

8) Receive complete information about your diagnosis, treatment and prognosis.

9) Receive all the information that you need to give informed consent for any proposed procedure or treatment. This information shall include the possible risks and benefits of the procedure or treatment.

10) Receive all the information you need to give informed consent for an order not to resuscitate. You also have the right to designate an individual to give this consent for you if you are too ill to do so. If you would like additional information, please ask for a copy of the pamphlet "Do Not Resuscitate Orders—A Guide for Patients and Families."

11) Refuse treatment and be told what effect this may have on your health.

12) Refuse to take part in research. In deciding whether or not to participate, you have the right to a full explanation.

13) Privacy while in the hospital and confidentiality of all information and records regarding your care.

14) Participate in all decisions about your treatment and discharge from the hospital. The hospital must provide you with a written discharge plan and written description of how you can appeal your discharge.

15) Review your medical record without charge and obtain a copy of your medical record for which the hospital can charge a reasonable fee. You cannot be denied a copy solely because you cannot afford to pay.

16) Receive an itemized bill and explanation of all charges.

17) Complain without fear of reprisals about the care and services you are receiving and to have the hospital respond to you and, if you request it, a written response. If you are not satisfied with the hospital's response, you can complain to the New York State Health Department. The hospital must provide you with the Health Department telephone number.

HOSPITALS MUST PROVIDE PATIENTS (INCLUDING INPATIENTS, OUTPATIENTS AND EMERGENCY SERVICE PATIENTS) WITH A COPY OF THEIR RIGHTS. HOSPITALS MUST ALSO PROVIDE ASSISTANCE TO PATIENTS TO UNDERSTAND AND EXERCISE THEIR RIGHTS.

10 NYCRR 405.7, 405.7(a)(1), 405.7(a)(2)

Department of Health
(212) 613-4855
Hotline: (800) 837-9018

Courtesy of St. Barnabas Hospital, Bronx, NY.

REFERENCE

Joint Commission on Accreditation of Healthcare Organizations (1994). *The Joint Commission: 1995 Accreditation Manual for Hospitals. Volume I: Standards.* Oakbrook Terrace, IL: JCAHO.

54
FIFTY FOUR

Administration of Medications

Fatima Ramos

OVERVIEW:

Standard of Care
Patient Care Outcome
Standard of Practice
Medication Orders
Transcribing Orders to the MAR
Transcribing Single, STAT, and Pre-op
    Orders

PRN Medications
Administration of Medications
Procedure
Continuous Quality Improvement

STANDARD OF CARE

All psychiatric patients admitted to the hospital will have their medication orders transcribed to the Medication Administration Record (MAR) in a timely manner and will have medications administered to them according to valid medication orders. See Box 54-1 for a sample medication administration record.*

PATIENT CARE OUTCOME

Patients will receive medication in a safe, effective, and efficient manner.

STANDARD OF PRACTICE

The nurse, and when indicated the unit clerk, transcribe medication orders to the MAR. The orders are validated by a registered nurse (RN). Medications are administered by the nurse according to valid medication orders.

MEDICATION ORDERS

Medication administration begins with written orders. They include the patient's name, diagnosis, drug allergies, adverse drug reactions, drug name, dosage, frequency, route and special instructions, prescriber's signature and printed name, written clearly. See Box 54-2 for a sample physician's order sheet, the form used for ordering medications.

(Text continues on page 452)

*The forms in this chapter are courtesy of St. Barnabas Hospital, Bronx, New York.

BOX 54-1: Sample Medication Administration Record

ST. BARNABAS HOSPITAL
BRONX, NY · DEPARTMENT OF NURSING
MEDICATION ADMINISTRATION RECORD

	ADDRESSOGRAPH HERE

DIAGNOSES _Schizophrenia, Chronic, Undiff. type_

ALLERGIC TO: NKA   DATE 12/12/94

Legend
Omitted Doses (use red pen):
Document in Medication Omission Record

1. NPO
2. Off-Unit
3. I.V. Out
4. Pt. Refused
5. Other

PAGE __1__ OF ____

ORDER DATE / EXP. DATE	STANDING MEDICATIONS / MED-DOSE-FREQ-ROUTE	DATE / HOUR	12/12 INIT.	12/13 INIT.	12/14 INIT.	12/15 INIT.	12/16 INIT.	12/17 INIT.	12/18 INIT.	12/19 INIT.	12/20 INIT.
FR 12/12/94 12/19 R.N. INIT.	Haldol 5 mg po. H.S.	9 pm	FR	4							
R.N. INIT.											
R.N. INIT.											
R.N. INIT.											
R.N. INIT.											

INJECTION CODES:

RT = RIGHT THIGH	RA = RIGHT ARM	LU = LEFT UPPER GLUTEAL	↑RAB = UPPER RIGHT ABDOMEN	↑LAB = UPPER LEFT ABDOMEN
LT = LEFT THIGH	LA = LEFT ARM	RU = RIGHT UPPER GLUTEAL	↓RAB = LOWER RIGHT ABDOMEN	↓LAB = LOWER LEFT ABDOMEN

BOX 54-2: Sample Physician's Order Sheet

ST. BARNABAS HOSPITAL
PHYSICIAN'S ORDERS

ADDRESSOGRAPH HERE

1. All orders must include date, time, prescriber's signature, printed name and beeper number.
2. Begin a new section for each set of orders. A set of orders may require more than one section. Prescriber must sign each section.

Diagnosis *Schizophrenia, chronic, undiff. type*

Drug Allergies *NKA*

Date & Time	DO NOT USE THIS SHEET UNLESS A RED NUMBER SHOWS → ◯	USE BLACK BALLPOINT PEN ONLY	W.C. Sig., Date, Time	R.N. Sig., Date, Time
12/12/94	ADMIT TO SERVICE OF XXX MD		12/12/94-1330pm	12/12/94-1pm
	DIAGNOSIS *above*			
	OLD CHART TO UNIT:			
	DIET: *regular*			
	ALLERGIES:			
	VITAL SIGNS AS PER UNIT ROUTINE			
	CALL MD FOR T > 100.0 (oral), BP > 150/100 OR < 100/50, P > 100 or < 60			
	WEIGHT ON ADMISSION AND ONCE PER WEEK			
	IMMEDIATE RISKS (CIRCLE APPROPRIATE WORDS)			
	SUICIDE ATTEMPT OR SELF-INJURY: NOT SIGNIFICANT / SIGNIFICANT			
	ASSAULT: NOT SIGNIFICANT / SIGNIFICANT			*Fatima Ramos RN*
	FALLS: NOT SIGNIFICANT / SIGNIFICANT			
	SPECIAL OBSERVATION: (CIRCLE ONE) ARMS LENGTH / CONTINUOUS / FREQUENT		XXX	
	LABS, SMA6, CREATININE, ALK, PHS, TOTAL BIL., SGPT, SGOT, T3, T4, TSH			
	CBC WITH DIFF, STOOL GUIAC x 1 IF 50 YEARS OLD OR OLDER			
	RPR (VDRL)			
	U/A – IF CONTINENT			
	URINE FOR DRUG SCREENING			
	URINE FOR PREGNANCY IF FEMALE UNDER 50 YRS. OLD (STAT)			
	ECG IF OLDER THAN 35 YRS. OLD			
	MEDICATIONS:			
	STANDING MEDICATIONS:			
	PPD 5 TU 0.1 CC I.D. (UNLESS TESTED WITHIN SIX MONTHS)			
	Haldol 5mg P.O. H.S.			
	FOR AGITATION OR AGGRESSIVE BEHAVIOR			
	ADMINISTER PO: *Haldol 1mg P.O. q8h PRN agitation*			
	IF PO REFUSED, ADMINISTER IM: *Haldol 1mg IM q8h PRN*			
	aggressive behavior			

PRESCRIBER SIGNATURE XXX MD	PRINT NAME XXX MD	BEEPER NUMBER XXX

AUTHORIZATION IS GIVEN TO DISPENSE MEDICATION BY NON-PROPRIETARY NAME AS DETERMINED BY THE PHARMACY AND THERAPEUTICS COMMITTEE. A NON-FORMULARY REQUEST FORM IS REQUIRED IF MEDICATIONS ARE NOT INCLUDED IN THE FORMULARY.

PHYSICIAN'S ORDER

TRANSCRIBING ORDERS TO THE MAR

When transcribing orders to the MAR the nurse:

1. Uses the addressograph plate to affix the patient's name and medical record number.
2. Enters the patient's DSM-IV diagnosis by name and number.
3. Enters in red ink any known allergies.
4. Enters the patient's date of admission.
5. Enters the page number.
6. Dates MAR for 9 consecutive days upon transcription of first medication.
7. Enters the medication order date and expiration date in the column provided on the left side of the MAR.
8. Writes own initials to the left of order date column to verify orders after reviewing transcription, if it was done by a unit clerk or LPN.
9. Enter in the standing medication column, the name of the drug, dose, frequency, route, and special instructions if applicable.
10. Enters in the HOUR vertical column the time the medication is to be given by beginning with the earliest hour after midnight. A new line is used for each hour a dose is to be given. Midnight, morning, noon, and afternoon are identified by using mid, A.M., noon, and P.M. Each medication order has six lines. The same medication with different doses and times may be entered in the six lines. However, this must be legible to prevent administration errors.
11. Draws an X through the boxes for the days medication IS NOT to be administered.
12. Provides one space below line of initials, horizontally, to note vital signs that are to be taken prior to administration of indicated medications. Among these may be antidepressants, antipsychotics, benzodiazepines, cardiac medication, and others.
13. Documents omitted medication doses by placing the appropriate code number, circled (found on the legend at the start of the form) in red ink, above initials in the appropriate box.
14. Signs the order form after orders are transcribed, with time and date on the right side of the form for each applicable section. In case orders are transcribed by someone other than the RN, orders and transcription must be reviewed as reflected by RN's signature, time, and date.
15. Sends a copy of the physician's orders to the pharmacy.

TRANSCRIBING SINGLE, STAT, AND PRE-OP ORDERS

1. For single and STAT medications the nurse enters the date and time to be given. The nurse who gives the medication enters own initials at the time medication is given. See Box 54-3.
2. For preoperative orders the nurse writes "pre-op" next to the medication order, and the time the medication is to be given. The nurse who gives the medication enters own initials at the time medication is given.
3. Intravenous therapy is recorded in this section at the time the nurse hangs the bag.

PRN MEDICATIONS

PRN medications are recorded by entering:

1. The PRN medication order date and the expiration date. Nurse's initials are to be entered at the time the transcription is reviewed. See Box 54-4.
2. The name of the drug, dosage, route, frequency, and any special instructions in the appropriate space.
3. The date, time, nurse's initials, and site, when indicated, at the time medication is given.

BOX 54-3: Sample Medication Administration Record for Single, STAT, Pre-Op Orders

ORDER DATE	NURSE INIT.	MED-DOSE-ROUTE	TO BE GIVEN			ORDER DATE	NURSE INIT.	MED-DOSE-ROUTE	TO BE GIVEN		
			DATE	TIME	NURSE INIT.				DATE	TIME	NURSE INIT.
12/12	FR	PPD Stud. 1cc 10	12/12	7 pm	FR						

---

4. Reorder and expiration dates in the shaded area or second column on the left of form.
5. The nurse's initials in the reorder initial box on the left of the form, after reviewing reorder and expiration dates.
6. Identification of initials placed in the MAR. Nurses, unit clerks, and others authorized to write in the MAR must initial and print name and title in the space provided.

ADMINISTRATION OF MEDICATIONS

The nursing responsibilities in administering medication follow the nursing process (Taylor, 1984, p. 502).

Assessment   The nurse makes a complete assessment of the patient's drug history at the time of admission or later as part of a medication work-up. Areas to be assessed include the patient's
1. Prior and current experiences with prescription and nonprescription drugs
2. Reactions to various medications taken previously
3. Attitudes about medication

Planning   Before the patient is started on medication, the nurse begins teaching the patient and family about:
1. The purpose of the medication
2. Possible side effects
3. The patient's responsibilities while taking the medication

If the decision is made to have the patient self-administer the medication, more detailed instruction is necessary.

Implementation
1. Generally speaking, in inpatient settings, the nurse administers the medication. Prior to the administration of a drug the nurse must have a thorough knowledge of

BOX 54-4: Sample Medication Administration Record for PRN Medication

ORDER DATE / EXP. DATE	REORDER DATE / EXP. DATE	MED-DOSE-FREQ-ROUTE	P.R.N. MEDICATION — DOSES GIVEN							
FR RN INIT. 12/12/94 / RECORD INIT. 12/19/94		Haldol 1mg po Q8 hr. p.r.n. for agitation	DATE 12/13							
			TIME 1 pm.							
			SITE po							
			INIT FR							
FR RN INIT. 12/12/94 / RECORD INIT. 12/19/94		Haldol 1mg IM Q8 hr. p.r.n. for aggressive behavior	DATE							
			TIME							
			SITE							
			INIT							

INITIAL IDENTIFICATION

INITIAL	PRINT NAME, TITLE	INITIAL	PRINT NAME, TITLE	INITIAL	PRINT NAME, TITLE
1 FR	FATIMA RAMOS RN	5		9	
2		6		10	
3		7		11	
4		8		12	

the drug's absorption, destruction, biotransformation, and excretion. The nurse must also be aware of the therapeutic range, dosage schedule, and effects of the drug, including contraindications.

2. The nurse must be technically skilled in administering drugs orally, subcutaneously, and intramuscularly. It is rarely necessary to administer drugs intravenously in a psychiatric setting.

3. If the patient refuses to take the prescribed medication, the nurse has additional responsibilities. In most states, the patient has the right to refuse medication. The nurse must be familiar with the state's mental health code as it relates to giving patients medication against their will in an emergency situation. When a patient refuses medication, the nurse always documents this in the patient record and notifies the physician.

BOX 54-5: Sample Medication Omission Record

MEDICATION OMISSION RECORD
Every Entry Must Be Dated & Signed

DATE	HOUR	REMARKS
12/13	9 pm	Patient refused 9pm Haldol 5mg po medication Dr xx notified. Patient calm. F. Ramos, RN

Evaluation   The nurse evaluates the patient's response to the medication, including behavior, symptom reduction, side effects, tolerance, and attitude about taking the medication. This evaluation is an important part of the nurse's responsibility because many times several types of medication are tried before the right medication is found.

PROCEDURE

The nurse carries out the following steps in giving patients medication (Taylor, 1984, p. 505):

1. The nurse makes sure the medication label on the container corresponds with the MAR for each patient prior to dispensing the medication.
2. Medication is placed in appropriate medication cups and given to the patient.
3. Before administering medication, the nurse identifies each patient by checking the name band and asking the patient's name.
4. The nurse makes certain the patient receives and takes the medication at the time it is given. The patient is not allowed to carry off the medication to take later, nor is the medication left at the bedside.
5. If the patient refuses to take medication, the nurse indicates this on the patient's medication omission record with the reason and informs the physician. (See Box 54-5.) In some settings, the medication is returned to the pharmacy, and in others, unused medication is destroyed.
6. The nurse indicates medications administered at other times (for example, prn) in the patient record.
7. After medication is administered, the nurse initials and signs the patient's MAR before administering medication to the next patient.

CONTINUOUS QUALITY IMPROVEMENT

The clinical nurse manager and appointed members of the unit's quality improvement committee monitor assurance of standards in administration of medication and promote improvement in medication administration.

REFERENCE

Taylor, C. M. (1984). Administration of medications. In S. Lego (ed.), *The American Handbook of Psychiatric Nursing* (pp. 501–505). Philadelphia: J. B. Lippincott.

BIBLIOGRAPHY

Joint Commission on Accreditation of Healthcare Organizations (1994). *The Joint Commission: 1995 Accreditation Manual for Hospitals. Volume I: Standards.* Oakbrook Terrace, IL: JCAHO.

55
FIFTY FIVE

Special Observation

Fatima Ramos

OVERVIEW:

Standard of Care
Patient Care Outcomes
Standard of Practice
Levels of Special Observation

Routine Observation
Nursing Assessment
Nursing Interventions
Continuous Quality Improvement

STANDARD OF CARE

All psychiatric patients accepted for inpatient admission must be assessed to determine a need for special observation. In acute inpatient settings, often all newly admitted patients are placed on a determined level of special observation, such as "frequent observation," for the first 24 hours to promote a safe environment.

PATIENT CARE OUTCOMES

1. Patients will experience a safe and therapeutic environment in the inpatient unit.
2. Patients will not harm themselves or others.

STANDARD OF PRACTICE

Psychiatric nurses, psychiatrists, and other qualified staff gather assessment data to determine patients' needs for special observation. Psychiatric nurses, mental health workers, and psychiatric nursing attendants receive education, preferably from a psychiatric clinical nurse specialist, prior to being assigned to monitor psychiatric patients requiring special observation.

LEVELS OF SPECIAL OBSERVATION

Frequent Observation Patients requiring frequent observation are checked on by staff every 15 minutes. Usually patients are placed on this level of observation for the first 24 hours after admission. After 24 hours, patients are reassessed for the need to continue or discontinue this level of observation. In many hospitals, frequent observation is initiated by a psychiatric nurse without requiring a physician's order. However, there are hospitals where a physician's order is required to initiate or to discontinue this level of observation. Frequent observation is implemented when assessment of patients indicates the need for close observation by the nursing staff.

Continuous Observation Patients requiring continuous observation must be visually monitored by staff at all times. It is not unusual for one staff member to observe more than one patient on this level of observation in an area designated for patients who benefit from decreased stimuli. Remote television cameras may be another option used

457

to monitor patients on continuous observation. In most hospitals, physicians must assess the patients' need for continuous observation in a specified time frame. When a physician is not available to assess patients to determine the need for continuous observation, a psychiatric nurse may initiate the intervention and later obtain an order from the physician. Reassessment of patients is done daily.

One-to-One (1:1) Observation   Patients requiring 1:1 observation must be visually monitored at all times by one staff member observing one patient. In most hospitals, this intervention requires a physician's order; however, a psychiatric nurse is able to initiate the intervention without an order in an emergency. Most hospitals have a protocol specifying how often patients must be reassessed by a physician. Reassessment of patients is done at least daily.

Arm's Length Observation   For patients requiring arm's length observation, the above 1:1 observation procedure is instituted and, in addition, the staff member monitoring the patient must be within arm's length of the patient. This level of observation is usually implemented with patients who are highly self-destructive or suicidal and who are able to tolerate the proximity of staff members. A physician's order and reassessment are usually required daily.

ROUTINE OBSERVATION

Inpatient psychiatric units are required to have a method of monitoring all patients. In most hospitals, all patients are visually observed at least once every half hour around the clock. A written record of whereabouts of patients is kept. A physician's order is usually not required; however, admission orders may indicate it as "routine observation."

NURSING ASSESSMENT

During a psychiatric nursing admission assessment, or at any time during hospitalization, nurses reassess patients to determine their need for special observation and identify a plan of care accordingly (JCAHO, 1994).

NURSING INTERVENTIONS

Psychiatric nurses implement and supervise others in the implementation of special observation and routine observation. Documentation of patients on special observation is recommended for every shift or every 8 hours. At least weekly multidisciplinary team plans and nursing care plans are revised.

CONTINUOUS QUALITY IMPROVEMENT

The clinical nurse manager and appointed members of the unit's quality improvement committee monitor assurance of standards and promote improvement in observation of patients.

REFERENCE

Joint Commission on Accreditation of Healthcare Organizations (1994). *The Joint Commission: 1995 Accreditation Manual for Hospitals. Volume I: Standards.* Oakbrook Terrace, IL: JCAHO.

56
FIFTY SIX

Suicide Precautions

Fatima Ramos

OVERVIEW:

Standard of Care	Nursing Interventions
Patient Care Outcomes	Levels of Observation
Standard of Practice	Continuous Quality Improvement
Nursing Assessment	

STANDARD OF CARE

Psychiatric patients admitted for inpatient treatment who are deemed to be suicidal at the time of admission or any time thereafter will be placed on suicidal precautions to prevent them from injuring themselves.

PATIENT CARE OUTCOMES

1. Patients will not harm themselves or others.
2. Patients will explore nondestructive alternative ways of coping with stress, anxiety, or depression.

STANDARD OF PRACTICE

Psychiatric nurses implement or supervise the implementation of suicide precautions to promote safety and prevent injury to patients.

NURSING ASSESSMENT

Upon admission to an inpatient psychiatric unit, patients are assessed by psychiatric nurses for current and past history of suicidal ideation. If psychiatric nurses or other qualified clinicians identify patients to be at risk for suicide or self-destructive behavior, they must be assessed further to determine specifics such as whether:

1. Patients are experiencing passive suicidal thoughts and will not act on the thoughts or they are at risk for impulsively acting on suicidal thoughts.
2. Patients are experiencing active suicidal thoughts with a known or unknown plan.
3. Patients have a history of suicidal gestures and have chosen means to harm themselves that prove to be progressively more threatening to their life. (See Chapter 1 for Psychiatric Nursing Assessment and Chapter 24 for The Client Who Is Suicidal.)

NURSING INTERVENTIONS

Without delay, psychiatric nurses implement special observation of patients who are at risk for harming themselves or attempting suicide. In such a case, nurses may initiate suicidal precautions prior to obtaining a physician's order. Most acute inpatient hospital programs have policies dictating that nurses or other qualified staff inform the psychiatrist without delay to further evaluate patients who are at a significant risk for self-destructive behavior or attempting suicide. When indicated, the physician writes an order for a special level of observation and suicide risk or precautions. Nurses will then implement or assign others to implement procedures to ensure suicide precautions. A multidisciplinary team meeting is held, including the individual patient and family, to decide the most effective interventions to address the patient's safety needs. Other measures implemented at the same time suicide precautions are initiated and thereafter may include:

1. Requiring patients to change into hospital clothing or pajamas while being observed by a qualified staff member.
2. Checking through patients' belongings and their rooms to look for potentially harmful objects or contraband. If found, contraband items must be removed and disposed of appropriately.
3. Restricting patients from leaving the unit and from having visitors to ensure safety. However, this is usually a team decision, unless patients' safety is imminently at risk.
4. Closely monitoring visits and searching packages for contraband items including:
   - belts
   - glass objects
   - matches
   - cigarettes
   - sharp objects
   - shoelaces
   - weapons
   - alcohol
   - drugs
   - substances that if ingested may cause harm, such as nailpolish remover
5. Closely monitoring patients during meals, and restricting them from using certain utensils such as knives (see Styron, 1990).
6. Encouraging patients to talk about their self-destructive and suicidal ideation instead of acting out.
7. Using deescalation techniques such as time-out in their room or in the quiet room, where patients benefit from decreased stimuli. Time-out may be 15 minutes to 1 hour or longer. Usually a staff member closely monitors these patients as per level of observation indicated.
8. Using medication such as benzodiazepines or neuroleptics on a standing or prn basis, to help patients through the acute period of time, usually in combination with an antidepressant (see Chapter 67).
9. Using seclusion only when other less restrictive measures have been unsuccessful.
10. Using restraints only when other less restrictive measures have been unsuccessful.
11. Reassessing patients on suicide precautions daily. A physician's order may be required daily or upon change in the patient's condition.
12. Documenting in the progress notes, daily or at the close of every shift, and updating the multidisciplinary treatment plan or nursing care plan.

LEVELS OF OBSERVATION

Patients in need of suicide precautions will be placed on one of four levels of observation (see Chapter 55):

1. *Routine observation:* This level of observation is indicated for all patients on an inpatient unit. Patients who have been on special levels of observation progressively

advance to routine observation, usually prior to attaining off-unit privileges or out-of-hospital passes. Patients who have chronic suicidal thoughts without acute symptoms may be placed on routine observation, unless there is evidence to otherwise increase the level of observation.

2. *Frequent observation* (15-minute checks): This level of observation is indicated for patients who have expressed passive suicidal ideation and have agreed to approach staff to talk when they feel they may act on their suicidal thoughts or feel unsafe. This level of observation may also be beneficial for chronic self-destructive patients who do not intend to kill themselves.

3. *Continuous observation* (visual monitoring): This level of observation is indicated for patients expressing
   - Passive suicidal ideation who do not agree to approach staff when they feel unsafe.
   - Passive suicidal ideation who do not feel safe without staff supervision.
   - Active suicidal ideation with or without a plan, who are not severely psychotic or disorganized and in need of a higher level of observation.

   When implementing this level of observation, nurses monitor or supervise others who monitor patients constantly.

4. *One-to-one observation:* This level of observation is indicated:
   - When patients express active suicidal ideation with a plan and show determination in carrying out the plan as soon as they are not observed.
   - When patients who are not verbalizing their suicidal ideation are known to have made recent suicide gestures.
   - When patients show disorganized behavior and may inadvertently harm themselves.
   - When patients who are depressed and psychotic hear voices telling them to kill themselves, or who, for example, believe the devil wants them to die. These patients pose a high risk for attempting suicide while in an acute state.

5. *Arm's-length observation:* This level of observation is indicated for patients who are actively suicidal and have either harmed themselves already or have made a substantial gesture that could potentially cause serious injury or death. This level of observation may also be indicated for patients who constantly engage in self-destructive behavior owing to a medical condition, such as organic brain pathology.

CONTINUOUS QUALITY IMPROVEMENT

The clinical nurse manager and appointed members of the unit's quality improvement committee monitor assurance of standards and promote improvement in patient care delivery for suicidal patients.

REFERENCES

Joint Commission on Accreditation of Healthcare Organizations (1994). *The Joint Commission: 1995 Accreditation Manual for Hospitals. Volume I: Standards.* Oakbrook Terrace, IL: JCAHO.

Styron, W. (1990). *Darkness Visible.* New York: Random House.

FIFTY SEVEN

Homicide/Aggression Precautions

Fatima Ramos

OVERVIEW:

Standard of Care
Patient Care Outcomes
Standard of Practice
Nursing Assessment
Frequent Observation

Continuous Observation
Least Restrictive Alternative
Documentation
Continuous Quality Improvement

STANDARD OF CARE

Psychiatric patients deemed to be homicidal or aggressive at the time of admission or any time thereafter will be placed on homicide/aggression precautions to prevent them from injuring themselves or others and to promote their safety.

PATIENT CARE OUTCOMES

1. Patients will not harm themselves or others.
2. Patients will establish a therapeutic relationship with at least one member of the therapeutic treatment team.

STANDARD OF PRACTICE

Psychiatric nurses implement or supervise the implementation of homicide/aggression precautions to prevent injury to patients and others, and to promote a safe environment.

NURSING ASSESSMENT

Upon admission to an inpatient psychiatric unit, patients are thoroughly assessed for past and current history of homicide ideation or aggressive and violent behavior toward others and property. When patients are identified to be homicidal or potentially violent, they are placed on homicide/aggression precautions. The level of observation is determined by the extent of the potential for violence. Patients are reassessed daily for appropriate level of observation. Movement from one level to another may require a physician's order. In an emergency, nurses may move patients from frequent to continuous observation without an order.

FREQUENT OBSERVATION

Frequent observation (see Chapter 55) is used when patients:
1. Have a history of homicidal or assaultive behavior

2. Experience passive homicidal or aggressive thoughts but are comfortable approaching staff when they think they might act on these thoughts
3. Experience active homicidal or aggressive thoughts but are comfortable approaching staff when they think they might act on these thoughts
4. Have made verbal threats toward other patients or staff
5. Exhibit unpredictable behavior

CONTINUOUS OBSERVATION

Continuous observation (see Chapter 55) is used when patients:
1. Experience passive homicidal or aggressive thoughts but are *not* comfortable or willing to discuss these with staff
2. Experience active homicidal or aggressive thoughts but are *not* comfortable or willing to discuss these with staff
3. Exhibit behaviors such as:
   - Verbally threatening others
   - Clenched fists
   - Paranoid or suspicious behavior
   - Hallucinations of an aggressive nature
   - Delusions of an aggressive nature
   - Angry facial expression
4. Act aggressively toward other patients or staff

LEAST RESTRICTIVE ALTERNATIVE

Nurses always choose the least restrictive alternative in managing homicidal or aggressive behavior, while maintaining safety. The alternatives moving from least restrictive to most restrictive are:
1. Frequent observation and communication about thoughts and feelings with a staff member
2. Continuous observation and communication about thoughts and feelings with a staff member
3. Medication
4. Seclusion
5. Restraints

Regardless of level of observation, the nurse is always available to talk with patients about any of their aggressive thoughts and feelings.

DOCUMENTATION

Documentation includes:
1. Detailed description of the patient's behavior
2. Precautions that were instituted
3. Nurse–patient communication
4. Daily reassessment of precautions
5. Evaluation of patient's response to interventions

CONTINUOUS QUALITY IMPROVEMENT

The clinical nurse manager and appointed members of the unit's quality improvement committee monitor assurance of standards and ways in which nursing care delivery might be improved.

BIBLIOGRAPHY

Joint Commission on Accreditation of Healthcare Organizations (1994). *The Joint Commission: 1995 Accreditation Manual for Hospitals. Volume I: Standards.* Oakbrook Terrace, IL: JCAHO.

Elopement Precautions

Fatima Ramos

<table>
<tr><td>OVERVIEW:</td><td>Standard of Care</td><td>Nursing Interventions</td></tr>
<tr><td></td><td>Patient Care Outcomes</td><td>Procedure</td></tr>
<tr><td></td><td>Standard of Practice</td><td>Continuous Quality Improvement</td></tr>
<tr><td></td><td>Nursing Assessment</td><td></td></tr>
</table>

STANDARD OF CARE

Psychiatric patients admitted for inpatient treatment may be placed on elopement precautions at the time of admission or at any time throughout their hospitalization. Elopement precautions are a set of interventions aimed at preventing patients from leaving or escaping from the hospital without valid notice.

PATIENT CARE OUTCOMES

1. Patients will remain safe in the inpatient unit.
2. Patients will individually establish a therapeutic relationship with at least one member of the treatment team.

STANDARD OF PRACTICE

Psychiatric nurses implement or supervise the implementation of elopement precautions to prevent patients from leaving or escaping the hospital. Prior to being allowed to leave the hospital, patients have a valid written pass or discharge order, and in some cases patients have gained privileges to leave the hospital. Patients placed on elopement precautions do not have privileges to leave the hospital or the inpatient unit.

NURSING ASSESSMENT

When a psychiatric nurse collects data that indicate patients are at risk for escaping or leaving the inpatient unit without valid notice, the nurse initiates the procedure for elopement precautions without delay. The nurse then conducts a thorough assessment of the patient by interviewing the patient and staff.

NURSING INTERVENTIONS

A psychiatric nurse initiates the procedure for elopement precautions as soon as it is determined necessary. The physician, the nursing supervisor, and sometimes hospital security and the family are then notified. Under certain circumstances, the police may also be notified. A multidisciplinary team meeting is held, including the patient, to address the patient's care needs and to decide the most effective interventions and appropriate protocol. The psychiatric nurse initiating the elopement precautions procedure must communicate this clearly with other staff verbally and in writing, usually via shift report. Documentation of patients requiring elopement precautions is recommended at least every shift. Nurses are careful to talk with patients at any time about their desire to leave the hospital, and to reassure them about the importance of remaining in the hospital for treatment.

PROCEDURE

Patients assessed to be in need of elopement precautions may be placed on one of three levels of observation:

1. Frequent observation
2. Continuous observation
3. 1:1 observation

Other interventions may include:

1. Requiring patients to change into bedclothes supervised by staff
2. Inspecting or checking patients' belongings and room for keys and potentially harmful objects
3. Requiring patients to wear bedclothes or pajamas only while on precautions
4. Identifying patients on precautions in the census sheet and flow sheet or record used to document observation of patients

CONTINUOUS QUALITY IMPROVEMENT

The clinical nurse manager and other members of the unit's quality improvement committee will monitor incidents of elopement and effective use of precautions, as well as ways to improve quality of patient care.

REFERENCE

Joint Commission on Accreditation of Healthcare Organizations (1994). *The Joint Commission: 1995 Accreditation Manual for Hospitals. Volume I: Standards.* Oakbrook Terrace, IL: JCAHO.

59

FIFTY NINE

Fall Precautions

Fatima Ramos

OVERVIEW:

Standard of Care
Patient Care Outcome
Standard of Practice

Nursing Assessment
Nursing Interventions
Continuous Quality Improvement

STANDARD OF CARE

Patients admitted for inpatient treatment at risk for falls are placed on the appropriate level of fall precautions.

PATIENT CARE OUTCOME

Patients will be protected from falls in a safe environment using the least restrictive interventions.

STANDARD OF PRACTICE

The psychiatric nurse places patients at risk for falls on the appropriate level of fall precautions upon admission and any time thereafter to meet patient care needs.

NURSING ASSESSMENT

On admission psychiatric patients' risk for falls must be assessed thoroughly and reassessed as needed. Assessment includes:
1. Gait and balance assessment (see Box 59-1)
2. Vital signs, i.e., assessment of orthostatic blood pressure and pulse, respirations, and temperature
3. Mental status assessment to determine the following risk factors:
   a. Confusion
   b. Disorientation to person, place, and time
   c. Inability to understand or to follow directions
   d. Marked memory and judgment impairment
4. Physical and other risk factor assessment (see Box 59-2)

NURSING INTERVENTIONS

The nurse analyzes the data collected in the assessment and selects the appropriate level of fall precautions (see Table 59-1). Patients identified to be at risk for falls are placed on a specific level of fall precautions. Depending on hospital policy, a physician's order may or may not be required to place patients on fall precautions with specific level identified. The multidisciplinary treatment plan may be sufficient to identify a patient on fall precautions. For example, a patient treatment plan may state that a patient is on "Fall Precautions Level II." In addition:

BOX 59-1: Gait and Balance Assessment

Check applicable space below

1. Patient sits in a chair without difficulty ☐
      with difficulty ☐

2. Patient stands and remains in place for 30 seconds without difficulty ☐
      with difficulty ☐

3. Patient walks across the room and turns around without difficulty ☐
      with difficulty ☐

4. Patient is able to return to chair and sit in it without difficulty ☐
      with difficulty ☐

Notes: Patients experiencing difficulty may have loss of balance, swaying, lurching, falling, or holding onto furniture or wall for support.

Document findings of patient's gait and balance assessment in the admission assessment profile and in the reassessment notes.

BOX 59-2: Assessment Form for Risk Factors for Falls

1. ____ Seizure disorder

2. ____ Decreased mobility

3. ____ Nocturia, urgency, and incontinence

4. ____ Over 70 years of age

5. ____ Status post ECT

6. ____ Sight impairment

7. ____ History of falls

8. ____ On a drug/alcohol withdrawal protocol

9. ____ Complaints of dizziness/ lightheadedness

10. ____ Use of ambulatory devices (walker, cane, crutches, wheelchair, orthopedic leg)

11. ____ Use of restraining devices (vest, siderails, and others)

12. ____ Specify other: _____
      _____

---

1. At the time of admission or soon thereafter, patients are given a tour of surroundings and an orientation to unit routines.
2. The patient unit, especially walkways, is kept free of clutter.
3. Patients identified to be at risk for falls are assessed upon admission and reassessed at least weekly thereafter.
4. Patients needing support devices are encouraged to use the devices appropriately.

CONTINUOUS QUALITY IMPROVEMENT

The clinical nurse manager and members of the unit's Quality Improvement Committee monitor data collection on patient falls and investigate each event to improve patient care delivery.

TABLE 59-1
Nursing Assessment and Intervention Levels with
Patients at Risk of Falling

ASSESSMENT	INTERVENTION
Level 1 • Patients have trouble with balance and have an unsteady gait, sometimes with dizziness. • Patients have one of the risk factors listed in Box 59-2.	• Help with walking, dressing, use of bathroom, arranging meal trays. • Place patient on frequent observation.
Level 2 • Patients have trouble with balance and an unsteady gait, sometimes with dizziness. • Patients have one of the risk factors listed in Box 59-2. • Patients experience mild to marked mental status impairment.	• Help with walking, dressing, use of bathroom, arranging meal trays. • Provide cloth rubber-soled bedroom slippers. • Teach patients with dizziness owing to orthostatic changes to sit up slowly and to rest a short time before standing and walking. • Move patient close to the nurse's station and post above suggestions by bed. • Place patient on continuous observation.
Level 3 • Patients have marked difficulty with gait and balance, sometimes with dizziness. • Patients have two or more of the risk factors listed in Box 59-2. • Patients experience severe mental status impairment and may be confused.	• All of the above. • Reorient patient as needed. • Place patient on 1:1 or arm's length observation.

BIBLIOGRAPHY   Joint Commission on Accreditation of Healthcare Organizations (1994). *The Joint Commission: 1995 Accreditation Manual for Hospitals. Volume I: Standards.* Oakbrook Terrace, IL: JCAHO.

60
SIXTY

Use of Seclusion and Restraints

Fatima Ramos

OVERVIEW:

Standard of Care
Patient Care Outcomes
Standard of Practice
Assessment

Phases of Nursing Intervention
Seclusion
Restraints
Continuous Quality Improvement

STANDARD OF CARE

In a hospital setting, psychiatric patients who present a danger to themselves or others may require emergency interventions such as *seclusion* and *restraints* when other less restrictive interventions have proven to be unsuccessful.

PATIENT CARE OUTCOMES

Patient will be maintained in a safe environment where:
1. The therapeutic process or medications are used to maintain control of homicidal or suicidal thoughts and feelings.
2. Seclusion or restraints are used only in emergencies.

STANDARD OF PRACTICE

Psychiatric nurses and other members of the therapeutic team attempt to manage aggressive or self-destructive behavior with the therapeutic relationship or medication. When these measures fail, they use seclusion or restraints in a safe, nonthreatening manner.

ASSESSMENT

Psychiatric nurses and other members of the therapeutic team receive education about assessment and therapeutic interventions used to deescalate patients who become aggressive or violent toward themselves or others. In emergencies psychiatric nurses initiate and carry out the use of seclusion and restraints without first attaining doctor's orders. Depending on regulatory codes and hospital policy, a psychiatrist may be required to further assess the need for seclusion or restraints and write orders. The nurse manager for the unit or a member of nursing administration may require immediate notification for the purpose of continuous quality improvement. Psychiatric nurses will also make a determination about patient care needs for patients requiring a language or a sign translator or requiring alternative care standards owing to retardation.

PHASES OF NURSING INTERVENTION

The psychiatric nurse considers three phases in the treatment of patients exhibiting aggressive and violent behavior toward themselves and others.

Phase I Proactive approach to attempt to deescalate behavior that might become dangerous to patients and others. This should occur prior to implementation of seclusion and restraints. (See Table 60-1.)

TABLE 60-1
Proactive Approaches in the Nursing Care of Psychiatric Patients Manifesting Aggressive Behavior

PATIENT BEHAVIOR	NURSING INTERVENTION
Patients raise their voices, use profane language, make threats to destroy property, kick the wall, spill food, and so forth.	The psychiatric nurse communicates with the individual patient in an empathic manner by: 1. Acknowledging that patient is upset. 2. Encouraging patient to talk about thoughts and feelings. 3. Exploring acceptable ways of dealing with anger and frustration. 4. If it is evident the patient cannot express thoughts and feelings, the patient is encouraged to go into a quiet area of the unit, alone or with special observation, to have time out away from others. When possible, intervention outlined in (3) is followed.

Phase II Active approach using seclusion and restraints to manage emergencies to prevent harm to patients and others. (See Box 60-1.)

BOX 60-1: Responding to a Psychiatric Emergency

1. Staff members are summoned to the scene.
2. A nurse takes charge, assigning tasks to other team members and providing direction throughout the emergency.
3. Other patients are cleared from the area and a staff member remains with them to allay their anxiety.
4. One nurse only communicates reassuringly with the aggressive patient throughout the emergency, as communication with a number of staff members may increase the patient's anxiety.
5. One staff member immobilizes each limb, keeping it close to the body, and the patient is carried to the seclusion room or to a restraint-ready bed.
6. Team members leave the area when dismissed by the leader.
7. A nurse documents the emergency process in the patient's record.
8. Team members attend a postemergency conference to discuss and evaluate the event, with a view toward improving emergency care.

Phase III Postactive approach to include debriefing of patient with staff, nursing documentation in the progress record, or automated data entry and quality improvement.

SECLUSION

Description Patients are confined in a small secured room with a soft, thin, indestructible mattress and no furniture. Seclusion may require either a nurse's or a physician's order in compliance with regulatory state mental health codes. The seclusion room must meet regulatory mental health standards that include size of a single-bedded room, adequate ventilation and temperature, wall surface without sharp edges, ceiling surface without exposed grid or hooks, a safety-installed camera, a corner plastic surveillance mirror, and a safety door that locks with a Plexiglas window at eye level. The room must always be cleaned between each patient use.

Contraindications Seclusion may not be indicated as an appropriate intervention for patients with the following conditions:
1. Mental retardation or developmental arrest
2. Inability to ambulate or placement on fall precautions
3. Cardiac ailment or complaints of chest pain
4. Seizure disorder
5. History of self-inflicting injury such as head-banging
6. High-risk pregnancy and third-trimester pregnancy
7. Fever
8. Respiratory distress

Nursing Intervention See Table 60-2 for nursing interventions and rationales with patients in seclusion.

TABLE 60-2
Nursing Care of Patients Placed in the Seclusion Room

NURSING INTERVENTION	RATIONALE
1. Prior to initiation of seclusion, the procedure and purpose of seclusion are explained to the patient, preferably by the staff assigned as the communicator.	1. To help decrease the patient's anxiety and maintain the therapeutic process.
2. The psychiatric nurse assuming the leadership role remains in the area to direct the procedure using the team approach.	2. To provide direction to trained staff who may be summoned from other departments or units.
3. The patient is escorted or, if necessary, carried into the seclusion room as a "whole unit" by the assigned staff.	3. Once the decision for use of seclusion is made, the psychiatric emergency team stays with the patient until the patient is safely escorted or carried to seclusion.
4. The patient's limbs are kept close to the body.	4. To prevent injury to the patient and staff.
5. Vital signs are taken.	5. To assess if patient's blood pressure is too low to tolerate medication.
6. Medication is administered intramuscularly.	6. To calm patient.
7. The patient is usually helped by staff to change into hospital pajamas or into the patient's own pajamas. This will allow staff to search the patient and belongings.	7. To assure the patient is free of contraband or objects that might be used to harm self or others.

(Continued)

TABLE 60-2 *(continued)*

NURSING INTERVENTION	RATIONALE
8. The communicator reiterates to the patient in simple clear language the procedure while in seclusion and the patient's expected behavior prior to and after leaving the seclusion room.	8. To provide support, decrease the patient's anxiety, and encourage the patient to use self-control.
9. The leader or charge nurse assigns a qualified staff member to special observation of the patient for the duration of seclusion. Depending on state law and hospital protocol, patients may be either on 15-minute checks or continuous observation.	9. To ensure safety, provide reassurance, and monitor the patient's condition. The patient must be visible to staff either every 15 minutes or continuously via a surveillance camera.
10. Seclusion is interrupted at least hourly by a team of staff. A registered professional nurse conducts an assessment of the patient that includes vital signs and mental status. Hydration, food, toileting, hygiene, and prn medication may be offered at this time if indicated. The nurse evaluates the need for continuation of seclusion.	10. To ensure safety and physical well-being and assess further need for seclusion.
11. Only authorized staff may unlock the seclusion room to allow the patient to leave except when patients need to be evacuated from the unit, such as in case of a fire.	11. To ensure effectiveness and efficiency of patient care.
12. Upon reassessment of patient, a registered nurse discontinues seclusion before the physician's order expires.	12. To provide least restrictive environment.
13. Episodes of seclusion must be followed by a debriefing of the patient and staff. Patients are asked what methods of calming work best for them and their preferences in acceptable deescalation techniques by staff.	13. To facilitate understanding of how future situations might be better handled.
14. Upon termination of seclusion, patients are encouraged to gradually return to the milieu.	14. To gradually normalize patients' behavior and to reassure patients they will be able to maintain self-control.
15. Nursing documentation must include (a) seclusion flow sheet, (b) nurse-written or automated documentation regarding events that led to use of seclusion, alternative interventions attempted and patient's responses, and time.	15. To comply with federal/state regulations.

Documentation See Box 60-2 for a sample physician's order sheet and Box 60-3 for a sample seclusion room flow sheet.

RESTRAINTS

Description When seclusion is considered inadequate as a way of protecting a patient and managing aggressive behavior, patients are placed in physical or mechanical devices used to involuntarily contain movement. According to the New York State Office of Mental Health Final Recommendations on the Use of Restraint and Seclusion, the move is toward "reduction of the use of all types of restraint" (New York State Office of Mental Health, 1994). Four-point restraints of leather or Velcro materials are the most widely used restraining devices in inpatient psychiatric units. To use these devices safely, psychiatric units are equipped with restraint-ready beds.

BOX 60-2: Sample Physician's Order Sheet for Seclusion or Restraints

ST. BARNABAS HOSPITAL
PHYSICIAN'S ORDERS

ADDRESSOGRAPH HERE

1. All orders must include date, time, prescriber's signature, printed name and beeper number.
2. Begin a new section for each set of orders. A set of orders may require more than one section. Prescriber must sign each section.

Diagnosis

Drug Allergies

Date & Time	DO NOT USE THIS SHEET UNLESS A RED NUMBER SHOWS ⟶ ◯	USE BLACK BALLPOINT PEN ONLY	W.C. Sig., Date, Time	R.N. Sig., Date, Time
	SECLUSION/RESTRAINTS			
	SECLUSION OR TYPE OF RESTRAINT:			
	INDICATION:			
	STARTING AND ENDING TIME:			
	ALTERNATIVES ATTEMPTED:			
	PHYSICAL DISTRESS RULED OUT:			
	INDICATIONS FOR REMOVAL:			
	SPECIAL INSTRUCTIONS:			

PRESCRIBER SIGNATURE	PRINT NAME:	BEEPER NUMBER

AUTHORIZATION IS GIVEN TO DISPENSE MEDICATION BY NON-PROPRIETARY NAME AS DETERMINED BY THE PHARMACY AND THERA-PEUTICS COMMITTEE. A NON-FORMULARY REQUEST FORM IS REQUIRED IF MEDICATIONS ARE NOT INCLUDED IN THE FORMULARY.

PHYSICIAN'S ORDER
PHARMACY COPY

Courtesy St. Barnabas Hospital, Bronx, NY.

BOX 60-3: Sample Seclusion Room Flow Sheet

ST. BARNABAS HOSPITAL
PSYCHIATRIC UNIT

SECLUSION ROOM FLOWSHEET

Observations and interventions are entered on this
sheet every 15 minutes by staff assigned to
observe patients.

ADDRESSOGRAPH HERE

DATE: _____

Name and title of staff initiating seclusion: _____

Name and physician notified: _____

Census: _____

Name of Nursing Supervisor notified: _____

# of Staff Present: _____

Patient gowned: _____   Patient searched: _____

Alternatives attempted prior to use of seclusion: _____

Care of Patient in Seclusion

TIME	VITAL SIGNS QIHR	MEDICATION DISPENSED	FLUID/FOOD	TOILETING	HYGIENE	REST	SLEEP	COMMENTS: RESPONSE TO MEDICATION/ BEHAVIORS OBSERVED	STAFF INIT.
									RN
									RN

Courtesy St. Barnabas Hospital, Bronx, NY.

Nursing Intervention See Table 60-3 for nursing interventions with patients in restraints.

Documentation See Box 60-2 for a sample physician's order sheet. Nurses document patients' responses to restraints in the restraint flow sheet. See Box 60-4.

TABLE 60-3
Nursing Care of Patients in Four-Point Restraints

NURSING INTERVENTION	RATIONALE
1. The nurse explains the procedure and purpose of restraints to the patient while in view of team members and remains with the patient to provide reassurance.	1. To allay the patient's anxiety and to communicate clearly to the patient and staff what will be happening
2. The leader provides direction to escort or carry the patient into a restraint-ready bed, preferably in the patient's room.	2. To provide safety for the patient and others
3. The patient is helped into bed. While one or two staff members apply the restraints, an adequate number of staff immobilize the patient, taking care to avoid physical discomfort for the patient. Restraints are applied to all four extremities to hold the patient without causing physical pain.	3. To provide safety and comfort for the patient and others
4. The patient may then be body searched for contraband and materials that may cause harm.	4. To provide safety for the patient and others
5. Vital signs are taken prior to administration of medication.	5. To be sure the patient's blood pressure is high enough to tolerate medication
6. The patient is given medication intramuscularly.	6. To calm patient
7. The nurse assigns a qualified staff member to observe the patient continuously and care for the patient.	7. To be sure the patient is safe and that bodily needs are met
8. State mental health codes will determine the duration of restraints and persons needing notification of the use of restraints. The unit chief or medical director and the clinical nurse manager must be notified for the purpose of continuous quality improvement.	8. To ensure compliance with standards and continuously improve the quality of care

9. At least hourly, the nurse:
   a. Conducts an assessment of the patient that includes vital signs, respiratory status, circulation and skin checks, and mental status.
   b. Provides relief from restraints by releasing one limb at a time and providing active range of motion exercises.
   c. Provides hydration, food, and toileting.
   d. Evaluates need for continuation of restraints.
	9. To ensure safety and physical well-being and assess further need for restraints

10. If restraints are no longer needed, the nurse releases the patient from restraints before the physician's order expires.	10. To provide least restrictive environment
11. The use of restraints must be followed by a debriefing of individual patients and staff. Patients are asked about methods of calming that work best for them and preferences in acceptable deescalation techniques used by staff.	11. To reduce patient's anxiety and provide information for future planning
12. Upon termination of restraints, patients are encouraged to gradually return to the milieu.	12. To gradually normalize patients' behavior and to reassure patients they will be able to maintain self-control

13. Nursing documentation must include:
   a. Four-point restraint flow sheet
   b. Nurse's written or automated documentation regarding:
     • Events that led to the use of restraints
     • Alternative interventions attempted and patient's responses
     • Time of initiation and time of discontinuation of restraints, patient's mood, affect, and psychomotor behavior
	13. To comply with federal/state regulations

BOX 60-4: Sample Restraint Flow Sheet

ST. BARNABAS HOSPITAL
PSYCHIATRIC UNIT

ADDRESSOGRAPH HERE

FOUR-POINT RESTRAINTS FLOWSHEET

Observations and interventions are entered on this
sheet every 15 minutes by staff assigned to
observe patients.

DATE: _____

Name and title of staff initiating 4-point restraints: _____

Name and physician notified: _____   Census: _____

Name of Nursing Supervisor notified: _____   # of Staff Present: _____

Patient gowned: _____   Patient searched: _____

Alternatives attempted prior to use of restraints: _____

Care of Patient in 4-Point Restraints

TIME	VITAL SIGNS QIHR	MEDICATION DISPENSED	FLUID/FOOD	TOILETING	HYGIENE	REST	SLEEP	RANGE OF MOTION EXERCISES QIHR	COMMENTS: RESPONSE TO MEDICATION/ BEHAVIORS OBSERVED	STAFF INIT.
										RN
										RN

Courtesy St. Barnabas Hospital, Bronx, NY.

CONTINUOUS QUALITY IMPROVEMENT

A psychiatric nurse manager or designee meets with the Continuous Quality Improvement Committee to reassess nursing procedures for seclusion and restraints.

REFERENCE

New York State Office of Mental Health (1994). *Final Recommendations on the Use of Restraints and Seclusion*. Albany, NY: The Office of Mental Health.

BIBLIOGRAPHY

Joint Commission on Accreditation of Healthcare Organizations (1994). *1995 Accreditation Manual for Hospitals. Volume I: Standards*. Oakbrook Terrace, IL: JCAHO.

61

SIXTY ONE

Electroconvulsive Therapy

Linda M. Fitzsimons
Fatima Ramos

OVERVIEW:

Standard of Care
Patient Care Outcome
Standard of Practice
Description
Background
Indications for Use
Special Populations
Contraindications

Pre-ECT Teaching
Equipment and Medications
Nursing Interventions
Treatment Monitoring
Recovery
Side Effects
Postictal Agitation
Continuous Quality Improvement

STANDARD OF CARE

Patients will receive safe and effective electroconvulsive therapy (ECT) in a protective environment.

PATIENT CARE OUTCOME

Patients will achieve the therapeutic effects of ECT with a minimum of anxiety.

STANDARD OF PRACTICE

The ECT nurse and physician, psychiatric nurses, and other qualified professionals make efforts to determine that ECT is warranted and implemented using the most effective and safe protocols.

DESCRIPTION

After more than 50 years and despite decades of controversy, electroconvulsive therapy (ECT) remains a major treatment for specific psychiatric disorders. In the United States, ECT is usually administered three times a week. The total number of treatments given during a course varies, with the average being nine. The techniques for administering ECT have improved considerably since its introduction and ECT helps 70–90% of depressed people who receive it.

ECT is administered to produce a profound antidepressant, antipsychotic, or antimanic therapeutic effect, through elicitation of an artificially induced grand mal seizure. During the ECT procedure, a small amount of electrical current is passed to the brain. ECT can be administered either bilaterally or unilaterally. With bilateral ECT, stimulus electrodes are placed in a frontotemporal position, symmetrically on both sides of the head. With right unilateral ECT, one electrode is in the same frontotemporal position as with bilateral ECT. The second electrode is typically placed over the ipsilateral hemisphere.

The electrical current induces a generalized grand mal seizure that affects brain centers controlling mood, appetite, and sleep. ECT is believed to correct the biochemical abnormalities that underlie severe depressive illness. A seizure alone is not sufficient to produce the desired therapeutic effect. A combination of factors including electrode placement and stimulus dosage is fundamental to achieving the effective therapeutic response. Until recently, standard practice dictated administering the same electrical dose to virtually all patients. It has recently been shown that the effect of stimulus intensity on efficacy is not associated with absolute electrical dose administered, but rather, whether the electrical dosage substantially exceeded the patient's individual seizure threshold.

BACKGROUND

In 1934, Laszlo Meduna, through intramuscular injections of camphor, deliberately induced generalized grand mal seizures, with the intent to treat psychoses (primarily schizophrenia). During the next decade, Metrazol was frequently used to chemically elicit seizures in patients with psychiatric disorders. Electroconvulsive therapy (ECT) was introduced by Cerletti and Bini in 1938. The clinical use of ECT greatly diminished with the introduction of psychotropic medications in the late 1950s. The 1980s saw the beginning of a new era in ECT research as a growing awareness of the limitations, safety issues, and side effects of psychotropic medications became apparent. Convulsive therapy is the somatic treatment with the longest continuous history of use in psychiatry (Abrams, 1992).

INDICATIONS FOR USE

Diagnostic indications are:

1. *Major depressive disorder:* ECT is mainly reserved for, but is not limited to, cases of major depressive disorder (all subtypes) and bipolar disorder, depressed, with one or more of the following characteristics:
   a. Failure to respond to adequate pharmacological treatment
   b. Presentation of severe symptomatology (e.g., severe major depression with suicidality, psychotic depression, debilitating psychiatric illness requiring a prompt antidepressant response)
   c. Previous optimal response to ECT, as ascertained by history
   d. Complicating medical conditions (e.g., heart disease, narrow-angle glaucoma) that could be worsened by psychotropic medications
   e. Adverse reactions to psychotropic medications (e.g., neuroleptic malignant syndrome, delirium, urinary retention, paralytic ileus) that contraindicate their use
2. *Mania:* ECT is also indicated for the treatment of mania (all subtypes). Reasons for referral should include one of the following:
   a. Ineffectiveness of pharmacological treatment strategies
   b. Prior optimal response to ECT
   c. Severe psychopathology requiring prompt intervention, e.g., manic delirium
3. *Schizophrenia:* ECT is sometimes indicated for the treatment of schizophrenia. Reasons for referral should include one of the following:
   a. Catatonia
   b. Prominent affective symptomatology
   c. Prior history of favorable response to ECT
   d. Ineffectiveness of pharmacological treatment strategies

SPECIAL POPULATIONS

1. *Elderly:* ECT may be used in the elderly, regardless of age. While there is some increased risk, particularly in those with preexisting cardiac abnormalities, there are no specific policies to alter the usual procedures for ECT. Appropriate modifications to decrease risk should be determined on a case-by-case basis by the ECT team.

2. *Pregnancy:* ECT is safe in all trimesters of pregnancy, and may pose less risk to the fetus than treatment with most psychotropic medications. Obstetric consultation should be obtained prior to ECT in all pregnant patients, and recommendations followed.

3. *Obsessive-compulsive disorder and Parkinson's disease:* The effectiveness of ECT in obsessive-compulsive disorder and in the short-term benefit of movement disorder in Parkinson's diseases remains uncertain.

CONTRAINDICATIONS

The contraindications for ECT should be considered relative rather than absolute. The American Psychiatric Association's Task Force Report (1990) on the practice of electroconvulsive therapy cites conditions in which the use of ECT would be associated with substantial risk and likelihood of serious morbidity or mortality. In each case, the expected benefits must be weighed against the possible risks. These specific conditions associated with increased risk include:

1. Space-occupying cerebral lesion, or other conditions associated with increased intracranial pressure
2. Recent intracerebral hemorrhage
3. Substantial anesthetic risk
4. Retinal detachment
5. Pheochromocytoma
6. Recent myocardial infarction with unstable cardiac function
7. Bleeding or otherwise unstable vascular aneurysm or malformation

PRE-ECT TEACHING

See Box 61-1 for a guide to pretreatment teaching.

BOX 61-1: Pre–Electroconvulsive Therapy Teaching

The nurse informs patients of the following facts and listens to their responses, answering any questions they may have:

1. ECT is a commonly used treatment for their disorder.

2. A low-voltage current is passed to the brain, but it causes no harm and no pain.

3. They will be asleep during the treatment.

4. Before the treatment they will:
   - have no food or drink after midnight
   - refrain from smoking in the morning
   - empty their bladder just before the treatment
   - have an IV line started

5. When they awaken they may be confused, but this feeling will pass in a few hours.

6. They may have a headache but will be given some medicine to stop it.

7. They may have temporary memory loss, and may want to write down important phone numbers, appointments, and so forth, before the treatment.

8. They will want to postpone any major decisions until a few weeks after their course of treatment ends.

A written instruction sheet with this information is provided to patients and their significant others.

EQUIPMENT AND MEDICATIONS

See Table 61-1 for a list of equipment and medications that are available during ECT.

TABLE 61-1
Equipment, Medications, Supplies, and Rationales for ECT

EQUIPMENT, MEDICATIONS, AND SUPPLIES	RATIONALE
1. ECT treatment device	1. Used to deliver electrical stimulus
2. ECG monitoring device	2. Used for essential cardiovascular monitoring
3. BP monitoring apparatus and stethoscope	3. Used to monitor hemodynamic changes
4. Oxygen delivery system and oxygen masks	4. Used to ensure oxygenation
5. Suction apparatus	5. Used to reduce copious secretions
6. Defibrillator	6. Used for emergency termination of atrial or ventricular fibrillation
7. EEG monitoring device	7. Provides accurate representation of seizure activity and duration
8. Pulse oximetry equipment	8. Measures oxygen saturation and airway management
9. Airways	9. Used for ventilatory dysfunction
10. Rubber mouth guards/bite blocks	10. Protects teeth and oral structures
11. IV bags/infusion sets	11. Used for intravenous access
12. Acetone/alcohol	12. Cleans skin prior to electrode placement
13. Gauze pads/tape	13. Promotes aseptic environment
14. Assorted syringes and needles	14. Used to administer medications
15. ECG/EEG electrodes and leads	15. Provides connection for cardiac and ictal monitoring
16. Electrode paste/gel	16. Improves current conduction and prevents temporal burns
17. ECG/EEG recording paper	17. Used for hard copy of cardiac and ictal activity
18. Emergency crash cart	18. Used for access to medications and supplies for emergencies
19. Anesthetic agent, e.g., Brevital	19. Provides brief anesthesia effect
20. Muscle relaxant, e.g., succinylcholine	20. Modifies motor seizure activity
21. Anticholinergic agent, e.g., atropine	21. Reduces risk of vagally mediated bradycardia; decreases salivary secretions
22. Diazepam (Valium)	22. Terminates prolonged seizure; relieves postictal agitation
23. Beta-blocking agents, e.g., esmolol	23. Controls cardiac and hemodynamic irregularities
24. Nitroglycerin	24. Treats arrhythmia

NURSING INTERVENTIONS

See Table 61-2 for nursing interventions before, during, and after ECT.

TABLE 61-2
Nursing Interventions and Rationales During ECT Treatments

NURSING INTERVENTION	RATIONALE
Pretreatment	
1. Ensure the patient has been kept NPO	1. Reduces possibility of vomiting and aspiration
2. Record vital signs	2. Provides baseline; alerts team to problems
3. Reassure patient	3. Reduces anxiety
4. Have patient void	4. Prevents voiding during treatment
5. Help patient onto stretcher	5. Ensures safety and promotes reassurance
6. Check patient's head for pins and jewelry and ensure hair is clean and dry	6. Prevents interference with electrical current
7. Remove jewelry, contact lenses, and hearing aids	7. Prevents interference with electrical current, loss of jewelry, lens, and hearing aid
8. Remove dentures or partial plate	8. Prevents aspiration; protects dentures and mouth
9. Apply ECG electrodes, begin baseline monitoring and connect patient to pulse oximeter	9. Establishes physiological monitoring
10. Insert IV line or help with procedure	10. Provides intravenous access
11. Check treatment orders to be sure they are recorded and complete	11. Ensures that physician's order required for each treatment is documented
12. Help with placement of bite block	12. Protects mouth and oral structures
13. Place BP cuff on extremity, and before succinylcholine is given, inflate cuff above patient's systolic BP	13. Occludes passage of muscle relaxant into extremity, facilitating observation of motor seizure
During Treatment	
1. Observe motor seizure in client and gently protect extremities	1. Ensures safety and prevents possible injury
2. Record time of motor seizure	2. Keeps record of length of motor seizure
Posttreatment	
1. Remove BP cuff from extremity	1. Permits normal circulation
2. After seizure ends, monitor BP and pulse every 1–2 minutes for 5 minutes, until a downward trend is observed	2. Determines if BP has returned to baseline within 5 minutes as it should
3. Remove EKG, EEG, and pulse oximeter	3. Promotes orientation and comfort
4. Call patient's name and begin to orient	4. Reduces anxiety
5. Offer reassurance regarding confusion and disorientation	5. Reduces anxiety and fear
6. Communicate to unit nurse any untoward incidents or effects of treatment	6. Ensures continuity of care

TREATMENT MONITORING

Two techniques are used simultaneously to monitor seizure duration during the ECT treatment:

1. The duration of the *motor* seizure is determined with the "cuff" technique. The flow of muscle relaxant to the limb (usually a wrist or foot) is prevented by inflating a blood pressure cuff substantially above the anticipated systolic pressure prior to relaxant infusion of succinylcholine. The cuff is deflated within a few seconds following seizure termination. The duration of motor seizure is recorded.

2. Seizure activity *in the brain* is monitored by electroencephalography, which should be continued until there is clear evidence that paroxysmal activity has terminated. Cardiac monitoring using a minimum of three leads is conducted during each treatment, and vital signs are monitored before, during, and following each ECT treatment until stabilization of ECT-related changes occurs. Interventions for cardiovascular and hemodynamic changes are conducted by the anesthesiologist in consultation with the ECT treatment team. Oxygen saturation should be near 100% during the procedure and monitored by oximetry.

RECOVERY

During the recovery period an anesthesiologist or nurse anesthetist monitors the patient:

1. Oxygenation is maintained by forced pressure, until resumption of adequate spontaneous respiration.

2. The teeth and hypopharynx are examined and secretions removed by suction, if necessary.

3. Monitoring of vital signs continues every 1–2 minutes until stabilization and return of consciousness.

4. After initial resumption of spontaneous respiration, consciousness, and orientation following the treatment, the patient is transported via stretcher into the recovery area.

5. Vital signs are taken every 15 minutes or more frequently if indicated, until the patient is stable.

6. Under the surveillance of the recovery room nurse, the patient is observed until significant reorientation occurs.

7. It is the responsibility of the ECT treatment team to manage any complications that arise.

8. Personnel subsequently responsible for posttreatment care, e.g., unit staff, are advised of specific problems presented by individual patients.

9. The condition of the patient, including vital signs and reaction to treatment, are documented by the ECT nurse and any adverse conditions are verbally communicated to the unit nurse.

SIDE EFFECTS

Headache, disorientation, and memory complaints appear to be the most common subjective side effects reported by patients during an ECT course. Nausea, tiredness, and muscle aches, which are reported less frequently, have been found to represent persistent somatic symptoms of depression rather than side effects of the treatment (Devanand & Fitzsimons, 1995). Complaint of headache is usually relieved with Tylenol or nonsteroidal anti-inflammatory drugs. Other less common side effects such as nausea may occur for up to 2 or 3 hours and then resolve. Patients often experience some memory loss following the completion of the treatments. This memory loss should gradually reverse itself over the course of several weeks, but some patients may never remember events that occurred during the weeks or months of hospitalization. ECT has a cumulative effect, and as patients progress through their ECT course, their cognition will most likely show signs of disturbance. Patients may ask about brain damage from ECT. It is important for nurses to be aware and to reassure patients that these cognitive side effects are transient and that scientific evidence concerning ECT, as it is done today, strongly indicates brain damage does not occur.

POSTICTAL AGITATION

Approximately 5–10% of patients receiving ECT develop a hyperactive delirium upon emergence from anesthesia, typically characterized by marked motor restlessness and agitation, incoherence, disorientation, and a fluctuating level of consciousness. Nurses should take precautions to safeguard the intravenous line in the event that medication is required to resolve the episode. Postictal agitation is a phenomenon that may last from a few minutes to an hour following seizure elicitation. In more severe cases, intravenous diazepam (Valium) in doses ranging from 2.5 mg to 20 mg is usually sufficient to treat this condition. In rare instances, higher doses of diazepam may be required. In patients with mild agitation, supportive management including reduction of external stimuli, quiet reassurances without undue bodily restraint, and continued reorientation usually suffice, until the patient is alert. Patients are never left alone during this period.

CONTINUOUS QUALITY IMPROVEMENT

The psychiatric nurse manager or designee leads the team to systematically assess and improve patient care delivery before, during, and after ECT.

REFERENCES

Abrams, R. (1992). *Electroconvulsive Therapy* (2nd ed.). New York: Oxford University Press.

American Psychiatric Association (1990). *The Practice of ECT: Recommendations for Treatment, Training, and Privileging*. A Task Force Report of the American Psychiatric Association. Washington, DC: American Psychiatric Press.

Devanand, D. P., & Fitzsimons, L. (1995). Subjective side effects during electroconvulsive therapy. *Convulsive Therapy, 11* (4), 232–240.

BIBLIOGRAPHY

Joint Commission of Accreditation of Health Care Organizations (1994). *1995 Accreditation Manual for Hospitals. Volume 1: Standards*. Oakbrook Terrace, IL: JCAHO.

Sackeim, H. A. (1988). Mechanisms of action of electroconvulsive therapy. In R. E. Hales & J. Frances (eds.), *Annual Review of Psychiatry*, vol. 7 (pp. 436–457). Washington, DC: American Psychiatric Press.

Sackeim, H. A., Prudic, J., Devanand, D. P., Kiersky, J., Fitzsimons, L., Coleman, E., & Settembrino, J. (1993). Effects of stimulus intensity and electrode placement on efficacy and cognitive effects of electroconvulsive therapy. *New England Journal of Medicine, 328*, 839–846.

62
SIXTY TWO

Teaching Self-Medication

Fatima Ramos

OVERVIEW:	Standard of Care	Nursing Interventions
	Patient Care Outcome	Patient and Family Education
	Standard of Practice	The Medication Group
	Nursing Assessment	Continuous Quality Improvement

STANDARD OF CARE

Patients in an inpatient setting requiring psychopharmacotherapy are educated about their medication as soon as they are ready to learn.

PATIENT CARE OUTCOME

Patients will learn about their medications to promote independence and reduce relapse.

STANDARD OF PRACTICE

Psychiatric nurses educate patients, their families, and significant others regarding psychopharmacotherapy.

NURSING ASSESSMENT

Psychiatric nurses assess and reassess patients to identify their level of readiness to learn about their medications. Nurses determine if patients may benefit from a medication group learning experience or an individualized experience, selecting the most effective medication educational experience for each patient. When appropriate, families and their significant others are included in the learning process.

NURSING INTERVENTIONS

Psychiatric nurses encourage patients to actively participate in individualized or group education regarding their medication treatment. Patients are usually given written information to reinforce individual or group educational experiences. The written material includes:
1. Name of medication
2. Specific symptoms medication will help eliminate
3. Usual dosage and time it is taken
4. Side effects
5. Usual treatment course

Table 62-1 shows nursing interventions and rationales for teaching self-medication.

TABLE 62-1
Teaching Self-Medication

NURSING INTERVENTION	RATIONALE
1. Meet with patient as soon as patient is ready to discuss goals for self-administration of medication.	1. To prepare patients who will be responsible for taking their own medications after discharge
2. Encourage patient to discuss any fears or concerns about taking medications.	2. To decrease anxiety and improve continuity of patient care
3. Provide medication education so patient will be able to state the following: • name of medication(s) • reasons for taking medication • exact dose of medication • appropriate time to take medication • probable course of psychopharmacotherapy • a wish to change the medication regimen will first be discussed with health care provider prior to any changes • a favorite way to remember to take medication on time • importance of informing other health care providers of medication treatment	3. To promote effective patient care delivery by encouraging independence and responsibility for own treatment
4. Provide patient with written medication information materials that can easily be understood.	4. To reinforce teaching experience
5. Schedule a time when patient can demonstrate technique for self-medication.	5. To demonstrate learning
6. Review step-by-step procedure prior to demonstration and observe patient throughout.	6. To decrease anxiety and increase knowledge of correct self-medication procedure
7. Ensure that patient takes all scheduled medication. Patients may at first practice self-medication with one or two medications; however, it is important to emphasize taking all prescribed medication on time.	7. To decrease anxiety and increase knowledge of correct self-medication procedure
8. Chart medications as received by patient in the medication administration record.	8. To follow usual recording procedure and to avoid medication errors
9. Document patient's response to teaching and reinforce as required.	9. To evaluate progress and reinforce teaching as required, for quality improvement purposes

PATIENT AND FAMILY EDUCATION

It is still a great challenge to ensure that psychiatric patients (especially those with propensity to become psychotic) take medication according to the prescribed regimen. Therefore, this topic must be discussed with patients and their significant others. Furthermore, patients and significant others must be encouraged to take an active role in patients' treatment after discharge from the hospital. (See Chapter 65 for the 24 steps in psychoeducation about medications.)

THE MEDICATION GROUP

Patients meet one to two times per week in a medication group as soon as the primary nurse and the nurse leading the group determine patients are ready to participate. Slides or posters are used to display pertinent information in an easy and clear form. Some programs may offer these groups in various languages depending on patient care needs and language skills of the nurses. Sessions may include:

1. Important facts about medications (see Chapter 65)
2. Antipsychotic medications (see Chapter 66)
3. Antidepressant medications (see Chapter 67)
4. Mood stabilizing medications (see Chapter 68)
5. Antianxiety and hypnosedative medications (see Chapter 69)

The medication group meets for 1 hour and is led by a psychiatric nurse and, when possible, a clinical pharmacist. Questions are encouraged, as well as any thoughts and feelings patients have about taking medications. Between groups patients are encouraged to talk to their primary nurses about their medication name, dose, and times. In the course of the group, patients learn (Sargent, 1984):

1. The reason for the medication
2. The importance of taking medication as prescribed
3. The length of time it takes for symptoms to return if medication is stopped
4. The side effects of the medications and how to treat them
5. Why and how medications may be changed
6. Where prescriptions can be filled
7. How much medications cost
8. How to ask for generic medication
9. How to keep track of the times that medications were taken
10. How to handle questions about medications from employers, co-workers, and friends
11. The effect of alcohol and illicit drugs ingested with medications
12. What foods and over-the-counter medications to avoid with certain medications
13. How long medications will be needed

The client may remain in the medication group throughout the hospital stay, but is ready to begin learning to self-administer medications when it is demonstrated that the client knows:

1. Name of medication and benefits
2. Dose
3. Time of day for each medication
4. Side effects
5. How to open bottle with safety cap
6. Why the previous points are important to know

CONTINUOUS QUALITY IMPROVEMENT

The psychiatric clinical nurse manager or designee leads the team to systematically assess and improve patient education in self-medication.

REFERENCE

Sargent, N. (1984). Teaching self-medication. In S. Lego (ed.), *The American Handbook of Psychiatric Nursing* (pp. 536–538). Philadelphia: J. B. Lippincott.

BIBLIOGRAPHY

Joint Commission on Accreditation of Health Care Organizations (1994). *1995 Accreditation Manual for Hospitals. Volume 1: Standards.* Oakbrook Terrace, IL: JCAHO.

63
SIXTY THREE

Documentation

Fatima Ramos
Susan L. Glodstein

OVERVIEW:

Standard of Care
Patient Care Outcomes
Standard of Practice
Components of the Patient Care Record
Guidelines for Recording Data
Admission Assessment/Legal Status
Interdisciplinary Treatment Plan

Daily Progress Notes
   Frequency
Reassessment
Patient/Family Education
Rating Scales
Discharge Note
Continuous Quality Improvement

STANDARD OF CARE

Patients have a patient care record with documented evidence of assessment; identified patient care needs; a treatment plan with goals, objectives, and strategies on how to effectively meet patient care needs; reassessment; patient care outcomes; discharge criteria; and a plan for continuity of care in an interdisciplinary and collaborative environment.

PATIENT CARE OUTCOMES

Documentation of satisfactory results related to comprehensive interdisciplinary and collaborative patient care delivery will be recorded.

STANDARD OF PRACTICE

Psychiatric professional registered nurses efficiently document evidence of providing comprehensive interdisciplinary and collaborative care to patients.

COMPONENTS OF THE PATIENT CARE RECORD

The patient's care record contains confidential written or automated information used for communication, coordination, evaluation, accountability, and improvement of patient care. The format for the patient care record follows:
1. Admission assessment/legal status
2. Multidisciplinary care plan
3. Daily progress notes
4. Reassessment
5. Patient/family education
6. Rating scales

7. Diagnostic data
8. Discharge notes

GUIDELINES FOR RECORDING DATA

1. Patient care records are legal documents and are kept confidential.
2. The patient's name and hospital identification number are included on each page (each entry if automated).
3. Data are legibly recorded as soon as possible to prevent distortion of facts.
4. Entries are dated and timed.
5. Facts and observations are reported objectively without passing judgment.
6. Abbreviations are used only when approved by the hospital.
7. The use of slang and coded language is avoided, unless it is a direct quote from a patient.
8. Entries are legibly signed with proper identified professional title.

ADMISSION ASSESSMENT/LEGAL STATUS

A thorough nursing assessment is included along with documentation of admission legal status.

INTERDISCIPLINARY TREATMENT PLAN

The interdisciplinary care plan includes the following:
1. Identification of patient and care providers. The primary nurse and the nurse therapist are identified along with other members of the interdisciplinary team.
2. Description of patient's initial participation and collaboration in the development of care plan.
3. Dates the care plan is reviewed and revised with description of patient's participation and approval of primary therapist or physician.
4. List of patient's assets or strengths and problems or care needs.
5. Measurable and observable goals and objectives with dates written, assigned discipline (to focus work with patient), and date of achieved goals and objectives.
6. Interventions—i.e., approaches and modalities to be used to facilitate favorable patient care outcomes.
7. Diagnoses as per the DSM-IV (Axes 1–5).

See Box 63-1 for a sample interdisciplinary treatment plan.

DAILY PROGRESS NOTES

Daily progress notes provide a concise record of the patient's response to the care plan and a way to communicate assessment, plans, interventions, and the patient's responses and relevant progress. Entries may include biological, psychosocial, and spiritual responses as well as any unique occurrences related to patient or care.

FREQUENCY

1. Newly admitted patients should have a nursing note each shift (days, evenings, and nights) for the first 24 hours of hospitalization.
2. Patients placed on frequent, continuous, 1:1, arm's length, and other special observation should also have a nursing note each shift.
3. Nursing notes should be written whenever significant events occur, such as prn/stat medication, time-out, physiological problems, seclusion, restraints, and so forth.
4. Patients on routine observation and without significant occurrences should have one nursing note per 24 hours.

BOX 63-1: Sample Interdisciplinary Treatment Plan

Date: 6/1/95   INTERDISCIPLINARY TREATMENT PLAN   Page: A1

Axis I:	ICD No.	Axis IV Stressors
Maj. depr., sing. epis, severe, without psychotic feat.	*296.23*	*Conflictual Relationships Family Discord*

Axis II:	ICD No.	Axis V
Axis II deferred	*0.00*	**Current GAF:** *20*

Axis III Dx: None

Highest GAF: *50*

Assets	Problem	Date Active	Date Resolved
Domicile *Employment* *Good physical health* *Intelligence*	*Depressed Mood* *Suicidal Ideas/Impulses*	*6/1/95* *6/1/95*	

Date	Legal Status	Expiration
6/5/95	*VOL*	*8/3/95*

Review Date	Participation
6/8/95	*Pt. unable to collaborate in treatment planning*

Problem: *Depressed Mood*

Objective:	Term	Date Achieved
Attends and participates in 2 activities daily (group therapy, movement group)	*Short term*	
Eats 3 balanced meals a day (1800 kcal)	*Short term*	
Mood will be free of depressive features in 2 weeks	*Short term*	
Sleeping 6–8 hours a night	*Short term*	
Will state 3 alternative strategies for managing stress	*Long term*	
Will state 3 feelings related to having a mental illness	*Long term*	
Will remain in outpatient treatment for 1 year	*Long term*	

Methods: *Activity Therapy Groups daily (AT)*
     Fluoxetine 20mg po QD (MD)
     Group Therapy 3 times a week (RN),
     Individual Therapy 3 times a week (CNS)

Problem: *Suicidal Ideas/Impulses*

Objective:	Term	Date Achieved
Absence of suicide attempts	*Short term*	
Cessation of suicidal impulses	*Short term*	
Will state 2 alternatives to inflicting harm to self	*Short term*	
Will immediately notify staff of suicidal thoughts or impulses	*Short term*	
Will state 3 plans for the future	*Long term*	

Methods: *Staff will assess patient at arms length (RN)*
     Staff will contract with patient not to hurt self (CNS, RN)
     Primary RN will meet with patient every shift to discuss issues (RN)

Primary Nurse: *Fatima Ramos, RN, MS, CS*
Primary Therapist: *Susan L. Glodstein, MS, RN, C*
Social Worker: *Iris Gordon*
Activities Therapist: *Carol Gaffney*
Other:

From St. Barnabas Hospital, Bronx, NY. Reprinted with permission.

The format for a daily note is as follows:
1. Date and time of note
2. Patient status (routine or special observation)
3. Description of mood and affect including suicidal and homicidal ideation when indicated
4. Description of patient's behavior
5. Nursing interventions including patient/family education
6. Patient's responses in general or specific to a particular intervention or modality of care
7. The nurse's signature and title at the end of the entry

See Box 63-2 for a sample daily progress note.

BOX 63-2: Sample Daily Progress Note

5-23-95   *Mr. Hall remains on continuous observation for suicidal ideation. Patient stated he continues to think about taking his life, but he would not attempt anything while in the hospital. He described his mood to be sad. His affect is flat. Patient is reclusive and evasive. He requires a great deal of encouragement to shower, dress, and take nourishments. Patient was able to use the time to talk about his thoughts and feelings during the usual 1:1 primary nurse–patient interaction. Patient continues to express lack of self-worth. He stated that antianxiety medication works to keep him calm. Written information regarding his medication was given to patient. Patient will remain on continuous observation.*

Fatima Ramos, RN, MSN, CS

REASSESSMENT

According to the Joint Commission on Accreditation of Health Care Organizations (JCAHO, 1994), patients must be reassessed frequently throughout the hospitalization. Reassessment of psychiatric patients should be documented as needed or at least once per week to update the patient care plan. The format for reassessment is as follows:
1. *Status of patient in relation to goals or objectives:* specific description regarding accomplishment or lack of accomplishment of goals set for the week or limited time period
2. *Goals/objectives:* at least one or two new goals or objectives or a revision of previous goals/objectives to become more relevant to patient's care needs
3. *Approaches/modalities:* nursing interventions to help patient attain goals/objectives, to progress toward favorable patient care outcomes and discharge
4. *Patient/family education:* educational needs such as problem-solving skills, constructive ways to deal with anger, and so forth
5. *Discharge planning:* needs such as reduction of anxiety about leaving the hospital, need to learn self-medication

PATIENT/FAMILY EDUCATION

The JCAHO regards patient/family education as a very important function of patient care delivery. Documentation of assessment, planning, interventions, and evidence of favorable outcomes must be easily identified. Psychiatric nurses document identified educational needs such as education about mental illness, symptoms, medication, individual psychotherapy, group psychotherapy, support groups, and other resources available to help patients and their families cope with psychiatric conditions or mental illness.

RATING SCALES

Standardized psychiatric rating scales are commonly used to collect admission assessment and reassessment data.

DISCHARGE NOTE

The psychiatric nurse is usually the member of the interdisciplinary team to see patients off the unit and may escort them off hospital premises. A discharge note must include:
1. Date and time of patient's discharge
2. Description of patient's mood, affect, and behavior
3. Whether patient left unaccompanied or accompanied and by whom
4. Patient's mode of transportation and destination
5. Belongings, prescriptions, appointments, and directions given to patient
6. Patient's statement, if any, regarding discharge
7. Nurse's signature and title

CONTINUOUS QUALITY IMPROVEMENT

The psychiatric clinical nurse specialist/nurse manager or designee leads the team to systematically assess and improve documentation of patient care delivery.

REFERENCE

Joint Commission on Accreditation of Health Care Organizations (1994). *1995 Accreditation Manual for Hospitals. Volume 1: Standards*. Oakbrook Terrace, IL: JCAHO.

64
SIXTY FOUR

Discharge Planning

Fatima Ramos

OVERVIEW:

Standard of Care	Interventions
Patient Care Outcome	Patient and Family Education
Standard of Practice	Documentation
Assessment of Patients and Families	Discharge Forms
The Multidisciplinary Care Plan	Continuous Quality Improvement

STANDARD OF CARE

Discharge planning is a component of comprehensive care and is carried out to provide continuity of care.

PATIENT CARE OUTCOME

Nurses, other team members, and patients will participate in developing a comprehensive discharge plan.

STANDARD OF PRACTICE

Psychiatric professional registered nurses identify patients' discharge needs and plan and implement care in an interdisciplinary and collaborative form to promote continuity of care.

ASSESSMENT OF PATIENTS AND FAMILIES

To plan for discharge with patients, nurses use the following data (St. Germain, 1984):

Objective Data
1. Demographic information
2. Medical history
3. Nursing history
4. Psychosocial/financial history
5. Current status
   a. Diagnosis
   b. Behavioral manifestations, level of functioning

Subjective Data
1. Patients' perceptions of their needs and problems
2. Patients' perceptions of their support system
3. Patients' and families' expectations of the hospital

4. Patients' plans for discharge and goals after discharge

THE MULTI-DISCIPLINARY CARE PLAN

A multidisciplinary patient care conference is held usually 1–3 days after admission. This conference is a forum in which the patient's care needs are shared and discussed with the patient. Goals are identified and a course of patient care with a plan for discharge is formulated with agreement of set target dates. This process may take longer for very acute care patients and those with difficult care needs.

INTERVENTIONS

The patients' and families' active participation from the start increases follow-through with the discharge plan. With the patients' consent, the nurse or social worker contacts appropriate community services available and accessible to patients and their families. Services to be contacted may include the following:

1. Outpatient psychotherapy resources such as mental health clinics, private practitioners such as psychiatric clinical nurse specialists, social workers, psychologists and other qualified psychotherapists
2. Structured day-treatment programs
3. Mental illness and chemical addiction (MICA) programs
4. Structured or partially assisted living residential programs
5. Chemical addictions rehabilitation programs
6. SRO (single-room occupancy) hotels or boarding homes
7. Shelters
8. Other places to live

Patients and their families are kept abreast of discharge plans and progress throughout hospitalization because this is usually a source of anxiety.

PATIENT AND FAMILY EDUCATION

Emphasis is placed on the importance of follow-through with outpatient care. As much as possible a connection with outpatient care is initiated by patients and their families before discharge by encouraging a visit to the site or an appointment with an outpatient care provider. Verbal and written information regarding symptoms, mental illness, support groups, and medication is provided to patients and their families.

DOCUMENTATION

Documentation reflects the ongoing progression of the discharge planning such as summaries of interdisciplinary conferences, dates, interactions with patients regarding discharge plans, outcome of contact with outpatient programs and residence resources, and so forth.

DISCHARGE FORMS

1. Referral forms are completed when appropriate in transfer of patients to other facilities (St. Germain, 1984).
    *   Written communications between hospital and outside agencies are made.
    *   Referral forms are similar to the discharge summaries written in the patient care record. They include summaries of patients' progress, based on assessment of needs and problems and treatment provided, as well as recommendations to ensure continuity of care.
2. Discharge forms are filled out in triplicate and the original is given to patients and their families. (See Box 64-1 for a sample discharge form.)

BOX 64-1: Sample Discharge Form

ST. BARNABAS HOSPITAL

Third Ave. & 183rd St., Bronx, NY 10457-2594   (718) 960-9000

ADDRESSOGRAPH HERE

DEPARTMENTS:

Psychiatry, Nursing, Social Work, Activity Therapy, Psychology

1. DISCHARGE:

Date: _____   Time: _____

Accompanied by: _____   Mode of transportation: _____

After discharge, the patient will be living at: _____

Phone number(s) for follow-up contact: Day _____   Eve _____

2. FOLLOW-UP APPOINTMENTS

Fordham Tremont Mental Health Center

☐ CCU ☐ CTP

2250 Ryer Ave.
Bronx, NY 10457
Tel: (718) 960-0661

Person to see: _____

Date: _____ Time: _____

☐ Psychosocial ☐ DTU

1910 Arthur Ave.
Bronx, NY 10457
Tel: (718) 960-0400

Person to see: _____

Date: _____ Time: _____

☐ Bronx Community College

University Ave. & West 181st St.
Bronx, NY 10453
Tel: (718) 220-6163

Person to see:

Date: Time: _____

☐ Other

Agency: _____
Address: _____
Telephone: _____

Person to see:

Date: Time: _____

St. Barnabas Hospital

☐ Outpatient Alcohol/Drug Services

4422 3rd Ave. (Mills Bldg. 3rd Fl)
Bronx, NY 10457
Tel: (718) ____-_____

Person to see: _____

Date: _____ Time: _____

☐ Medical Center

183rd & 3rd Ave.
Bronx, NY 10457
Tel: (718) 960-6430

Person to see:

Date: Time: _____

☐ Primary Care Clinic

470 East Fordham Rd.
Bronx, NY 10458
Tel: (718) 960-3800

Person to see:

Date: Time: _____

3. DIET INSTRUCTIONS:

_____

4. OTHER INSTRUCTIONS:

_____

5. MEDICATION TO BE TAKEN AT HOME:

Medicine	Dose	Frequency	Route	Reason
_____	_____	_____	_____	_____
_____	_____	_____	_____	_____
_____	_____	_____	_____	_____
_____	_____	_____	_____	_____

Allergies: _____

Enough medicine is being prescribed to last until _____

You will need to go to your appointments to get more, before you run out. If you allow yourself to run out of medications, you may get sick.

☐ I understand and accept these recommendations. I have been given, and understand, reasons for these recommendations, and the possible side effects of the medications.

☐ I understand that my medications may affect my ability to drive.

☐ I understand the manner HIV is transmitted and the precautions helpful in preventing the spread of AIDS.

☐ I understand the danger of taking illegal drugs and alcohol.

Date: _____

_____
Patient's Signature

_____
Psychologist Signature

_____
Activity Therapist Signature

_____
C.S.W. Signature

_____
R.N. Signature

_____
M.D. Signature

From St. Barnabas Hospital, Bronx, NY. Reprinted with permission.

CONTINUOUS QUALITY IMPROVEMENT

The psychiatric clinical nurse specialist/nurse manager or designee leads the team to systematically assess, evaluate, and improve discharge planning for psychiatric patients.

REFERENCES

St. Germain, L. (1984). Discharge planning. In S. Lego (ed.), *The American Handbook of Psychiatric Nursing* (pp. 539–541). Philadelphia: J. B. Lippincott.

Joint Commission on Accreditation of Health Care Organizations (1994). *1995 Accreditation Manual for Hospitals. Volume 1: Standards.* Oakbrook Terrace, IL: JCAHO.

PART SIX

Psychopharmacology

65

SIXTY FIVE

General Nursing Roles in Psychopharmacology

Susan L. W. Krupnick

OVERVIEW:

Introduction
Neuroscience: Brain and Behavior
    Integration
Psychopharmacology Guidelines for
    Psychiatric–Mental Health Nurses

Goal
Psychoeducation
Monitoring Treatment
Future Directions in
    Psychopharmacologic Treatment

INTRODUCTION

A powerful revolution has occurred since the mid-1950s in the treatment of psychiatric disorders. With the presentation of neuropsychopharmacology, medications were introduced that treat the symptoms of specific psychiatric disorders. At the same time, their actions in the brain provide models that clarify and define the underlying pathophysiology of these disabling disorders. The past 20 years of neuroscience research have further fueled this revolution and have significantly increased our understanding of the biobehavioral matrix of psychiatric illness. The scientific advances of the past decade and into the 1990s, referred to as the Decade of the Brain, are rapidly changing the understanding of the human brain, psychiatric illness, and specific biochemical treatment of these disorders. Psychiatric nurses have integrated the important neuroscience findings in concert with psychopharmacologic advances into their clinical nursing practice to ensure safe, responsible, and effective care of people with psychiatric illness.

In contemporary treatment psychological and psychopharmacologic models are highly compatible. When used in a combination or matrix model the clinical outcomes are positive and powerful in enhancing quality of life for both the client and family and improving functional status.

The psychiatric nurse has an integral role in helping clients incorporate psychopharmacologic medications into their treatment plan to recover and maintain mental health and well-being, while attempting to prevent or minimize negative sequelae and identify early symptoms of relapse. The psychiatric nurse at both the generalist and advanced practice level is responsible for the following:

1. Assessing the therapeutic effects of medication
2. Identifying adverse reactions early
3. Knowing therapeutic dosages to age range (child, adult, geriatric)

4. Documenting administration and biobehavioral responses
5. Instructing the client and family members
6. Managing side effects aggressively

Advanced practice psychiatric nurses, either clinical nurse specialists (CNSs) or nurse practitioners (NPs), in most states have prescriptive authority. The inclusion of prescriptive authority is based on the state nurse practice act in conjunction with state and federal regulations governing prescriptions. Advanced practice psychiatric nurses apply neurobiological, psychopharmacological, psychological, and physiological knowledge to all aspects of the therapeutic process. Additionally, the advanced practice psychiatric nurse educates other nurses and health care providers about the appropriate use of psychopharmacologic agents.

NEUROSCIENCE: BRAIN AND BEHAVIOR INTEGRATION

The brain is a mass of tissue consisting of several billion neurons that coordinate behavior by electrochemical activity. The high metabolic rate of the brain facilitates its functions of processing, sorting, analyzing, integrating, and retrieving information. Brain metabolism can be quickly and severely altered when cerebral blood flow is compromised.

Behavior is the expression of brain function and the mind and is a complex interplay between people and their environment. Current research studies are indicating that genetics and neuroendocrine mechanisms have an influence on behavior.

The most abundant type of nerve cell is the conducting neuron, which generates and transmits nerve impulses. Propagation of electrochemical impulses from neuron to neuron is the basic mechanism for nervous system activity. During this transmission process, specific neurochemicals called neurotransmitters are released. These neurochemicals diffuse across the synaptic cleft and attach to specific receptor sites to initiate the impulse at the next neuron. Upon the completion of impulse transfer, some of the neurotransmitter remains in the synaptic cleft. The remaining neurotransmitter can either be broken down by enzyme processes or reabsorbed into the presynaptic membrane by a reuptake process.

These neurotransmitter processes of degradation or reuptake can be inhibited or enhanced by the action of psychotropic medications. A specific psychopharmacologic medication may either increase or decrease the degradation or reuptake of the neurotransmitter to alter its functional activity and equilibrate or normalize the neurotransmitter level. The subsequent regulatory effect alleviates the targeted behavioral symptoms of psychiatric illness. See Table 65-1 for biochemical neurotransmitters and their effects.

There are specific classes of neurotransmitters including the following:
1. Biogenic amines (monoamines)
   a. Catecholamines
   b. Indolamines
2. Acetylcholine
3. Amino acids
4. Peptides

Many psychiatric disorders are hypothesized to be caused by either an excess or deficit of a specific neurotransmitter. Medications can affect the process of cell-to-cell "communication" at the synapse by several different mechanisms:
1. *Blockade:* The neurotransmitter is prevented from binding to the postsynaptic receptor.

TABLE 65-1
Biochemical Neurotransmitters, Functions, and Effects of Excess or Deficit

NEUROTRANSMITTERS	MAJOR FUNCTION	EFFECTS OF EXCESS	EFFECTS OF DEFICIT
Biogenic Amine: Catecholamines			

Dopamine
 	
• Precursor = tyrosine
  Subtypes:
    D_1
    D_{2a}
    D_{2b}
    D_3
    D_4
    D_5
	• Thinking
	• Decision-making
	• Responding with reward-seeking behaviors
	• Fine muscle movements
	• Integration of thoughts and emotions
	• Stimulation of the hypothalamus to release hormones affecting thyroid, adrenal, and sex hormones
		Mild:
		• Helps with creativity
		• Helps with problem-solving
		• Helps with generalization to situations
		• Helps spatial ability
		Severe:
		• Disorganized thinking
		• Loose associations
		• Disabling compulsions
		• Tics
		• Stereotypic behaviors
			Mild:
			• Poor impulse control
			• Poor spatial ability
			• Inability to have abstract thinking
			Severe:
			• Parkinson's disease
			• Endocrine changes
			• Movement disorders

Norepinephrine • Only 1% of all neurotransmitter content • Precursor = dopamine • Measured in urine as MHPG	• Alertness • Ability to focus attention • Ability to be oriented • Priming of nervous system for "fight or flight" • Arousal of senses • Ability to learn • Increased memory • Awareness • Stimulation of sympathetic nervous system	• Anxiety • Hyperalertness • Paranoia • Loss of appetite	• Dullness • Low energy • Depression
Biogenic Amine: Indolamines			

Serotonin (5-HT)
• Opposite to norepinephrine
• Precursor = tryptophan
• Measured in urine as 5-HIAA
  Subtypes:
    $5HT_1$
      $5HT_{1a}$
      $5HT_{1b}$
      $5HT_{1c}$
      $5HT_{1d}$
    $5T_2$
    $5HT_3$
    $5HT_4$
	• Inhibition of activity and behavior
	• Increased sleep time
	• Reduces aggression, play, sexual and eating activity
	• Regulation of
	    temperature
	    sleep cycle
	    pain perception
	    mood states
	• Precursor to melatonin, which plays a role in circadian rhythms, some depressions, light–dark cycles, jet lag, female reproductive cycle, seasonal skin pigment changes
		• Sedation
		• Marked increase in metabolites leading to hallucinations
			• Irritability
			• Hostility
			• Depression
			• Sleep disturbance

(Continued)

TABLE 65-1 *(continued)*

NEUROTRANSMITTERS	MAJOR FUNCTION	EFFECTS OF EXCESS	EFFECTS OF DEFICIT
Acetylcholine			
Acetylcholine • Precursor = choline	Preparation for action • Conservation of energy • Attention • Memory • Defense or aggression • Thirst • Sexual behavior • Mood regulation • REM sleep • Stimulation of parasympathetic nervous system • Control of muscle tone by a balance with dopamine in the basal ganglia	• Self-consciousness • Overinhibition • Anxious depression • Psychophysiological complaints • Depression	• Lack of inhibition • Poor recent memory • Alzheimer's disease • Euphoria • Parkinson's disease • Antisocial behavior • Manic behavior • Speech blockage
Amino Acids			
GABA (gamma-aminobutyric acid) • Precursor = glutamic acid • Generalized inhibitor of interneural transmission	• Reduction of aroused aggression, anxiety, and excitation	• Anticonvulsant reaction • Sedation • Impaired recent memory	• Irritability • Seizures • Huntington's disease • Epilepsy
Glutamate	• Rapid-acting excitation • Intermediate transmitter activity	• Irritability	• Sedation
Aspartate	• Rapid-acting excitation • Intermediate transmitter activity	• Irritability	• Sedation
Glycine	• Inhibition • Excitation • Impulse modulation	• Sedation	• Irritability
Peptides			

Endorphins (Endogenous opioid peptides)
• Counteract the impact of physical and psychological stress and re-establish the organism's homeostasis
	• Alteration of the emotional implications of a painful experience
	• Involvement in
	  reward
	  feeding
	  growth
	  consolidation of memory
		• Insensitivity to pain
		• Movement disorder similar to catatonia
		• Auditory hallucinations
		• Impaired memory
			• Hypersensitivity to pain and stress
			• Inability to experience pleasure

2. *Blocked reuptake:* The presynaptic cell does not reabsorb the neurotransmitter adequately, leaving more neurotransmitter in the synapse, which enhances or prolongs its action.

3. *Interference with storage vesicles:* The neurotransmitter is either released again into the synapse (↑ neurotransmitter) or is released to metabolizing enzymes (↓ neurotransmitter).

4. *Precursor chain interference:* The process that makes the neurotransmitter is either enhanced or disrupted.

5. *Release:* More neurotransmitter is released into the synapse from the storage vesicles in the presynaptic cell.
6. *Synaptic enzyme interference:* Less neurotransmitter is metabolized, making more available in the synapse.

Current and future neuropsychopharmacology research is focused on a more definitive understanding of neuropsychiatric illness so that psychopharmacologic medications can be developed that have increased specificity. This specificity might in turn decrease the unwanted side effects that result when actions of the medication are exerted on areas of the body that are not related to the psychiatric illness.

PSYCHOPHARMACOLOGY GUIDELINES FOR PSYCHIATRIC–MENTAL HEALTH NURSES

Contemporary psychiatric–mental health nursing has its foundations in the integration and application of information from behavioral, biological, social, and neurosciences. Presently these fields are dramatically expanding, requiring nurses to continually incorporate the most current research findings into psychiatric–mental health practice. Therefore, the American Nurses Association organized a task force to address the issue of psychopharmacology in psychiatric nursing (American Nurses Association, 1994a). The task force developed a monograph that details psychopharmacology guidelines for psychiatric–mental health nurses. A brief overview of these guidelines include:

○ *Neurosciences:* "Commensurate with level of practice, the psychiatric–mental health nurse integrates current knowledge from the neurosciences to understand etiological models, diagnostic issues and treatment strategies for psychiatric illness" (American Nurses Association, 1994b, p. 41).

○ *Psychopharmacology:* "The psychiatric–mental health nurse involved in the care of patients who have been prescribed psychopharmacologic agents demonstrates knowledge of psychopharmacologic principles, including pharmacokinetics, pharmacodynamics, drug classification, intended and unintended effects with related nursing implications" (American Nurses Association, 1994b, p. 42).

○ *Clinical management:* "The psychiatric–mental health nurse applies principles from the neurosciences and psychopharmacology to provide safe and effective management of clients being treated with psychopharmacologic agents. Clinical management includes assessment, diagnosis, and treatment considerations" (American Nurses Association, 1994b, p. 42).

1. Assessment includes:
   • Physical assessment
   • Neuropsychiatric assessment
   • Psychosocial assessment
   • Psychopharmacological assessment
2. *Diagnosis:* "Psychiatric–mental health nurses have the knowledge, skills and ability to utilize appropriate nursing, psychiatric and medical diagnostic classification systems to guide psychopharmacologic management of clients with mental illness" (American Nurses Association, 1994b, p. 11).
3. "*Treatment:* Psychiatric–mental health nurses participate actively in the treatment of clients with mental illness. They integrate prescribed psychopharmacologic interventions during the following phases of treatment:
   • Initiation
   • Stabilization

- Maintenance
- Discontinuation and follow-up"

(American Nurses Association, 1994b, pp. 44–45)

Psychiatric–mental health nurses are integral health care providers throughout the continuum of client care, in diverse practice settings including psychiatric mobile outreach programs, psychiatric crisis services, inpatient services, community-based services, and psychiatric home care programs. The psychiatric–mental health nurse needs current research knowledge to provide comprehensive care to these vulnerable client populations, while actively collaborating with health care providers across the continuum of care to provide ongoing care. Throughout the chapters describing psychopharmacology, the clinical management guidelines are based on a collaborative model of care.

GOAL

The goal of clinical management of psychopharmacologic interventions is to promote psychophysiologic stability that facilitates the attainment of psychological, social, and spiritual growth, thereby enhancing the quality of clients' lives and improving their health.

The psychiatric nurse develops a partnership with the client and family members to create a holistic and continuous treatment system that empowers the client to actively participate in the decision-making process related to psychopharmacologic intervention. Specific elements in the clinical management of clients receiving psychopharmacologic interventions include:

- Client advocacy
- Collaboration
- Efficacy and active monitoring of treatment progress
- Education, both nurse and client focused
- Adherence to legal and ethical standards

PSYCHOEDUCATION

Psychiatric–mental health nurses educate the client and family members so that the client is fully informed regarding care, gives consent, and uses the knowledge to participate in the process of pharmacotherapy. The educational process includes preparation and actual practice for the client/family members in self-medication. This includes mobilizing outreach systems to provide in-home care to continue the learning process of self-medication.

The goal of this psychoeducational process is to prepare the client or family members to correctly administer the prescribed medications, monitor for desired effect, as well as side effect(s), and institute specific side-effect management interventions. This psychoeducational process starts on inpatient units but must continue through the outpatient and home care settings.

Upon the completion of the teaching process the client/family members will be able to:

1. Identify the specific medication(s) by name (generic/brand) and appearance.
2. Identify the target symptoms to be reduced by stating the purpose of medication.
3. State the specific symptoms that will be affected by medication. For example:
   - Reduce or eliminate voices
   - Reduce false beliefs
   - Decrease tension, anger, unusual or "bad" thoughts
   - Improve concentration and the ability to more clearly express oneself
   - Reduce fear, confusion, or agitation
   - Help control impulsive or aggressive behavior

- Stabilize mood by reducing feelings of depression or mania
- Help promote sleep
- Improve memory and clarify thinking

4. Properly administer or apply each medication initially with direct supervision or coaching with movement to independent function.
5. Correctly perform necessary techniques and procedures before taking the medication, such as:
   - Pulse check
   - Blood pressure check
   - Glucose monitoring
   - Cleaning of skin area if topical or intramuscular application
6. Demonstrate ability to properly care for devices or instruments used to administer medication.
7. Identify specific side effects of each medication.
8. Collaboratively develop with the health care provider an *aggressive* side-effect management plan. See Table 65-2 for side-effect management strategies.

TABLE 65-2
Psychotropic Medication: Side-Effect Management Strategies

SYSTEM	SIDE EFFECTS	CLASS OF DRUG*	NURSING INTERVENTIONS
Cardiovascular	Orthostatic hypotension	APS TCA MAOI ACH	Instruct the client to rise slowly from a lying to sitting or standing position. Keep side rails up for hospitalized clients. Suggest they call for assistance when getting up until they have learned to manage the problem. Suggest elastic or support stockings. Instruct the client to avoid hot showers or baths, since they may cause vasodilation and aggravate the problem. Monitor the blood pressure when drug therapy is started and during periods of dosage adjustment.
	Tachycardia	TCA ACH LITH	Monitor the pulse two to four times daily until stable. Withhold the dose if the resting pulse before a dose is 110 or greater (follow institutional policy regarding this). Teach the client/family to record the pulse regularly at home. Instruct the client to avoid excessive caffeine intake.
Endocrine and metabolic	Weight gain	APS TCA MAOI	Weigh the client weekly; instruct the client to monitor and record weight at home on a weekly basis. Provide dietary instruction about nutritious but low-calorie meal planning. Help in the development of a regular exercise program.
	Hyperglycemia and hypoglycemia	TCA APS	Monitor blood sugar carefully and frequently in diabetic clients. Consult physician or nurse practitioner about modifications in prescribed diet, insulin dose, or dose of oral hypoglycemic agent as necessary.

(Continued)

*Code: APS = antipsychotic; TCA = tricyclic; MAOI = monoamine oxidase inhibitor; ACH = anticholinergic; LITH = lithium; SSRI = selective serotonin reuptake inhibitor; SSNRI = selective serotonin–norepinephrine reuptake inhibitor; BENZ = benzodiazepines

TABLE 65-2 *(continued)*

SYSTEM	SIDE EFFECTS	CLASS OF DRUG	NURSING INTERVENTIONS
Endocrine and metabolic (continued)	Increased or decreased libido; changes in ability to ejaculate or maintain erection	APS TCA LITH SSRI SSNRI	Conduct sexual history. Provide emotional support to client and spouse as appropriate. Alter the drug dose or switch medications. Collaborate with physician or nurse practitioner to consider treatment with yohimbine (Yocon), an α_2-adrenergic antagonist, or neostigmine (Prostigmin) 7.5–15 mg 30 minutes before sexual intercourse.
	Menstrual irregularities Amenorrhea Galactorrhea False pregnancy	APS TCA	Refer women for gynecological exam if appropriate. Advise the use of birth control measures to avoid unplanned pregnancy.
Gastrointestinal	Gastric irritation	TCA LITH	Alter the prescribed times for taking doses to coincide with meals. Decrease the size of the dose and administer more frequently. Change the medication form (for example, switch to liquid from tablets).
	Anorexia	SSRI SSNRI	Instruct client to do daily "food journal."
	Nausea/vomiting	SSRI SSNRI TCA	Administer medication with meals. Decrease dose. Collaborate with physician in considering cisapride 5 mg BID for nausea from SSRI.
Hematological	Leukopenia Thrombocytopenia	TCA	Continue to monitor closely.
	Agranulocytosis	TCA APS	Discontinue drug immediately. Manage medically. Educate about reverse isolation. Try medication from different chemical structural group.
Hepatic	Jaundice: • ↑ Temperature • Malaise • Abnormal liver function tests • Abdominal pain	APS TCA	Discontinue medication. Switch to another chemical structural group. Monitor liver function tests. Instruct in high-protein/carbohydrate diet.
Neurological	Drowsiness and sedation	APS TCA MAOI ACH BENZ SSRI	Caution the client to avoid driving or other dangerous activities requiring mental alertness until the degree of drowsiness can be evaluated. (With some medications or with some clients drowsiness may be a desirable effect.) Increase the nighttime dose or give the entire day's dosage at bedtime if daytime drowsiness persists. (Persistent drowsiness may indicate the need to change the medication or dose; this requires careful clinical judgment. Drowsiness may lessen with time. Encourage the client to continue the medication for several weeks at least.)
Neurological	Anticholinergic dry mouth†	APS TCA MAOI ACH SSRI	Encourage the client to take frequent sips of water or other beverages; because weight gain is often a problem, low-calorie beverages are preferred. Suggest that the client suck on hard candy or mints or chew gum; low-calorie or sugarless forms are preferred. Frequent toothbrushing or rinsing the mouth with a pleasant mouthwash or other solution may help eliminate a bad taste in the mouth. Commercially prepared saliva substitutes are available; consult a pharmacist.

TABLE 65-2 *(continued)*

SYSTEM	SIDE EFFECTS	CLASS OF DRUG	NURSING INTERVENTIONS
Neurological (continued)	Constipation†	APS TCA MAOI ACH	Monitor and record the frequency of bowel movements. Encourage the client to increase the dietary intake of bran, fresh fruits, or prunes. Collaborate with nutritionist. Have the client increase fluid intake to 2500–3000 ml per day if not contraindicated by other medical conditions. Encourage the client to increase level of activity (walking or engaging in other forms of exercise) within any functional limits. Consult with the physician or nurse practitioner about prescribing stool softeners or bulk-forming agents.
	Blurred vision†	APS TCA MAOI ACH BENZ	Caution the client to avoid driving or operating hazardous equipment until the blurring clears. If blurred vision persists, notify physician or nurse practitioner, since it may indicate a need to change drugs or reduce dosages. Encourage client to see an ophthalmologist.
	Urinary retention†	APS TCA	Although this side effect is possible at any age, it is more prevalent in the elderly, the immobilized, and in men with enlarged prostate glands. Monitor intake and output. Assess client for difficulty voiding, subjective complaints of incomplete bladder emptying. Notify physician or nurse practitioner if retention is suspected; catheterization may be necessary. Suggest the client void before taking ordered doses of medication. Teach the client to notify the health care provider if retention is suspected.
	Anticholinergic diaphoresis	TCA SSRI	Maintain adequate fluid intake (usually over 2500–3000 ml/day) depending on cardiopulmonary function. Assess for electrolyte imbalance and monitor serum electrolytes. Encourage good hygiene. Suggest cotton clothing.
	Seizures	APS TCA	Decrease dose. Change to a high-potency antipsychotic.
	Insomnia	SSRI SSNRI	Administer medication early in the day. Lower the dose. Instruct the client in sleep hygiene measures. Decrease or delete caffeine.

† Collaborate with physician or nurse practitioner to consider use of 1% solution of pilocarpine (a cholinergic agonist) as a mouthwash three times a day or bethanechol (Urecholine, Myotonachol) 10–30 mg OD-BID (cholinergic agonist).

9. Describe what specific action to implement if a dose of medication is missed.
10. Identify psychophysiologic effects of not taking medications or abrupt discontinuation of medications.
11. List the signs and symptoms of medication toxicity from possible iatrogenic or self-induced overdose.
12. Identify any food/nutrient/medication (prescribed or illicit) interactions of each medication. See Table 65-3 for the effect of specific dietary substances and Table 65-4 for alterations in neurotransmitter functions resulting from drugs or foods.

TABLE 65-3
Psychotropic Medications: Effects of Specific
Dietary Substances and Chemicals

MEDICATION CLASS	FOOD/CHEMICAL	EFFECTS
Antidepressants (cyclics)	Alcohol Abscorbic acid Coffee/tea	Sedation, drowsiness ↑ Elimination Uneven absorption
Antianxiety (anxiolytics)	Alcohol Caffeine Nicotine	↑ Sedation, cumulative effects ↓ Effectiveness ↓ Sedation effect of benzodiazepines
Antipsychotics	Alcohol Ascorbic acid Caffeine Nicotine	↑ Sedation ↓ Absorption of fluphenazine (↓ effectiveness of antipsychotic) ↑ Drug threshold of antipsychotics ↓ Sedation effect of chlorpromazine
Lithium	Caffeine Sodium	↑ Lithium elimination Sudden ↓ in caffeine ingestion may precipitate lithium toxicity ↑ Lithium elimination Low-sodium diet causes retention of lithium and toxicity
Monoamine oxidase inhibitors (nonbenzamide)	Alcohol High tyramine/tryptophan foods Alcohol • Beer, wines Broad beans Aged cheese • Camembert • Edam • Cheddar Beef/chicken livers Orange pulp Pickled/smoked fish, poultry, or meats Packaged soups Yeast vitamin supplements Meat extracts (Marmite, Bovril) Summer sausage Moderately high tyramine foods (1–2 servings/day permitted) Avocados Bananas Eggplant Plums Raisins Spinach Soy sauce Sour cream Tomatoes Yogurt	Neurotoxicity, irritability Tyramine-induced hypertensive crisis: *Signs and symptoms:* headache, stiff neck, sweating, nausea and vomiting, ↑ blood pressure *Treatment* consists of immediate medical care • Nifedipine (Procardia) 10 mg • Alpha-adrenergic blocker such as phentolamine (Regitine) • Chlorpromazine (Thorazine)

TABLE 65-4
Alterations in Neurotransmitter Function

DRUG/SUBSTANCE	ACETYLCHOLINE	ADENOSINE	DOPAMINE	ENDORPHIN	GABA	NOREPINEPHRINE	SEROTONIN
Alcohol	—	—	↑ ↓	—	—	—	—
Amphetamine	—	—	↑	—	↑	—	↑
Barbiturates	—	—	—	—	↑	—	—
Benzodiazepine	—	—	—	—	↑	—	—
Caffeine	—	—	—	—	—	—	—
Chocolate	—	—	—	—	—	—	↑
Cocaine	—	—	↑	—	↓	↑	—
Hallucinogens	—	↑	↑	↑	—	—	↓
Marijuana	—	—	↑	—	—	—	—
Nicotine	↓	—	↑	—	—	—	—
PCP	↑ ↓	—	↑	↑	↑	↑	↑
Sugar	—	—	—	↑	—	—	↑

Compiled from Bloom, F. E., & Kupfer, D. J. (1995). *Psychopharmacology: The Fourth Generation of Progress.* New York: Raven Press.

13. Describe proper storage of medication(s).
14. Discuss an individual plan to remember the medication regimen (e.g., medication box organizers, written list or chart, computer reminders, wristwatch alarm reminder).
15. Acknowledge risks of taking expired medications, sharing medications, or taking someone else's medications.
16. Identify their designated pharmacy.
17. Describe and demonstrate their ability to successfully obtain prescribed medications.
18. Collaborate with health care provider(s) to develop a simplified written schedule of their medications including:
    • Name of medication (brand and generic)
    • Dose
    • Purpose
    • Time of administration
19. Keep a written schedule of medications with them in a purse or wallet.
20. Identify and use insurance, community, or pharmaceutical company (patient assistance program) resources for medication reimbursement.
21. Discuss the need to have a medication alert device or computerized system for an information safeguard.
22. Collaborate with a health care provider(s) to design a medication chart for home use that includes a picture or actual sample of each medication for quick identification, especially if the client has some learning difficulties or a language barrier.
23. Review written materials specific to their medication(s) with inpatient health care providers, and take written material home to reinforce learning. Written information is language specific to client/family.
24. Use audiocassette tapes with above information particularly if the client or family member in the caregiver role is blind.

MONITORING TREATMENT

Monitoring the trajectory of illness response and the effects, including side effects of psychopharmacologic agents, requires that the psychiatric–mental health nurse in collaboration with the client/family develop a clearly defined response plan. This intervention plan includes defining conditions that require changes in dosages or medications. See Box 65-1 for a symptom checklist.

BOX 65-1: Client-Focused Symptom Checklist

Client's name _____   Age: _____

Date: _____   Baseline   Y   N

Follow-up after initiation of psychotropic   Y   N

24 hours after initiation ☐   3 days after initiation ☐

1 week after initiation ☐   weekly evaluation ☐

Psychotropic medications: _____

Do you have any of the following symptoms? Yes No	Are they uncomfortable? Yes No	If yes, how uncomfortable? 1–3*
Always hungry		
Blurred vision		
Body stiff or rigid		
Bruising easier		
Constipation		
Decreased sexual interest		
Diarrhea		
Different menstruation		
Difficulty in swallowing		
Diminished appetite		
Dizziness/lightheadedness		
Drowsiness		
Dry mouth, throat, or nose		
Edema		
Excessive sleeping		
Faint		
Fluid discharge from breast		
Frequent or difficult urination		
Headache		
Increased sweating		
Increased thirst		
Insomnia		
Jaundice		
Lack of energy		
Nausea or vomiting		
Nervousness		
Poor memory		
Rapid or pounding heart		
Ringing in the ears		
Skin rash		
Slurred speech		
Sores in mouth		
Stiff tongue		
Swollen breasts		
Tremors, shakes, jitters		
Unsteady gait		
Upset stomach		
Weight gain		
Weird dreams/nightmares		

*Scale: 1 = Minimal discomfort; 2 = Moderate discomfort; 3 = Severe discomfort

The identification of additional and alternative/complementary strategies that may be beneficial to clients and may fit within their belief and value system must be considered or researched. This is important especially when the client or family introduces the potential technique. Table 65-5 provides guidelines for enhancing medication compliance.

TABLE 65-5
Guidelines for Enhancing Medication Regimen Compliance

NURSING INTERVENTION	RATIONALE
1. Assess for and identify client-specific risk factors for noncompliance. • Continuity of care is lacking. • Cultural barriers exist. • Treatment providers devalue psychopharmacology. • Medication is expensive. • The client is not a "partner" in the medication treatment plan. • Family/environmental stress is not well managed. • Family support is lacking. • A history of noncompliance has not been investigated. • There is inadequate client and family education concerning treatment. • Health care provider is insensitive to beliefs and wishes of the client concerning treatment. • The daily dosing schedule is complex. • The client is taking many drugs. • The client's lifestyle is restricted. • Signs and symptoms recur. • Remission of target signs and symptoms takes place. • Side-effect management is inadequate. • The client is socially isolated. • The client is stigmatized. • The client is a substance abuser. • The client is suicidal. • The client has unmet and unrealistic expectations of medication benefits versus risk of side effects.	Identifying risk factors for potential or suspected noncompliance from the client's perspective will help nurses target areas of conflict or difficulty. Psychoeducation and community-based follow-up can be directed at these specific issues rather than the provocative label of "noncompliant."
2. Teach client and family about prescribed medication.	Compliance is fostered and enhanced when clients are viewed as partners in the treatment program. Client compliance is a complex and multifaceted issue for the nurse, client, and family.
3. Collaborate with client to develop strategies to incorporate medication-taking into daily routine.	Compliance is an outcome of a client making *informed* choices that help in mastering the challenges of the illness.
4. Instruct client/family about importance of focused side-effect management.	Side effects and financial cost are two risk factors that clients frequently state made them stop the medication.
5. Encourage active participation of family members in education about client's medication while discussing the need of their support.	Incorporating the family members in medication education sessions provides opportunities to further identify family stressors and potential caregiver strain. Allows family members the opportunity to ask, learn, be heard and supported in their learning needs.

FUTURE DIRECTIONS IN PSYCHOPHARMACOLOGIC TREATMENT

Psychiatric–mental health nurses can expect several new psychopharmacologic medications to be released, even as this book goes to press. Presently there are several hundred psychopharmacologic agents being investigated in the United States. These include antidepressants, antipsychotics, and nootropics or metabolic enhancers. Nootropics are proposed to alleviate the symptoms of mental aging and cerebral insufficiency. Currently one available medication that is used specifically to treat the mild to moderate dementia changes related to Alzheimer's is tacrine (Cognex). (See Box 65-2.)

BOX 65-2: Tacrine (Cognex)

Chemical structural group: Nootropic
    synthetic acetylcholinesterase inhibitor

Mechanism of action: Tacrine has been shown to increase presynaptic acetylcholine release through blocking slow K channels while increasing postsynaptic monoaminergic stimulation by interfering with norepinephrine and serotonin uptake.

Dose: 10 mg po QID for 6 weeks
    Incremental titration: 10 mg up to therapeutic range of 40 mg QID (160 mg daily)

Side effects: ataxia, anorexia, diarrhea, vomiting, nausea, bradycardia in clients with sick sinus syndrome

Laboratory monitoring required: Liver function tests

The focus of future psychopharmacologic medications for the debilitating Alzheimer's disease is the development of specific agents that interfere with the neurodegenerative process of the illness. The "ideal" cholinesterase would have the following characteristics: a long enough half-life to permit one dose per day, minimal peripheral side effects and toxicity, good absorption, and effective central nervous system penetration.

Psychiatric–mental health nurses are in crucial positions to contribute to these research efforts, either by direct involvement in clinical drug trials or by direct clinical practice with clients receiving these new medications. In these roles the psychiatric nurse must remember the importance of effective evaluation of these medications, determining the advantages and disadvantages of a new medication as compared to the existing standard medications in specific relationship to their clients' psychophysiologic needs, reactions, and preferences.

The psychiatric–mental health nurse in collaboration with the client, family, and medical psychiatry team members will address these areas as they consider initiating pharmacologic treatment with a new medication. In comparison to the older medication:

1. Is the mechanism of action more specific to the desired psychobiological outcome?
2. Is the onset of action quicker?
3. Is the side effect profile "better" and acceptable to the client/family?
4. Are there no or few long-term adverse effects?
5. Are there minimal medication or food/nutrient interactions?
6. What is the wide margin of safety related to abuse, addiction, and suicide potential?
7. Are there several administration routes?

8. Is there a low profile of discontinuation problems?
9. Is the medication cost-effective?

Although cost-effectiveness is the last question on the list, in the managed health care arena it can be a significant determining factor. Therefore, it is imperative that psychiatric–mental health nurses know the cost of current psychopharmacologic intervention. The newest medication that is specific for the client and has been effective during inpatient care will not be helpful if the client cannot afford it upon discharge. Clients may stop taking the medication if they do not have prescription coverage, or if their particular plan will not cover the prescribed medication, or if they do not have enough money to pay other bills and purchase their medication.

Collaborative partnerships with the client/family and team members will diminish the effects of the above financial issues and increase the probability of a successful psychopharmacologic outcome.

REFERENCES

American Nurses Association (1994a). Psychiatric mental health nursing psychopharmacology project. *ANA Task Force on Psychopharmacology.* Washington, DC: American Nurses Association.

American Nurses Association (1994b). *Psychopharmacology Guidelines for Psychiatric Mental Health Nurses.* Washington, DC: American Nurses Association.

Bloom, F. E., & Kupfer, D. J. (1995). *Psychopharmacology: The Fourth Generation of Progress.* New York: Raven Press.

BIBLIOGRAPHY

Andreasen, N. C. (1984). *The Broken Brain: The Biological Revolution in Psychiatry.* New York: Harper and Row.

Becker, P., & Jamieson, A. (1992). Common sleep disorders in the elderly: Diagnosis and treatment. *Geriatrics, 47* (3), 41–42, 45–48, 51–52.

Benca, R., Obermey, W., Thisted, R., & Gillin, C. (1992). Sleep and psychiatric disorders. *Archives of General Psychiatry, 49* (8), 651–668.

Bergeron, R., & Blier, P. (1994). Cisapride for the treatment of nausea produced by selective serotonin reuptake inhibitors. *American Journal of Psychiatry, 151* (7), 1084–1086.

Bezchlibnyk-Butler, K., & Jeffries, J. (1994). *Clinical Handbook of Psychotropic Drugs* (2nd ed.). Toronto: Hogrefer Huber Publishers.

Cleary, C., Dever, A., & Schweizer, E. (1992). Psychiatric inpatients' knowledge of medication at hospital discharge. *Hospital and Community Psychiatry, 43* (2), 140–144.

Cohen, S. (1988). *The Chemical Brain.* Minneapolis, MN: CompCare.

Collins-Colon, T. (1990). Do it yourself: Medication management for community based clients. *Journal of Psychosocial Nursing and Mental Health Services, 28* (6), 25–29.

Coudreaut-Quinn, E. A., Emmons, M. A., & McMorrow, M. J. (1992). Self medication during inpatient psychiatric treatment. *Journal of Psychosocial Nursing and Mental Health Services, 30* (12), 32–36.

Dalack, G. W., Glassman, A. H., Rivelli, S., Covey, L., & Sterner, F. (1995). Mood, major depression and fluoxetine response in cigarette smokers. *American Journal of Psychiatry, 152* (3), 398–403.

Dowling, J. E. (1992). *Neurons and Networks: An Introduction to Neuroscience.* Cambridge, MA: Harvard University Press.

Gitlin, M. (1994). Psychotropic medications and their effects on sexual function: Diagnosis, biology and treatment approaches. *Journal of Clinical Psychiatry. 55* (9), 406–413.

Goff, D. C., Henderson, D. C., & Amico, E. (1992). Cigarette smoking in schizophrenia: Relationship to psychopathology and medication side effects. *American Journal of Psychiatry, 149,* 1189–1194.

Gray, G. E., & Gray, L. K. (1989). Nutritional aspects of psychiatric disorders. *Journal of the American Dietetic Association. 8* (10), 1492–1498.

Keltner, N. L., & Folks, D. G. (1992). Culture as a variable in drug therapy. *Perspectives in Psychiatric Care, 28* (1), 33–36.

Kirmer, D. (1988). Caffeine use and abuse in psychiatric clients. *Journal of Psychosocial Nursing and Mental Health Services, 26* (11), 20–25.

Lin, K. M., Poland, R. E., & Nakasaki, G. (1993). *Psychopharmacology and Psychobiology of Ethnicity.* Washington, DC: American Psychiatric Association Press.

Lund, V. E., & Frank, D. I. (1991). Helping the medicine go down. Nurse's and patient's perceptions about medication compliance. *Journal of Psychosocial Nursing and Mental Health Services, 29* (7), 6–9.

McEnany, G. W. (1991). Psychobiology and psychiatric nursing: A philosophical matrix. *Archives in Psychiatric Nursing, 5* (5), 255–261.

McEnany, G. W. (1992). Psychobiology. In H. S. Wilson & C. R. Kneisel (eds.), *Psychiatric Nursing* (4th ed.). Menlo Park, CA: Addison-Wesley Publishing Co.

Mulaik, J. S. (1992). Noncompliance with medication regimens in severely and persistently mentally ill schizophrenic patients. *Issues in Mental Health Nursing, 13* (3), 219.

Pennebaker, D. F., & Riley, J. (1995). Psychopharmacological therapy. In D. Antai-Ontag (ed.), *Psychiatric Nursing: Biological and Behavioral Concepts.* Philadelphia: W. B. Saunders Co.

Shulman, K. I., Walker, S. E., MacKenzie, S., & Knowles, S. (1989). Dietary restriction, tyramine, and the use of monoamine oxidase inhibitors. *Journal of Clinical Psychopharmacology, 9* (6), 397–402.

Smith, G. R., & Knice-Ambinder, M. (1989). Promoting medication compliance in clients with chronic illness. *Holistic Nursing Practice, 4* (1), 70–77.

Talley, S., & Brooke, P. (1992). Prescriptive authority for psychiatric clinical nurse specialists: Framing the issues. *Archives of Psychiatric Nursing, 6D* (2), 71–82.

66
SIXTY SIX

Antipsychotic Medications

Susan L. W. Krupnick

OVERVIEW:

Introduction
Indications
Chemical Structural Groups
Method of Action
Target Symptoms
Dosage

Side-Effect Profile
Monitoring Treatment
   Initiation Phase
   Stabilization Phase
   Maintenance Phase

INTRODUCTION

Antipsychotic medication is the general term that refers to a now diverse group of pharmacological agents that are effective in the symptomatic treatment of psychoses. These medications have also been referred to as major tranquilizers or neuroleptics. The specific central nervous system action of these medications became known as ataractic and neuroleptic. Neuroleptic refers to the neurological aspects of these medications, demonstrated by the extrapyramidal and parkinsonian effects, whereas the term antipsychotic is more commonly used as it describes the actual desired effects of these medications.

INDICATIONS

Antipsychotic medications are used with:
1. Agitation in acute deliria or dementia
2. Bipolar disorder
3. Delusional disorder
4. Drug-induced psychoses
5. Organic psychoses
6. Other acute psychoses
7. Pervasive developmental disorders with severe agitation or aggression
8. Psychotic depression
9. Schizophrenia
10. Severe anxiety that is unresponsive to all other treatments
11. Severe dyscontrol or psychosis associated with personality disorders
12. Tourette's disorder

CHEMICAL STRUCTURAL GROUPS

Antipsychotic medications are categorized according to the following groups:
1. Phenothiazines
2. Thioxanthenes
3. Butyrophenones

4. Benzisoxazoles
5. Dihydroindolones
6. Diphenylbutylpiperidines
7. Dibenzoxazepines
8. Dibenzodiazepines
9. Benzamides

METHOD OF ACTION

These medications affect the levels of a variety of brain neurotransmitters, specifically dopamine, histamine, norepinephrine, and serotonin, at the receptor sites. Sites of action include both central nervous system (limbic, reticular activating system, extrapyramidal) and peripheral nervous system. The newer antipsychotic agents clozapine and nisperidone more selectively block specific central dopamine neurotransmitter receptors.

TARGET SYMPTOMS

Antipsychotic drugs help to relieve:
1. Agitation (severe)
2. Anorexia related to psychosis
3. Blunted affect
4. Combativeness
5. Confusion
6. Delusions
7. Extreme sensitivity to environmental stimuli
8. Feelings of unreality
9. Hallucinations
10. Hyperactivity
11. Ideas of reference
12. Insomnia related to psychosis
13. Paranoia/suspiciousness
14. Social withdrawal
15. Terror
16. Uncontrollable hostility
17. Uncontrollable negativism
18. Uncontrollable rage
19. Unclear or racing thoughts
20. Verbal threats and aggressiveness

DOSAGE

See Table 66-1 for dosage of antipsychotic medications.

SIDE-EFFECT PROFILE

See Table 66-2 for the side effects of antipsychotic medications.

MONITORING TREATMENT

Prior to initiating treatment:
1. Collaborate with medical–psychiatric team members to conduct a thorough medical evaluation including a comprehensive medical history, complete physical assessment, and focused neurological examination, with specific attention to:
   - Heart rate
   - Blood pressure
   - Ophthalmological examination
   - Assessment of extrapyramidal signs and symptoms

TABLE 66-1
Antipsychotic Medication Doses

GENERIC NAME	BRAND NAME	DOSE FORMS (mg)	INITIAL DOSES (mg/day)	RANGES (mg/day)	PRN (mg/po)	PRN (mg/IM)	GERIATRIC DOSE RANGE (mg/day)
PHENOTHIAZINES *Aliphatics*							
Chlorpromazine	Thorazine	t:10/25/50/100/200 SR:30/75/150/200/300 o:30 mg/ml, 100 mg/ml p:25 mg/ml s:10 mg/5 ml sp:25/100	200–1600	25–2000	25–100	25–50	25–200
Piperidines							
Mesoridazine	Serentil	t:10/25/50/100 o:25 mg/ml p:25 mg/ml	75–300	30–400	10–100	25	75–200
Thioridazine	Mellaril / Mellaril-S	t:10/15/25/50/100/ 150/200 o:30 mg/ml, 100 mg/ml su:25 mg/5 ml, 100 mg/5 ml	150–300	40–800	20–200	N/A	25–200
Piperazines							
Fluphenazine	Permitil / Prolixin	t:1/2.5/5/10 o:5 mg/ml e:0.5 mg/ml o:5 mg/ml p:2.5 mg/ml	2.5–20	1–30	0.5–10	1–5	2–10
Fluphenazine decanoate	Prolixin Decanoate	p:25 mg/ml	25	6.5–100	—	—	6.25–12.5*
Perphenazine	Trilafon	t:2/4/8/16 o:16 mg/5 ml p:5 mg/ml	16–32	4–64	4–8	5–10	4–48
Trifluoperazine	Stelazine	t:1/2/5/10 o:10 mg/ml p:2 mg/ml	6–50	2–80	5–10	1–2	2–15
BUTYROPHENONES							
Haloperidol	Haldol	t:0.5/1/2/5/10/20 o:2 mg/ml p:5 mg/ml	2–40	1–100	0.5–5	2–5	1–6
Haloperidol decanoate	Haldol decanoate	p:50 mg/ml, 100 mg/ml	50–100	50–300	—	—	—
THIOXANTHENES							
Chlorprothixene	Taractan	t:10/25/50/100 o:100 mg/5 ml p:25 mg/2 ml	50–200	30–600	25–100	25–50	—
Thiothixene	Navane	c:1/2/5/10/20 o:5 mg/ml p:2/5 mg/ml	2–5	6–30	2–20	2–4	2–15
DIPHENYLBUTYLPIPERIDINES							
Pimozide	Orap	t:2 mg	1–2	1–20	N/A	N/A	—
DIBENZOXAZEPINE							
Loxapine	Loxitane Loxitane-C Loxitane-IM	c:5/10/25/50 o:25 mg/ml p:50 mg/ml	20–50	60–200	10–60	12.5–50	—
DIHYDROINDOLONES							
Molindone	Moban	t:5/10/25/50/100 o:20 mg/ml	50–100	15–200	5–75	N/A	85–190
DIBENZODIAZEPINES							
Clozapine	Clozaril	t:25/100	25–50	30–900	—	N/A	200–300
BENZISOXAZOLES							
Risperidone	Risperdal	t:1/2/3/4	1–2	4–6† 4–16	—	N/A	1–4

c = capsules; e = elixir; o = oral concentrate; p = parenteral concentrate; s = syrup; sp = suppository; SR = sustained release spansules; su = suspension; t = tablets; N/A = not available

*Every 2–3 weeks   †Maximal effect was generally seen in a range of 4–6mg/day. Doses > 6mg were associated with more EPS.

TABLE 66-2
Side-Effect Profile of Antipsychotic Medications

GENERIC NAME	BRAND NAME	SIDE EFFECTS			
		SEDATIVE	EPS	HYPO-TENSIVE	ANTI-CHOLINERGIC
PHENOTHIAZINES					
Aliphatics					
Chlorpromazine	Thorazine	+++	++	+++	+++
Piperidines					
Thioridazine	Mellaril	+++	+	+++	+++
Mesoridazine	Serentil	+++	+	+++	+++
Piperazines					
Trifluoperazine	Stelazine	+	+++	++	+
Perphenazine	Trilafon	++	++	++	++
Fluphenazine	Prolixin, Permitil	+	+++	+	+
Acetophenazine	Tindal	++	++	+	+
THIOXANTHENES					
Chlorprothixene	Taractan	+++	++	+++	+++
Thiothixene	Navane	+	+++	++	+
BUTYROPHENONES					
Haloperidol	Haldol	+	+++	+	+
DIHYDROINDOLONES					
Molindone	Moban	++	+	+	++
DIBENZOXAPINES					
Loxapine	Loxitane	++	++	++	++
DIBENZOXAZEPINES					
Clozapine	Clozaril	+++	+	++	+++
DIPHENYLBUTYLPIPERIDINES					
Pimozide	Orap	+	+++	+	+
BENZISOXAZOLES					
Risperidone	Risperdal	++	+	++	++

Key: + = Least; ++ = Moderate; +++ = Most

2. Collaborate with medical–psychiatric team members to ensure that a complete laboratory and test evaluation is conducted including:
   - CBC with differential
   - Liver function tests (LFTs)
   - Renal function tests
   - Electrocardiogram (ECG) for males over 30 years old, females over 40 years old
3. Collaborate in the selection of an appropriate antipsychotic medication (see Box 66-1) based on the side effect profile, risk–benefit ratio, history of prior successful use by the client or related family members, and identification of target symptoms.
4. Inform and instruct the client and family member of risk factors and common side effects, especially the risk of tardive dyskinesia.
5. Provide written educational material to reinforce instruction.

6. Document completely all instruction in the medical record, including client and family member responses and concerns about initiating antipsychotic medication therapy.
7. Obtain signature on informed consent form for administering psychotropic medication if this is required in the policy statement of the institution or by the state.
8. Use a baseline symptom checklist to identify symptoms the client is already experiencing. (Refer to Client-Focused Symptom Checklist in Chapter 65, Box 65-1.)
9. Complete an initial risk assessment for extrapyramidal symptoms (EPS). The risk management tool described in Box 66-1 provides an excellent objective assessment tool for identifying potential EPS.

BOX 66-1: The Risk Management Tool for Extrapyramidal Symptoms (EPS)

PATIENT-SPECIFIC RISKS

Risk Factor	Criteria	Points
☐ Age	> 55	3
	40–55	2
	< 40	1
☐ Sex	Female	2
	Male	1
	Male < 30	2
☐ History	Exposure to ECT	1
	Previous EPS	2
☐ Diagnosis	Organic Brain Syndrome	3
	Schizoaffective and/or affective disorder	1
	Total	_____

Interpretation of totals

_____	Low predisposition for EPS	2–5
_____	High predisposition for EPS	6–8
_____	Extreme predisposition for EPS	9–12

AGENT-SPECIFIC RISKS

High-potency medication	4
Moderate-potency medication	3
Low-potency medication	2
Exposure > 60 days	2
Exposure > 2 years	3
Depot injections	2
Two or more antipsychotic agents	2
Total	_____

Interpretation of totals

_____	Low risk	2–5
_____	Moderate risk	6–8
_____	Extreme risk	> 8

(Continued)

BOX 66-1 *(continued)*

TREATMENT-SPECIFIC RISKS FOR EPS

Risk Factor	Points
No prophylaxis, and no PRN for anti-EPS medication	5
No prophylaxis, written order for PRN EPS medication	3
Prophylactic medication for EPS, but no PRN order	2
Prophylaxis and PRN coverage	1
PRN of antipsychotics > 5 times/week	4
PRN of antipsychotics 3–5 times/week	3
PRN of antipsychotics 2–5 times/week	2
Ratio of antipsychotic PRNs to anti-EPS, > 3:1	4
Total	____

Interpretation of totals

Low treatment risk	1–4
High treatment risk	5–8
Severe treatment risk	8–13

TOTAL—RISK DESIGNATIONS FOR EPS

Risk Factor	Points
Low	4–15
High	16–21
Extreme	> 21

From: Blair, D. T. (1990). Risk management for extrapyramidal symptoms. *Quality Review Bulletin* (March), 116–124. Used with permission.

INITIATION PHASE

1. Initiate antipsychotic medication in a low dosage and monitor the client's targeted symptom complex response in relation to occurrence of side effects.
2. Consult with medical–psychiatric team members to consider the benefit of initiating anticholinergic medication for prophylaxis of EPS. This is especially important when initiating antipsychotic medications of high potency, or if the client is younger than 40 years of age. See Table 66-3 for a description of EPS and Tables 66-4 and 66-5 for details about anticholinergic medications. These medications are indicated when the client experiences:
   - Akathisia
   - Dystonia
   - Pseudoparkinsonism (including akinesia)
   It must be kept in mind that geriatric patients are sensitive to these medications. Also, anticholinergic medications are capable of producing euphoria and have potential for abuse.
3. Closely monitor an increase of the dosage until targeted symptoms improve while side effects are tolerable and managed effectively and aggressively to maintain dose titration.
4. Closely monitor for adverse reactions; continue use of the risk management tool to assess for EPS changes from baseline assessment.

TABLE 66-3
Types of Extrapyramidal Symptoms/Syndromes

SYMPTOM/SYNDROME	ONSET	CLINICAL COURSE	RISK FACTORS/GROUPS
Akathisia: A need to move	5–60 days	Muscular discomfort Motor, inner-driven restlessness Restless legs May be misdiagnosed as an increase in anxiety Can persist if not treated with anticholinergics	20–50% of patients Elderly women
Akinesia (Parkinsonism): Tremors, rigidity, and bradykinesias	5–30 days	Can occur throughout treatment Responds to a reduction in neuroleptic agents to lowest *effective* level or an anticholinergic agent	12–45% of patients Elderly women
Dystonia: Rigidity in muscles that control posture, gait, or ocular movement	1–5 days	Acute, spasmodic, and painful muscle rigidity and contraction Responds to IM or IV antiparkinsonian medication	Young males
Neuroleptic Malignant Syndrome (NMS)	Days–weeks, usually 24–72 hours	Muscular rigidity, tremors, impaired ventilation, muteness, altered consciousness, and autonomic hyperactivity Mortality rate 11–30% Responds to discontinuation of antipsychotic and anticholinergic agents Drug treatment may include bromocriptine and dantrolene	0.5–2.4% of patients 80% are less than 40 years old. Affects twice as many men as women. Usually occurs with high-potency neuroleptic medications
"Rabbit" Syndrome (Perioral Tremor): Rapid up movements that mimic a rabbit	Months–years	Occurs late in neuroleptic treatment and responds well to anticholinergic agents	4% of patients who are untreated with anticholinergic agents
Tardive Dyskinesia (TD): Tardive means late appearing; Dyskinesia refers to abnormal voluntary skeletal movements	6–24 months	Usually affects the muscles of the mouth and face Signs include lip smacking, grinding the teeth, rolling or protruding tongue	15–25% of patients (range 0.5–60%) Women, elderly, and patients with affective disorders

STABILIZATION PHASE

1. Maintain a treatment dosage for 2–4 weeks to ensure an adequate treatment trial.
2. Use sedative medications or beta blockers for agitation, rather than adding prn doses to the daily dose. This practice of prn's may adjust the daily received dose beyond a therapeutic or beneficial level.
3. Avoid polypharmacy. Using concomitant or augmented medication therapy that is focused on targeted symptoms requires vigilant monitoring of effect versus side effect versus interaction effect.

MAINTENANCE PHASE

1. Gradually reduce the maintenance dosage after stabilization of the targeted symptoms.
2. Reevaluate the administered dosage on at least a weekly basis.

TABLE 66-4
Anticholinergic Medications Used in
Pharmacological Intervention of EPS

		SYMPTOMS				
GENERIC NAME	BRAND NAME	AKATHISIA	AKINESIA	DYSTONIA	RIGIDITY	TREMOR
Amantadine	Symmetrel	2	3	2	3	2
Benztropine	Cogentin	2	2	3	3	2
Biperiden	Akineton	1	2	1	2	1
Diazepam	Valium	2	0	3	2	0
Diphenhydramine	Benadryl	2	1	2	1	2
Lorazepam	Ativan	2	0	0	0	0
Procyclidine	Kemadrin	1	2	2	2	1
Propranolol	Inderal	3	0	0	0	0
Trihexyphenidyl	Artane	2	2	2	2	1

Key: 0 = no effect; 1 = slight effect; 2 = moderate effect; 3 = good effect

TABLE 66-5
Anticholinergic Medications

GENERIC NAME	BRAND NAME	DOSE FORMS	ORAL DOSES	IM/IV DOSES	MECHANISM
Amantadine	Symmetrel	c:100 mg s:50 mg/5 ml	100 mg BID-TID	—	Dopaminergic agent
Benztropine	Cogentin	t:0.5/1/2 mg i:1 mg/ml	1–3 mg BID	1–2 mg	Anticholinergic
Biperiden	Akineton	t:2 mg p:5 mg/ml	2 mg BID-QID	2 mg	Anticholinergic
Bromocriptine*	Parlodel	t:2.5 mg c:5 mg	5–50 mg	—	Dopaminergic
Dantrolene*	Dantrium	c:25/50/100 mg	50 mg BID	—	Muscle relaxant
Diazepam	Valium	t:2/5/10 mg i:5 mg/ml	5 mg TID	5–10 mg	GABAminergic
Diphenhydramine	Benadryl	c:25/50 mg	p:10 mg/ml, 50 mg/ml	25–50 mg TID-QID	25–50 mg
Lorazepam	Ativan	t:0.5/1/2 mg p:2/4 mg/ml	1–2 mg TID	—	GABAminergic
Procyclidine	Kemadrin	t:5	2.5–5 mg TID	—	Anticholinergic
Trihexyphenidyl	Artane	t:2/5 mg SR:5 mg e:2 mg/5 ml	2–5 mg TID	—	Anticholinergic

Key: c = capsules; e = elixir; i = injection; p = parenteral; s = syrup; SR = sustained release sequels; t = tablets
*Used in the treatment of neuroleptic malignant syndrome (NMS).

3. Educate the client and family regarding the importance of antipsychotic medications to maintain symptom reduction and improved functional status.
4. Educate the client and family about early recognition of symptom relapse.
5. Initially assess and use follow-up evaluations to identify EPS using objective rating scales such as:
   a. Abnormal Involuntary Movement Scale (AIMS)
   b. Clamps Abnormal Movement Scale
   c. Simpson Neurological Rating Scale

6. Encourage client to use the symptom checklist to identify changes in symptoms. (See Box 65-1.)
7. Collaborate with colleagues to determine if the clinical response is positive or inadequate. If the response is determined inadequate, a plasma level of the antipsychotic medication must be obtained. This can help assess compliance or abnormal medication metabolism. See Table 66-6 for the therapeutic plasma levels for specific antipsychotics.
8. Discuss with clients their compliance in taking the medications; if compliance is *not* the reason for a subtherapeutic level, then an increase in the antipsychotic medication is needed.
9. Monitor the client for effect versus side effect. If there is no improvement after an additional adequate trial of 2–4 weeks, the antipsychotic medication should be tapered gradually and substituted with another antipsychotic from a different chemical class.

TABLE 66-6
Therapeutic Plasma Levels of Specific Antipsychotic Medications

ANTIPSYCHOTIC MEDICATION	THERAPEUTIC PLASMA LEVELS (mg/ml)
Chlorpromazine (Thorazine)	100–400
Clozapine (Clozaril)	141–204
Fluphenazine (Prolixin)	0.1–3.0
Fluphenazine decanoate (Prolixin)	0.05–2.7
Haloperidol (Haldol)	2–20
Perphenazine (Trilafon)	0.8–2.4
Thioridazine (Mellaril)	1.0–1.5
Thiothixene (Navane)	2–15
Trifluoperazine (Stelazine)	1–2.3

REFERENCE

Blair, D. T. (1990). Risk management for extrapyramidal symptoms. *Quality Review Bulletin* (March), 116–124.

BIBLIOGRAPHY

Ayd, F. J. (1994). Risperidone (Risperdal): A unique antipsychotic. *International Drug Therapy, 29* (1), 2, 5–10.
Blair, D. T., & Dauner, A. (1992). Dangerous consequences: Induced tardive akathisia. *Journal of Psychosocial Nursing and Mental Health Services, 30*(3), 41–43.
Blair, T., & Dauner, A. (1993). Neuroleptic malignant syndrome: Liability in nursing practice. *Journal of Psychosocial Nursing and Mental Health Services, 31* (2), 5–12.
Dickey, W. (1991). The neuroleptic malignant syndrome. *Progress in Neurobiology, 36* (5) 425–436.
Dillon, N. B. (1992). Screening system for tardive dyskinesia: Development and implementation. *Journal of Psychosocial Nursing and Mental Health Services, 30* (10) 3–7.
Gomez, G. E., & Gomez, E. G. (1990). The special concerns of neuroleptic use in the elderly. *Journal of Psychosocial Nursing and Mental Health Services, 28* (1), 7–14.
Jaretz, N., Flowers, E., & Milsap, L. (1992). Clozapine: Nursing care considerations. *Perspectives in Psychiatric Care, 28* (3), 19–24.
Kane, J. M. (ed.) (1993). *Risperidone: Major Progress in Antipsychotic Treatment.* Oxford, England: Oxford Clinical Communications.
Kaplan, H. I., & Sadock, B. J. (1993). *Pocket Handbook of Psychiatric Drug Treatment.* Philadelphia: Williams & Wilkins.
Keltner, N. L., & Folks, D. G. (1993). *Psychotropic Drugs.* St Louis: C. V. Mosby.

Lin, K. M., Poland, R. E., & Nakasaki, G. (1993). *Psychopharmacology and Psychobiology of Ethnicity.* Washington, DC: American Psychiatric Press.

Littrell, K., & Magill, A. M. (1993). The effect of clozapine on pre-existing tardive dyskinesia. *Journal of Psychosocial Nursing and Mental Health Services, 31* (9), 14–18.

Lohr, J. B., & Caligiuri, M. P. (1992). Quantitative instrumental measurement of tardive dyskinesia: A review. *Neuropsychopharmacology, 6* (4), 231–239.

Stern, R. G., Kahn, R. S., & Davidson, M. (1993). Predictors of response to neuroleptic treatment in schizophrenia. *Psychiatric Clinics of North America, 16* (2), 313–338.

SIXTY SEVEN

Antidepressant Medications

Susan L. W. Krupnick

OVERVIEW:

Introduction
Indications
Chemical Structural Groups
Method of Action

Target Symptoms
Dosage
Side-Effect Profile
Monitoring Treatment

INTRODUCTION

The 1950s signaled an important time in the historical development of psychopharmacologic approaches to treating depression. Monoamine oxidase inhibitors (MAOIs) were serendipitously discovered as a "side effect" when treating tubercular patients with iproniazid. These patients' general well-being and mood improved while taking the iproniazid.

Simultaneously the first tricyclic antidepressant (TCA), imipramine, was initially tested for antipsychotic symptoms. Although it clearly had no positive effect on psychotic symptoms, the symptoms of depression improved. Then in the late 1950s imipramine was marketed for its antidepressant actions. Several more selective and specific medications have been developed through neurobiological research over the last four decades since the initial TCAs were developed. Research into the neurobiological correlates of depression has ushered in several new discoveries that have markedly improved treatment options for the approximately 11–12 million Americans who suffer from this potentially incapacitating disorder.

INDICATIONS

Antidepressant medications are indicated to treat the following disorders:
1. Bipolar disorder, depressed
2. Depression in the medically ill and elderly
3. Dysthymic disorder
4. Major depression
5. Obsessive–compulsive disorder
6. Panic attacks
7. Schizoaffective disorder, depressed
8. Treatment-resistant depression

CHEMICAL STRUCTURAL GROUPS

Antidepressant medications are grouped as follows:
1. Tricyclic agents (TCAs): tertiary amines; secondary amines
2. Tetracyclic agents
3. Triazolopyridines
4. Aminoketones
5. Monoamine oxidase inhibitors (MAOIs)
6. Selective serotonin reuptake inhibitors (SSRIs)
7. Selective serotonin–norepinephrine reuptake inhibitors (SSNRIs)

METHOD OF ACTION

Tricyclic Agents Block the reuptake of norepinephrine or serotonin, desensitize post-synaptic receptors, reregulate an abnormal receptor–neurotransmitter relationship, promote a downregulation of activity by decreasing beta-adrenergic receptor sensitivity to norepinephrine (Downregulation Theory).

Tetracyclic Agents Block the reuptake of serotonin and some norepinephrine; limited anticholinergic effect.

Monoamine Oxidase Inhibitors MAO is the enzyme that catalyzes the breakdown of various amines: epinephrine, norepinephrine, serotonin, and dopamine. Inhibition of MAO results in an increased concentration of these amines in the synaptic cleft. It is believed that the MAO inhibitor antidepressant effect is a result of increased availability of CNS norepinephrine and serotonin.

Selective Serotonin Reuptake Inhibitors Selectively inhibit serotonin uptake without significantly altering normal epinephrine uptake mechanism. Their action is more specific, while the side effect profile is more narrow.

Selective Serotonin–Norepinephrine Reuptake Inhibitors Presynaptically enrich the synapse with serotonin while also inhibiting norepinephrine reuptake in the presynaptic area. Postsynaptically block $5HT_2$ receptor stimulation.

CNS Stimulants (Psychostimulants) Directly release catecholamines into synaptic clefts and onto postsynaptic receptor sites. Block the reuptake of catecholamines, thereby prolonging action. Act on MAO enzymes to slow down metabolism. Generally used with the medically ill and elderly when exhibiting failure to thrive.

TARGET SYMPTOMS

Antidepressants act to reduce:
1. Anergia
2. Anhedonia (loss of pleasure)
3. Anorexia
4. Concentration difficulties
5. Guilt
6. Helplessness
7. Hopelessness
8. Increase or loss of appetite
9. Insomnia or hypersomnia
10. Loss of energy
11. Loss of sex drive
12. Preoccupation with death

13. Psychomotor agitation
14. Psychomotor retardation
15. Sad or anxious mood

DOSAGE   See Table 67-1 for identification of chemical groups and specific medications with therapeutic doses and geriatric doses.

TABLE 67-1
Antidepressant Medication Doses

GENERIC NAME	BRAND NAME	DOSE FORMS (mg)	THERAPEUTIC DOSES (mg/day)	RANGES (mg/day)	GERIATRIC DOSES (mg/day)
TRICYCLICS					
Amitriptyline	Elavil	t:10/25/50/75/100/150 p:10 mg/ml	75–300	24–450	Start 10 25–50
	Endep	t:10/25/50/75/100/150			
Amoxapine	Asendin	t:25/50/100/150	200–400	50–600	100–150
Clomipramine	Anafranil	c:25/50/75	125–300	25–500	Start 10 50–150
Doxepin	Sinequan	c:10/25/50/75/100/150 o:10 mg/ml	150–300	25–300	Start 10 10–75
	Adapin	c:10/25/50/75/100/150			
Imipramine	Tofranil	c:10/25/50 p:25 mg/2 ml	150–300	25–300	Start 10
	Janimine	t:10/25/50			25–100
Imipramine pamoate	Tofranil-PM (sustained release)	c:75/100/125/150			
Trimipramine	Surmontil	c:25/50/100	150–300	25–300	Start 10 25–100
Desipramine	Norpramin Pertofrane	t:10/25/50/75/100/150 c:25/50	150–300	25–400	Start 10 25–100
Nortriptyline	Pamelor	c:10/25/50/75 o:10 mg/5 ml	75–150	20–200	Start 10 25–100
	Aventyl	c:10/25			
Protriptyline	Vivactil	t:5/10	30–60	10–60	Start 5 5–20
MONOAMINE OXIDASE INHIBITORS (MAOIs)					
Hydrazines					
Phenelzine	Nardil	t:15	45–60	45–90	Start 7.5 15–45
Benzamides					
Moclobemide	Aurorix	t:100/150/300	300–450	150–600	—
Nonhydrazines					
Tranylcypromine	Parnate	t:10	20–40	10–60	Start 5 10–40
AMINOKETONE					
Bupropion	Wellbutrin	t:75/100	225–450	100–450	75–450
TETRACYCLIC					
Maprotiline	Ludiomil	t:25/50/75	150–225	25–225	Start 10 25–75
TRIAZOLOPYRIDINE					
Trazodone	Desyrel	t:50/100/150/300	200–600	50–600	Start 25 25–200

(Continued)

TABLE 67-1 *(continued)*

GENERIC NAME	BRAND NAME	DOSE FORMS (mg)	THERAPEUTIC DOSES (mg/day)	RANGES (mg/day)	GERIATRIC DOSES (mg/day)
SELECTIVE SEROTONIN REUPTAKE INHIBITORS (SSRI)					
Fluoxetine	Prozac	c:10/20 l:20mg/5ml	20	20–120	Start 5 5–20
Paroxetine	Paxil	t:20/30	20	20–50	Start 10 20–40
Sertraline	Zoloft	t:50/100	50–150	50–200	Start 50 50–150
Fluvoxamine	Luvox	t:50/100	100	50–300	Start 50 50–150
SELECTIVE SEROTONIN/NOREPINEPHRINE REUPTAKE INHIBITORS (SSNRIs)					
Venlafaxine	Effexor	t:25/37.5/50/75/100	75–225	150–375	—
Nefazodone	Serzone	t:100/150/200/250	200	300–600	Start 100 100–400
CNS STIMULANTS					
Dextroamphetamine	Dexedrine	t:5/10 SR-sp:5/10/15 e:5mg/ml	10–20	5–40	10–15
Methylphenidate	Ritalin Ritalin-SR	t:5/10/20 SR-t:20	20–30	20–80	10–30
Pemoline	Cylert	t:18.75/37.5/75	56.25–75	37.5–112.5	—

c = capsule; l = liquid; t = tablet; o = oral; p = parenteral
*Not available in United States at present time.

SIDE-EFFECT PROFILE   See Table 67-2 for a side-effect profile of antidepressant medications.

MONITORING TREATMENT

Prior to initiating antidepressant medication:
1. Collaborate with medical–psychiatry service members to complete a thorough medical evaluation with specific focus on:
   a. Cardiovascular assessment including an EKG
   b. Comprehensive thyroid status assessment (TFTs)
   c. Liver function tests (LFTs)
2. Collaborate with the medical–psychiatry service members in the selection of appropriate medication based on:
   a. History of present illness
   b. Specific target signs and symptoms
   c. Basis of side effect profile:
      • Stimulating versus sedating effects
      • Cardiovascular effect
      • Anticholinergic effect
   d. History of previous positive versus negative response
3. Instruct the client and family members of benefits and risks of selected medication. Teach and provide information on serotonin syndrome if on an SSRI. Serotonin syndrome is a medication-induced syndrome that has been attributed to excessive stimulation of the serotonergic system. This syndrome occurs with clients treated concurrently with a combination of two or more serotonergic medications such as fluoxetine or an MAOI with trazodone. It can also occur in clients who take only one SSRI. See Box 67-1 for characteristics and treatment.

TABLE 67-2
Side-Effect Profiles of Antidepressant Medications

GENERIC NAME	BRAND NAME	SIDE EFFECTS			
		SEDATIVE	ANTI-CHOLINERGIC	HYPO-TENSIVE	CARDIAC
TRICYCLICS					
Amitriptyline	Elavil Endep	+++	+++	+++	+++
Amoxapine	Asendin	++	++	++	+
Clomipramine	Anafranil	++	++	++	++
Doxepin	Sinequan Adapin	+++	+++	++	++
Imipramine	Tofranil Janimine	++	++	+++	+++
Imipramine Pamoate	Tofranil-PM (sustained release)	++	++	+++	+++
Trimipramine	Surmontil	+++	+++	++	+++
Desipramine	Norpramin Pertofrane	++	++	++	+
Nortriptyline	Pamelor	++	++	+	++
Protriptyline	Aventyl Vivactil	+	++	++	+++
MONOAMINE OXIDASE INHIBITORS (MAOI)					
Hydrazines					
Isocarboxazid	Marplan	+	+	++	O
Phenelzine	Nardil	+	+	++	O
Benzamides					
Moclobemide		O	O	+	O
Nonhydrazines					
Tranylcypromine	Parnate	+	+	+	O
AMINOKETONE					
Bupropion	Wellbutrin	?	+	+	+
TETRACYCLIC					
Maprotiline	Ludiomil	++	++	++	++
TRIAZOLOPYRIDINE					
Trazodone	Desyrel	++	?	+++	+
SELECTIVE SEROTONIN REUPTAKE INHIBITORS (SSRI)					
Fluoxetine	Prozac	?	+	+	+
Paroxetine	Paxil	?	+	+	+
Sertraline	Zoloft	O	O	O	O
Fluvoxamine	Luvox	+	O	O	O
SELECTIVE SEROTONIN-NOREPINEPHRINE REUPTAKE INHIBITORS (SSNRI)					
Nefazodone	Serzone	+	+	+	+
Venlafaxine	Effexor	+	+	+*	++

Key: ? = Questionable; O = None; + = Minimal; ++ = Moderate; +++ = Most
*Reports of dose-dependent sustained increases in blood pressure.

4. Provide both client and family member with specific written material related to selected medication.
5. Explain that there may be a delay in the desired therapeutic response as well as the common side effects.

Initiation Phase

1. Initiate and carefully increase the dose of the antidepressant medication gradually while monitoring the effect versus side effect.

BOX 67-1: Identifying Characteristics and Treatment of Serotonin Syndrome

Characteristics:	Early Phase	Agitation
		Confusion
		Diaphoresis
		Diarrhea
		Flushing
		Lethargy
		Myoclonic jerks
		Restlessness
		Tremors
	Middle Phase	Hypertension
		Hypertonicity
		↑ Myoclonus
		Rigor
	Late Phase	Acidosis
		DIC
		Respiratory failure
		Renal failure
		Rhabdomyolysis

Treatment: Early identification!
Discontinue serotonergic medications
Emergency medical treatment to support physiological
recovery:
  Cooling blankets for hyperthermia
  Clonazepam for myoclonus
  Chlorpromazine IM for hyperthermia and sedation
  Nifedipine for hypertension
  $5HT_{1a}$ antagonists and beta blockers

2. If there is no therapeutic response after 1 week within the therapeutic dose range, gradually increase the dose to the maximum recommended dose.
3. Monitor client behavioral response, therapeutic medication levels, and EKG (when appropriate); if no therapeutic response, adjust dose to obtain positive response.
4. Actively participate with medical–psychiatry team members to consider augmentation strategies or a change to another first-line antidepressant for a severely depressed client who has achieved only a partial response to antidepressant treatment.

Maintenance Phase
1. Monitor EKG and therapeutic medication levels weekly.
2. Collaborate with the client in completing symptom checklist to determine the client's perception of response to medication.
3. Maintain treatment for at least 4–6 months symptom-free in the case of a first-time depressive episode.
4. Instruct the client and family member(s) about long-term antidepressant treatment for recurrent disease.

BIBLIOGRAPHY

Cram, G. E. (1957). Iproniazid (Marsilid) phosphate, a therapeutic agent for mental disorders and debilitating disease. *Journal of Psychiatric Research, 8* (2), 142–152.

Depression Guideline Panel (1993). *Depression in Primary Care: Volume I, Detection and Diagnosis.* Clinical Practice Guidelines. Number 5. Rockville, MD: U.S. Department of Health and Human Services. Agency for Healthcare Policy and Research Publication No. 93-0551.

DeVance, C. L. (1990). *Fundamentals of Monitoring Psychoactive Drug Therapy.* Baltimore: Williams & Wilkins.

Fawcett, J., Kravitz, H. M., Zajecka, J. M., & Schall, M. R. (1991). CNS stimulant potentiation of monoamine oxidase inhibitors in treatment-refractory depression. *Journal of Clinical Psychopharmacology, 11* (21), 127–139.

Fitton, A., Faulds, D., & Goa, K. L. (1992). Moclobemide: A review of its pharmacological properties and therapeutic use in depressive illness. *Drugs, 43* (4), 561–596.

Frank, E., Kupfer, D. J., Perle, J., Carnes, C., Jarreh, D. B., Mallinger, A. G., Those, M. E., McEachran, A. B., & Grechocinski, J. (1990). Three year outcomes for maintenance therapies in recurrent depression. *Archives of General Psychiatry, 47* (12), 1093–1099.

Freeman, C. P., Trimble, M. R., Deakin, J. F. W., Stokes, T. M., & Ashford, J. J. (1994). Fluvoxamine or clomipramine in the treatment of obsessive compulsive disorder: A multicenter, randomized, double blind, parallel group comparison. *Journal of Clinical Psychiatry, 55* (7), 301–305.

Gitlin, M. (1994). Psychotropic medications and their effect on sexual function: Diagnosis, biology, and treatment approaches. *Journal of Clinical Psychiatry, 55* (9), 406–413.

Khan, A., Fabre, L. F., & Rudolph, R. (1991). Venlafaxine in depressed outpatients. *Psychopharmacology Bulletin, 27* (2), 141–144.

Preskorn, S. H., & Burke, M. (1992). Somatic therapy for major depressive disorder: Selection of an antidepressant. *Journal of Clinical Psychiatry, 53* (supplement), 5–18.

Rosenberg, P. B., Ahmed, I., & Hurwitz, S. (1991). Methylphenidate in depressed medically ill patients. *Journal of Clinical Psychiatry, 52* (6), 263–267.

Salzman, C. (ed.) (1992). *Clinical Geriatric Psychopharmacology* (2nd ed.). Baltimore: Williams & Wilkins.

Satel, S. L., & Nelson, J. C. (1989). Stimulants in the treatment of depression: A critical overview. *Journal of Clinical Psychiatry, 50* (7), 241–249.

Sternbach, H. (1991). The serotonin syndrome. *American Journal of Psychiatry, 148* (6), 705–713.

Woods, S. W., Tesar, G. E., Murray, G. B., & Cassem, N. H. (1986). Psychostimulant treatment of depressive disorders secondary to medical illness. *Journal of Clinical Psychiatry, 47* (1), 12–15.

Yager, J. (1986). Bethanechol chloride can reverse erectile and ejaculatory dysfunction induced by tricyclic antidepressants and mazindol. Case Report. *Journal of Clinical Psychiatry, 47* (4), 210–211.

Zajecka, J., Fawcett, J., Schaff, M., Jeffriess, H., & Guy, C. (1991). The role of serotonin in sexual dysfunction. *Journal of Clinical Psychiatry, 52* (2), 66–68.

68
SIXTY EIGHT

Mood-Stabilizing Medications

Susan L. W. Krupnick

OVERVIEW:

INTRODUCTION

The psychopharmacologic treatment of mania began with an observation by Cade, a physician, in 1949 that the calming effect of lithium in animals was also extended to humans with manic-depressive illness (Cade, 1949). Clinical investigations followed that conclusively demonstrated that lithium was effective in preventing recurrence of mania. The impact of this medication has been profound for clients experiencing bipolar disorder, their families, and society. Additional medications from different chemical structural classes and with apparently different mechanisms of actions have also been found effective in the prophylaxis and treatment of mania. These medications include specific anticonvulsants, calcium channel blockers, alpha-adrenergic agonists, and beta-adrenergic receptor blockers.

INDICATIONS

Mood-stabilizing medications are indicated in the treatment of:
1. Aggressive behaviors
2. Acute mania
3. Unipolar or bipolar depressions
4. Rapid cycling
5. Symptoms secondary to complex partial seizures
6. Schizoaffective disorder

CHEMICAL STRUCTURAL GROUPS

Mood-stabilizing medications fall into the following groups:

1. Lithium
   - Lithium carbonate
   - Lithium citrate
2. Anticonvulsants
   - Carbamazepine (CBZ)
   - Clonazepam
   - Valproic acid (VPA)
3. Calcium channel blockers
4. Alpha-adrenergic blockers
5. Beta-adrenergic receptor blockers

METHOD OF ACTION

Lithium Precise mechanisms of action are unknown, but it is hypothesized that lithium ions substitute for the sodium ion in neurons. This normalizes the ability of the neuron to release, inactivate, and respond to neurotransmiters, thereby correcting an ion exchange abnormality.

Anticonvulsants

1. *Carbamazepine:* inhibits kindling, a process that accelerates behavioral and convulsive responses from a repetition of same stimulus
2. *Clonazepam:* Useful in acute mania, its apparent antimanic effect could be secondary to sedation
3. *Valproic acid:* Has antikindling, anticonvulsant, and GABA-ergic effects

TARGET SIGNS AND SYMPTOMS

See Box 68-1 for symptoms of mania and depression warranting treatment.

BOX 68-1: Symptoms of Mania and Depression

Mania	*Depression*
Assaultive/threatening behavior	Anhedonia
Catatonia	Anorexia or increased appetite
Distractibility	Constipation
Euphoria	Decreased libido
Expansiveness	Fatigue
Flight of ideas	Guilt
Grandiosity	Helplessness
Hallucinations	Hopelessness
Hypergraphia	Irritability
Hypersexuality	Motor retardation
Ideas of reference	Pessimism
Irritability	Poor concentration
Lability with depression	Sadness
Manipulativeness	Self-reproach
Motor hyperactivity	Sleep disturbance (insomnia or hypersomnia)
Persecutory and religious delusions	Slowed thinking
Pressured speech	Somatic complaints
Sleep disturbance (decreased sleep)	Suicidal ideation
	Weight change

DOSAGE   See Table 68-1 for information about each mood-stabilizing medication.

SIDE EFFECTS   See Table 68-2 for a comparison of side effects of lithium, carbamazepine, and valproic acid.

MONITORING TREATMENT WITH LITHIUM

PRETREATMENT PHASE

Prior to initiating lithium treatment:

1. Collaborate with medical–psychiatry team members to conduct a comprehensive medical evaluation. Consider factors predictive of lithium responsiveness. See Box 68-2.
2. Ensure that appropriate medical laboratory evaluations are completed and evaluate clinical laboratory studies in relation to renal, thyroid, cardiac, carbohydrate, and hematologic function. Include in the pretreatment lithium laboratory assessment:
   Renal function studies
   - Blood urea nitrogen (BUN)
   - Creatinine: 24-hour creatinine clearance and protein
   - Electrolytes
   - Fluid deprivation test
   - Urinalysis

TABLE 68-1
Mood-Stabilizing Medications

GENERIC NAME	BRAND NAME	DOSE FORMS (mg)	DOSE RANGE	USUAL PLASMA LEVEL (mEq/L)	PLASMA LEVEL RANGE (mEq/L)	ELDERLY PLASMA LEVEL (mEq/L)
LITHIUM						
Lithium carbonate	Eskalith Eskalith CR Lithane Lithobid	t:300 c:300 t:450 t:300	Acute mania 1500–2100 mg Maintenance 900–1200 mg	Acute 0.8–1.2 Maintenance 0.6–1.0	0.5–1.5 0.46–1.2	0.6–0.8 0.3–0.6
Lithium citrate	Cibalith-S	s:300/5 ml				

			STARTING DOSE (mg/day)	THERAPEUTIC DOSES (mg/day)	DOSE RANGE (mg/day)	PLASMA LEVELS (μg/ml or ng/ml)
ANTICONVULSANTS						
Carbamazepine	Tegretol Mazepine	t:100/200 susp:100 mg/5 ml	400	800–1200	200–1800	8–12 μg/ml
Clonazepam (acute mania)	Klonopin	t:0.5/1/2	1–2	4–16	0.5–40	20–80 ng/ml
Valproic acid	Depakene Depakote	c:250 s:250 mg/5ml t:125/250/500	500	100–1500	1000–3000	50–100 μg/ml
CALCIUM CHANNEL BLOCKERS						
Verapamil	Isoptin Calan Verelan	t:40/80/120 ER:120/180/240 cap:120/180/240 p:2.5 mg/mll	120	360–480	240–480	100–300 ng/ml
ALPHA₂-ADRENERGIC AGONIST						
Clonidine	Catapres	t:0.1/0.2/0.3	0.2	0.2–0.8	0.2–1.2	—
BETA-ADRENERIC RECEPTOR BLOCKAGE						
Propranolol	Inderal	t:10/20/40/60/80/90 ER:60/80/120/160 conc:80 mg/5ml p:1mg/ml solution:4 mg/ml, 8 mg/ml	100	100–640	100–640	50–100 ng/ml

TABLE 68-2
Comprehensive Side-Effect Comparison of Lithium,
Carbamazepine, and Valproic Acid

SYSTEM SIDE EFFECT	LITHIUM	CARBAMAZE-PINE	VALPROIC ACID
Cardiovascular			
Congestive heart failure	−	+	−
Dizziness	+	+	R
Faintness	+	+	−
Hypotension	−	+	−
Hypertension (can be aggravated)	−	+	−
Central Nervous System			
Ataxia	+	+	R
Anxiety	−	−	R
Cogwheeling	+	−	−
Confusion	+	+	R
Depression	−	R	R
Dysarthria	+	+	R
Hallucinations	−	+	−
Headache	+	+	R
Hypersomnia	+	−	−
Incoordination	+	+	R
Increased alertness	−	−	+
Insomnia	+	−	−
Jerking limbs	+	+	−
Memory impairment	+	−	−
Muscle or leg cramps	+	+	−
Paresthesia	+	R	R
Restlessness	+	−	−
Rigidity	+	−	−
Sedation	−	+	+
Seizures	+	−	−
Tremor	+	R	R
Weakness	+	−	+
Gastrointestinal			
Anorexia	R	+	−
Abdominal cramps	+	+	+
Constipation	−	+	R
Diarrhea	+	+	R
Dry mouth	+	+	−
Edema	+	−	R
Hepatitis	−	+	+
Increased appetite	+	−	R
Nausea/vomiting	+	+	+
Pancreatitis	−	+	+
Weight gain	+	−	+
Weight loss	R	+	−
Genitourinary			
Acute urinary retention	−	R	−
Nephrogenic diabetes insipidus	+	−	−
Polyuria	+	−	R
Polydipsia	+	−	R
Urinary frequency	+	+	−

(Continued)

TABLE 68-2 *(continued)*

SYSTEM SIDE EFFECT	LITHIUM	CARBAMAZE-PINE	VALPROIC ACID
Hematologic			
Agranulocytosis	−	+	+
Anemia	−	+	R
Leukopenia	−	+	R
Bruising	−	+	+
Petechiae	−	+	+
Integumentary			
Alopecia	+	R	+
Photosensitivity	−	+	+
Pruritus	R	+	+
Pruritic rash (allergy)	+	+	+
Vision			
Blurred vision	+	+	−
Diplopia	−	+	R
Nystagmus	−	−	R

Key: + = present; − = absent; R = rare

Compiled from: Maxmen, J. S. (1991). *Psychotropic drugs: Fast facts.* New York: W. W. Norton; Calabrese, J. R., Bowden, C., & Woyshville, M. J. (1995). Lithium and the anticonvulsants in the treatment of bipolar disorder. In F. E. Bloom & D. J. Kupfer (eds.), *Psychopharmacology: The Fourth Generation of Progress* (pp. 1099–1111). New York: Raven Press.

Thyroid function studies
- Antithyroid antibodies
- T_3 RU (resin uptake)
  - T_4 RIA (radioimmunoassay)
  - T_4 FTI (free thyroxine index)
  - TSH (thyroid-stimulating hormone)
  - Serum calcium ion value

Cardiac function
  - Assessment of any history or symptoms of cardiac disease, especially hypertension, and diuretic use
  - EKG

Carbohydrate metabolism function
  - FBS (fasting blood sugar)
  - Baseline weight
  - History of diabetes mellitus

Hematologic function: Complete blood count with differential
Reproductive function: Pregnancy test in childbearing women

3. Instruct client and family members about the use of lithium including effect, side effects, need for ongoing therapeutic medication monitoring, and early signs or symptoms of lithium toxicity. If the client is pregnant or considering pregnancy, educate her and her family about effects on the fetus.

INITIATION PHASE

1. Initiate lithium therapy at 300 mg twice a day and monitor closely while increasing by 300 mg every 3–4 days.
2. Ensure that lithium levels are obtained 12 hours after the last dose twice a week.

BOX 68-2: Predictive Factors in Lithium Treatment Response

Positive Responders

"Classical mania"

Acute, elated, moderate episodes without psychotic features

Depressive episode to euthymia and then mania has a better response than depression to mania

Family history of mania or bipolar illness

History of treatment compliance

Positive family member response to lithium

Prior manic episode

Negative Responders

Anxiety

Bipolar disorder secondary to medical disorder

Bipolar type II females

Mixed states

Obsessive features

Onset after 40

Rapid cycling

Comorbid substance abuse

Compiled from: Goodwin, F. R., & Jamison, K. R. (1990). *Manic-Depressive Illness*. New York: Oxford University Press; Calabrese, J. R., Bowden, C., & Woyshville, M. J. (1995). Lithium and the anticonvulsants in the treatment of bipolar disorder. In F. E. Bloom & D. J. Kupfer (eds.), *Psychopharmacology: The Fourth Generation of Progress* (pp. 1100–1101). New York: Raven Press.

STABILIZATION PHASE

1. The dose is increased until mood stabilization is achieved and the therapeutic blood level range is 0.6–1.4 mEq/L for adult clients. For geriatric clients or those with medical illness a therapeutic range is 0.6–0.8 mEq/L.
2. Monitor the client for agitation in acute mania. If acute mania symptoms persist, then concomitant therapy with antipsychotic medications may be considered.
3. Observe for a reduction in acute manic symptoms while monitoring for the side effects of lithium.
4. Instruct client and family members in side effect and nutritional management. Provide written educational material to reinforce learning.
5. Collaborate with medical–psychiatric team members to consider addition of carbamazepine if client is unresponsive to lithium alone.

MAINTENANCE PHASE

1. Monitor psychophysiologic and behavioral responses to lithium.
2. After the client has a positive response to medication regimen, the maintenance lithium dose is usually reduced but maintained in a therapeutic blood level range.
3. Collaborate with client, family, and medical–psychiatry team members to schedule and monitor specific laboratory studies.
   Renal function studies every 3–6 months
   - BUN
   - Creatinine
   - Fluid deprivation test
   Thyroid studies every 6 months
   - TSH

Cardiac function
- EKG—I month after stable lithium level and then biannually if no cardiac difficulties
- Carbohydrate metabolism studies biannually
     FBS
     Urine for ketones
- Hematologic function studies
Lithium levels monitored every 1–3 months (or more frequently if necessary)
4. Closely monitor client for medication response versus side effect and watch for early symptoms of lithium toxicity in the "warning range" of 1.2–1.5 mEq/L. In this range the risk of developing lithium toxicity can rise rapidly, especially in the elderly and medically compromised client.
5. If client develops lithium toxicity, when appropriate after recovery, interview client and family to identify reasons for lithium toxicity and develop a health teaching plan to increase compliance.

LITHIUM TOXICITY

See Table 68-3 for the assessment and management of lithium toxicity.

MONITORING TREATMENT WITH ANTICONVULSANTS

PRETREATMENT PHASE

Prior to initiating treatment:
1. Collaborate with medical–psychiatry team members to conduct a comprehensive medical evaluation.
2. Ensure that appropriate medical laboratory evaluations are completed and evaluate clinical laboratory studies as follows:
   Carbamazepine (Tegretol)
   - CBC with differential (especially platelets and reticulocyte)
   - Electrolytes
   - EEG
   - EKG
   - Liver function tests (LFTs)
   - Pregnancy test (childbearing women)
   Valproic acid and derivatives
   - CBC with differential
   - EEG
   - Liver function tests (LFTs)
   - Serum determination of concomitant antiepileptic drugs
   - Prothrombin time (PT)
   - Partial thromboplastin time (PTT)
   - Thyroid function tests
   - Total protein, serum albumin
   - Pregnancy test in childbearing women
3. Collaborate with medical–psychiatry team members in selecting appropriate anticonvulsant agent.
4. Instruct client and family members of desired effect, side effects, and importance of monitoring serum levels.
5. Initiate medication as follows: carbamazepine (CBZ) at 200 mg twice a day, or valproic acid (VPA) at 250 mg twice a day.
6. Monitor for effect versus side effect.

TABLE 68-3
Lithium Toxicity: Assessment and Management

ASSESSMENT OF SIGNS AND SYMPTOMS	LITHIUM LEVEL	MANAGEMENT STRATEGIES
"Warning range"	1.2–1.5 mEq/L	• Monitoring closely for any symptoms • Redraw lithium level • Emphasize maintenance of salt & water during hot weather or exercise

Mild to moderate toxicity
Gastrointestinal:
   Abdominal pain
   Dryness of mouth
   Vomiting
Neurological:
   Ataxia
   Dizziness
   Lethargy or excitement
   Muscle weakness
   Nystagmus
   Slurred speech
	1.5–2.0 mEq/L	• Have clients contact their treating healthcare provider or go to hospital psychiatric crisis unit or emergency room. Hospitalize or use 24-hour observation bed
		• Discontinue lithium
		• Instruct client to ingest fluids
		• Conduct physical examination, neurological and mental status assessment
		• Monitor vital signs
		• Order laboratory studies

Moderate to severe toxicity
Gastrointestinal:
   Anorexia
   Diarrhea
   Persistent nausea and vomiting
Neurological:
   Blurred vision
   Cardiac disturbances
   Choreoathetoid movements
   Clonic limb movements
   Coma
   Convulsions
   Delirium
   EEG changes
   Increased deep tendon reflexes
   Muscle fasiculations
   Stupor
   Syncope
	2.0–2.5 mEq/L	• Use above strategies and hospitalize client
		• Order lithium level, serum electrolytes, renal function tests
		• Order EEG
		• Order EKG
		• Provide vigorous hydration
		• Adjust electrolyte imbalances with IV fluids
		• *If acute ingestion:*
		   □ Obtain residual gastric contents by emesis or gastric lavage
		   □ Increase gastric content absorption with activated charcoal
		   □ Offer supportive measures

Severe lithium toxicity
Cardiac failure:
   Conduction abnormalities
   Dysrhythmias
   Hypotension
Metabolic:
   Increased temperature
Neurological:
   Generalized convulsions
   Impaired consciousness
Renal:
   Oliguria
   Renal failure
Possible death
	> 2.5 mEq/L	• As above
		• Order lithium levels every 3 hours
		• > 4.0 mEq/L or if life-threatening clinical presentation start hemodialysis
		• Repeat hemodialysis every 6–10 hours to manage rebound peaks in serum lithium

Compiled from: Rosse, R. B., Grese, A. A., Deutsch, S. I., & Morihisa, J. M. (1989). *Laboratory Diagnostic Testing in Psychiatry.* Washington, DC: American Psychiatric Press Inc; Silver, J. M., Yudovsky, S. C., & Hurowitz, G. I. (1994). Psychopharmacology and ECT. In R. E. Hales, S. C. Yudofsky, & J. A. Talbolt (eds.), *Textbook of Psychiatry* (2nd ed.) (pp. 897–1008). Washington, DC: American Psychiatric Press.

STABILIZATION PHASE

1. Collaborate in the decision-making process to increase CBZ dose by 200 mg or VPA dose by 250 mg at 3–5-day intervals.
2. Ensure that serum levels are obtained and reviewed every week until therapeutic levels are attained as follows: CBZ 8–12 μg/ml; VPA 50–100 ng/ml.

MAINTENANCE PHASE

1. Monitor levels every month for the first 3 months after initiation of treatments. If stabilized, monitor every 3 months.
2. Instruct client and family about importance of hematologic monitoring if on carbamazepine.
3. If client is taking carbamazepine, obtain CBC with differential every 2 weeks for the first 2 months, and if no alterations, then monitor every 3 months.
4. Instruct client and family about importance of liver function monitoring when on CBZ or VPA.
5. Obtain and monitor the following liver function studies every month for the first 2 months of treatment; if no alterations, then every 3 months.
   - SGOT
   - SGPT
   - LDH
   - Alkaline phosphatase
6. Instruct client and family to watch for petechiae, pallor, unusual weakness, elevated temperature, or signs of infection.

REFERENCES

Cade, J. S. K. (1949). Lithium salts in the treatment of psychotic excitement. *Medical Journal of Australia. 2*, 349–353.

Calabrese, J. R., Bowden, C., & Woyshville, M.J. (1995). Lithium and the anticonvulsants in the treatment of bipolar disorder. In F. E. Bloom & D. J. Kupfer (eds.), *Psychopharmacology: The Fourth Generation of Progress* (pp. 1100–1101). New York: Raven Press.

Goodwin, F. R., & Jamison, K. R. (1990). *Manic-Depressive Illness.* New York: Oxford University Press.

Maxmen, J. S. (1991). *Psychotropic Drugs: Fast Facts.* New York: W. W. Norton.

Rosse, R. B., Giese, A. A., Deutsch, S. I., & Morihisa, J. M. (1989). *Laboratory Diagnostic Testing in Psychiatry.* Washington, DC: American Psychiatric Press.

Silver, J. M., Yudovsky, S. C. & Hurowitz, G. I. (1994). Psychopharmacology and ECT. In R. E. Hales, S. C. Yudofsky, & J. A. Talbolt (eds.), *Textbook of Psychiatry* (2nd ed.) (pp. 897–1008). Washington, DC: American Psychiatric Press.

BIBLIOGRAPHY

Dilsaver, S. C., Swann, A. C., Shouib, A. M., & Bowers, T. C. (1993). The manic syndrome: Factors which may predict a patient's response to lithium, carbamazepine and valproate. *Journal of Psychiatry and Neuroscience, 18* (2), 61–66.

Dubovsky, S. L. (1994). Geriatric neuropsychopharmacology. In C. E. Coffey & J. L. Cummings (eds.), *Textbook of Geriatric Neuropsychiatry* (pp. 595–632). Washington, DC: American Psychiatric Press.

Garza-Trevins, E. S., Overall, J. E., & Hollister, L. E. (1992). Verapamil versus lithium in acute mania. *American Journal of Psychiatry, 149* (11), 121–122.

Gerner, R. H., & Stanton, A. (1992). Algorithm for patient management of acute manic states: Lithium, valproate or carbamazepine? *Journal of Clinical Psychopharmacology, 12* (1), supplement, 57S–63S.

Glod, C. A., & Mathieu, J. (1993). Expanding uses of anticonvulsants in the treatment of bipolar disorder. *Journal of Psychosocial Nursing and Mental Health Services, 31* (5), 37–39.

Hales, R. E., Yudofsky, S. C., & Talbott, J. A. (1994). *Textbook of psychiatry* (2nd ed.). Washington, DC: American Psychiatric Press.

Sachs, G. S., Rosenbaum, J. F., & Jones, L. (1990). Adjunctive clonazepam for maintenance treatment of bipolar affective disorder. *Journal of Clinical Psychopharmacology, 106* (1), 42–47.

Token, M., Castillo, J., Baldessarini, C. Z., Zarote, C., & Kando, J. C. (1995). Blood dyscrasias with carbamazepine and valproate: A pharmacoepidemiological study of 2,228 patients at risk. *American Journal of Psychiatry, 152* (3), 413–418.

69

Antianxiety and Hypnosedative Medications

Susan L. W. Krupnick

OVERVIEW:

Introduction
Antianxiety Medications
    Indications
    Chemical Structural Groups
    Method of Action
    Target Signs and Symptoms
    Dosage
    Monitoring Treatment

Hypnosedative Medications
    Indications
    Chemical Structural Groups
    Method of Action
    Target Signs and Symptoms
    Dosage
    Monitoring Treatment

INTRODUCTION

Antianxiety medications, specifically the benzodiazepines, are the most widely prescribed and used medications. The first benzodiazepine, chlordiazepoxide (Librium), was marketed in 1960. Diazepam (Valium) was on the market 3 years later.

Benzodiazepines are very effective for the alleviation of acute anxiety while retaining efficacy over time. Clients with a history of anxiety are likely to need long-term pharmacological intervention; therefore, close monitoring of treatment response is necessary.

Benzodiazepines are referred to as antianxiety agents, anxiolytics, or mild tranquilizers. Benzodiazepines are also classified as hypnosedative or sedative–hypnotics. A sedative medication reduces daytime activity, diminishes excitement, and usually has a quieting effect. A hypnotic drug produces drowsiness and facilitates the onset and maintenance of sleep.

The benzodiazepines have become the hypnosedative medications of first choice. They have a higher therapeutic index and a wider margin of safety than most of the other hypnosedative medications such as barbiturates and nonbarbiturate compounds.

ANTIANXIETY MEDICATIONS

INDICATIONS

Antianxiety medications are used to treat:
1. Generalized anxiety disorder
2. Bipolar disorder
3. Panic disorder

4. Akathisia (restlessness and uncontrolled movement)
5. Abstinence withdrawal syndromes
6. Emergency care of drug-induced and psychotic agitation

CHEMICAL STRUCTURAL GROUPS

Antianxiety medications fall into two groups:
1. Benzodiazepines
2. Azapirone

METHOD OF ACTION

Benzodiazepine Anxiolytics Benzodiazepine anxiolytics bind to specific receptor sites that are associated with gamma-aminobutyric acid (GABA) binding sites and chloride channels. Benzodiazepine binding increases the affinity of the GABA receptor for GABA, therefore increasing the flow of chloride ions into the neurons. Recent neuroscience research has determined two subtypes of CNS benzodiazepine receptors (omega receptors): BZ_1 and BZ_2. BZ_1 receptors are believed to be important in the mediation of sleep, while BZ_2 receptors are implicated in cognition, memory, and motor control.

Azaspirone Anxiolytics In contrast to the benzodiazepine anxiolytics, azaspirone anxiolytics have no effect on the GABA receptor mechanism. They act as an agonist or partial agonist on serotonin type 1_A receptors, which produce the anxiolytic effect. Some evidence is reported that there is influence on dopaminergic neurons also.

TARGET SIGNS AND SYMPTOMS

Box 69-1 shows the psychosocial and the somatic signs and symptoms that warrant treatment with antianxiety medications.

DOSAGE

See Table 69-1 for antianxiety medication doses.

MONITORING TREATMENT

Pretreatment Phase
1. Collaborate with the medical–psychiatry team members in completing a comprehensive medical evaluation with specific focus on:
   - Thyroid status
   - Caffeine intake
   - Nicotine intake
   - Current medications
2. Collaborate with the client to identify psychosocial factors that contribute to or precipitate anxiety.
3. Conduct a thorough assessment of client and family system history of addictive illness and previous abuse of prescription medications.
4. Instruct both client and family members concerning effect and side effects of selected medication.
5. Provide both client and family members with written information concerning medication.

Initiation Phase
1. Initiate benzodiazepines at a low dose.

BOX 69-1: Target Signs and Symptoms Treated with Antianxiety Medications

Psychosocial/Behavioral
Anxiety
Apprehensiveness
Amotivational behavior
Compulsiveness
Distractibility
Fearfulness
Feelings of dread
Frustration
Impaired judgement
Intolerance
Nervousness
Overconcern
Panic
Phobias
Preoccupation
Repetitive motor behavior
Tension
Worry

Somatic
Anorexia
Backache/pain
"Butterflies in stomach"
Chest discomfort
Diaphoresis/sweating
Dizziness/lightheadedness
Dyspnea
Dry mouth
Faintness
Fatigue
Headaches
Hyperventilation
Muscle tension/pain
Nausea
Palpitations
Paresthesia
Sexual disturbance
Shortness of breath
Stomach pain
Tachycardia/"skipped beats"
Tremulousness
Urinary/bowel frequency
Vomiting

TABLE 69-1
Antianxiety Medication Doses

GENERIC NAME	TRADE NAME	DOSAGE FORMS (mg)	ADULT DOSE RANGE	GERIATRIC DOSE
Benzodiazepines				
Alprazolam	Xanax	t:0.25/0.5/1/2	0.5–4.0	Start 0.25 0.25–2.0
Chlordiazepoxide	Librium	t:5/10/25 c:5/10/25 p:100 mg/ampule	15–100	Start 5 20–40
Clonazepam	Klonopin	t:0.5/1/2	0.5–20	Start 0.25 0.25–2
Clorazepate	Tranxene	t:3.75/7.5/11.25/15/22.5 c:3.75/7.5/15	7.5–60	Start 3.75 7.5–30
Diazepam	Valium	t:2/5/10 p:5 mg/ml	2–60	Start 2 2–10
	Valrelease	c: (ER) 15		
Halazepam	Paxipam	t:20/40	60–160	Start 5 10–40
Lorazepam	Ativan	t:0.5/1/2 p:2 mg/ml, 4 mg/ml	2–6	Start 0.5 0.5–4.0
Oxazepam	Serax	t:15 c:10/15/30	30–120	Start 10 10–90
Prazepam	Centrax	t:10 c:5/10/20	20–60	Start 5 10–15
Azaspirone				
Buspirone	BuSpar	t:5/10	15–60	Start 5 5–30

2. Monitor psychophysiologic responses while slowly increasing medication every 3–4 days until sedation or therapeutic effect is attained.
3. Reinforce medication teaching, especially concerning sedative properties, performance impairment, potential for dependence properties, and interaction with alcohol and drugs.

Maintenance Phase

1. Collaborate with the client to determine degree of effect on anxiety.
2. Reevaluate the need for continued anxiolytic medication.
3. Encourage the client to use daily symptom checklist to evaluate and monitor medication response.
4. Reinforce instructions with the client not to discontinue anxiolytics abruptly.
5. Instruct the client and family about benzodiazepine discontinuance syndrome signs and symptoms. See Table 69-2.

TABLE 69-2
Benzodiazepine-Discontinuance Syndrome Symptoms

SYMPTOM CATEGORY	TYPE OF SYMPTOMS	SEVERITY OF SYMPTOMS	CLINICAL COURSE
Rebound	Return of original diagnostic symptoms	More than original symptoms	Rapid onset Temporary
Recurrence	Same as the original diagnostic symptoms	Same	Insidious gradual onset Does not disappear with time.
Abstinence–withdrawal	New symptoms presentation Early symptoms: • Agitation • Anxiety* • Anorexia • Blurred vision • Dizziness • Headache • Insomnia* • Nausea • Restlessness* • Tremulousness • Tinnitus • Vertigo Late symptoms: • Confusion • Diarrhea • Hallucinations • Hypotension • Hyperthermia • Myoclonus • Psychosis • Seizures *During first several days of discontinuance	Variable	Early and late symptom presentation Duration 2–4 weeks Can be protracted greater than 4 weeks

Termination of Benzodiazepine Therapy
1. Collaborate with medical–psychiatry team, client, and family to *taper* medication when anxiety symptoms have been effectively treated.
2. Collaborate with health care providers and client to design a written taper schedule, gradually decreasing anxiolytic dose by 10% of *daily* dose per week for clients on treatment longer than 3 months.

HYPNOSEDATIVE MEDICATIONS

INDICATIONS
Hypnosedative medications are used for insomnia.

CHEMICAL STRUCTURAL GROUPS
Hypnosedative medications fall into three groups:
1. Benzodiazepines
2. Barbiturates
3. Nonbarbiturate compounds

METHOD OF ACTION

Benzodiazepines Benzodiazepines depress subcortical levels of the central nervous system (CNS), particularly the limbic system, and reticular formation. They potentiate the effects of the inhibitory neurotransmitter gamma-aminobutyric acid (GABA), thereby producing a calming effect.

Barbiturates Barbiturates depress the central nervous system (CNS). They interfere with transmission through the reticular formation concerned with arousal. They cause an imbalance in inhibitory and facilitatory mechanisms that influence the cerebral cortex and reticular formation.

Nonbarbiturate Compounds The exact mechanism is not clearly known, although there is depression of the central nervous system owing to an increase in the threshold of the arousal centers in the brain stem.

TARGET SIGNS AND SYMPTOMS
Signs and symptoms that warrant treatment with hypnosedatives include:
1. Difficulty falling asleep
2. Difficulty staying asleep
3. Not feeling rested after sleeping

DOSAGE
See Table 69-3 for hypnosedative medication doses.

MONITORING TREATMENT

Pretreatment Phase
1. Collaborate with medical–psychiatry team members in a comprehensive medical and psychiatric evaluation to determine the impact of medical or psychiatric disorders on sleep.
2. Conduct a sleep history assessment including usual sleep rituals.
3. Encourage the client to complete a sleep–wake log.
4. Instruct the client in sleep hygiene techniques.
5. Ensure specific laboratory studies have been completed and evaluated.

TABLE 69-3
Hypnosedative Medication Doses

GENERIC NAME	BRAND NAME	DOSE FORMS (mg)	USUAL DOSES (mg)	DOSE RANGES (mg)	WHEN TO TAKE BEFORE BED-TIME (hours)	GERIATRIC DOSE (mg)
BENZODIAZEPINES						
Estazolam	ProSom	t:1/2	1	1–2	0.5	0.5
Flurazepam	Dalmane	c:15/30	15–30	15–30	0.5	15
Quazepam	Doral	t:7.5/15	7.5–15	7.5–15	1.5	7.5
Temazepam	Restoril	c:7.5/15/30	15–30	7.5–30	1–2	7.5–15
Triazolam	Halcion	t:0.125/0.25	0.25	0.125–0.5	0.5	0.125
IMIDAZOPYRIDINE						
Zolpidem	Ambien	t:5/10	10	5–20	0.5	5–10
BARBITURATES						
Amobarbital	Amytal	p:250/500	65–200	65–200	0.5	65
Aprobarbital	Alurate	e:40 mg/5ml	40–160	40–160	0.5	40
Butabarbital	Butisol	t:15/30/50/100 e:30 mg/5ml	50–100	50–100	0.5	50
Pentobarbital	Nembutal	c:50/100 su:30/60/120/200 p:50 mg/ml	100	50–200	0.5	50
Phenobarbital	Luminal	t:16/32/100 Many generic doses	100–200	15–600	1	16
Secobarbital	Seconal	c:30/50/100 su:30/60/120/200 p:50 mg/ml	100–200	100–200	0.25	50
NON-BARBITURATE COMPOUNDS						
Chloral hydrate	Noctec	c:250/500 s:500 mg/5ml	500–1500	500–2000	0.5	500
Ethchlorvynol	Placidyl	c:200/500/750	500–750	500–1000	0.5	500

c = capsules; e = elixir; p = parenteral; s = syrup; su = suppository; t = tablets

- CBC with differential
- Renal function
- Sleep disorder assessment (when indicated)

6. Instruct the client and family members in effect and side effects of selected hypnosedative medication.
7. Discontinue substances that disrupt sleep, such as caffeine and alcohol.

Initiation Phase

1. Initiate hypnosedative medication at low dose.
2. Monitor sleep pattern response and any "hangover effect" or other side effects.
3. Slowly increase dose level to therapeutic range while monitoring sleep response.

Maintenance Phase

1. Monitor psychophysiologic responses to hypnosedative medication.
2. Conduct sleep checks to ascertain if client is sleeping; check for restlessness, frequent position changes, and frequent awakenings.
3. Instruct and practice sleep hygiene strategies with client.
4. Instruct and practice relaxation techniques with client.

5. Discuss plans for a scheduled taper of hypnosedative medications.
6. Obtain and monitor laboratory studies to assess renal and hematological function when necessary.
7. Assess and monitor client for these symptoms:
   - Amnesia
   - Falls
   - Fractures
   - Hangover
   - Hypnosedative withdrawal
   - Rebound insomnia
   - Respiratory ailments

BIBLIOGRAPHY

American Psychiatric Association Task Force (1990). *Benzodiazepine Dependence, Toxicity and Abuse.* Washington, DC: American Psychiatric Association.

Ashton, H. (1991). Protracted withdrawal syndromes from benzodiazepines. *Journal of Substance Abuse Treatment, 8* (1–2), 19–28.

Hewlett, W. A., Vinogradov, S., & Agras, W. S. (1992). Clonazepam treatment of obsessions and compulsions. *Journal of Clinical Psychiatry, 51* (4), 158–161.

Mendelson, W. B. (1992). Clinical distinction between long-acting and short-acting benzodiazepines. *Journal of Clinical Psychiatry, 53* (no. 12, supplement), 4–7.

Nino-Murcia, G. (1992). Diagnosis and treatment of insomnia and risks associated with lack of treatment. *Journal of Clinical Psychiatry, 53* (no. 12, supplement), 43–47.

Peden, J. G. (1993). Benzodiazepine use of the medicine/psychiatry interface. *Psychiatric Annals, 23* (6), 301–309.

Roger, M., Attali, P., & Coquelin, J. P. (1993). Multicenter, double-blind, controlled comparison of zolpidem and triazolam in elderly patients with insomnia. *Clinical Therapeutics, 15* (1), 127–136.

Roth, T., & Roehrs, R. (1992). Issues in the use of benzodiazepine therapy. *Journal of Clinical Psychiatry, 53* (6), 14–18.

Roy-Byrne, P. P., & Cowley, D. S. (eds.) (1991). *Benzodiazepines in Clinical Practice: Risks and Benefits.* Washington, DC: American Psychiatric Press.

Tunnicliff, G., Eison, A. S., & Taylor, D. D. (1991). *Buspirone: Mechanisms and benefits.* Washington, DC: American Psychiatric Association Press.

Wenzel, S. P., Burke, W. J., et al. (1993). Use of benzodiazepines in the elderly. *Psychiatric Annals, 23* (6), 325–331.

Wysowski, D. K., & Baum, C. (1991). Outpatient use of prescription sedative–hypnotic drugs in the United States 1970–1989. *Archives of Internal Medicine, 151* (9), 1779–1783.

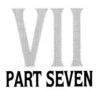

PART SEVEN

Special Issues in Psychiatric Nursing

70
SEVENTY

Legal Issues in Psychiatric–Mental Health Nursing

Rose Eva Bana Constantino

OVERVIEW:

Introduction
Sources of the Law
Types of Law
Tort Law
   Intentional Torts
   Quasi-intentional Torts
   Unintentional Torts
Types of Psychiatric Commitment
Application for Involuntary Emergency
   Examinations and Treatment
Justification for Involuntary Treatment
Competence

Constitutional Parameters
Patients' Rights
Informed Consent
Right to Refuse Treatment
Duty of Therapist to Warn Third Parties
Confidentiality
HIV Infection and the Law
Reporting Child Abuse
Legal Alternatives of Adult Abuse
   Victims
Impaired Nurses

INTRODUCTION

Psychiatric–mental health nurses are constantly challenged by theories, laws, regulations, and standards of practice and must be vigilant about the legal ramifications of their nursing care. The state and federal governments' interest in the care of the mentally ill is undeniably complex. Psychiatric–mental health care has been more carefully examined by the courts than any other aspect of the health care system, partly because of the legal and ethical issues raised by involuntary treatments and involuntary civil commitment.

SOURCES OF THE LAW

Northrop and Kelly (1987) describe the four sources of law:

> *1. Common law derives from earlier decisions of the court (legal precedent or stare decisis), custom, and tradition. Tort law was developed from common law. Past decision of the courts becomes law and should be followed when a court confronts the same question in a new case. Common law has important ramifications for nursing practice.*
>
> *2. Constitutional law derives from the Constitution and the Supreme Court's interpretation of the Constitution, which cannot be overruled by statute.*

3. Statutory law derives from statutes enacted or codified by the legislative branch of the government.

4. Administrative law derives from regulations promulgated by administrative agencies authorized by statutes. (pp. 13–20)

TYPES OF LAW

Northrop and Kelly (1987) describe two types of law:

1. **Substantive** defines the substance or content of the law, which may be categorized as civil, administrative, and criminal (p. 22).

2. **Procedural** governs the procedure or rules employed to create, implement, or enforce the substantive law. The procedural aspects of the litigation of a civil case are filing a complaint by the plaintiff, service of the complaint to the defendant, pretrial proceedings, discovery, the trial, and the appeal (p. 20).

TORT LAW

Civil liability for nursing practice falls in the area of tort law. Torts may be intentional, quasi-intentional, or unintentional.

INTENTIONAL TORTS

Intentional torts involve injurious acts to person or property. The following are common law recognized intentional torts (Northrup & Kelly, 1987):

Battery is an unpermitted and intentional contact with a person's body or anything connected to the body such as clothing, cane, or object in hand, even when the person is asleep, unconscious, or under anesthetics.

Assault is an apprehension or mental disturbance of the personal integrity of immediate harmful or offensive contact. Actual contact is not an element of assault; therefore, this cause of action is frequently joined with battery.

False imprisonment is an intentional restraint of the plaintiff's movement caused by the defendant's words, actions, and gestures. The plaintiff must be aware of the confinement.

Intentional infliction of emotional distress is an interference of the plaintiff's peace of mind caused by the defendant's extreme and outrageous conduct. The conduct need not be directed to the plaintiff. A third person present who is known by the defendant to be present and suffers emotional distress while observing the extreme and outrageous conduct will recover from the defendant.

PMH nurses may be involved as plaintiffs, defendants or witnesses.

QUASI-INTENTIONAL TORTS

Quasi-intentional torts protect a plaintiff's interests in reputation, privacy, and freedom from unfounded legal action. The following are common law recognized quasi-intentional torts (Northrup & Kelly, 1987):

Defamation is made up of two torts: slander or oral communication and libel or written communication. Intent and malice are elements in defamation. In defamation, truth is a defense.

Malicious prosecution is used to recover damages caused by the defendant's acts of bringing an action or a proceeding. The plaintiff must prove that the proceeding was terminated in her favor, the proceeding was initiated without probable cause, the action was brought with malice, and actual damages were sustained.

Interference with or invasion of the right to privacy is comprised of four separate causes of action protecting a person's interest in and right to privacy:
1. appropriation of name and likeness, such as when a plaintiff's name, picture, or likeness is used without consent for a business purpose by the defendant;
2. intrusion upon solitude or seclusion, including physical intrusion or invasion of one's home or hospital room or eavesdropping;
3. public disclosure of private facts; and
4. false light in a public eye.

Breach of confidentiality includes the disclosure of a confidential physcian–patient privileged communication by a nurse.

PMH nurses may be involved as plaintiffs, defendants, or witnesses.

UNINTENTIONAL TORTS

Professional Negligence   Negligence is an unintentional tort that involves harm resulting from the failure of a person to conduct himself or herself in a reasonable and prudent manner. To establish a claim of professional negligence against the nurse, the plaintiff must introduce proof of the existence of the four elements necessary for a professional negligence action (Northrop & Kelly, 1987). A dismissal of the plaintiff's claim of negligence against the nurse may result if any one of these elements is not established. The four elements, the law, and an example are shown in Table 70-1.

TABLE 70-1
Elements of Negligence, the Law, and Examples in Psychiatric–Mental Health Nursing

ELEMENTS OF NEGLIGENCE	THE LAW	EXAMPLE
1. Duty	1. The law imposes a higher duty of care upon those who hold themselves out as professionals. In *Fraijo v. Hartland Hospital* (1979) the California Appellate Court set forth that one who undertakes to perform the services of a professional nurse, whether gratuitously or for money, is under a legal duty to use that reasonable degree of skill, knowledge, and care ordinarily possessed by nurses acting under similar circumstances (Northrop & Kelly, 1987).	1. A schizophrenic patient developed total paralysis of the left leg after the nurse administered a psychotropic medication intramuscularly and hit the patient's sciatic nerve.
2. Breach of duty	2. An act or omission of an act by a nurse may constitute a breach of the standard or duty of care (Northrop & Kelly, 1987).	2. The nurse breached the standard or duty of care by acting unreasonably in not accurately measuring the safe site "upper, outer quadrant" of the patient's left buttocks before administering the medication.
3. Proximate cause	3. The plaintiff must introduce proof that the breach of duty by the nurse was the proximate cause or the legal cause of the plaintiff's injury (Northrop & Kelly, 1987).	3. There was no other previous, intervening or superseding cause of the patient's paralysis of the left leg but for the nurse's action.
4. Damages	4. If there is no damage, there is no recovery under a negligence theory. The threat or possibility of future harm is not sufficient proof of damages. Proof of actual loss or damage must be shown (Northrop & Kelly, 1987).	4. The measure of money damages is based on the medical costs the patient has or will incur to treat, rehabilitate, and prevent further deterioration of the leg. Future loss of patient's earning capacity and care is calculated.

Special Negligence Doctrine   See Table 70-2 for the elements, the law, and an example.

Presumptions in Negligence

1. *Res ipsa loquitur:* a kind of circumstantial evidence that gives rise to an inference in presumption of negligence, which literally means "the thing speaks for itself" (e.g., a patient suffered a foot-drop after the nurse applied a four-point restraint).
2. *Violation of statute or presumption of negligence or negligence per se:* A plaintiff may obtain a presumption of negligence if the nurse's violation of a statute or regulation is the proximate cause of the plaintiff's injury. Before the courts will apply the presumption of negligence, the statute must be designed to protect a class of persons,

TABLE 70-2
Elements of Special Negligence Doctrine, the Law, and
Examples in Psychiatric–Mental Health Nursing

ELEMENTS OF SPECIAL NEGLIGENCE DOCTRINE	THE LAW	EXAMPLE
1. Master/servant or respondeat superior	1. A variation of vicarious liability wherein the law imputes negligence to certain persons who have not committed any negligent act because of their relationship with a negligent actor. The act must be within the scope of the employment and the kind that the employee was employed to perform within the limits of time and space with a purpose to serve the employer (Northrop & Kelly, 1987).	1. A patient successfully strangulated himself in his room using the drawstrings of his pajamas. The psychiatric hospital employer is liable for the psychiatric nurse's negligent act of failing to remove the drawstrings from the patient's pajama bottoms.
2. Independent contractor–agent	2. The law does not impute liability on the hospital if the nurse is considered an independent contractor wherein the hospital has no control over the nurse's conduct. But if the nurse is acting as a physician's agent, vicarious liability for the agent's negligence should be imposed upon the physician (Northrop & Kelly, 1987).	2. Liability will not be imputed on the psychiatric hospital if the nurse, in performing negligent conduct, is not employed by the hospital or the hospital has no control over the nurse's action, unless the hospital was negligent in selecting the nurse, or in some way ratified or authorized the negligent conduct.
3. Captain of the ship and borrowed servant	3. This doctrine is applicable in surgery cases where the nurse employed by the hospital becomes the temporary servant of the surgeon. The surgeon as the captain of the ship is deemed liable for the negligent act of the nurse (Northrop & Kelly, 1987).	3. Psychiatric–mental health nurses employed by a hospital become a "borrowed servant" when they moonlight for a nurse-managed psychiatric home health care center. The center becomes the captain of the ship and is deemed liable in any negligent act of the nurse.
4. Ostensible agency	4. The law imputes liability in the hospital for the acts of the nurse who is not employed by the hospital if the circumstances imply a general representation to the public that the nurse was an employee of the hospital and the patient relied on that representation in submitting to the nurse's care. Unless there is evidence that the patient knew or should have known that the nurse was not an employee when treatment was given, the law will imply an agency relationship and the hospital will also be found liable (Northrop & Kelly, 1987).	4. Although untested to date, a psychiatric–mental health nurse who owns a nurse-managed psychiatric outpatient center and maintains a psychiatric hospital's home health care on a contractual referral basis may imply an ostensible agency relationship with a hospital so that the law will make the hospital liable for the negligent action of the nurse-managed center. These decisions are made on a case-by-case basis.

the plaintiff must be a member of the class of persons, and the plaintiff's injury must be the kind that the statute or regulation is designed to prevent. Nurses, therefore, should look to their state practice acts to determine what duties of care are statutorily prescribed (Northrop & Kelly, 1987).

TYPES OF PSYCHIATRIC COMMITMENT

1. Informal Commitment   Competent individuals can admit themselves to a facility for voluntary treatment and discharge themselves on short notice without fear of being involuntarily committed.

2. Voluntary Commitment   A facility can admit a competent individual for voluntary treatment, but can demand that certain requirements be satisfied before the individual can be discharged. The institution retains the right to involuntary commitment proceedings instead of discharging the patient.

3. Third-Party Commitment   A person other than the proposed patient who has authority by virtue of an established legal relationship with that person (e.g., a guardian) can seek the proposed patient's voluntary or involuntary civil commitment. Laws governing third-party commitment vary somewhat depending on whether the proposed patient is an adult or a minor.
- *Adults:* A legal guardian or a parent with guardianship powers can consent to have the ward/adult child civilly committed. Depending on the jurisdiction and circumstances, the commitment may be either voluntary or involuntary. When voluntary commitment is sought, the guardian can withdraw consent and initiate a process leading to discharge unless involuntary commitment proceedings are instituted. Involuntary commitment is effected if consent is withdrawn. Some type of proceeding, either administrative or judicial, must be held before discharge will be granted.
- *Minors:* A parent or legal guardian can consent, subject to administrative review as established in *Parham v. J.R.* (1979), to have a child civilly committed. As in the commitment of an adult, the commitment of a minor can be either voluntary in that the parent's withdrawal of consent will lead to discharge, or involuntary in that discharge depends on an administrative or legal proceeding.

4. Short-Term Commitment   This type of involuntary commitment is characterized by the relatively short duration between patients being taken into custody and their being released or held over for extended commitment. Depending on the jurisdiction, short-term commitments may be limited statutorily to periods ranging from 24 hours to 30 days (Parry, 1993). Short-term commitments also may be divided into three different subtypes based on their substantive purposes:
- *Emergency commitment* applies when a person's mental condition poses an immediate danger to self or others.
- *Commitment for observation or evaluation* is used to observe, examine, or evaluate a respondent pursuant to extended commitment proceedings.
- *Temporary commitment* is a stop-gap or interim measure used before extended proceedings can be held.

5. Extended Commitment   Under this procedure, patients are subject to long-term or in some cases indefinite involuntary commitment to inpatient facilities, but only after the most rigorous substantive and procedural due process requirements are met.

6. Outpatient Commitment   This process is used to involuntarily commit a patient to an outpatient facility. Depending on the statutory scheme and circumstances involved, the process may be similar to preventive detention or may be a less restrictive alternative to inpatient hospitalization (e.g., day treatment, where the patient attends treatment during the day and goes home at night, or night treatment, where the patient comes to the treatment center at night).

7. Criminal Commitment   A person who remains in the control of the criminal justice system may be subject to involuntary inpatient or outpatient treatment. Depending on the circumstances, treatment may occur in facilities run by either the mental health or the criminal justice authorities. Generally, four subtypes of criminal commitment exist.
- *Pretrial detention* occurs when a defendant who has been accused of a crime but has not been adjudicated incompetent to stand trial is treated involuntarily.
- *Commitment of persons found incompetent to stand trial* occurs when persons who are found incompetent to stand trial are committed for treatment until they regain their competency or they cannot be held any longer without violating due process.
- *Insanity acquittal* occurs when defendants who are found not guilty by reason of insanity are committed to treatment facilities until they are no longer mentally disabled and dangerous.
- *Posttrial commitment* occurs when defendants are committed involuntarily to treatment facilities while serving their sentences.

8. Recommitment   This procedure is for renewing involuntary extended commitments in either the civil or the criminal system. Generally, the same standards used for the original commitment apply. In a criminal context, the burden of proof may shift to the patient/inmate.

APPLICATION FOR INVOLUNTARY EMERGENCY EXAMINATIONS AND TREATMENT	In the Commonwealth of Pennsylvania, an application form must be completed by the person who believes that the patient is in need of involuntary emergency examination and treatment. A notice of intent to file a petition for extended involuntary treatment must be completed by a member of the treatment team.
JUSTIFICATION FOR INVOLUNTARY TREATMENT	Generally, an application for involuntary treatment must be completed by a member of a treatment team for all commitment types when the patient refuses voluntary treatment or the treatment team considers the patient unable to decide on a voluntary treatment. Justification for involuntary treatment may include one or all of the following items:

1. Patient was violent and aggressive in the emergency room.
2. Patient was in an acute medical crisis in the emergency room.
3. Patient has a history of becoming violent when hospitalized.
4. Patient is unable to sign informed consent.
5. Patient has continually signed out of hospital against medical advice.
6. Patient has continually refused prescribed treatment, i.e., medication
7. Other; specify.

COMPETENCE	A determination of competence to make treatment decisions should closely follow any decision to involuntarily commit a respondent, unless the respondent already has been adjudicated incompetent. If an incompetent respondent does not already have a guard-

ian, a guardian should be appointed. Involuntarily committing a respondent is not in itself a determination that the respondent is incompetent to make treatment decisions. Nor is a determination of some other type of incompetency the same as incompetency to make treatment decisions (Parry, 1994). State probate courts have jurisdiction to make the finding of incompetence and to appoint a guardian or conservator. Competence to take care of self or property does not require faultless decision making but does require the ability to understand the consequences of actions and decisions (Smith-Hurd, 1987). If the client is found incompetent, the state may appoint a:

1. *Conservator,* who confers authority only over property or estate of the client.
2. *Guardian,* who confers authority over both person and property of the client. Civilly committed clients are presumed competent to give informed consent or, conversely, to refuse treatment unless there is a judicial determination that the client is incapable of making treatment decisions.

CONSTITUTIONAL PARAMETERS

The U.S. Constitution is the one set of principles that is legally and morally binding for all Americans. Thus, constitutional principles should provide the foundation upon which any civil commitment system is built and implemented. Moreover, the Constitution's requirements provide the minimum standards necessary to satisfy substantive and procedural due process. Constitutional principles with an impact on commitment include (Parry, 1994):

1. *Right to treatment:* Patients who are involuntarily committed have a right to treatment minimally necessary to prevent or reduce illness (*Donaldson v. O'Connor,* 1974).
2. *Dangerousness:* Dangerousness is a constitutional requirement for civil commitment (*Zinermon v. Burch,* 1990).
3. *Criminal commitment:* Criminals cannot be committed or held in mental health facilities without the same due process as anyone else facing civil commitment (*Baxtrom v. Herold,* 1966).
4. *Least restrictive alternative:* Patients have a right to treatment that intrudes minimally on their personal liberties (*In re Devine,* 1991).
5. *Commitment of minors:* Parents or guardians may have mentally ill minors voluntarily or involuntarily committed (*Parham v. J.R.,* 1979).
6. *Informed consent:* Patients being committed voluntarily must be deemed competent to make an admission decision. Otherwise, involuntary procedures must be instituted. Informed consent includes statements on risks and benefits, costs and payments, confidentiality, right to refuse or end hospitalization, and voluntary consent.
7. *Procedural due process:* The State must provide clear and convincing evidence of a patient's need for commitment. The U.S. Supreme Court has never decided whether right to counsel is constitutionally required, but case law and state statutes firmly establish this right (Parry, 1993).
8. *Equal protection:* Adults with *mental retardation* can be committed to a mental health facility when clear and convincing evidence has been found of the need. However, proof beyond a reasonable doubt is required if the patient is mentally ill.

PATIENTS' RIGHTS

The courts have established specific legal rights pertaining to the mentally ill:

General Legal Rights

1. Right to adequate treatment and that confinement for treatment not generate into punishment (Parry, 1994).

2. Criteria for treatment (*Baxtrom v. Herold,* 1966).
   a. Humane psychological and physical environment
   b. Qualified staff in sufficient numbers
   c. Individualized treatment plans
3. Right to release: Nondangerous civilly committed persons must be provided with an opportunity for treatment beyond custodial care or they have a right to be released (*O'Connor v. Donaldson,* 1975).
4. Right to aftercare: Every client must have an individualized posthospitalization plan. Hospitals must adopt a functional approach to discharge planning, with emphasis on linkage with community mental health and social service agencies (Parry, 1994).

Legal Rights for Inpatients

1. Treatment with dignity and respect, all civil rights that have not been specifically curtailed by order of court.
2. Unrestricted and private communication inside and outside the facility including the following rights to:
   a. Peaceful assembly and to join with other patients to organize a body of, or participate in, patient government when patient government has been determined to be feasible by the facility.
   b. Be assisted by any advocate of choice in the assertion of rights and to see a lawyer in private at any time.
   c. Make complaints and to have complaints heard and adjudicated promptly.
   d. Receive visitors of patients' own choice at reasonable hours unless the treatment team has determined in advance that a visitor or visitors would seriously interfere with treatment or welfare.
   e. Receive and send unopened letters and to have outgoing letters stamped and mailed. Incoming mail may be examined for good reason in patients' presence for contraband. Contraband means specific property that entails a threat to health and welfare or to the hospital community.
   f. Have access to telephones designated for patient use.
3. Impartial access to treatment or accommodations that are available or medically indicated, regardless of race, color, religious creed, handicap, ancestry, national origin, age, sex, or sources of payment for care.
4. Practice the religion of choice or to abstain from religious practices.
5. Keep and use personal possessions, unless it has been determined that specific personal property is contraband. The reasons for imposing any limitation and its scope must be clearly defined, recorded, and explained to the patient. Patients have the right to sell any personal article they make and keep the proceeds from its sale.
6. Handle personal affairs including making contracts, holding a driver's license or professional license, marrying or obtaining a divorce, and writing a will.
7. Participate in the development and review of their treatment plans.
8. Receive treatment in the least restrictive setting within the facility necessary to accomplish the treatment goals.
9. Be discharged from the facility as soon as they no longer need care and treatment.
10. Not to be subjected to any harsh or unusual treatment.
11. Request and receive information regarding their total bill for services. Receive timely notification prior to termination of eligibility for reimbursement by any third-party payer for the cost of care.

12. Be discharged from the facility if involuntarily committed in accordance with civil court proceedings and not receiving treatment, if patient is not dangerous to self or others and can survive safely in the community.

13. Be paid for any work that benefits the operation and maintenance of the facility in accordance with existing federal wage and hour regulations.

14. Request access to medical records and to appeal or submit patient's comments to be included as part of the record.

15. Receive a copy of any consent signed during treatment, and have a copy kept in the record.

16. Indicate advance directives or living wills and receive information about future medical treatments in the event that medical illness makes patient unable to communicate wishes directly.

17. Refuse to participate in a research project after it has been thoroughly explained.

18. File a grievance and appeal to ensure that the patient rights enunciated in federal and state regulations are safeguarded and disputes resulting therefrom are resolved promptly and fairly.

INFORMED CONSENT

Psychiatric–mental health nurses are often involved in research studies, particularly clinical drug trials. In these situations patients may give informed consent following:

1. A fair explanation of the procedures to be followed, together with their purposes, including identification of any procedure that is experimental.

2. A description of any attendant discomforts and risks reasonably expected.

3. A description of any benefits reasonably expected.

4. An offer to answer any inquiries concerning the procedure.

5. Instruction that the client is free to withhold or withdraw consent and to discontinue participation at any time.

6. A disclosure of any appropriate alternative procedures that may be advantageous for the client.

7. A reasonable description of any controlled substances and any other drugs to be used, and their anticipated effects and interactions.

RIGHT TO REFUSE TREATMENT

Nurses are sometimes faced with situations involving a patient's refusal of medications or other treatments. The right to refuse treatment is not absolute. Most statutes provide that medications and treatments can be given if they are needed to prevent serious harm to the patient. Without a client's informed consent, facilities may not use involuntary seclusion, mechanical restraint, or forced psychotropic medication, except in an emergency situation to protect the safety of the client or others, and when delay could result in significant deterioration of the client's mental health. In an emergency, a qualified physician must find that the possibility of side effects is less serious than the need to prevent violence and that there are no less restrictive alternatives (Parry, 1994). A guardian may consent to force medication or other treatment in nonemergency situations.

DUTY OF THERAPIST TO WARN THIRD PARTIES

A duty to warn third parties exists when a therapist determines, or pursuant to the standards of the profession *should* determine, that the client presents a serious physical danger to another person. The protection of privilege ends where public peril begins (*Tarasoff v. Regents of University of California,* 1976).

TABLE 70-3
Legal Issues Involving HIV and Psychiatric–Mental Health Nursing

ISSUE	THE LAW
1. Involuntary HIV testing of psychiatric patients	1. Consent from the psychiatric patient must be sought to test blood for HIV. Substitute decision-making only applies to children age 13 or younger and to involuntarily committed adult psychiatric patients (Lo, 1989).
2. Involuntary confinement of a psychiatric patient who is HIV-positive and having sex with other patients	2. Knowing transmission of HIV through sexual contact is prohibited by law. The institution has the legal means to prohibit such contact. The Illinois Supreme Court held that a statute prohibiting a person from knowingly transmitting HIV was constitutional (*Illinois v. Russel*, 1994).
3. Duty to warn the partner of a psychiatric patient who is HIV-positive	3. In 1988, New York and California enacted laws permitting notification of contacts of HIV persons. These laws require that the informant persuade the patient to allow notification without disclosing the identity of the patient. Alternatively, public health officials may be asked to notify contacts. Recent statutes, however, do not require notification, encouraging voluntary notification (Lo, 1989).
4. Disclosure of a psychiatric patient's HIV status by the nurse to an unauthorized person	4. The Arkansas Supreme Court held that a nurse who disclosed information about a man's HIV test to an unauthorized third party did not constitute medical malpractice (*Wyatt v. St. Paul Fire & Marine Insurance Co.*, 1994).
5. Psychiatric nurses' refusal to care for an HIV-positive psychiatric patient	5. In general, nurses have no legal duty to care for HIV-positive psychiatric patients. However, moral obligation, employment contracts, and professional and ethical standards may impose some authority to obligate the nurse to care for HIV-positive patients.
6. Psychiatric nurses' duty to inform employer of HIV status	6. While HIV-positive psychiatric nurses have a moral obligation to inform their employer of their HIV status, their right to privacy should be balanced with the risk of infection to co-workers or patients who come under their care.
7. Nurses' claims for emotional distress caused by exposure to AIDS or needlestick	7. In *Tischler v. Dimenna* (1994), a New York court recognized claims for emotional distress caused by exposure to AIDS. Moreover, the Montana Supreme Court held that the State Worker's Compensation Act provided the exclusive remedy for a former employee who developed a fear of AIDS after being punctured by a needle (*Blythe v. Radiometer America, Inc.*, 1993).

CONFIDENTIALITY

Access to Records   It is the responsibility of the facility and the professional to keep all information, records, and correspondence confidential and to allow access to them only:
1. Upon a judicial order compelling discharge
2. When the patient requests they be given to an attorney or other health care provider
3. To be used to enable the patient to receive third-party reimbursement for services

Privilege
1. Specifically refers to the relationship of a particular professional to a client and provides the client with protection against the release of any information obtained through the relationship.
2. Each state defines which professionals are privileged and whether privilege is absolute.
3. Communication with nurses in psychotherapy relationships generally is not privileged.
4. Privilege is generally granted to communication with psychiatrists, licensed psychologists, clergy, and attorneys, except:

    a. To place or retain the client in a hospital

    b. Under court examination, when the client has been informed that the examination would not be privileged

    c. When the client cites mental or emotional condition as a claim or defense in any court proceeding (except a child custody case)

    d. In a child custody case in which mental condition bears significantly on the client's suitability to provide care

HIV INFECTION AND THE LAW

HIV/AIDS has led to many legal issues in psychiatric–mental health nursing. See Table 70-3 for some of these issues and the law pertaining to each.

REPORTING CHILD ABUSE

All 50 states and the District of Columbia have enacted statutes requiring nurses to report cases or suspected cases of child abuse to child welfare agencies. Failure to do so may result in suspension of license.

LEGAL ALTERNATIVES OF ADULT ABUSE VICTIMS

Adults who are suffering abuse may seek legal protection from the courts by filing a Protection from Abuse (PFA) petition (Protection from Abuse Act, 1994).

IMPAIRED NURSES

If a nurse has clear and convincing evidence that a peer comes to work chemically impaired, the nurse has an obligation to report the incident to a supervisor. If after following the established institutional channels of communication the situation persists, the nurse has an obligation to report the incident to the State Board of Nursing. In most jurisdictions, nurses are responsible for seeking the rehabilitation program necessary to treat their impaired status to protect the patients, the institution, and the public from harm.

REFERENCES

Baxtrom v. Herold, 383 U.S. 107 (1966).

Blythe v. Radiometer America, Inc., 866 P.2d 218 (Mont. Sup. Ct. 1993).

Donaldson v. O'Connor, 493 F.2d 507 (5th Cir. 1974).

Fraijo v. Hartland Hospital, 160 Cal. Rptr. 246, 252 (Cal. App. 1979).

Illinois v. Russel, 630 N.E.2d 794 (Ill. Sup. Ct. 1994).

In re Devine, 572 N.E.2d 1238, 15 MPDLR 455 (Ill. App. Ct. 1991).

Lo, B. (1989). Clinical ethics and HIV-related illnesses: Issues in treatment and health services. In W. LeVee (ed.), *New Perspectives on HIV-Related Illnesses: Progress in Health Services Research* (pp. 170–179). Washington, DC: U.S. Dept. of Health and Human Services.

Northrop, C., & Kelly, M. (1987). *Legal Issues in Nursing.* St. Louis: Mosby.

O'Connor v. Donaldson, 442 U.S. 563, 576 (1975).

Parham v. J.R., 442 U.S. 584, 3 MDLR 231 (1979).

Parry, J. (1993). Mental health law. In M. G. MacDonald, R. M. Kaufman, A. M. Capron, & I. M. Birnbaum (eds.), *Treatise on Health Law* (pp. 20–64). New York: Bender.

Parry, J. (1994). Involuntary civil commitment in the 90s: A constitutional perspective. *Mental and Physical Disabilities Law Reporter, 18* (3), 320–328.

Protection from Abuse Act 1994, 23 Pa. C.S. §§ 6101–6118.

Smith-Hurd (1987). Illinois Annotated Statutes. Chapter 91 1/2, § 3-607.

Tarasoff v. Regents of University of California, 17 C.3d 425 (Cal. 1976).

Tischler v. Dimenna, 609 N.Y.S.2d 1002 (N.Y. Sup. Ct. 1994).

Wyatt v. St. Paul Fire & Marine Ins. Co., 868 S.W.2d 505 (Ark. Sup. Ct. 1994).

Zinermon v. Burch, 110 S.Ct. 975 (1990), 14 MPDLR 116.

BIBLIOGRAPHY

Applebaum, P. S. (1994). *Almost a Revolution: Mental Illness Law and the Limits of Change.* New York: Oxford University Press.

71
SEVENTY ONE

Ethical Issues in Psychiatric–Mental Health Nursing

Carol Taylor

OVERVIEW:

Introduction
Approaches to Bioethics
  Principle-Based Approach
  The Care Perspective
Advocacy Challenges
  Identifying and Supporting the
    Appropriate Decision Maker
  Helping Clients Realize Health Goals
  Preventing and Resolving Ethical Conflict

Specific Ethical Issues
  Ensuring Informed Consent
  Enrolling Subjects in Clinical Trials
  Implementing Controversial Therapies
  Counseling Clients Who Are Suicidal
  Advocating for Marginalized Clients
Psychotherapy

INTRODUCTION

Ethical competence is a core competence of psychiatric–mental health (PMH) nurses. Box 71-1 shows the American Nurses Association Code for Nurses (1985). See Appendix A for the practice standard that delineates nursing's ethical responsibilities. Advocacy is a particularly challenging role for psychiatric–mental health nurses because of the increasing scarcity of mental health resources and the unique vulnerabilities of many psychiatric–mental health clients.

APPROACHES TO BIOETHICS

PRINCIPLE-BASED APPROACH

This popular approach to bioethics (Beauchamp & Childress, 1994) derives its moral action guides from four principles of obligation grounded in common morality.

1. *The Principle of Respect for Autonomy:* To respect an autonomous agent is to acknowledge that person's right to hold views, to make choices, and to take actions based on personal values and beliefs. It requires more than obligations of nonintervention because it includes obligations to maintain autonomous choice in others while allaying fears and other conditions that destroy or disrupt their autonomous actions. For example, the PMH nurse respects the client's decision to refuse medications without frightening the client into reversing the decision.

562

BOX 71-1: The American Nurses Association Code for Nurses

1. The nurse provides services with respect for human dignity and the uniqueness of the client, unrestricted by considerations of social or economic status, personal attributes, or the nature of health problems.

2. The nurse safeguards the client's right to privacy by judiciously protecting information of a confidential nature.

3. The nurse acts to safeguard the client and the public when health care and safety are affected by the incompetent, unethical, or illegal practice of any person.

4. The nurse assumes responsibility and accountability for individual nursing judgments and actions.

5. The nurse maintains competence in nursing.

6. The nurse exercises informed judgment and uses individual competence and qualifications as criteria in seeking consultation, accepting responsibilities, and delegating nursing activities to others.

7. The nurse participates in activities that contribute to the ongoing development of the profession's body of knowledge.

8. The nurse participates in the profession's efforts to implement and improve standards of nursing.

9. The nurse participates in the profession's efforts to establish and maintain conditions of employment conducive to high-quality nursing care.

10. The nurse participates in the profession's effort to protect the public from misinformation and misrepresentation and to maintain the integrity of nursing.

11. The nurse collaborates with members of the health professions and other citizens in promoting community and national efforts to meet the health needs of the public.

Reprinted with permission from *Code for Nurses with Interpretive Statements.* Copyright 1985, American Nurses Association, Washington, DC.

---

2. *The Principle of Nonmaleficence:* This principle asserts an obligation not to inflict harm intentionally. For example, the PMH nurse does not "punish" clients for deviant behavior.

3. *The Principle of Beneficence:* Positive beneficence requires the provision of benefits. Utility requires that benefits and drawbacks be balanced. For example, the advanced-practice PMH nurse balances the potential benefits and drawbacks of hospitalizing a client.

4. *The Principle of Justice:* What is just is what is fair, equitable, and appropriate in light of what is due or owed to a person. The term *distributive justice* is used broadly to refer to the distribution of all rights and responsibilities in society. For example, the advanced-practice PMH nurse advocates for a system of health care that effectively meets the needs of the homeless.

The principle-based approach to bioethics obligates health care professionals to act in ways that are respectful of a person's autonomy, beneficial, and just. Limitations of popular versions of this approach to bioethics include:

1. Lack of a unifying moral theory
2. Reduction of ethics to "hard cases" (quandary ethics)
3. Devaluation of everyday ethical concerns
4. Communication of the false notion that all actions justified by a principle are equally "correct"

THE CARE PERSPECTIVE

The care perspective (Taylor, 1993) calls attention to the *character* of moral agents as well as to their *actions.* Challenging a reductionistic–mechanistic approach to health care and health care ethics that "objectifies" clients, it directs attention to the reality of particular clients viewed in the context of their life narratives. Characteristics of this perspective include:

1. Centrality of the caring relationship
2. Promotion of the dignity and respect of clients as people
3. Acceptance of particular client and health care professional variables (beliefs, values, relationships) as morally relevant factors in health care decision-making
4. Norms of responsiveness and responsibility
5. Redefinition of fundamental moral skills

Limitations of this perspective include the underdevelopment of caring as a concept and the reality of caring's "dark side"—that is, difficulty balancing care for others with appropriate self-care, potential harsh abuse of client autonomy in the name of caring, and so forth.

ADVOCACY CHALLENGES

Advocacy is a moral commitment to respect the autonomy of others and to facilitate their exercise of self-determination. It is linked to a basic belief that the freedom to choose in light of goods is a fundamental human right that promotes dignity and well-being. Advocacy responsibilities of caregivers committed to helping clients realize their health goals are as follows (see also Box 71-2).

IDENTIFYING AND SUPPORTING THE APPROPRIATE DECISION MAKER

1. General Rules of Thumb
   - Persons with intact decision-making capacity are self-determining. They have the moral and legal right to consent to, and equally to decline, any and all medically indicated treatment options.
   - The last competent decision of persons who are variably incapacitated holds.
   - Incapacity does not, of itself, cause clients to lose the right to be self-determining. Decisions for incapacitated clients who at one time possessed decision-making capacity should reflect their identity, decisional history, and moral norms. Their surrogates are to use a *substituted judgment* standard when making decisions for these clients. (For example, a client who was adamantly opposed to having electroshock therapy slipped into a catatonic stupor. Her doctors wanted to use ECT, but her sister advocated against it on her behalf.)
   - A surrogate decides for a never competent client using a *best interests* standard. Since the values and interests of this person are not known, decisions are based on a more general sense of what is in the client's best interests.

2. Important Clarifications
   - Criteria for decision-making capacity include (1) ability to comprehend information relevant to the decision at hand; (2) ability to deliberate in accord with own

BOX 71-2: Advocacy Responsibilities

Identifying and Supporting the Decision Maker

1. Determine and document the client's decision-making capacity.

2. Protect the right of clients with intact decision-making capacity to be self-determining.

   a. Facilitate communication and documentation of the client's preferences.

   b. Anticipate the treatment decisions that will most likely have to be made and initiate discussion of preferences.

   c. Help in the preparation of advance directives for treatment.

3. Promote authentic autonomy; authentic decisions reflect the individual's identity, decisional history, and moral norms.

4. Identify and reduce coercive influences that are interfering with autonomous decision making.

5. Help clients who wish to delegate health care decision making to identify an appropriate proxy decision maker.

6. Support the proxy decision maker; clarify the proxy's role.

7. Identify limits to client/proxy autonomy and limits to caregiver autonomy.

Helping Clients Realize Health Goals

1. Make sure clients understand their condition and related diagnostic and therapeutic options.

2. Assess whether or not clients understand the probable consequences of each of their options (including the option of nontreatment).

3. Encourage communication among all those involved in the decision to be made: client, family, health care professionals, religious leader, etc.

4. Allow clients to verbalize their feelings.

5. Help clients assess their options in relation to their beliefs, values, interests, goals.

6. Ensure that all interventions are consistent with the overall goal of therapy.

7. Ensure that the client's bio-psycho-social-spiritual needs are addressed.

8. Ensure continuity of care as clients are transferred among services intrainstitutionally and interinstitutionally.

9. Weigh the moral relevance of third-party interests, e.g., family, caregivers, institution, society; note the special vulnerabilities of select groups of clients such as the homeless, those with histories of deficient self-care behaviors, the uninsured, etc.

Preventing and Resolving Ethical Conflict

1. Establish that preventing and resolving ethical conflict falls within the authority of all health care professionals engaged in the care of a client.

2. Facilitate timely communication among all those involved in decision making: one-on-one meetings, periodic meetings of the client, family, and interdisciplinary team to clarify goals and treatment plan.

3. Develop awareness of, and responsiveness to, conscious and unconscious sources of conflict.

4. Document pertinent information on the client record.

5. Use appropriate resources such as an ethics consultant or the institutional ethics committee to resolve ethical conflict.

---

values/goals; and (3) ability to communicate with caregivers (Hastings Center, 1987).

- Limitations to autonomy include (1) harm to specific, identifiable third parties; (2) violation of the morals of the health care professional; (3) violation of internal morality of the profession; and (4) therapeutic privilege.

- Criteria for valid surrogate or proxy include (1) must be competent; (2) must know the client and the client's values to the extent that this is possible; (3) no undue conflict of interest; and (4) no serious emotional conflict.

HELPING CLIENTS REALIZE HEALTH GOALS

Nurses play an important role in helping clients and families make decisions by encouraging discussion about both the effectiveness and benefit/burden ratio of proposed therapy.

A treatment is effective to the degree that it reverses the natural progression of the disease/disorder or alleviates an important symptom. This is an objective determination to the extent that nursing and medicine are objective sciences. What complicates many decisions about psychiatric treatment options are uncertainties about clinical effectiveness.

A treatment is beneficial if it advances the overall interests of the client. Whether or not the benefits of proposed therapy outweigh the burdens is a subjective determination that can only be made by the client or by those who know the client well.

PREVENTING AND RESOLVING ETHICAL CONFLICT

Nurses play an important role in preventing ethical conflict by identifying potential sources of conflict and initiating mediation before the problem escalates. Interpersonal competence is essential to successful mediation. An ethics work-up tool that will facilitate analysis of ethical conflict is shown in Box 71-3.

BOX 71-3: The Ethics Work-Up for Nurses

The ability to work up the ethical aspects of a case is an essential part of clinical reasoning. The emphasis in the ethics work-up is on a sensible progression from the facts of the case to a morally sound decision. This ethics work-up or a similar version may be used by a variety of health professionals, such as physicians, nurses, social workers, etc. With some adjustments, it may also be used by laypersons. However, this ethics work-up is intended for use by nurses, with special emphasis on the role and responsibilities of nurses. It is understood that nurses will collaborate with other parties, principally other members of the health care team, clients, and family members when using this work-up.

Using the five principal steps of the ethics work-up, health professionals holding a variety of philosophical and religious positions regarding ethics can share a basic framework for thinking about and discussing morally troubling cases:

1. **What are the facts?** It is vitally important to clarify the facts of the case to anchor the decision. These facts are both medical and social. For example, both an estimate of prognosis and an understanding of the client's home situation are often relevant to an ethical decision.
   Persons involved (Who?)
   Diagnosis, prognosis, therapeutic options (What?)
   Chronology of events, time constraints on decision (When?)
   Medical setting (Where?)
   Reasons supporting claims, goals of current care (Why?)

Nurses may be instrumental in ensuring that the client/family and other nonmedical health professionals understand the medical facts and that the health care team understands pertinent nonmedical information about the client and family.

2. **What is the issue?** It is necessary to identify the specific ethical issue in the case. The issue may not be ethical, but rather a diagnostic problem or a simple miscommunication.

3. **Frame the issue:** Some health professionals will explore the issue using only one moral approach. Others will eclectically employ a variety of approaches. But no matter what one's underlying moral orientation, the ethical issue at stake in a given case can be framed in terms of several broad areas of concern, representing aspects of the case that may be in ethical conflict. It is therefore useful, if somewhat artificial, to dissect the case apart along the lines of the following areas of concern:

   a. Identify the appropriate decision maker(s).

   b. Apply the criteria to be used in reaching clinical decisions.
      (1) *The specific biomedical good of the client:* One should ask, What will advance the biomedical or clinical good of the client? What are the medical/psychological/mental health options and likely outcomes?
      (2) *The broader goods and interests of the client:* The nurse focuses the interdisciplinary team's attention on the broad aspects of the

BOX 71-3 *(continued)*

client's good, i.e., the client's dignity, religious faith, other valued beliefs, life goals, relationships, and the particular good of the client's choice.

(3) *The goods and interests of other parties:* Health professionals must also be attentive to the goods and interests of others, e.g., in the distribution of resources. One should ask, What are the concerns of other parties (family, health care professionals, health care institution, law, society, etc.) and what differences do they make morally in the decisions that must be made about this case? In deciding about an individual case, however, these concerns should generally not be given as much importance as that afforded the good of the individual client whom health professionals have pledged to serve.

The caregiving team explains the treatment options to the client/surrogates and if indicated makes a recommendation. The client/surrogate makes an uncoerced, informed decision. Limits to client/surrogate autonomy include the bounds of rational health care, the probability of direct harm to identifiable third parties, and violation of the consciences of involved health care professionals. In problematic cases the interdisciplinary team may meet to ensure consistency in their recommendations to the client/surrogate(s).

c. Establish the nurse's (nursing's) moral/professional obligations. Nurses must decide what they owe the client as well as themselves, the

health care team, the health care institution, and other third parties. Conflicts may exist.

4. **Decide:** In nursing ethics, as in all other aspects of nursing, a decision must be made. There is no simple formula. The answer will require clinical judgment, practical wisdom, and moral argument. Nurses must ask themselves, "What should I do? Where can I get help?" They must analyze the data, reflect on the data morally, and draw a conclusion, while prepared to explain the decision and the moral reasons for it. Sources of justification include:

a. The nature of the nurse–client relationship; compatibility of recommended course of action with aims of nursing (internal morality of profession).

b. Approaches to ethical inquiry: principle-based ethics, virtue-based ethics, feminist/caring/existentialist ethics, casuistry, theological ethics.

c. Grounding and source of ethics: philosophical (based in reason), theological (based in faith), sociocultural (based in custom).

5. **Critique:** It is important to be able to critique the decision that has been made by considering its major objections and then by either responding adequately to them or changing the decision. The nurse should also seek colleagues' opinions when time permits. Some cases can even be taken to an ethics committee for further reflection. Retrospective analysis is also useful in preparing for the next time such a situation is encountered.

Used with the permission of the Georgetown University Center for Clinical Bioethics.

SPECIFIC ETHICAL ISSUES

ENSURING INFORMED CONSENT

Obtaining informed consent is the responsibility of the health care professional who is performing the procedure or treatment for which consent is being sought. Nursing's responsibility is often simply to confirm that an informed, voluntary consent has been obtained. At other times, nurses may be responsible for obtaining consent for select nurse-managed therapies. Beauchamp and Childress (1994) identify the following elements of informed consent:

Threshold Elements (Preconditions)
1. Competence to understand and decide
2. Voluntariness in deciding

Information Elements
3. Disclosure of material information

4. Recommendation of a plan
5. Understanding of items 3 and 4

Consent Elements
6. Decision in favor of a plan
7. Authorization of the chosen plan

Nurses are often involved in controversies about how much clients should be told about the risks and benefits of therapies, including drugs, devices, and other treatments. In this situation, they must make decisions based on ethical concerns, rather than the self-interest of researchers or administrators.

ENROLLING SUBJECTS IN CLINICAL TRIALS

When consent is obtained for participation in research, disclosures should include the aims, methods, anticipated benefits and risks of the research, any anticipated inconvenience or discomfort, and the subjects' right to withdraw from the research at any point.

Nursing responsibilities include:
1. Working with the interdisciplinary team to evaluate the client's decision-making capacity
2. Ensuring that disclosure, understanding (risk/benefit ratio), and voluntariness are adequate; identifying subtle sources of coercion
3. Making sure that subjects understand they can withdraw their consent at any time, even after the research is begun
4. Remaining a consistent advocate for the client, cultivating sensitivity to how a research agenda can compromise the client care agenda

IMPLEMENTING CONTROVERSIAL THERAPIES

Whenever nurses are asked to implement controversial therapies, such as the use of placebos or therapies of unproven benefit for the condition being treated, ECT, or controversial behavior control therapies, the following nursing responsibilities hold:
1. Initiating a discussion with the caregiving team about the reasons for initiating the controversial therapy, challenging any reasons (convenience to the caregivers, increased knowledge, etc.) that do not serve the immediate interests of the client. The nurse ensures that the client/proxy decision maker understands the potential benefits and risks of the proposed "therapeutic" regimen.
2. Closely monitoring the client's responses to the regimen if implemented and reporting any adverse effects to the team.
3. Reminding all involved nurses that their primary role is to be an advocate for the client and that their primary consideration is the client's well-being.

COUNSELING CLIENTS WHO ARE SUICIDAL

The public's increasing acceptance of the notion that individuals have the right to determine the time and manner of their dying and the right to suicide assistance if desired is confronting all health care professionals with new moral challenges. Special responsibilities of psychiatric–mental health nurses include:
1. Participating in the debate about rational suicide—i.e., can suicide be a free and rational choice, or are there always unresolved emotional issues that if addressed would result in individuals no longer wanting to end their lives? Are there situations, e.g., terminal AIDS, when clients have the right to end their lives early?

2. Participating in the public debate about the advisability of legalizing assisted suicide and aid in dying; nursing's intimate experience of the human realities underlying this debate can inform the public debate.
3. Continuing to work with the interdisciplinary team to develop effective counseling strategies for clients who believe ending their life is the only way to resolve their problems.
4. Counseling clients who are suicidal.

ADVOCATING FOR MARGINALIZED CLIENTS

Many of the clients who need psychiatric care are marginalized. Abandoned by their families and society, they frequently lack the support systems available to most of us. Moral pitfalls for psychiatric–mental health nurses operate at two extremes: an unrealistic commitment to being a savior or rescuer or a decision to completely distance themselves from the human plight of those whose needs are overwhelming. Appropriate nursing responses include:

1. Periodically checking one's "responsiveness meter" to ensure that indifference is not interfering with these clients receiving appropriate care
2. Initiating attempts to creatively discuss problems with the interdisciplinary team, identifying what is at the root of problematic behaviors
3. Identifying and tapping available resources
4. Making the system work for these clients; participating in policy development
5. Critically evaluating biases that interfere with these clients receiving optimal care, for example, discouraging the capricious prejudicial labeling of clients as "borderline" and then rejecting them either overtly or subtly

PSYCHOTHERAPY

When psychiatric–mental health nurses conduct psychotherapy, the following ethical principles apply (see also Chapter 50 for ethical dilemmas involving managed care):

1. Nurses do not enter into sexual relationships with clients.
2. Nurses do not enter into business relationships with clients.
3. Nurses do not enter into social relationships with clients.
4. Nurses seek supervision when ethical dilemmas arise.
5. In the event that the client can no longer pay the agreed-upon fee, the nurse:
   - Reduces the fee, or
   - Refers the client to another therapist, supplying three names, and giving the client ample time to terminate.
6. Nurses respect client confidentiality.

REFERENCES

American Nurses Association (1985). *Code for Nurses with Interpretive Statements* (EDMNA, Appendix C, p. 266). Kansas City, MO: American Nurses Association.
Beauchamp, T., & Childress, J. (1994). *Principles of Biomedical Ethics* (4th ed.). New York: Oxford University Press.
Hastings Center (1987). *Guidelines on the Termination of Life-Sustaining Treatment and the Care of the Dying.* Bloomington, IN: Indiana University Press.

BIBLIOGRAPHY

American Nurses Association (1994). *Guidelines on Reporting Incompetent, Unethical, or Illegal Practices.* Washington, DC: American Nurses Association.
Appelbaum, P. S. (1994). *Almost a Revolution: Mental Health Law and the Limits of Change.* New York: Oxford University Press.
Benjamin, M., & Curtis, J. (1992). *Ethics in Nursing* (3rd ed.). New York: Oxford University Press.
Bloch, S., & Chodoff, P. (1991). *Psychiatric Ethics* (2nd ed.). New York: Oxford University Press.

Conwell, Y., & Caine, E. D. (1991). Rational suicide and the right to die. *New England Journal of Medicine, 325* (15), 1100–1103.

Edwards, R. B. (ed.). (1982). *Psychiatry and Ethics.* Buffalo, NY: Prometheus Books.

Group for the Advancement of Psychiatry (1990). *A Casebook in Psychiatric Ethics.* New York: Brunner-Mazel.

Jonsen, A. R., Siegler, M., & Winslade, W. J. (1992). *Clinical Ethics* (3rd ed.). New York: Macmillan Publishing Co.

Pellegrino, E. D., & Thomasma, D. C. (1988). *For the Patient's Good: The Restoration of Beneficence in Health Care.* New York: Oxford University Press.

President's Commission for the Study of Ethical Problems in Medicine and Biomedical and Behavioral Research (1982). *Making Health Care Decisions: The Ethical and Legal Implications of Informed Consent in the Patient–Practitioner Relationship.* Washington, DC: President's Commission.

Ross, J. W., Bayley, C. B., Michel, V., & Pugh, D. (1986). *Handbook for Hospital Ethics Committees.* Chicago: American Hospital Publishing.

Ross, J. W., Glaser, J. W., Rasinski-Gregory, D., Gibson, J. M., & Bayley, C. (1993). *Health Care Ethics Committees: The Next Generation.* Chicago: American Hospital Publishing.

Sullivan, M. D., & Youngner, S. J. (1994). Depression, competence, and the right to refuse lifesaving medical treatment. *American Journal of Psychiatry, 151,* 971–978.

Taylor, C. (1993). Nursing ethics: The role of caring. *AWHONN's Clinical Issues in Perinatal and Women's Health Nursing, 4* (4), 552–560.

SEVENTY TWO

Cultural Issues in Psychiatric–Mental Health Nursing

Kem Betty Louie

INTRODUCTION

Ethnic background is one factor that determines the way people experience their environment, develop values and attitudes as well as a sense of security, and set goals and expectations. The meaning of behavior varies according to the norms and rules of each culture and subculture. Cultural groups vary in the incidence and symptoms of mental illness. Though there are basic symptoms of mental illness that appear the same in all cultures, variations in the symptoms show the influence of culture. Studies have shown that the content and choice of sense organs in expressing hallucinations vary from culture to culture. For example, auditory hallucinations are observed more frequently in Western countries, whereas in non-Western countries people tend to exhibit more visual, olfactory, and tactile hallucinations (Al-Issa, 1978). It is postulated that in non-Western cultures, visual and other senses are more culturally emphasized as a means of communication and contact with the social environment than these senses are in Western societies. Psychosomatic illness also varies from culture to culture (Shorter, 1994). With this borne in mind, the determination of mental illness should be based on mental state and not social behavior.

Behaviors that are ambiguous or unfamiliar to the nurse may not be necessarily indicative of a psychiatric disorder. If health planning and treatment are to be effective, consideration of the client's cultural beliefs, attitudes, values, and goals must be assessed. Although clients come from a specific culture or subculture, individual variations exist and therefore nurses are cautioned against stereotyping clients or families. By the same token, differences can occur within broad racial groups. For example, within the Asian American/Pacific Islander category, differences are seen in the way Japanese, Chinese, and Vietnamese clients may display mental illness or difficulties in living.

PREDICTED DEMOGRAPHICS IN THE UNITED STATES

Based on the 1990 census, the following changes are projected for the year 2000 (U.S. Department of Commerce, Bureau of the Census, 1992):
1. Percentage of Caucasians will drop to 72%.
2. Percentage of African Americans will increase to 13.1%.
3. Percentage of Hispanics will increase to 11.3%.
4. Percentage of American Indians and Asian American/Pacific Islanders will increase to 4.3%.

Six million immigrants will enter the United States in this decade, and most will settle on the East and West coasts.

CULTURAL SENSITIVITY

Cultural sensitivity refers to the nurse's ability to be aware of and respect the client's values and lifestyles even when these differ from the nurse's own. Before nurses can transmit an open and nonjudgmental attitude toward ethnic clients, they must understand and develop insight into their own cultural belief systems. Otherwise, they are apt to unwittingly transmit negative feelings, attitudes, and values to the client, causing anxiety and discomfort.

CULTURAL COMPETENCE

Cultural competence is a multidimensional concept involving various aspects of knowledge, attitude, and skills. Nurses are expected to be culturally competent as well as sensitive in caring for clients from different cultural and ethnic backgrounds.

Table 72-1 shows a framework for cultural sophistication (Orlandi, 1992). The various aspects of knowledge, attitude, and skill development of cultural competence range from high to low. Cultural competence includes self-knowledge, multicultural education, and empathy (Jenkins, 1993).
1. *Self-knowledge* requires the awareness of perceptions of one's own culture, including personal biases and stereotypes. Pinderhughes (1989, p. 27) suggests responding to several questions to further explore thoughts and feelings about one's own culture:
   a. What was your first experience with feeling different?
   b. What are your earliest images of race or color? What information were you given about how to deal with racial issues?

TABLE 72-1
Cultural Sophistication Framework

	CULTURALLY INCOMPETENT	CULTURALLY SENSITIVE	CULTURALLY COMPETENT
Cognitive Dimension	Oblivious	Aware	Knowledgeable
Affective Dimension	Apathetic	Sympathetic	Committed to change
Skills Dimension	Unskilled	Lacking some skills	Highly skilled
Overall Effect	Destructive	Neutral	Constructive

Orlandi, M. (1992). Cultural sophistication framework. In M. Orlandi, R. Weston, & L. Epstein, *Cultural Competence for Evaluators* (OSAP Cultural Competence Series). DHHS Pub. (ADM) 92-1884, U.S. Government Printing Office.

     c. Discuss your experiences as a person having or lacking power in relation to the following: ethnicity, racial identity, class identity, gender identity.

2. *Multicultural education* requires attending programs on cross-cultural issues of mental health in addition to workshops provided to learn more about the historical, social, and acculturation problems of diverse groups.

3. *Empathy* is a genuine feeling for people whose cultural background is different from the nurse, and requires the nurse to view the situation from the perspective of the client.

CULTURAL ASSESSMENT

A guide to a cultural assessment is presented in Table 72-2. These items serve only as a guide and should be incorporated in a nursing history.

TABLE 72-2
Guide to Cultural Assessment

	EXAMPLE
Ethnicity	
Identify the following: specific cultural group and subgroup, degree of identification with group, citizenship or immigrant status, and length of time in this country.	Chinese, a student in this country for 3 years, states she is Buddhist.
Identify the language: 1. Language usually spoken in public and at home (include dialect) 2. Fluency in English 3. Degree of comfort in giving information (disclosure) 4. Nonverbal communication (gestures, posture, eye movements)	Speaks "broken" English in public and Toy Shan Chinese at home. Client is hesitant to give information regarding her illness. Answers questions literally. Speaks in a low voice and does not maintain eye contact with interviewer.
Family Constellation	
Identify the: 1. Type of family structure, matriarchal or patriarchal 2. Members in the family/household, gender, and sibling rank	States that her father is head of the household. There are five members in her family, her husband, mother-in-law, son, and daughter. Client is the oldest of three children.
Diet and Nutritional Preferences	
Identify the following: 1. Ethnic food preferences 2. Food taboos 3. Any special food preparations	Enjoys oriental foods, will not eat cold or raw foods.
Health and Illness Beliefs	
• How does the client perceive this hospital admission? • What is believed to be the cause of the illness? • How is the condition usually treated in this group?	Has difficulty expressing her emotions. States she is tired all the time and is unable to sleep. She is not doing well in her studies. She has taken herbal medicines and has not found them effective. She believes that there is an imbalance in her body.

PSYCHOLOGICAL TESTS

Psychological tests should be interpreted flexibly, keeping in mind the following:

1. *The norms of the test:* What is the normal range of scores for this client, taking into consideration the age, sex, culture, and diagnosis? The standard norms of this test may not be applicable to this client.

2. *The client's view of the test-taking situation:* Does the client view this situation as a threat, a challenge, or a humiliating situation?

3. *The client's responses to the specific items or answers:* Does the client understand clearly what is being asked? Ethnic clients may answer the questions literally or give responses they think the interviewer wants to hear.

INTERVIEWING

When interviewing ethnic clients, nurses should bear in mind the following:

1. Clients may expect an initial period of polite exchange or small talk before getting down to business. Direct questioning about their problems may be considered offensive and rude. For example, greeting the Asian American client who holds strong traditional values with "How is your family?" instead of "How are you?" acknowledges the client's strong family bonds (Sue & Sue, 1990).

2. Communication barriers can occur because of cultural differences in the connotative and denotative meaning of words and phrases. For example, a client may say, "The devil is behind these walls." The denotative or common meaning of devil is a demon or evil spirit. The connotative meanings of a devil may include a wicked or cruel person, an unhappy person, or in the African American culture, a select group of people or a woman.

3. Display of emotions and expressions of emotions may be different in various cultures. For example, what may be called hysteria in one ethnic group may be a display of genuine, appropriate expression of love in another.

4. Time orientations including tempo or speed of conversation vary among cultural groups. Interrupting clients before they have finished a thought is considered insulting in many cultures.

5. Nonverbal facial and body gestures and expressions, as well as social distance, are culturally interpreted. The nurse's own verbal and nonverbal expression may influence the client's responses.

6. Content within the assessment form that is biased toward middle-class values and beliefs can cause misunderstanding or hostility.

7. Developing rapport and trust may be difficult. For example, mistrust or reserved behavior when speaking with strangers may be the typical response in African American or Asian American cultures and need not indicate hostility.

8. Information from secondary sources such as family, friends, and others may be collected to understand the total situation.

USE OF TRANSLATORS

The need for translators or interpreters is fairly common for non-English-speaking clients. Interpreters may be professionals, local volunteers, relatives, or friends (Konut, 1975). When using an interpreter it is helpful to:

1. Explain the reason for the interview and the type of questions to the interpreter. This information will help the interpreter elicit general or literal responses, essays or short answers from the client.

2. Introduce the interpreter to the client and family. If possible, allow some time for them to be acquainted.

3. Speak directly to the client and allow the interpreter to translate. Do not interrupt the interpreter or client when either is speaking.
4. After the interview, spend some time with the interpreter to share information about the nonverbal communication and ease of obtaining information from the client.
5. Whenever possible, arrange for clients to speak to the same interpreter each time they are being interviewed.

MENTAL STATUS ASSESSMENT

Information obtained from the mental health assessment includes four areas that are particularly culturally sensitive:

1. *Affect or emotional state:* For example, certain Asian Americans and American Indians respond automatically in a passive and quiet manner. Other groups may respond with hostility and aggression.
2. *General intellectual level:* Clients' intelligence is often judged by their ability to use factual information in a comprehensive manner. This is difficult to assess if the client has had little or no education.
3. *Reasoning and judgment:* The values of many cultural groups are different from white American middle-class values. Differences in reasoning and judgment may be merely differences in values. For example, an Asian American client may attempt suicide to "save face" in the family or community.
4. *Abstract thinking:* The content and terms must be within the client's cultural understanding. The client's response to proverbs such as "A rolling stone gathers no moss" may not be indicative of the client's inability to think abstractly, but rather of unfamiliarity with the proverb.

NURSING INTERVENTIONS

To deliver culturally sensitive and competent care to clients, the nurse uses strategies tailored to ethnic clients in general and to specific groups. See Table 72-3 for overall nursing interventions and rationales, and Table 72-4 for specific information about three ethnic groups. Subgroups and individual groups will exist within this outline. These cultural groups were chosen because they represent beliefs and values that generally are different from the larger American society.

Nursing care includes a psychiatric, functional, and physical assessment, with a focus on somatic complaints (Flaskerud, 1987). Clients from some cultural groups express their distress and emotional conflicts through physical illness. Treatment should be problem- or situation-centered. Clients and families are taught about the nature of the illness or problem and about the remission of symptoms.

TRANSFERENCE

It is important that nurses become aware of the possible transference clients may have toward the culturally different therapist. Feelings and attitudes such as viewing the nurse therapist as an authority figure, as oppressive, or as a racist should be explored.

COUNTER-TRANSFERENCE

Because nurses may have unconscious ethnic prejudices, they must be carefully attuned to any unusual or irrational thoughts and feelings while counseling ethnic clients. These thoughts and feelings range from expecting clients to adopt mainstream white American middle-class values to denying the influence of race upon their own personality development.

TABLE 72-3
Nursing Interventions and Rationales with Ethnic Clients

INTERVENTION	RATIONALE
1. Use the client as a primary cultural informant.	1. Ethnic clients are generally aware of the differences between the dominant culture and their own cultural group.
2. Understand the perception and meaning of the identified behaviors for the client and family.	2. Culture is an important determinant in the expression of behaviors.
3. Establish therapeutic goals and plan of care within a cultural context. Develop distinct and flexible approaches to care.	3. Individualized care is a goal of nursing. A plan of care that takes into consideration the cultural aspects of clients increases their cooperation in implementing the plan.
4. Set up groups of clients with the same ethnic background to reduce situational crises and expand the range of coping patterns.	4. Clients from the same ethnic group can help each other to understand and anticipate the normal patterns and stresses of individual and community living by sharing these problems in group situations.
5. Collaborate and consult with community leaders and organizations.	5. For many cultural groups, the neighborhood is thought of as their extended family. Additional information can be sought there.

TABLE 72-4
Cultural Information and Therapeutic Strategies

VALUES AND BELIEFS	ACCEPTED CAUSE OF MENTAL ILLNESS	TRADITIONAL SOLUTIONS	COPING PATTERNS	THERAPEUTIC STRATEGIES
African Americans				
Family unity, loyalty, assertive behavior, religion, work and achievement, predominantly matriarchal, extended family	Environmental hazards, oppression, racism, divine punishment, impaired relationships	Family, church, friends, root doctors	Low disclosure, hostility, open expression of pain, withdrawal	Address specific problems, immediate goals and needs rather than abstract matters, deal with transference and countertransference
Puerto Ricans				
Sense of dignity, respect and deference to authority figures; *machismo;* patriarchal family structure, extended family important; "voices" and "visions"	*Mal ojo* (evil eye), evil spirits and forces, punishment by God and envious others	Folk healers, spiritualists, family	Low disclosure, open expression of pain	Deal with language barrier, specific matters that are problem-focused, include father and other family members in therapy
Asians				
Respect and deference to authority figures, maintenance of self-control, patriarchal family, social sensitivity	The individual, divine punishment, imbalance of the yin and yang	Folk healers, herbalists	Low disclosure, reserve, avoid confrontation, physical complaints are more acceptable than emotional problems	Approach problems subtly; concrete behavior-oriented solutions are preferred, approach is formal, include family in discussion of goals and therapeutic plans

Adapted from a grid designed by Murillo-Rhodes, I. Downstate University, New York, New York. Reprinted with permission.

POTENTIAL PROBLEMS IN THERAPY

Four factors that may interfere with the therapeutic treatment of ethnic clients have been identified (Pedersen, 1988):

1. *Mismatching therapist and client:* Research shows that therapist and client of similar ethnicity or social class are better able to effect therapeutic outcomes than those of differing ethnicity and social class.

2. *Lack of credibility of the therapist:* Therapists who do not know the norms, beliefs, and values of the cultural group will not appear credible. The therapist must also be able to experience a variety of roles in the therapeutic relationship, such as a change agent or ombudsman.

3. *Cultural misunderstanding:* The therapist may confuse the client's appropriate cultural response with a neurotic transference, as in the case of aggressive or passive behavior.

4. *Clients' expectations versus those of the therapist:* Therapy should help clients find the most personally satisfying solution to their own problems, apart from what the therapist may see as a solution. The therapist must guard against imposing goals based on the therapist's and not the client's culture. When working with the culturally different client the therapist must decide to what extent to focus on the difference and to what extent the therapist should emphasize the universal human attributes of the clients. One point of view is the therapist guides clients to change to fit into the environment or mainstream of the client's dominant culture. The more common point of view is that the therapist helps clients to adjust to the situation, with a view toward eventually changing it for the better.

REFERENCES

Al-Issa, I. (1978). Sociocultural factors in hallucinations. *International Journal of Social Psychiatry, 167,* 24–27.

Flaskerud, J. H. (1987). A proposed protocol for culturally relevant nursing psychotherapy. *Clinical Nurse Specialist, 1,* 150–157.

Jenkins, Y. M. (1993). Diversity and social esteem. In J. L. Chin, V. DeLa Cancela, & Y. M. Jenkins (eds.), *Diversity in Psychotherapy: The Politics of Race, Ethnicity and Gender* (pp. 45–64). Westport, CT: Praeger.

Konut, S. A. (1975). Guidelines for using interpreters. *Hospital Progress, 56,* 39–41.

Orlandi, M. A. (1992). Defining cultural competence: An organizing framework. In M. A. Orlandi, R. Weston, & L. G. Epstein (eds.), *Cultural Competence for Evaluators* (OSAP Cultural Competence Series, pp. 293–296). Washington, DC: U.S. Government Printing Office, DHHS Pub. No. (ADM) 92-1884.

Pedersen, P. (1988). *A Handbook for Developing Multicultural Awareness.* Alexandria, VA: American Association for Counseling and Career Development.

Pinderhughes, E. B. (1989). *Understanding Race, Ethnicity and Power.* New York: Free Press.

Shorter, E. (1994). *From the Mind to the Body: The Cultural Origins of Psychosomatic Symptoms.* New York: The Free Press.

Sue, D. W., & Sue, D. (1990). *Counseling the Culturally Different.* New York: John Wiley & Sons.

U.S. Department of Commerce, Bureau of the Census (1992). *Statistical Abstract of the United States: 1992* (112th ed.). Washington, DC: U.S. Government Printing Office.

BIBLIOGRAPHY

Atkinson, D., Morten, G., & Sue, D. (eds.) (1989). *Counseling American Minorities: A Cross-Cultural Perspective.* Dubuque, IA: W. C. Brown.

Bednar, R., Wells, M., & Person, S. (1989). *Self-Esteem: Paradoxes and Innovations in Clinical Theory and Practice.* Washington, DC: American Psychological Association.

Beeber, L., Hendrix, M., Taylor, C., & Wykle, M. (1993). The challenge of diversity. *Journal of Psychosocial Nursing and Mental Health Services, 31* (8), 23–28.

Boyd-Frankin, N. (1989). *Black Families in Therapy.* New York: Guilford.

Brislin, R. W., & Yoshida, T. (1993). *Improving Intercultural Interactions.* Newbury Park, CA: Sage Publications.

Burlew, A. K. H., Banks, A. C., McAdoo, H. P., & Azibo, D. (eds.) (1992). *African American Psychology.* Newbury Park, CA: Sage.

Campinha-Bacote, J. (1988). Culturological assessment: An important factor in psychiatric consultation–liaison nursing. *Archives of Psychiatric Nursing, 2* (4), 244–248.

Campinha-Bacote, J. (1994). Cultural competence in psychiatric mental nursing: A conceptual model. *Nursing Clinics of North America, 29* (1), 1–8.

Capers, C. (1994). Mental health issues and African-Americans. *Nursing Clinics of North America, 29* (1), 57–64.

Chin, J., De La Cancela, V., & Jenkins, Y. (eds.) (1993). *Diversity in Psychotherapy: The Politics of Race, Ethnicity and Gender.* Westport, CT: Praeger.

Chung, R., & Kagawa-Singer, M. (1993). Predictors of psychological distress among Southeast Asian refugees. *Social Science and Medicine, 36* (5), 631–639.

Comas-Diaz, L. (1989). Culturally relevant issues for Hispanics. In V. R. Koslow & E. Salett (eds.), *Crossing Cultures in Mental Health.* Washington, DC: Society for International Educational Training and Research.

Comas-Diaz, L., & Griffith, E. (eds.) (1988). *Clinical Guidelines in Cross-Cultural Mental Health.* New York: John Wiley & Sons.

Comas-Diaz, L., & Jacobsen, F. M. (1991). Ethnocultural transference and countertransference in the therapeutic dyad. *American Journal of Orthopsychiatry, 61* (8), 392–402.

Cravener., P. (1992). Establishing a therapeutic alliance across cultural barriers. *Journal of Psychosocial Nursing and Mental Health Services, 30* (12), 10–14, 37–38.

Crowley, J., & Simmons, S. (1992). Mental health, race and ethnicity: A retrospective study of the care of ethnic minorities and whites in a psychiatric unit. *Journal of Advanced Nursing, 17* (9), 1078–1087.

Cushner, K., & Brislin, R. W. (1995). *Intercultural Interactions.* Newbury Park, CA: Sage.

Dana, R. (ed.) (1988). *Multicultural Assessment Perspectives of Professional Psychology.* Needham Heights, MA: Allyn & Bacon.

de Leon Siantz, M. (1994). The Mexican-American migrant farmworker family: Mental health issues. *Nursing Clinics of North America, 29* (1), 65–72.

Donnelly, P. (1992). The impact of culture on psychotherapy: Korean clients' expectations in psychotherapy. *Journal of the New York State Nurses Association, 23* (2) 12–15.

Flaskerud, J. (1986). The effects of culture compatible intervention on the utilization of mental health services by minority clients. *Community Mental Health Journal, 22,* 127–141.

Flaskerud, J. (1987). A proposed protocol for culturally relevant nursing psychotherapy. *Clinical Nurse Specialist, 1* (4) 150–157.

Flaskerud, J., & Soldevilla, E. (1986). Filipino and Vietnamese clients: Utilizing an Asian mental health center. *Journal of Psychosocial Nursing and Mental Health Services, 24* (8), 32–36.

Fulani, L. (ed.) (1988). *The Psychopathology of Everyday Racism and Sexism.* New York: Harrington Press.

Gaines, A. D. (ed.) (1992). *Ethnopsychiatry: The Cultural Construction of Professional and Folk Psychiatries.* Albany, NY: State University of New York Press.

Gustafson, M. (1989). Western voodoo: Providing mental health care to Haitian refugees. *Journal of Psychosocial Nursing and Mental Health Services, 27* (12), 22–25.

Halpern, D. (1993). Minorities and mental health. *Social Science and Medicine, 36* (5), 597–607.

Ho, M. (1987). *Family Therapy with Ethnic Minorities.* Beverly Hills, CA: Sage Publications.

Hu, T., Snowden, L., Jerrell, J., & Nguyen, T. (1991). Ethnic populations in public mental health: Services choice and level of use. *American Journal of Public Health, 81* (11), 1429–1434.

Jackson, M. (1991). Counseling Arab Americans. In C. Lee & B. Richardson (eds.), *Multicultural Issues in Counseling: New Approaches to Diversity.* Alexandria, VA: American Association for Counseling and Development.

Keltner, B. (1993). Native American children and adolescents: Cultural distinctiveness and mental health needs. *Journal of Child and Adolescent Psychiatric and Mental Health Nursing, 6* (4), 18–23.

Knab, S. (1986). Polish Americans: Historical and cultural perspectives of influence in the use of mental health services. *Journal of Psychosocial Nursing and Mental Health Services, 24* (1), 31–34.

Landis, D., & Bhagat, R. S. (1995). *Handbook of Intercultural Training.* Newbury Park, CA: Sage.

Lawson, W. (1986). Racial and ethnic factors in psychiatric research. *Hospital and Community Psychiatry, 37* (1), 50–54.

Lipson, J. (1993). Afghan refugees in California: Mental health issues. *Issues in Mental Health Nursing, 14* (4), 411–423.

Locke, D. (1992). *Increasing Multicultural Understanding.* Newbury Park, CA: Sage Publications.

Long, C. (1986). Cultural considerations in the assessment and treatment of intrafamilial abuse. *American Journal of Orthopsychiatry, 56* (1), 131–136.

Long, K. (1986). Suicide intervention and prevention with Indian adolescent populations. *Issues in Mental Health Nursing, 8* (3), 247–253.

Matsuoka, J. (1990). Differential acculturation among Vietnamese refugees. *Social Work, 35,* 341–345.

McGoldrick, M. (1991). Irish mothers. *Journal of Feminist Family Therapy, 2* (2), 3–8.

McGoldrick, M. (1994). The ache for home. *Family Therapy Networks.* July/Aug., 38–94.

Meleis, A. (1992, Spring). Cultural diversity research. *Communicating Nursing Research, 25,* 151–173.

Minratho, M. (1985). Breaking the race barrier. The white therapist in interracial psychotherapy. *Journal of Psychosocial Nursing and Mental Health Services, 23* (8), 19–24.

Padilla, A. M. (1994). *Hispanic Psychology: Critical Issues in Theory and Research.* Newbury Park, CA: Sage.

Paniagua, F. A. (1994). *Assessing and Treating Culturally Diverse Clients: A Practical Guide.* Newbury Park, CA: Sage.

Pederson, P. (1988). *A Handbook for Developing Multicultural Awareness.* Alexandria, VA: American Association for Counseling and Career Development.

Pickwell, S. (1989). The incorporation of family primary care for Southeast Asian refugees in a community-based mental health facility. *Archives of Psychiatric Nursing, 3* (3), 173–177.

Ponterotto, J. G., & Alexander, C. (1995). *Handbook of Multicultural Counseling.* Newbury Park, CA: Sage.

Reeves, K. (1986). Hispanic utilization of an ethnic mental health center. *Journal of Psychosocial Nursing and Mental Health Services, 24* (2), 23–26.

Ridley, C. R. (1994). *Overcoming Unintentional Racism in Counseling and Therapy.* Newbury Park, CA: Sage.

Ruiz, D. (1990). *Handbook of Mental Health and Mental Disorder Among Black Americans.* New York: Greenwood Press.

Saba, G., Career, B., & Hardy, K. (1991). *Minorities and Family Therapy.* New York: Haworth.

Schwartz, D. (1985). Caribbean folk beliefs and Western psychiatry. *Journal of Psychosocial Nursing and Mental Health Services, 23* (11), 26–30.

Sue, D. (1990). *Counseling the Culturally Different* (2nd ed.). New York: John Wiley.

Sue, S., & Zane, H. (1987). The role of culture and cultural techniques in psychotherapy. *American Psychologist, 39,* 1234–1235.

Tyler, F., Brome, D., & Williams, J. (1991). *Ethnic Validity, Ecology, and Psychotherapy.* New York: Plenum Press.

Watson, J. (1990). Caught between two cultures . . . psychiatric care for people from ethnic minorities. *Nursing Times, 86* (39), 66–68.

Williams, C. (1990). Biopychosocial elements of empathy: A multidimensional model. *Issues in Mental Health Nursing, 11* (2), 155–173.

SEVENTY THREE

Women's Issues in Psychiatric–Mental Health Nursing

Suzanne Lego

OVERVIEW:

Introduction
Female Development
Female Versus Male Disorders
Premenstrual Syndrome
Self-Defeating Personality Disorder
Paraphiliac Coercive Disorder

Menopause
Sexism in Psychiatry
Gender Factors in Psychotherapy
    Female Clients with Male Therapists
    Male Clients with Female Therapists

INTRODUCTION

In the past decade increasing emphasis has been placed on the role of gender in the development of mental disorders and the role of sexism in its treatment. Since the majority of mental patients are female, it is important for nurses to examine the issues of gender and sexism in the field.

FEMALE DEVELOPMENT

Freud's description of normal human development is based on what we now consider a "masculine" psychology. A central concept is the Oedipus conflict, which allows that castration anxiety evolves in little boys after seeing that girls, including their own mothers, lack a penis. The idea is set in motion that the female is deviant in that she lacks something biologically. Horney (1926) and Thompson (1942) along with others objected to the biological imperative, asserting that sociocultural influences reinforce feelings of inferiority in relation to men. Sullivan (1940) and the object relations theorists, moving even farther from Freud's biological drive theories, asserted that it was the mutual interaction between mother and infant that helped develop the child's sense of self.

We now know that gender differences in forming identity occur even before birth. Parents who know the gender of their children tend to decorate nurseries and to buy clothing with gender-specific colors. Newborns are treated in gender-specific ways. Girls are carried facing inward toward the mother more often and boys are carried facing the world. Baby girls who cry are seen as vulnerable and needy, while boys are often characterized as having lusty, aggressive cries. Mahler, Pine, and Bergman (1975) emphasized the importance of separation–individuation and rapprochement in the development of an autonomous self. We now know that boys are encouraged to separate and move out into the world, to be competitive and aggressive, while girls are encouraged to value connectedness and relatedness with others.

Kohut's (1971) self-psychology theory emphasized the importance of the relationship of self to other. Gilligan (1982), Miller (1976), and Surrey (1983) have described the "relational self" in women. Gilligan (1982) wrote about the differences in moral development between girls and boys. The male concept of right and wrong is typically based on the abstract principles of justice and laws. Women base moral judgment on principles of compassion and care. In a recent study of preadolescent girls, Brown and Gilligan (1992) found that a profound change occurs in girls as they reach a certain age. While they move through school days with confidence in their abilities, at around age 11 their self-doubt increases. Their overwhelming drive becomes a need to please and attract males. As females move through adolescence and into adulthood the desire for connectedness continues, as does their attraction to humanistic qualities, less valued in Western industrial society than the male qualities of disconnection, autonomy, and individual achievement (Jordan & Surrey, 1986).

When females enter marriage they are searching for something very different than are men. Women value intimacy, the ability to connect to one another, empathy, fidelity, and kindness to their nuclear families. Many men, on the other hand, want wives who are skilled lovers and who share their interests, believing that if they provide a good living for their families, they have fulfilled their obligations. Based on these differences, clients often reveal different sets of problems. Females often have low self-esteem, identity confusion, and fear of autonomy. Males, on the other hand, have problems resulting from an inability to recognize and discuss feelings, tending instead to act out.

FEMALE VERSUS MALE DISORDERS

Table 73-1 shows a list of disorders occurring more often in females than males and possible explanations. In general, women's disorders represent acting "in" while male disorders represent acting "out."

PREMENSTRUAL SYNDROME

While a small minority of women have premenstrual or menstrual problems, the vast majority do not. Feminists consider the elevation of these problems to classification as a psychiatric disorder a disservice to women. Many feminist writers in the mental health field have described the "manufacture of PMS," or as Carol Tavris (1989) calls it, the "medicalization of PMS." A number of reasons are given:

1. Research on PMS erupted in the 1970s when women moved into the work force in great numbers, posing a threat to men (Tavris, 1989).
2. Large grants for research are given to those who study a "disease" or "abnormality." Elevating PMS to this category elevated the careers of biomedical researchers (Tavris, 1989).
3. Drug companies support and encourage this movement as they seek to gain financially if women take pills each month (Parlee, 1987; Dumont, 1990).
4. Gynecologists who might be forced to close their obstetrical practices owing to the high cost of malpractice insurance, having "lost a traditional source of income, are turning to new patient groups and new diagnoses for replenishment" (Tavris, 1989, p. 143).

TABLE 73-1
Disorders That Occur More Often in Women
Than Men and Possible Explanations

DISORDER	POSSIBLE EXPLANATION
1. Borderline personality disorder	1. Many theorists believe the genesis for BPD occurs in the rapprochement subphase of the separation–individuation phase of development. It is more difficult for mothers to allow females to separate and be autonomous than it is for them to allow the same for male children. Females are socialized to be connected to others (Benjamin, 1986). In addition, psychiatric disorders were found to occur in 20% of women who had been abused as children. BPD and childhood abuse have been found to be related. See Chapter 28.
2. Depression	2. An American Psychological Association Task Force (1990) on women and depression gave the following reasons: • Avoidant, passive, dependent behavioral patterns; pessimistic, negative cognitive styles; and focusing too much on depressed feeling instead of action and mastery strategies • High rates of sexual abuse in childhood, so that depressive symptoms may be long-lasting symptoms of posttraumatic stress syndrome for many women • The burdens of marriage and child rearing, which fall much more heavily on women • Poverty in which women and children are vastly overrepresented
3. Postpartum depression	3. Though this disorder is largely attributed to female hormone changes, research has shown that it is more likely to occur in women who do not have help and support following the baby's birth (Tavris, 1989).
4. Bipolar disorder	4. Same as depression. Also, bipolar disorder has been hypothetically tied to rigid requirements for behavior that conform to parental expectations (Arieti, 1978). Females in our culture are subject to more rigid standards of behavior than are males.
5. Phobias	5. The most common fear in females is agoraphobia. Owing to a fear of moving out into the world, it seems symbolically appropriate.
6. Eating disorders	6. Again, females are held to much stricter standards of cultural expectations. In our culture "thin is good." Clients with eating disorders are often seen as: • Avoiding femininity, thus rebelling against growing up • Striving for perfection Both goals are consistent with female roles in the United States (Kaschak, 1992). See Chapter 27.
7. Dissociative identity disorder	7. This disorder is associated with severe trauma. Females are more vulnerable to trauma, and rather than act out, they act in. See Chapter 29.
8. Hysteria	8. Hysteria received its name from the Latin word for *uterus,* and has always been considered a female disorder. In Freud's Vienna it was thought to result from the repression of sexual feelings. Hysteria is another example of women acting "in," not "out," and often occurred in women who could not voice their opposition, instead becoming blind or paralyzed (Shorter, 1994).
9. Psychosomatic disorders	9. Edward Shorter has written a very scholarly chapter about the predominance of psychosomatic disorders in females (Shorter, 1994). He concludes that owing to social factors women are simply more unhappy than men. This unhappiness is expressed by the body, rather than acted out.

5. Psychiatrists who have moved from long-term psychotherapy to prescribing medications profit from a new "disorder" that the media has hyped (Tavris, 1989; Caplan, 1995).
6. "The language of PMS is empowering for women because it gives a medical and social reality to experiences that were previously ignored, trivialized, or misunderstood" (Tavris, 1989, p. 143), normal though they may be.

7. When the American Psychiatric Association (APA) first considered including this syndrome, which they called late luteal phase dysphoric disorder (LLPDD) in the DSM-III-R, a power struggle ensued between those who wanted it included and a strong group of feminist mental health professionals who did not want it included. The power struggle took on a life of its own (Caplan, 1995).

SELF-DEFEATING PERSONALITY DISORDER

Authors of the American Psychiatric Association's DSM III-R (1987) also proposed a diagnosis called self-defeating personality disorder (SDPD). Feminists again pressured the APA not to include it as they saw it as an example of blaming the victims, mostly women who had been abused as children and were currently in abusive relationships. Instead of seeing the behavior of women in these circumstances as a normal response to continued abuse, these psychiatrists saw their behavior as part of a psychiatric disorder. Critics feared the application of a psychiatric diagnosis would lead to simply "curing" the "patient" rather than addressing the social factors that play such a part in creating the situation, as has happened with depression. In addition, once ordinary behaviors created by the society are given a psychiatric diagnosis, they become institutionalized and more and more people develop the "symptoms" of the disorder (Caplan, 1995; Breggin, 1991; Kaminer, 1993; Shorter, 1994; Tavris, 1992; Stuhlmiller, 1995).

PARAPHILIAC COERCIVE DISORDER

The APA also proposed a diagnosis called paraphiliac rapism, later changed to paraphiliac coercive disorder, that received objection from feminist groups. The fear was that this medicalization of deviance would be used as a legal defense for rapists, allowing them to go to mental hospitals or therapy rather than being incarcerated. A psychiatric nurse, Dr. Claire Fagin, who was then president of the American Orthopsychiatric Association, sent a letter on March 29, 1986, to the APA protesting on behalf of the board of directors, expressing their objection to all three diagnoses (Caplan, 1995). None of the three diagnoses appears in the DSM-IV, largely owing to the courageous women who were willing to take on organized psychiatry.

MENOPAUSE

Menopause is another natural occurrence in women that has been medicalized, providing patients for doctors and profits for drug companies (Sheehy, 1991; Tavris, 1989). Psychiatric nurses must strike a balance between the extremes of seeing women who are in menopause as psychiatrically disturbed and the other extreme of seeing the women as psychosomatic whiners. Box 73-1 shows holistic treatments that can help women through the normal reactions and discomforts of menopause.

SEXISM IN PSYCHIATRY

Because most psychiatrists are male and most psychiatric patients are female, mental hospitals and other agencies tend to reinforce traditional male and female societal roles. Many writers have pointed out that the mental health system in the United States is patriarchal. In 1970, Broverman and colleagues published a now famous study showing that mental health professionals held very different standards of mental health for men than for women, and the standards for healthy men were essentially the same as for healthy adults. Other examples of sexism in psychiatry include:
1. "Clinicians, most of whom are men, all too often treat their patients, most of whom are women, as 'wives' and 'daughters' rather than as people" (Chesler, 1972, p. xxi).
2. Female victims of spousal abuse end up in mental hospitals far more often than their husbands who abuse them (Breggin, 1991).

BOX 73-1: Beneficial Holistic Behaviors During Menopause

Diet

- Dong quai, a Chinese herb containing plant sterols with estrogen-like effects
- Siberian ginseng for fatigue and depression
- Vitamins C and E to relieve hot flashes
- Primrose oil containing gamma-linolenic acid to mediate hormonal activity
- Avoidance of smoking, alcohol, coffee, as they raise acid levels in the blood
- Avoidance of carbonated sodas and beef, as they have high phosphorus content
- A diet high in vegetables, complex carbohydrates, fiber, fish, and vegetable protein such as tofu
- Foods high in calcium to prevent osteoporosis: milk, cream of wheat, barley, rice, oatmeal, yogurt, canned sardines, collards, parsley, dried figs, sunflower seeds

Exercise

- Kegal's exercises to prevent problems with bladder control (squeezing and releasing the vagina)
- Overall body exercise to increase bone density, circulation, and well-being

Acupuncture

- Thought to relieve hot flashes and sweats

Prayer, Biofeedback, Yoga, Meditation

- To relieve stress

From Sheehy, G. (1991). *Menopause: The Silent Passage.* New York: Random House; Cutler, W. B., Garcia, C., & Edwards, D. A. (1983). *Menopause: A Guide for Women and the Men Who Love Them.* New York: W. W. Norton.

---

3. Psychiatrists often suppress women's complaints with drugs or ECT (Breggin, 1991).
4. Women are far more likely to receive drugs and ECT than are men. Some argue that this is because they are more likely to be depressed. This does not explain why females were also far more likely to be lobotomized than were men (Breggin, 1991).

True life examples of sexism in mental health treatment are shown in Box 73-2. The second example shows the importance of regarding the client's delusions as life metaphors.

GENDER FACTORS IN PSYCHOTHERAPY

FEMALE CLIENTS WITH MALE THERAPISTS

This combination is the most common and the most controversial. Some beliefs about this arrangement are:

1. Male therapists may hinder female patients by being less alert to gender problems and gender role stereotypes (Shainess, 1983).
2. Male therapists are less likely to experience shame, and may miss it in their patients (Lewis, 1986).
3. The male therapist who has left his wife for a younger woman may find it difficult to be sympathetic or empathetic with the older woman who comes to him after her husband has done the same to her (Shainess, 1983).
4. Women may choose female therapists to avoid having to please men.
5. Women may fear erotic transference and countertransference. A study of psychiatrists conducted by Gartrell, Olarte, and Herman in 1986 revealed that of the

---

BOX 73-2: Actual Examples of Sexism in Mental Health Care in 1995

Private Practice

A 50-year-old woman entered therapy to try to figure out why she was unable for 17 years to leave a marriage that had been humiliating and demoralizing. When she told her husband, a physician, she had filed for divorce, he begged her repeatedly to start taking Prozac. He told her that her irrational act of seeking divorce was not her "fault"—it was a problem in her brain, and he did not hold her responsible. If only she would take the Prozac she'd "be happy again." He begged her to seek a second opinion. She went to see a psychiatrist who, to his credit, did not concur with the husband that she needed medication, but did patiently explain to her, in the same patronizing manner as her husband, that she should think of her family as a football team, and her husband as the quarterback.

A Psychiatric Hospital

A 60-year-old woman was admitted with "delusional behavior" and the diagnosis of bipolar disorder. On the unit she told the nurses her husband, a dentist, was very controlling, never allowing her to make any decisions. Though she had a college degree in psychology, she never worked and instead stayed home with her children. On the unit she had the following delusions: She "saw" her husband's car pull into the parking lot, but he never came up to the unit to visit. She knew it was his car because it had a small stuffed animal that said "Love Me" she had given him. The animal had fallen over but her husband had not bothered to set it upright. She also believed her grown children came to the hospital lot but did not come up to visit her. At times she believed her husband was dead. Her psychiatrist told her she had a "chemical imbalance" and placed her on medications. He said to her nurse, "Isn't her voice annoying?" and complained that she talked too much.

1057 male and 366 female psychiatrists who responded, 7.1% of males and 3% of females admitted to sexual contact with a patient during or after psychiatric treatment (Noël & Watterson, 1992).

6. Women may choose female therapists because they are looking for role models.

MALE CLIENTS WITH FEMALE THERAPISTS

Potential problems associated with this arrangement are:

1. In American culture inhibition of speech in front of women is strongly ingrained (Gornick, 1986).
2. Cultural roles also hold that men look at women, and women are looked at (Gornick, 1986).
3. Women are often looked at as the object of desire. When women are also therapists, symbolizing authority, male clients may find this paradox difficult to handle.
4. Men may interpret the natural tendency to feel vulnerable in therapy as evidence they are being "seduced" into merging again with their mothers.

REFERENCES

American Psychiatric Association (1987, 1994). *Diagnostic and Statistical Manual of Mental Disorders* (3rd ed. rev. and 4th ed.). Washington, DC: American Psychiatric Association.

American Psychological Association (1990). *Women and Depression: Risk Factors and Treatment Issues.* Washington, DC: American Psychological Association.

Arieti, S. (1978). Sociocultural factors, sociology of knowledge, and depression. In S. Arieti & J. Bemporad (eds.), *Severe and Mild Depression: The Psychotherapeutic Approach* (pp. 361–389). New York: Basic Books.

Benjamin, J. (1986). The alienation of desire: Women's masochism and ideal love. In J. L. Alpert (ed.), *Psychoanalysis and Women: Contemporary Reappraisals* (pp. 113–138). Hillsdale, NJ: The Analytic Press.

Breggin, P. R. (1991). *Toxic Psychiatry.* New York: St. Martin's Press.

Broverman, I. K., Broverman, D. M., Clarkson, F. E., Rosenkrantz, P. S., & Vogel, S. R. (1970). Sex-role stereotypes and clinical judgments of mental health. *Journal of Consulting and Clinical Psychology, 34* (1), 1–7.

Brown, L. M., & Gilligan, C. (1992). *Meeting at the Crossroads: Women's Psychology and Girls' Development.* Cambridge, MA: Harvard University Press.

Caplan, P. (1995). *They Say You're Crazy: How the World's Most Powerful Psychiatrists Decide Who's Normal.* Reading, MA: Addison-Wesley.

Chesler, P. (1972). *Women and Madness.* New York: Doubleday.

Cutler, W. B., Garcia, C., & Edwards, D. A. (1983). *Menopause: A Guide for Women and the Men Who Love Them.* New York: W. W. Norton.

Dumont, M. (1990). In bed together at the market: Psychiatry and the pharmaceutical industry. *American Journal of Orthopsychiatry, 60,* 484–485.

Gilligan, C. (1982). *In a Different Voice.* Cambridge, MA: Harvard University Press.

Gornick, L. (1986). Developing a new narrative: The woman therapist and the male patient. In J. L. Alpert (ed.), *Psychoanalysis and Women: Contemporary Reappraisals* (pp. 257–286). Hillsdale, NJ: The Analytic Press.

Horney, K. (1926). The flight from womanhood. In H. Kelman (ed.), *Feminine Psychology* (pp. 54–70). New York: Norton.

Jordan, J. V., & Surrey, J. L. (1986). The self-in-relation: Empathy and the mother–daughter relationship. In T. Bernay & D. W. Cantor (eds.), *The Psychology of Today's Woman: New Psychoanalytic Visions* (pp. 81–104). Hillsdale, NJ: The Analytic Press.

Kaminer, W. (1993). *I'm Dysfunctional, You're Dysfunctional: The Recovery Movement and Other Self-Help Fashions.* New York: Vintage Books.

Kaschak, E. (1992). *Engendered Lives: A New Psychology of Women's Experience.* New York: Basic Books.

Kohut, H. (1971). *The Analysis of the Self.* New York: International Universities Press.

Kramer, P. D. (1993). *Listening to Prozac.* New York: Viking.

Lewis, H. B. (1986). *Sex and the Superego: Psychic War in Men and Women,* rev. ed. Hillsdale, NJ: The Analytic Press.

Mahler, M. S., Pine, F., & Bergman, A. (1975). *The Psychological Birth of the Human Infant: Symbiosis and Individualism.* New York: Basic Books.

Miller, J. B. (1976). *Toward a New Psychology of Women.* Boston: Beacon Press.

Noël, B., & Watterson, K. (1992). *You Must Be Dreaming.* New York: Poseidon.

Parlee, M. B. (1987). Media treatment of premenstrual syndrome. In B. E. Ginsburg & B. F. Carter (eds.), *Premenstrual Syndrome.* New York: Plenum.

Shainess, N. (1983). Significance of match in sex of analyst and patient. *American Journal of Psychoanalysis, 43* (3), 205–217.

Sheehy, G. (1991). *Menopause: The Silent Passage.* New York: Random House.

Shorter, E. (1994). *From the Mind to the Body: The Cultural Origins of Psychosomatic Symptoms.* New York: The Free Press.

Stuhlmiller, C. M. (1995). The construction of disorders: Exploring the growth of PTSD and SAD. *Journal of Psychosocial Nursing, 33* (4), 20–23.

Sullivan, H. S. (1940). *Conceptions of Modern Psychiatry.* New York: Norton.

Surrey, J. (1983). *The Relational Self in Women.* Wellesley, MA.: Stone Center for Developmental Services and Studies.

Tavris, C. (1989). *The Mismeasurement of Women.* New York: Simon and Schuster.

Thompson, C. (1942). Cultural processes in the psychology of women. *Psychiatry, 4,* 331–339.

Appendices

Appendix A

Standards of Psychiatric–Mental Health Clinical Nursing Practice*

STANDARDS OF CARE

"Standards of Care" pertain to professional nursing activities that are demonstrated by the nurse through the nursing process. These involve assessment, diagnosis, outcome identification, planning, implementation, and evaluation. The nursing process is the foundation of clinical decision making and encompasses all significant action taken by nurses in providing psychiatric–mental health care to all clients.

Standard I. Assessment

THE PSYCHIATRIC–MENTAL HEALTH NURSE COLLECTS CLIENT HEALTH DATA.

Rationale

The assessment interview—which requires linguistically and culturally effective communication skills, interviewing, behavioral observation, database record review, and comprehensive assessment of the client and relevant systems—enables the psychiatric–mental health nurse to make sound clinical judgments and plan appropriate interventions with the client.

Measurement Criteria

1. The priority of data collection is determined by the client's immediate condition or need.
2. The data may include but are not limited to:
   a. ability to remain safe and not be a danger to oneself and others.
   b. client's central complaint, symptoms, or focus of concern.
   c. physical, developmental, cognitive, mental, and emotional health status.
   d. history of health patterns and illness.
   e. family, social, cultural, and community systems.
   f. daily activities, functional health status, substance use, health habits, and social roles, including work and sexual functioning.
   g. interpersonal relationships, communication skills, and coping patterns.
   h. spiritual or philosophical beliefs and values.
   i. economic, political, legal, and environmental factors affecting health.
   j. significant support systems, both available and underutilized.
   k. health beliefs and practices.
   l. knowledge, satisfaction, and motivation to change, related to health.
   m. strengths and competencies that can be used to promote health.
   n. other contributing factors that influence health.
3. Pertinent data are collected from multiple sources using various assessment techniques and standardized instruments as appropriate. Multiple sources of assessment data can include not only the client, but also family, social network, other health care providers, past and current medical record, and community agencies and systems (with consideration of the client's confidentiality).
4. The client, significant others, and interdisciplinary team members are involved in the assessment process to the extent possible.

*From A Statement on Psychiatric–Mental Health Clinical Nursing Practice and Standards of Psychiatric–Mental Health Clinical Nursing Practice (1994). Washington, DC: American Nurses Publishing. Reprinted with permission.

5. The client and significant others are informed of their respective roles and responsibilities in the assessment process and data analysis.
6. The assessment process is systematic and ongoing.
7. The data collection is based on clinical judgment to ensure that relevant and necessary data are collected.
8. The database is synthesized, prioritized, and documented in a retrievable form.

Standard II. Diagnosis

THE PSYCHIATRIC–MENTAL HEALTH NURSE ANALYZES THE ASSESSMENT DATA IN DETERMINING DIAGNOSES.

Rationale

The basis for providing psychiatric–mental health nursing care is the recognition and identification of patterns of response to actual or potential psychiatric illnesses and mental health problems.

Measurement Criteria

1. Diagnoses and potential problem statements are derived from assessment data.
2. Interpersonal, systemic, or environmental circumstances—that affect the mental well-being of the individual, family, or community—are identified.
3. The diagnosis is based on an accepted framework which supports the psychiatric–mental health nursing knowledge and judgment used in analyzing the data.
4. Diagnoses conform to accepted classification systems—such as North American Nursing Diagnosis Association (NANDA) Nursing Diagnosis Classification, *International Classification of Diseases* (WHO, 1993), and *The Diagnostic and Statistical Manual of Mental Disorders* (APA, 1987) used in the practice setting.
5. Diagnoses and risk factors are validated with the client, significant others, and other health care providers when appropriate and possible.
6. Diagnoses identify actual or potential psychiatric illness and mental health problems of clients pertaining to:
   a. the maintenance of optimal health and well-being and the prevention of psychobiologic illness.
   b. self-care limitations or impaired functioning related to mental and emotional distress.
   c. deficits in the functioning of significant biological, emotional, and cognitive systems.
   d. emotional stress or crisis components of illness, pain, and disability.
   e. self-concept changes, developmental issues, and life process changes.
   f. problems related to emotions such as anxiety, aggression, sadness, loneliness, and grief.
   g. physical symptoms that occur along with altered psychological functioning.
   h. alterations in thinking, perceiving, symbolizing, communicating, and decision making.
   i. difficulties in relating to others.
   j. behaviors and mental states that indicate the client is a danger to self or others or has a severe disability.
   k. interpersonal, systemic, sociocultural, spiritual, or environmental circumstances or events which have an effect on the mental and emotional well-being of the individual, family, or community.
   l. symptom management, side effects/toxicities associated with psychopharmacologic intervention and other aspects of the treatment regimen.
7. Diagnoses and clinical impressions are documented in a manner that facilitates the identification of client outcomes and their use in the plan of care and research.

Standard III. Outcome Identification

THE PSYCHIATRIC–MENTAL HEALTH NURSE IDENTIFIES EXPECTED OUTCOMES INDIVIDUALIZED TO THE CLIENT.

Rationale

Within the context of providing nursing care, the ultimate goal is to influence health outcomes and improve the client's health status.

Measurement Criteria

1. Expected outcomes are derived from the diagnoses.
2. Expected outcomes are client-oriented, therapeutically sound, realistic, attainable, and cost-effective.
3. Expected outcomes are documented as measurable goals.
4. Expected outcomes are formulated by the nurse and the client, significant others, and interdisciplinary team members, when possible.
5. Expected outcomes are realistic in relation to the client's present and potential capabilities.
6. Expected outcomes are identified with consideration of the associated benefits and costs.
7. Expected outcomes estimate a time for attainment.
8. Expected outcomes provide direction for continuity of care.
9. Expected outcomes reflect current scientific knowledge in mental health care.
10. Expected outcomes serve as a record of change in the client's health status.

Standard IV. Planning

THE PSYCHIATRIC–MENTAL HEALTH NURSE DEVELOPS A PLAN OF CARE THAT PRESCRIBES INTERVENTIONS TO ATTAIN EXPECTED OUTCOMES.

Rationale

A plan of care is used to guide therapeutic intervention systematically and achieve the expected client outcomes.

Measurement Criteria

1. The plan is individualized, tailored to the client's mental health problems, condition, or needs and it:
   a. identifies priorities of care in relation to expected outcomes.
   b. identifies effective interventions to achieve the outcomes.
   c. specifies interventions that reflect current psychiatric–mental health nursing practice and research.
   d. includes an education program related to the client's health problems, treatment, and self-care activities.
   e. indicates responsibilities of the psychiatric–mental health nurse and the client, and may include responsibilities for interdisciplinary team members to carry out the plan of care.
   f. gives direction for client-care activities delegated by the psychiatric–mental health nurse to other care providers.
   g. provides for appropriate referral and case management to insure continuity of care.
2. The plan is developed in collaboration with the client, significant others, and interdisciplinary team members, when appropriate.
3. The plan is documented in a manner that allows access to it by team members and modification of the plan as necessary.

Standard V. Implementation

THE PSYCHIATRIC–MENTAL HEALTH NURSE IMPLEMENTS THE INTERVENTIONS IDENTIFIED IN THE PLAN OF CARE.

Rationale

In implementing the plan of care, psychiatric–mental health nurses use a wide range of interventions designed to prevent mental and physical illness, and promote, maintain, and restore mental and physical health. Psychiatric–mental health nurses select interventions according to their level of practice. At the basic level, the nurse may select counseling, milieu therapy, self-care activities, psychobiological interventions, health teaching, case management, health pro-

motion and health maintenance, and a variety of other approaches to meet the mental health needs of clients. In addition to the intervention options available to the basic-level psychiatric–mental health nurse, at the advanced level the certified specialist may provide consultation, engage in psychotherapy, and prescribe pharmacologic agents where permitted by state statutes or regulations.

Measurement Criteria

1. Interventions are selected based on the needs of the client and accepted nursing practice.
2. Interventions are selected according to the psychiatric–mental health nurse's level of practice, education, and certification.
3. Interventions are implemented within the established plan of care.
4. Interventions are performed in a safe, ethical, and appropriate manner.
5. Interventions are documented.

Standard Va. Counseling

THE PSYCHIATRIC–MENTAL HEALTH NURSE USES COUNSELING INTERVENTIONS TO ASSIST CLIENTS IN IMPROVING OR REGAINING THEIR PREVIOUS COPING ABILITIES, FOSTERING MENTAL HEALTH, AND PREVENTING MENTAL ILLNESS AND DISABILITY.

Measurement Criteria

1. Counseling interventions—including communication and interviewing techniques, problem-solving skills, crisis intervention, stress management, relaxation techniques, assertiveness training, conflict resolution, and behavior modification—are documented.
2. Counseling reinforces healthy behaviors and interaction patterns and helps the client modify or discontinue unhealthy ones.
3. Counseling promotes the client's personal and social integration.

Standard Vb. Milieu Therapy

THE PSYCHIATRIC–MENTAL HEALTH NURSE PROVIDES STRUCTURES, AND MAINTAINS A THERAPEUTIC ENVIRONMENT IN COLLABORATION WITH THE CLIENT AND OTHER HEALTH CARE PROVIDERS.

Measurement Criteria

1. The client is familiarized with the physical environment, the schedule of activities, and the norms and rules that govern behavior and activities of daily living, as applicable.
2. Current knowledge of the effects of the client's environment is used to guide nursing actions.

3. The therapeutic environment is designed utilizing the physical environment, social structures, culture, and other available resources.
4. Communication among clients and staff supports an effective milieu.
5. Specific activities are selected that meet the client's physical and mental health needs.
6. Limits of any kind (e.g., restriction of privileges, restraint, seclusion, timeout) are used in a humane manner, are the least restrictive necessary, and are employed only as long as needed to assure the safety of the client and of others.
7. The client is given information about the need for limits and the conditions necessary for removal of the restriction, as appropriate.
8. The client and significant others are given the opportunity to ask questions and discuss their feelings and concerns about past, current, and projected use of various environments.

Standard Vc. Self-Care Activities

THE PSYCHIATRIC–MENTAL HEALTH NURSE STRUCTURES INTERVENTIONS AROUND THE CLIENT'S ACTIVITIES OF DAILY LIVING TO FOSTER SELF-CARE AND MENTAL AND PHYSICAL WELL-BEING.

Measurement Criteria

1. The self-care interventions assist the client in assuming personal responsibility for activities of daily living.
2. The self-care activities of daily living are appropriate for the client's age, developmental level, gender, sexual orientation, ethnic/social background, and education.
3. Self-care interventions are aimed at maintaining and improving the client's functional status.

Standard Vd. Psychobiological Interventions

THE PSYCHIATRIC–MENTAL HEALTH NURSE USES KNOWLEDGE OF PSYCHOBIOLOGICAL INTERVENTIONS AND APPLIES CLINICAL SKILLS TO RESTORE THE CLIENT'S HEALTH AND PREVENT FURTHER DISABILITY.

Measurement Criteria

1. Current knowledge of psychopharmacology and other psychobiological therapies are used to guide nursing action.
2. Psychopharmacological agents' intended actions, untoward effects, and therapeutic doses are monitored, as are blood levels where appropriate.
3. The client's responses to therapies serve as clinical indications of treatment effectiveness.

4. Nursing interventions are directed toward alleviating untoward effects of psychobiological interventions, when possible.
5. Opportunities are provided for the client and significant others to question, discuss, and explore the feelings about past, current, and projected use of therapies.
6. Nursing observations about the client's response to psychobiological interventions are communicated to other health providers.

Standard Ve. Health Teaching

THE PSYCHIATRIC–MENTAL HEALTH NURSE, THROUGH HEALTH TEACHING, ASSISTS CLIENTS IN ACHIEVING SATISFYING, PRODUCTIVE, AND HEALTHY PATTERNS OF LIVING.

Measurement Criteria

1. Health teaching is based on principles of learning.
2. Health teaching includes information about coping, interpersonal relations, mental health problems, mental disorders, and treatments and their effects on daily living, as well as information pertinent to physical status or developmental needs.
3. The nurse uses health teaching methods appropriate to the client's age, developmental level, gender, ethnic/social background, and education.
4. Constructive feedback and positive rewards reinforce the client's learning.
5. Practice sessions and experiential learning are used as needed.

Standard Vf. Case Management

THE PSYCHIATRIC–MENTAL HEALTH NURSE PROVIDES CASE MANAGEMENT TO COORDINATE COMPREHENSIVE HEALTH SERVICES AND ENSURE CONTINUITY OF CARE.

Measurement Criteria

1. Case management services are based on a comprehensive approach to the client's physical, mental, emotional, and social health problems.
2. Case management services are provided in terms of the client's needs and the accessibility, availability, quality, and cost-effectiveness of care.
3. Health-related services and more specialized care are negotiated as needed—on behalf of the client—with the appropriate agencies and providers.
4. Relationships with agencies and providers are maintained throughout the client's use of the health care services to ensure confidentiality of care.

5. The client's decisions related to the plan of care and treatment choices are supported, as appropriate.

Standard Vg. Health Promotion and Health Maintenance

THE PSYCHIATRIC–MENTAL HEALTH NURSE EMPLOYS STRATEGIES AND INTERVENTIONS TO PROMOTE AND MAINTAIN MENTAL HEALTH AND PREVENT MENTAL ILLNESS.

Measurement Criteria

1. Health promotion and disease prevention strategies are based on knowledge of health beliefs, practices, and epidemiological principles, along with the social, cultural, and political issues that affect mental health in an identified community.
2. Health promotion and disease prevention interventions are designed for clients identified as at-risk for mental health problems.
3. Consumer participation is encouraged in identifying mental health problems in the community and planning, implementing, and evaluating programs to address those problems.
4. Community resources are identified to assist consumers in using prevention and mental health care services appropriately.

Advanced Practice Interventions Vh–Vj

The following interventions (Vh–Vj) may be performed only by the certified specialist in psychiatric–mental health nursing.

Standard Vh. Psychotherapy

THE CERTIFIED SPECIALIST IN PSYCHIATRIC–MENTAL HEALTH NURSING USES INDIVIDUAL, GROUP, AND FAMILY PSYCHOTHERAPY, CHILD PSYCHOTHERAPY, AND OTHER THERAPEUTIC TREATMENTS TO ASSIST CLIENTS IN FOSTERING MENTAL HEALTH, PREVENTING MENTAL ILLNESS AND DISABILITY, AND IMPROVING OR REGAINING PREVIOUS HEALTH STATUS AND FUNCTIONAL ABILITIES.

Measurement Criteria

1. The therapeutic contract with the client is structured to include:
   a. purpose, goals, and expected outcomes.
   b. time, place, and frequency of therapy.
   c. fees and payment schedule.
   d. participants involved in therapy.
   e. confidentiality.
   f. availability and means of contacting therapist.
   g. responsibilities of both client and therapist.
2. Knowledge of personality theory, growth and development, psychology, psychopathology, social systems, small-group and family dynamics, stress and adaptation, and theories related to selected therapeutic methods is used, based on the client's needs.
3. Therapeutic principles are used to understand and interpret the client's emotions, thoughts, and behaviors.
4. The client is helped to deal constructively with thoughts, emotions, and behaviors.
5. Increasing responsibility and independence are fostered in the client to reinforce healthy behaviors and interactions.
6. Continuing of care is provided in therapist's absence.
7. Nursing care for the client's physical needs is referred to another provider when it is determined that such care provided by the therapist would impair the client/therapist relationship.

Standard Vi. Prescription of Pharmacologic Agents

THE CERTIFIED SPECIALIST USES PRESCRIPTION OF PHARMACOLOGIC AGENTS IN ACCORDANCE WITH THE STATE NURSING PRACTICE ACT, TO TREAT SYMPTOMS OF PSYCHIATRIC ILLNESS, AND IMPROVE FUNCTIONAL HEALTH STATUS.

Measurement Criteria

1. Prescriptive authority for pharmacologic agents is used only by those nurses who are qualified by education and experience and in accordance with the state nursing practice act or state and federal regulations.
2. Psychoactive pharmacologic agents are prescribed based on a knowledge of psychopathology, neurobiology, physiology, immunology, expected therapeutic actions, anticipated side effects, and courses of action for unintended or toxic effects.
3. Specific pharmacological agents are prescribed based on clinical indicators of the client's status, including the results of diagnostic and laboratory tests, as appropriate.
4. Information about intended effects, potential side effects of the proposed prescription, and alternative treatments is provided to the client.

Standard Vj. Consultation

THE CERTIFIED SPECIALIST PROVIDES CONSULTATION TO HEALTH CARE PROVIDERS AND OTHERS TO INFLUENCE THE PLANS OF CARE FOR CLIENTS, AND TO ENHANCE THE ABILITIES OF OTHERS TO PROVIDE PSYCHIATRIC AND MENTAL HEALTH CARE AND EFFECT CHANGE IN SYSTEMS.

Measurement Criteria

1. Consultation activities are based on models of consultation, systems principles, communication and interviewing techniques, problem-solving skills, change theories, and other theories as indicated.
2. A working alliance, based on mutual respect and role responsibilities, is established with the consultee.
3. The decision to implement the system change or plan of care remains the responsibility of the consultee.

Standard VI. Evaluation

THE PSYCHIATRIC–MENTAL HEALTH NURSE EVALUATES THE CLIENT'S PROGRESS IN ATTAINING EXPECTED OUTCOMES.

Rationale

Nursing care is a dynamic process involving change in the client's health status over time, giving rise to the need for new data, different diagnoses, and modifications in the plan of care. Therefore, evaluation is a continuous process of appraising the effect of nursing interventions and the treatment regimen on the client's health status and expected health outcomes.

Measurement Criteria

1. Evaluation is systematic and ongoing.
2. The client, significant others, and team members are involved in the evaluation process, as possible, to ascertain the client's level of satisfaction with care and evaluate the cost and benefits associated with the treatment process.
3. The client's responses to interventions are documented.
4. The effectiveness of interventions in relation to outcomes is evaluated.
5. Ongoing assessment data are used to revise diagnoses, outcomes, and the plan of care as needed.
6. Revisions in the diagnoses, outcomes, and the plan of care are documented.
7. The revised plan provides for continuity of care.

STANDARDS OF PROFESSIONAL PERFORMANCE

"Standards of Professional Performance" describe a competent level of behavior in the professional role, including activities related to quality of care, performance appraisal, education, collegiality, ethics, collaboration, research, and resource utilization. All psychiatric–mental health nurses are expected to engage in professional role activities appropriate to their education, position, and practice setting. Therefore, some standards or measurement criteria identify these activities.

While "Standards of Professional Performance" describe the roles of all professional nurses, there are many other responsibilities that are hallmarks of psychiatric–mental health nursing. These nurses should be self-directed and purposeful in seeking necessary knowledge and skills to enhance career goals. Other activities—such as membership in professional organizations, certification in specialty or advanced practice, continuing education, and further academic education—are desirable methods of enhancing the psychiatric–mental health nurse's professionalism.

Standard I. Quality of Care

THE PSYCHIATRIC–MENTAL HEALTH NURSE SYSTEMATICALLY EVALUATES THE QUALITY OF CARE AND EFFECTIVENESS OF PSYCHIATRIC–MENTAL HEALTH NURSING PRACTICE.

Rationale

The dynamic nature of the mental health care environment and the growing body of psychiatric nursing knowledge and research provide both the impetus and the means for the psychiatric–mental health nurse to be competent in clinical practice, to continue to develop professionally, and to improve the quality of client care.

Measurement Criteria

1. The psychiatric–mental health nurse participates in quality-of-care activities as appropriate to the nurse's position, education, and practice environment. Such activities can include:
   a. identification of aspects of care important for quality monitoring—e.g., functional status, symptom management and control, health behaviors and practices, safety, client satisfaction, and quality of life.
   b. identification of indicators used to monitor the effectiveness of psychiatric–mental health nursing care.
   c. collection of data to monitor quality and effectiveness of psychiatric–mental health nursing care.

   d. analysis of quality data to identify opportunities for improving psychiatric–mental health nursing care.
   e. formulation of recommendations to improve psychiatric–mental health nursing practice or client outcomes.
   f. implementation of activities to enhance the quality of psychiatric–mental health nursing practice.
   g. participation in interdisciplinary teams which evaluate clinical practice or mental health services.
   h. development of policies and procedures to improve quality psychiatric–mental health care.
2. The psychiatric–mental health nurse seeks feedback from the client and significant others about their satisfaction with care.
3. The psychiatric–mental health nurse uses the results of quality-of-care activities to initiate changes in psychiatric–mental health nursing practice.
4. The psychiatric–mental health nurse uses the results of quality-of-care activities to initiate changes throughout the mental health care delivery system, as appropriate.

Standard II. Performance Appraisal

THE PSYCHIATRIC–MENTAL HEALTH NURSE EVALUATES OWN PSYCHIATRIC–MENTAL HEALTH NURSING PRACTICE IN RELATION TO PROFESSIONAL PRACTICE STANDARDS AND RELEVANT STATUTES AND REGULATIONS.

Rationale

The psychiatric–mental health nurse is accountable to the public for providing competent clinical care and has an inherent responsibility as a professional to evaluate the role and performance of psychiatric–mental health nursing practice according to standards established by the profession and regulatory bodies.

Measurement Criteria

1. The psychiatric–mental health nurse engages in performance appraisal of own clinical practice and role performance with peers or supervisors on a regular basis, identifying areas of strength as well as areas for professional/practice development.
2. The psychiatric–mental health nurse seeks constructive feedback regarding own practice and role performance from peers, professional colleagues, clients, and others.
3. The psychiatric–mental health nurse takes action to achieve goals identified during performance appraisal and peer review, resulting in changes in practice and role performance.
4. The psychiatric–mental health nurse participates in peer review activities when possible.

Standard III. Education

THE PSYCHIATRIC–MENTAL HEALTH NURSE ACQUIRES AND MAINTAINS CURRENT KNOWLEDGE IN NURSING PRACTICE.

Rationale

The rapid expansion of knowledge pertaining to basic and behavioral sciences, technology, information systems, and research requires a commitment to learning throughout the psychiatric–mental health nurse's professional career. Formal education, continuing education, certification, and experiential learning are some of the means the psychiatric–mental health nurse uses to enhance nursing expertise and advance the profession.

Measurement Criteria

1. The psychiatric–mental health nurse participates in educational activities to improve clinical knowledge, enhance role performance, and increase knowledge of professional issues.
2. The psychiatric–mental health nurse seeks experiences and independent learning activities to maintain and develop clinical skills.
3. The psychiatric–mental health nurse seeks additional knowledge and skills appropriate to the practice setting by participating in educational programs and activities, conferences, workshops, and interdisciplinary professional meetings.
4. The psychiatric–mental health nurse documents own educational activities.
5. The psychiatric–mental health nurse seeks certification when eligible.

Standard IV. Collegiality

THE PSYCHIATRIC–MENTAL HEALTH NURSE CONTRIBUTES TO THE PROFESSIONAL DEVELOPMENT OF PEERS, COLLEAGUES, AND OTHERS.

Rationale

The psychiatric–mental health nurse is responsible for sharing knowledge, research, and clinical information with colleagues, through formal and informal teaching methods, to enhance professional growth.

Measurement Criteria

1. The psychiatric–mental health nurse uses opportunities in practice to exchange knowledge, skills, and clinical observations with colleagues and others.
2. The psychiatric–mental health nurse assists others in identifying teaching/learning needs related to clinical care, role performance, and professional advancement.

3. The psychiatric–mental health nurse provides peers with constructive feedback regarding their practices.

4. The psychiatric–mental health nurse contributes to an environment that is conducive to clinical education of nursing students, as appropriate.

Standard V. Ethics

THE PSYCHIATRIC–MENTAL HEALTH NURSE'S DECISIONS AND ACTIONS ON BEHALF OF CLIENTS ARE DETERMINED IN AN ETHICAL MANNER.

Rationale

The public's trust and its right to humane psychiatric–mental health care are upheld by professional nursing practice. The foundation of psychiatric–mental health nursing practice is the development of a therapeutic relationship with the client. The psychiatric–mental health nurse engages in therapeutic interactions and relationships which promote and support the healing process. Boundaries need to be established to safeguard the client's well-being and to prevent the development of intimate or sexual relationships.

Measurement Criteria

1. The psychiatric–mental health nurse's practice is guided by the *Code for Nurses*.

2. The psychiatric–mental health nurse maintains a therapeutic and professional relationship with clients at all times.

3. The psychiatric–mental health nurse maintains client confidentiality and appropriate professional boundaries.

4. The psychiatric–mental health nurse functions as a client advocate.

5. The psychiatric–mental health nurse delivers care in a nonjudgmental and nondiscriminatory manner sensitive to client diversity.

6. The psychiatric–mental health nurse identifies ethical dilemmas that occur within the practice environment and seeks available resources to help formulate ethical decisions.

7. The psychiatric–mental health nurse reports abuse of clients' rights, and incompetent, unethical, and illegal practices.

8. The psychiatric–mental health nurse participates in obtaining the client's informed consent for procedures, treatments, and research, as appropriate.

9. The psychiatric–mental health nurse discusses with the client the delineation of roles and the parameters of the relationship.

10. The psychiatric–mental health nurse carefully manages self-disclosure.

11. The psychiatric–mental health nurse does not promote or engage in intimate or sexual relationships with current clients.

12. The psychiatric–mental health nurse avoids sexual relationships with clients or former clients and recognizes that to engage in such a relationship is unusual and an exception to accepted practice.

Standard VI. Collaboration

THE PSYCHIATRIC–MENTAL HEALTH NURSE COLLABORATES WITH THE CLIENT, SIGNIFICANT OTHERS, AND HEALTH CARE PROVIDERS IN PROVIDING CARE.

Rationale

Psychiatric–mental health nursing practice requires a coordinated, ongoing interaction between consumers and providers to deliver comprehensive services to the client and the community. Through the collaborative process, different abilities of health care providers are used to solve problems, communicate, and plan, implement, and evaluate mental health services.

Measurement Criteria

1. The psychiatric–mental health nurse collaborates with the client, significant others, and health care providers in the formulation of overall goals, plans, and decisions related to client care and the delivery of mental health services.

2. The psychiatric–mental health nurse consults with other health care providers on client care, as appropriate.

3. The psychiatric–mental health nurse makes referrals—including provisions for continuity of care—as needed.

4. The psychiatric–mental health nurse collaborates with other disciplines in teaching, consultation, management, and research activities as opportunities arise.

Standard VII. Research

THE PSYCHIATRIC–MENTAL HEALTH NURSE CONTRIBUTES TO NURSING AND MENTAL HEALTH THROUGH THE USE OF RESEARCH.

Rationale

Nurses in psychiatric–mental health nursing are responsible for contributing to the further development of the field of mental health by participating in research. At the basic level of practice, the psychiatric–mental health nurse uses research findings to improve clinical care and identifies clinical problems for research study. At the advanced level, the psychiatric–mental health nurse engages and/or collaborates with others in the research process to discover, examine, and test knowledge, theories, and creative approaches to practice.

Measurement Criteria

1. The psychiatric–mental health nurse uses interventions substantiated by research as appropriate to the nurse's position, education, and practice environment.
2. The psychiatric–mental health nurse participates in research as appropriate to the nurse's position, education, and practice environment. Such activities can include:
   a. identification of clinical problems suitable for psychiatric–mental health nursing research.
   b. participation in data collection.
   c. participation in unit, organization, or community research committees or programs.
   d. sharing research activities with others.
   e. conducting research and disseminating findings.
   f. critiquing research for application to practice.
   g. using research findings in the development of policies, procedures, and guidelines for client care.
   h. consulting with research experts and colleagues as necessary.

Standard VIII. Resource Utilization

THE PSYCHIATRIC–MENTAL HEALTH NURSE CONSIDERS FACTORS RELATED TO SAFETY, EFFECTIVENESS, AND COST IN PLANNING AND DELIVERING CLIENT CARE

Rationale

The client is entitled to psychiatric–mental health care which is safe, effective, and affordable. As the cost of health care increases, treatment decisions must be made in such a way as to maximize resources and maintain quality of care. The psychiatric–mental health nurse seeks to provide cost-effective quality care by using the most appropriate resources and delegating care to the most appropriate, qualified health care provider.

Measurement Criteria

1. The psychiatric–mental health nurse analyzes factors related to safety, effectiveness, and cost when two or more practice options would result in the same expected client outcome.
2. The psychiatric–mental health nurse discusses benefits and cost of treatment options with the client, significant others, and other providers, as appropriate.
3. The psychiatric–mental health nurse assists the client and significant others in identifying and securing appropriate services available to address health-related needs.

4. The psychiatric–mental health nurse assigns tasks or delegates care based on the needs of the client and the knowledge and skills of the selected provider.
5. The psychiatric–mental health nurse participates in ongoing resource utilization review.

REFERENCES

American Nurses Association (1967). *Statement on psychiatric and mental health nursing practice.* Kansas City, MO: the Author.

American Nurses Association (1976). *Statement on psychiatric and mental health nursing practice.* Kansas City, MO: the Author.

American Nurses Association (1980). *Code for nurses.* Kansas City, MO: the Author.

American Nurses Association (1982). *Standards of psychiatric and mental health nursing practice.* Kansas City, MO: the Author.

American Nurses Association (1985). *Standards of child and adolescent psychiatric and mental-health nursing practice.* Kansas City, MO: the Author.

American Nurses Association (1990). *Standards of psychiatric consultation-liaison nursing practice.* Kansas City, MO: the Author.

American Nurses Association (1991a). *Nursing's agenda for health care reform.* Kansas City, MO: the Author.

American Nurses Association (1991b). *Standards of clinical nursing practice.* Kansas City, MO: the Author.

American Psychiatric Association (1987). *Diagnostic and statistical manual of mental disorders (third edition, revised).* Washington, DC: the Author.

Billings, C. V. (1993, February). The possible dream of mental health reformers. *The American Nurse, 25* (2), 5.

Haber, J., & Billings, C. 1993. Primary mental health care: A vision for the future of psychiatric–mental health nursing. *ANA Council Perspectives, 2* (2), 1.

Koldjeski, D. (1984). *Community Mental Health Nursing: Directions in Theory and Practice.* New York: John Wiley & Sons.

Krauss, J. (1993). *Health Care Reform: Essential Mental Health Services.* Washington, DC: American Nurses Publishing.

Lowery, B. J. (1992). Psychiatric nursing in the 1990s and beyond. *Journal of Psychosocial Nursing, 30,* 7–13.

McBride, A. B. (1990). Psychiatric nursing in the 1990s. *Archives of Psychiatric Nursing, IV* (1), 21–28.

Pothier, P. C., Stuart, G. W., Puskar, K., & Babich, K. (1990). Dilemmas and directions for psychiatric nursing in the 1990s. *Archives of Psychiatric Nursing, IV* (5), 284–291.

U.S. Department of Health and Human Services. U.S. Public Health Service (1990). *Healthy People 2000: National Health Promotion and Disease Prevention.* Washington, DC: U.S. Government Printing Office.

World Health Organization (1993). *International Classification of Diseases* (10th ed.). Geneva: the Author.

Worley, N. K., Drago, L., & Hadley, T. (1990). Improving the physical health–mental health interface for the chronically mentally ill: Could nurse case managers make a difference? *Archives of Psychiatric Nursing, IV* (2), 108–111.

Appendix B

DSM-IV Classifications, Axis I and II Categories and Codes*

Disorders Usually First Diagnosed in Infancy, Childhood, or Adolescence (49)

MENTAL RETARDATION (50)

Note: These are coded on Axis II.

317	Mild Mental Retardation (50)
318.0	Moderate Mental Retardation (50)
318.1	Severe Mental Retardation (50)
318.2	Profound Mental Retardation (50)
319	Mental Retardation, Severity Unspecified (51)

LEARNING DISORDERS (51)

315.00	Reading Disorder (51)
315.1	Mathematics Disorder (51)
315.2	Disorder of Written Expression (52)
315.9	Learning Disorder NOS (52)

MOTOR SKILLS DISORDER (53)

315.4	Developmental Coordination Disorder (53)

COMMUNICATION DISORDERS (54)

315.31	Expressive Language Disorder (54)
315.31	Mixed Receptive-Expressive Language Disorder (55)
315.39	Phonological Disorder (55)
307.0	Stuttering (56)
307.9	Communication Disorder NOS (57)

PERVASIVE DEVELOPMENTAL DISORDERS (57)

299.00	Autistic Disorder (57)
299.80	Rett's Disorder (59)
299.10	Childhood Disintegrative Disorder (60)
299.80	Asperger's Disorder (61)
299.80	Pervasive Developmental Disorder (62)

ATTENTION-DEFICIT AND DISRUPTIVE BEHAVIOR DISORDERS (63)

314.xx	Attention-Deficit/Hyperactivity Disorder (63)
.01	Combined Type
.00	Predominantly Inattentive Type
.01	Predominantly Hyperactive-Impulsive Type
314.9	Attention-Deficit/Hyperactivity Disorder NOS (65)
312.8	Conduct Disorder (66)
	Specify type: Childhood-Onset Type/Adolescent-Onset Type
313.81	Oppositional Defiant Disorder (68)
312.9	Disruptive Behavior Disorder NOS (69)

FEEDING AND EATING DISORDERS OF INFANCY OR EARLY CHILDHOOD (69)

307.52	Pica (69)
307.53	Rumination Disorder (70)
307.59	Feeding Disorder of Infancy or Early Childhood (70)

TIC DISORDERS (71)

307.23	Tourette's Disorder (71)
307.22	Chronic Motor or Vocal Tic Disorder (71)
307.21	Transient Tic Disorder (72)
	Specify if: Single Episode/Recurrent
307.20	Tic Disorder NOS (73)

*From American Psychiatric Association (1994). *Diagnostic and Statistical Manual of Mental Disorders* (4th ed.). Washington, DC: American Psychiatric Association. Reprinted with permission.

ELIMINATION DISORDERS (73)

—.—   Encopresis (73)

787.6   With Constipation and Overflow Incontinence (74)

307.7   Without Constipation and Overflow Incontinence (74)

307.6   Enuresis (Not Due to a General Medical Condition) (74)
         Specify type: Nocturnal Only/Diurnal Only/Nocturnal and Diurnal

OTHER DISORDERS OF INFANCY, CHILDHOOD, OR ADOLESCENCE (75)

309.21   Separation Anxiety Disorder (75)
         Specify if: Early Onset

313.23   Selective Mutism (76)

313.89   Reactive Attachment Disorder of Infancy or Early Childhood (77)
         Specify if: Inhibited type/Disinhibited Type

307.3   Stereotypic Movement Disorder (78)
         Specify if: With Self-Injurious Behavior

313.9   Disorder of Infancy, Childhood, or Adolescence NOS (79)

Delirium, Dementia, and Amnesic and Other Cognitive Disorders (81)

DELIRIUM (81)

293.0   Delirium Due to . . . *[Indicate the General Medical Condition]* (81)

—.—   Substance Intoxication Delirium *(refer to Substance-Related Disorders for substance-specific codes)* (82)

—.—   Substance Withdrawal Delirium *(refer to Substance-Related Disorders for substance-specific codes)* (83)

—.—   Substance Due to Multiple Etiologies *(code each of the specific etiologies)* (84)

780.09   Delirium NOS (85)

DEMENTIA (85)

290.xx   Dementia of the Alzheimer's Type, with Early Onset *(also code 331.0 Alzheimer's disease on Axis III)* (85)
  .10   Uncomplicated
  .11   With Delirium
  .12   With Delusions
  .13   With Depressed Mood
           Specify if: With Behavioral Disturbance

290.xx   Vascular Dementia (88)

  .40   Uncomplicated
  .41   With Delirium
  .42   With Delusions
  .43   With Depressed Mood
           Specify if: With Behavioral Disturbance

294.9   Dementia Due to HIV Disease *(also code 043.1 HIV infection affecting central nervous system on Axis III)* (90)

294.1   Dementia Due to Head Trauma *(also code 854.00 head injury on Axis III)* (90)

294.1   Dementia Due to Parkinson's Disease *(also code 332.00 Parkinson's disease on Axis III)* (90)

290.10   Dementia Due to Pick's Disease *(also code 331.1 Pick's disease on Axis III)* (90)

294.10   Dementia Due to Creutzfeldt-Jakob Disease *(also code 046.1 Creutzfeldt-Jakob disease on Axis III)* (90)

294.1   Dementia Due to . . . *[Indicate the General Medical Condition not listed above] (also code the general medical condition on Axis III)* (90)

—.—   Substance-Induced Persisting Dementia *(refer to Substance-Related Disorders for substance-specific codes)* (91)

—.—   Dementia Due to Multiple Etiologies *(code each of the specific etiologies)* (92)

294.8   Dementia NOS (93)

AMNESTIC DISORDERS (93)

294.0   Amnestic Disorder Due to . . . *[Indicate the General Medical Condition]* (93)
         Specify if: Transient/Chronic

—.—   Substance-Induced Persisting Amnestic Disorder *(refer to Substance-Related Disorders for substance-specific codes)* (94)

294.8   Amnestic Disorder NOS (94)

OTHER COGNITIVE DISORDERS (96)

294.9   Cognitive Disorder NOS (96)

Mental Disorders Due to a General Medical Condition Not Elsewhere Classified (97)

293.89   Catatonic Disorder Due to . . . *[Indicate the General Medical Condition]* (98)

310.1   Personality Change Due to . . . *[Indicate the General Medical Condition]* (99)
         Specify type: Labile Type/Disinhibited Type/Aggressive Type/Apathetic Type/Paranoid Type/Other Type/Combined Type/Unspecified Type

293.9   Mental Disorder NOS Due to . . . *[Indicate the General Medical Condition]* (100)

Substance-Related Disorders (103)

^a*The following specifiers may be applied to Substance Dependence:*

With Physiological Dependence/Without Physiological
    Dependence
Early Full Remission/Early Partial Remission
Sustained Full Remission/Sustained Partial Remission
On Agonist Therapy/In a Controlled Environment

The following specifiers apply to Substance-Induced Disorders as noted:

^IWith Onset During Intoxication/^WWith Onset During Withdrawal

ALCOHOL-RELATED DISORDERS (116)

Alcohol Use Disorders (116)

303.90   Alcohol Dependence^a (108)
305.00   Alcohol Abuse (112)

Alcohol-Induced Disorders (116)

303.00   Alcohol Intoxication (117)
291.8   Alcohol Withdrawal (118)
          Specify if: With Perceptual Disturbances
291.0   Alcohol Intoxication Delirium (82)
291.0   Alcohol Withdrawal Delirium (83)
291.2   Alcohol-Induced Persisting Dementia (91)
291.1   Alcohol-Induced Persisting Amnestic Disorder
          (94)
291.x   Alcohol-Induced Psychotic Disorder (157)
    .5   With Delusions^{I,W}
    .3   With Hallucinations^{I,W}
291.8   Alcohol-Induced Mood Disorder^{I,W} (184)
291.8   Alcohol-Induced Anxiety Disorder^{I,W} (215)
291.8   Alcohol-Induced Sexual Dysfunction^I (240)
291.8   Alcohol-Induced Sleep Disorder^{I,W} (266)
291.9   Alcohol-Related Disorder NOS (117)

AMPHETAMINE (OR AMPHETAMINE-LIKE)–RELATED DISORDERS (119)

Amphetamine Use Disorders (119)

304.40   Amphetamine Dependence^a (108)
305.70   Amphetamine Abuse^a (112)

Amphetamine-Induced Disorders (119)

292.89   Amphetamine Intoxication (120)
          Specify if: With Perceptual Disturbances
292.0   Amphetamine Withdrawal^a (112)
292.81   Amphetamine Intoxication Delirium (82)
292.xx   Amphetamine-Induced Psychotic Disorder (157)
    .11   With Delusions^I
    .12   With Hallucinations^I

292.84   Amphetamine-Induced Mood Disorder^{I,W} (184)
292.89   Amphetamine-Induced Anxiety Disorder^I (215)
292.89   Amphetamine-Induced Sexual Dysfunction^I
          (240)
292.89   Amphetamine-Induced Sleep Disorder^{I,W} (266)
292.9   Amphetamine-Related Disorder NOS (120)

CAFFEINE-RELATED DISORDERS (122)

Caffeine-Induced Disorders (122)

305.90   Caffeine Intoxication (123)
292.89   Caffeine-Induced Anxiety Disorder^I (215)
292.89   Caffeine-Induced Sleep Disorder^I (266)
292.9   Caffeine-Related Disorder NOS (122)

CANNABIS-RELATED DISORDERS (123)

Cannabis Use Disorders (123)

304.30   Cannabis Dependence^a (108)
305.20   Cannabis Abuse (112)

Cannabis-Induced Disorders (124)

292.89   Cannabis Intoxication (124)
          Specify if: With Perceptual Disturbances
292.81   Cannabis Intoxication Delirium (82)
292.xx   Cannabis-Induced Psychotic Disorder (157)
    .11   With Delusions^I
    .12   With Hallucinations^I
292.89   Cannabis-Induced Anxiety Disorder^I (215)
292.9   Cannabis-Related Disorder NOS (124)

COCAINE-RELATED DISORDERS (125)

Cocaine Use Disorders (125)

304.20   Cocaine Dependence^a (108)
305.60   Cocaine Abuse (112)

Cocaine-Induced Disorders (125)

292.89   Cocaine Intoxication (126)
          Specify if: With Perceptual Disturbances
292.81   Cocaine Intoxication Delirium (82)
292.0   Cocaine Withdrawal (128)
292.81   Cocaine Intoxication Delirium (82)
292.xx   Cocaine-Induced Psychotic Disorder (157)
    .11   With Delusions^I
    .12   With Hallucinations^I
292.84   Cocaine-Induced Mood Disorder^{I,W} (184)
292.89   Cocaine-Induced Anxiety Disorder^{I,W} (215)
292.89   Cocaine-Induced Sexual Dysfunction^I (240)
292.89   Cocaine-Induced Sleep Disorder^{I,W} (266)
292.9   Cocaine-Related Disorder NOS (126)

HALLUCINOGEN-RELATED DISORDERS (128)

Hallucinogen Use Disorders (128)

304.50 Hallucinogen Dependence[a] (108)
305.30 Hallucinogen Abuse (112)

Hallucinogen-Induced Disorders (128)

292.89 Hallucinogen Intoxication (129)
292.89 Hallucinogen Persisting Perception Disorder
        (Flashbacks) (130)
292.81 Hallucinogen Intoxication Delirium (82)
292.xx Hallucinogen-Induced Psychotic Disorder (157)
   .11   With Delusions[I]
   .12   With Hallucinations[I]
292.84 Hallucinogen-Induced Mood Disorder[I] (184)
292.89 Hallucinogen-Induced Anxiety Disorder[I] (215)
292.9   Hallucinogen-Related Disorder NOS (129)

INHALANT-RELATED DISORDERS (131)

Inhalant Use Disorders (131)

304.60 Inhalant Dependence[a] (108)
305.90 Inhalant Abuse (112)

Inhalant-Induced Disorders (131)

292.89 Inhalant Intoxication (132)
292.81 Inhalant Intoxication Delirium (82)
292.82 Inhalant-Induced Persisting Dementia (91)
292.xx Inhalant-Induced Psychotic Disorder (157)
   .11   With Delusions[I]
   .12   With Hallucinations[I]
292.84 Inhalant-Induced Mood Disorder[I] (184)
292.89 Inhalant-Induced Anxiety Disorder[I] (215)
292.9   Inhalant-Related Disorder NOS (132)

NICOTINE-RELATED DISORDERS (133)

Nicotine Use Disorder (133)

305.10 Nicotine Dependence[a] (108)

Nicotine-Induced Disorder (133)

292.0   Nicotine Withdrawal (133)
292.9   Inhalant-Related Disorder NOS (133)

OPIOID-RELATED DISORDERS (134)

Opioid Use Disorders (134)

304.00 Opioid Dependence[a] (108)
305.50 Opioid Abuse (112)

Opioid-Induced Disorders (134)

292.89 Opioid Intoxication (135)
        Specify if: With Perceptual Disturbances
292.0   Opioid Withdrawal (136)

292.81 Opioid Intoxication Delirium (82)
292.xx Opioid-Induced Psychotic Disorder (157)
   .11   With Delusions[I]
   .12   With Hallucinations[I]
292.84 Opioid-Induced Mood Disorder[I] (184)
292.89 Opioid-Induced Sexual Dysfunction[I] (240)
292.89 Opioid-Induced Sleep Disorder[I,W] (266)
292.9   Opioid-Related Disorder NOS (135)

PHENCYCLIDINE (OR PHENCYCLIDINE-LIKE)–RELATED DISORDERS (137)

Phencyclidine Use Disorders (137)

304.90 Phencyclidine Dependence[a] (108)
305.90 Phencyclidine Abuse (112)

Phencyclidine-Induced Disorders (137)

292.89 Phencyclidine Intoxication (138)
        Specify if: With Perceptual Disturbances
292.81 Phencyclidine Intoxication Delirium (82)
292.xx Phencyclidine-Induced Psychotic Disorder (157)
   .11   With Delusions[I]
   .12   With Hallucinations[I]
292.84 Phencyclidine-Induced Mood Disorder[I] (184)
292.89 Phencyclidine-Induced Anxiety Disorder[I] (215)
292.9   Phencyclidine-Related Disorder NOS (138)

SEDATIVE-, HYPNOTIC-, OR ANXIOLYTIC-RELATED DISORDERS (139)

Sedative, Hypnotic, or Anxiolytic Use Disorders (139)

304.10 Sedative, Hypnotic, or Anxiolytic Dependence[a]
        (108)
305.40 Sedative, Hypnotic, or Anxiolytic Abuse (112)

Sedative-, Hypnotic-, or Anxiolytic-Induced Disorders (139)

292.89 Sedative, Hypnotic, or Anxiolytic Intoxication
        (141)
292.0   Sedative, Hypnotic, or Anxiolytic Withdrawal
        (142)
        Specify if: With Perceptual Disturbances
292.81 Sedative, Hypnotic, or Anxiolytic Intoxication
        Delirium (82)
292.81 Sedative, Hypnotic, or Anxiolytic Withdrawal
        Delirium (83)
292.82 Sedative-, Hypnotic-, or Anxiolytic-Induced
        Persisting Dementia (91)
292.83 Sedative-, Hypnotic-, or Anxiolytic-Induced
        Persisting Amnesia Disorder (94)
292.xx Sedative-, Hypnotic-, or Anxiolytic-Induced
        Psychotic Disorder (157)

.11   With Delusions[I,W]

.12   With Hallucinations[I,W]

292.84   Sedative-, Hypnotic-, or Anxiolytic-Induced Mood Disorder[I,W] (184)

292.89   Sedative-, Hypnotic-, or Anxiolytic-Induced Anxiety Disorder[W] (215)

292.89   Sedative-, Hypnotic-, or Anxiolytic-Induced Sexual Dysfunction[I] (240)

292.89   Sedative-, Hypnotic-, or Anxiolytic-Induced Sleep Disorder[I,W] (266)

292.9   Sedative-, Hypnotic-, or Anxiolytic-Related Disorder NOS (141)

POLYSUBSTANCE-RELATED DISORDER (143)

304.80   Polysubstance Dependence[a] (143)

OTHER (OR UNKNOWN) SUBSTANCE–RELATED DISORDERS (143)

Other (or Unknown) Substance Use Disorders (144)

304.90   Other (or Unknown) Substance Dependence[a] (108)

305.90   Other (or Unknown) Substance Abuse (112)

Other (or Unknown) Substance–Induced Disorders (144)

292.89   Other (or Unknown) Substance Intoxication (113)
Specify if: With Perceptual Disturbances

292.0   Other (or Unknown) Substance Withdrawal (113)
Specify if: With Perceptual Disturbances

292.81   Other (or Unknown) Substance–Induced Delirium (82)

292.82   Other (or Unknown) Substance–Induced Persisting Dementia (91)

292.83   Other (or Unknown) Substance–Induced Persisting Amnestic Disorder (94)

292.xx   Other (or Unknown) Substance–Induced Psychotic Disorder (157)

.11   With Delusions[I,W]

.12   With Hallucinations[I,W]

292.84   Other (or Unknown) Substance–Induced Mood Disorder[I,W] (184)

292.89   Other (or Unknown) Substance–Induced Anxiety Disorder[I,W] (215)

292.89   Other (or Unknown) Substance–Induced Sexual Dysfunction[I] (240)

292.89   Other (or Unknown) Substance–Induced Sleep Disorder[I,W] (266)

292.9   Other (or Unknown) Substance–Related Disorder NOS (145)

Schizophrenia and Other Psychotic Disorders (147)

295.xx   Schizophrenia (147)

The following Classification of Longitudinal Course applies to all subtypes of Schizophrenia:

Episodic With Interepisode Residual Symptoms (*specify if:* With Prominent Negative Symptoms)/Episodic With No Interepisode Residual-Symptoms
Continuous (*specify if:* With Prominent Negative Symptoms)
Single Episode In Partial Remission (*specify if:* With Prominent Negative Symptoms)/Single Episode In Full Remission
Other or Unspecified Pattern

.30   Paranoid Type (149)
.10   Disorganized Type (149)
.20   Catatonic Type (149)
.90   Undifferentiated Type (150)
.60   Residual Type (150)

295.40   Schizophreniform Disorder (152)
Specify if: Without Good Prognostic Features/With Good Prognostic Features

295.70   Schizoaffective Disorder (152)
Specify type: Bipolar Type/Depressive Type

297.1   Delusional Disorder (153)
Specify type: Erotomanic Type/Grandiose Type/Jealous Type/Persecutory Type/Somatic Type/Mixed Type/Unspecified Type

298.8   Brief Psychotic Disorder (154)
Specify if: With Marked Stressor(s)/Without Marked Stressor(s)/With Postpartum Onset

297.3   Shared Psychotic Disorder (154)

293.xx   Psychotic Disorder Due to . . . *[Indicate the General Medical Condition]* (156)

.81   With Delusions
.82   With Hallucinations

——.—   Substance-Induced Psychotic Disorder *(refer to Substance-Related Disorders for substance-specific codes)* (157)
Specify if: With Onset During Intoxication/With Onset During Withdrawal

298.9   Psychotic Disorder NOS (159)

Mood Disorders (161)

Code current state of Major Depressive Disorder or Bipolar I Disorder in fifth digit:

1 = Mild
2 = Moderate
3 = Severe Without Psychotic Features
4 = Severe With Psychotic Features
    Specify: Mood-Congruent Psychotic Features/Mood-Incongruent Psychotic Features

5 = In Partial Remission
6 = In Full Remission
0 = Unspecified

The following specifiers apply (for current or most recent episode) to Mood Disorders as noted.

[a]Severity/Psychotic/Remission Specifiers/ [b]Chronic/ [c]With Catatonic Features/ [d]With Melancholic Features/ [e]With Atypical Features/ [f]With Postpartum Onset

The following specifiers apply to Mood Disorders as noted:

[g]With or Without Full Interepisode Recovery/ [h]With Seasonal Pattern/ [i]With Rapid Cycling

DEPRESSIVE DISORDERS (167)

296.xx	Major Depressive Disorder,	
.2x	Single Episode[a,b,c,d,e,f] (167)	
.3x	Recurrent[a,b,c,d,e,f,g,h] (168)	
300.4	Dysthymic Disorder (169)	

Specify if: Early Onset/Late Onset
Specify: With Atypical Features

311	Depressive Disorder NOS (171)

BIPOLAR DISORDERS (173)

296.xx	Bipolar I Disorder (173),
.0x	Single Manic Episode[a,c,f] (173)

Specify if: Mixed

.40	Most Recent Episode Hypomanic[g,h,i] (174)
.4x	Most Recent Episode Manic[a,c,f,g,h,i] (175)
.6x	Most Recent Episode Mixed[a,c,f,g,h,i] (176)
.5x	Most Recent Episode Depressed[a,b,c,d,e,f,g,h,i] (177)
.7	Most Recent Episode Unspecified[g,h,i] (178)
296.89	Bipolar II Disorder[a,b,c,d,e,f,g,h,i] (180)

Specify (current or most recent episode): Hypomanic/Depressed

301.13	Cyclothymic Disorder (181)
296.80	Bipolar Disorder NOS (182)
293.83	Mood Disorder Due to . . . *[Indicate the General Medical Condition]* (183)

Specify type: With Depressive Features/With Major Depressive-Like Episode/With Manic Features/With Mixed Features

———.— Substance-Induced Mood Disorder *(refer to Substance-Related Disorders for substance-specific codes)* (184)

Specify type: With Depressive Features/With Manic Features/With Mixed Features
Specify if: With Onset During Intoxication/With Onset During Withdrawal

296.90	Mood Disorder NOS (186)

Anxiety Disorders (199)

300.01	Panic Disorder Without Agoraphobia (201)
300.21	Panic Disorder With Agoraphobia (202)
300.22	Agoraphobia Without History of Panic Disorder (203)
300.29	Specific Phobia (203)

Specify type: Animal Type/Natural Environment Type/Blood-Injection-Injury Type/Situational Type/Other Type

300.23	Social Phobia (205)

Specify if: Generalized

300.3	Obsessive-Compulsive Disorder (207)

Specify if: With Poor Insight

309.81	Posttraumatic Stress Disorder (209)

Specify if: Acute/Chronic
Specify if: With Delayed Onset

308.3	Acute Stress Disorder (211)
300.02	Generalized Anxiety Disorder (213)
293.89	Anxiety Disorder Due to . . . *[Indicate the General Medical Condition]* (214)

Specify if: With Generalized Anxiety/With Panic Attacks/With Obsessive-Compulsive Symptoms

———.— Substance-Induced Anxiety Disorder *(refer to Substance-Related Disorders for substance-specific codes)* (215)

Specify if: With Generalized Anxiety/With Panic Attacks/With Obsessive-Compulsive Symptoms/With Phobic Symptoms
Specify if: With Onset During Intoxication/With Onset During Withdrawal

300.00	Anxiety Disorder NOS (217)

Somatoform Disorders (219)

300.81	Somatization Disorder (219)
300.81	Undifferentiated Somatoform Disorder (220)
300.11	Conversion Disorder (221)

Specify type: With Motor Symptom or Deficit/With Sensory Symptom or Deficit/With Seizures or Convulsions/With Mixed Presentation

307.xx	Pain Disorder (223)
.80	Associated With Psychological Factors
.89	Associated With Both Psychological Factors and a General Medical Condition

Specify if: Acute/Chronic

300.7	Hypochondriasis (224)

Specify if: With Poor Insight

300.7	Body Dysmorphic Disorder (225)
300.81	Somatoform Disorder NOS (226)

Factitious Disorders (227)

300.xx   Factitious Disorder (227)
   .16   With Predominantly Psychological Signs and Symptoms
   .19   With Predominantly Physical Signs and Symptoms
   .19   With Combined Psychological and Physical Signs and Symptoms
300.19   Factitious Disorder NOS (228)

Dissociative Disorders (229)

300.12   Dissociative Amnesia (229)
300.13   Dissociative Fugue (229)
300.14   Dissociative Identity Disorder (230)
300.6   Depersonalization Disorder (231)
300.15   Dissociative Disorder NOS (231)

Sexual and Gender Identity Disorders (233)

SEXUAL DYSFUNCTIONS (233)

The following specifiers apply to all primary Sexual Dysfunctions:

Lifelong Type/Acquired Type
Generalized Type/Situational Type
Due to Psychological Factors/Due to Combined Factors

Sexual Desire Disorders (233)

302.71   Hypoactive Sexual Desire Disorder (233)
302.79   Sexual Aversion Disorder (234)

Sexual Arousal Disorders (234)

302.72   Female Sexual Arousal Disorder (234)
302.72   Male Erectile Disorder (235)

Orgasmic Disorders (235)

302.73   Female Orgasmic Disorder (235)
302.74   Male Orgasmic Disorder (236)
302.75   Premature Ejaculation (236)

Sexual Pain Disorders (237)

302.76   Dyspareunia (Not Due to a General Medical Condition) (237)
306.51   Vaginismus (Not Due to a General Medical Condition) (237)

Sexual Dysfunction Due to a General Medical Condition (239)

625.8   Female Hypoactive Sexual Desire Disorder Due to . . . [Indicate the General Medical Condition] (239)

608.89   Male Hypoactive Sexual Desire Disorder Due to . . . [Indicate the General Medical Condition] (240)
607.84   Male Erectile Disorder Due to . . . [Indicate the General Medical Condition] (240)
625.0   Female Dyspareunia Due to . . . [Indicate the General Medical Condition] (240)
608.89   Male Dyspareunia Due to. . . [Indicate the General Medical Condition] (240)
625.8   Other Female Sexual Dysfunction Due to . . . [Indicate the General Medical Condition] (240)
608.89   Other Male Sexual Dysfunction Due to. . . [Indicate the General Medical Condition] (240)
———.—   Substance-Induced Sexual Dysfunction (refer to Substance-Related Disorders for substance-specific codes) (240)
     Specify if: With Impaired Desire/With Impaired Arousal/With Impaired Orgasm/With Sexual Pain
     Specify if: With Onset During Intoxication
302.70   Sexual Dysfunction NOS (242)

PARAPHILIAS (243)

302.4   Exhibitionism (243)
302.81   Fetishism (243)
302.89   Frotteurism (244)
302.2   Pedophilia (244)
     Specify if: Sexually Attracted to Males/Sexually Attracted to Females/Sexually Attracted to Both
     Specify if: Limited to Incest
     Specify type: Exclusive Type/Nonexclusive Type
302.83   Sexual Masochism (245)
302.84   Sexual Sadism (245)
302.3   Transvestic Fetishism (245)
     Specify if: With Gender Dysphoria
302.82   Voyeurism (246)
302.9   Paraphilia NOS (246)

GENDER IDENTITY DISORDERS (246)

302.xx   Gender Identity Disorder (246)
   .6   in Children
   .85   in Adolescents or Adults
     Specify if: Sexually Attracted to Males/Sexually Attracted to Females/Sexually Attracted to Both/Sexually Attracted to Neither
302.6   Gender Identity Disorder NOS (248)

302.9   Sexual Disorder NOS (249)

Eating Disorders (251)

307.1   Anorexia Nervosa (251)
     Specify type: Restricting Type; Binge-Eating/Purging Type

307.51   Bulimia Nervosa (252)
          Specify type: Purging Type/Nonpurging Type
307.50   Eating Disorder NOS (253)

Sleep Disorders (255)

PRIMARY SLEEP DISORDERS (255)

Dyssomnias (255)

307.42   Primary Insomnia (255)
307.44   Primary Hypersomnia (256)
          Specify if: Recurrent
347   Narcolepsy (257)
780.59   Breathing-Related Sleep Disorder (257)
307.45   Circadian Rhythm Sleep Disorder (258)
          Specify type: Delayed Sleep Phase Type/Jet Lag
          Type/Shift Work Type/Unspecified Type
307.47   Dyssomnia NOS (259)

Parasomnias (260)

307.47   Nightmare Disorder (260)
307.46   Sleep Terror Disorder (261)
307.46   Sleepwalking Disorder (261)
307.47   Parasomnia NOS (262)

SLEEP DISORDERS RELATED TO ANOTHER MENTAL DISORDER (263)

307.42   Insomnia Related to . . . *[Indicate the Axis I or Axis II Disorder]* (263)
307.44   Hypersomnia Related to . . . *[Indicate the Axis I or Axis II Disorder]* (264)

OTHER SLEEP DISORDERS (265)

780.xx   Sleep Disorder Due to . . . *[Indicate the General Medical Condition]* (265)
   .52   Insomnia Type
   .54   Hypersomnia Type
   .59   Parasomnia Type
   .59   Mixed Type
——.—   Substance-Induced Sleep Disorder *(refer to Substance-Related Disorders for substance-specific codes)* (266)
          Specify type: Insomnia Type/Hypersomnia Type/Parasomnia Type/Mixed Type
          Specify if: With Onset During Intoxication/With Onset During Withdrawal

Impulse-Control Disorders Not Elsewhere Classified (269)

312.34   Intermittent Explosive Disorder (269)
312.32   Kleptomania (269)
312.33   Pyromania (270)
312.31   Pathological Gambling (271)
312.39   Trichotillomania (272)
312.30   Impulse-Control Disorder NOS (272)

Adjustment Disorders (273)

309.xx   Adjustment Disorder (273)
   .0   With Depressed Mood
   .24   With Anxiety
   .28   With Mixed Anxiety and Depressed Mood
   .3   With Disturbance of Conduct
   .4   With Mixed Disturbance of Emotions and Conduct
   .9   Unspecified
          Specify if: Acute/Chronic

Personality Disorders (275)

Note: These are coded on Axis II.

301.0   Paranoid Personality Disorder (276)
301.20   Schizoid Personality Disorder (277)
301.22   Schizotypal Personality Disorder (278)
301.7   Antisocial Personality Disorder (279)
301.83   Borderline Personality Disorder (280)
301.50   Histrionic Personality Disorder (281)
301.81   Narcissistic Personality Disorder (282)
301.82   Avoidant Personality Disorder (283)
301.6   Dependent Personality Disorder (284)
301.4   Obsessive-Compulsive Personality Disorder (285)
301.9   Personality Disorder NOS (286)

Other Conditions That May Be a Focus of Clinical Attention (287)

PSYCHOLOGICAL FACTORS AFFECTING MEDICAL CONDITION (288)

316   . . . *[Specified Psychological Factor]* Affecting . . . *[Indicate the General Medical Condition]* (288)
          Choose name based on nature of factors:
          Mental Disorder Affecting Medical Condition
          Psychological Symptoms Affecting Medical Condition
          Personality Traits or Coping Style Affecting Medical Condition
          Maladaptive Health Behaviors Affecting Medical Condition
          Stress-Related Physiological Response Affecting Medical Condition

Other or Unspecified Psychological Factors
Affecting Medical Condition

MEDICATION-INDUCED MOVEMENT DISORDERS (289)

332.1	Neuroleptic-Induced Parkinsonism (290)
333.92	Neuroleptic Malignant Syndrome (290)
333.7	Neuroleptic-Induced Acute Dystonia (290)
333.99	Neuroleptic-Induced Acute Akathisia (291)
333.82	Neuroleptic-Induced Tardive Dyskinesia (291)
333.1	Medication-Induced Postural Tremor (291)
333.90	Medication-Induced Movement Disorder NOS (292)

OTHER MEDICATION-INDUCED DISORDER (292)

995.2	Adverse Effects of Medication NOS (292)

RELATIONAL PROBLEMS (292)

V61.9	Relational Problem Related to a Mental Disorder or General Medical Condition (293)
V61.20	Parent–Child Relational Problem (293)
V61.1	Partner Relational Problem (294)
V61.8	Sibling Relational Problem (294)
V62.81	Relational Problem NOS (294)

PROBLEMS RELATED TO ABUSE OR NEGLECT (294)

V61.21	Physical Abuse of Child (295) *(code 995.5 if focus of attention is on victim)*
V61.21	Sexual Abuse of Child (295) *(code 995.5 if focus of attention is on victim)*
V61.21	Neglect of Child (295) *(code 995.5 if focus of attention is on victim)*

V61.1	Physical Abuse of Adult (295) *(code 995.81 if focus of attention is on victim)*
V61.1	Sexual Abuse of Adult (296) *(code 995.81 if focus of attention is on victim)*

ADDITIONAL CONDITIONS THAT MAY BE A FOCUS OF CLINICAL ATTENTION (296)

V15.81	Noncompliance With Treatment (296)
V65.2	Malingering (296)
V71.01	Adult Antisocial Behavior (297)
V71.02	Child or Adolescent Antisocial Behavior (298)
V62.89	Borderline Intellectual Functioning (298) **Note:** This is coded on Axis II.
780.9	Age-Related Cognitive Decline (298)
V62.82	Bereavement (299)
V62.3	Academic Problem (299)
V62.2	Occupational Problem (300)
313.82	Identity Problem (300)
V62.89	Religious or Spiritual Problem (300)
V62.4	Acculturation Problem (301)
V62.89	Phase of Life Problem (301)

Additional Codes

300.9	Unspecified Mental Disorder (nonpsychotic) (303)
V71.09	No Diagnosis or Condition on Axis I (303)
V71.09	No Diagnosis on Axis II (304)
799.9	Diagnosis Deferred on Axis II (304)

Appendix C

Classification of Human Responses of Concern for Psychiatric–Mental Health Nursing Practice†

I. **HUMAN RESPONSE PATTERNS IN ACTIVITY PROCESSES**

1.1 *Motor Behavior*

   1.1.1 Potential for Alteration
      *1.1.1.1 Activity Intolerance
      1.1.1.2
   1.1.2 Altered Motor Behavior
      *1.1.2.1 Activity Intolerance
      1.1.2.2 Bizarre Motor Behavior
      1.1.2.3 Catatonia
      1.1.2.4 Disorganized Motor Behavior
      *1.1.2.5 Fatigue
      1.1.2.6 Hyperactivity
      1.1.2.7 Hypoactivity
      1.1.2.8 Psychomotor Agitation
      1.1.2.9 Psychomotor Retardation
      1.1.2.10 Restlessness

1.2 *Recreation Patterns*

   1.2.1 Potential for Alteration
      1.2.1.1
      1.2.1.2
   1.2.2 Altered Recreation Patterns
      1.2.2.1 Age Inappropriate Recreation
      1.2.2.2 Anti-social Recreation
      1.2.2.3 Bizarre Recreation
      *1.2.2.4 Diversional Activity Deficit
   1.2.99 Recreation Patterns NOS

1.3 *Self Care*

   1.3.1 Potential for Alteration in Self Care
   *1.3.2 Potential for Altered Health Maintenance
   1.3.3 Altered Self Care

   *1.3.3.1 Altered Eating
      1.3.3.1.1 Binge-Purge Syndrome
      1.3.3.1.2 Non-nutritive Ingestion
      1.3.3.1.3 Pica
      1.3.3.1.4 Unusual Food Ingestion
      1.3.3.1.5 Refusal to Eat
      1.3.3.1.6 Rumination
   *1.3.3.2 Altered Feeding
      *1.3.3.2.1 Ineffective Breast Feeding
   *1.3.3.3 Altered Grooming
   *1.3.3.4 Altered Health Maintenance
   *1.3.3.5 Altered Health Seeking Behaviors
      *1.3.3.5.1 Knowledge Deficit
      *1.3.3.5.2 Noncompliance
   *1.3.3.6 Altered Hygiene
   1.3.3.7 Altered Participation in Health Care
   *1.3.3.8 Altered Toileting
   *1.3.4 Impaired Adjustment
   *1.3.5 Knowledge Deficit
   *1.3.6 Noncompliance
   1.3.99 Self Care Patterns NOS

1.4 *Sleep/Arousal Patterns*

   1.4.1 Potential for Alteration
   *1.4.2 Altered Sleep/Arousal Patterns
      1.4.2.1 Decreased Need for Sleep
      1.4.2.2 Hypersomnia
      1.4.2.3 Insomnia
      1.4.2.4 Nightmares/Terrors
      1.4.2.5 Somnolence
      1.4.2.6 Somnambulism
   1.4.99 Sleep/Arousal Patterns NOS

†From O'Toole, A. W., & Loomis, M. E. (1989). Revision of phenomena of concern for psychiatric mental health nursing. *Archives of Psychiatric Nursing, 3* (5), 292–299. Reprinted with permission.
*Approved NANDA diagnoses.

2. HUMAN RESPONSE PATTERNS IN COGNITION PROCESSES

2.1 *Decision Making*

2.1.1   Potential for Alteration
2.1.2   Altered Decision Making
2.1.3   Decisional Conflict
2.1.99 Decision Making Patterns NOS

2.2 *Judgment*

2.2.1   Potential for Alteration
2.2.2   Altered Judgment
2.2.99 Judgment Patterns NOS

2.3 *Knowledge*

2.3.1   Potential for Alteration
*2.3.2   Altered Knowledge Processes
    2.3.2.1 Agnosia
    2.3.2.2 Altered Intellectual Functioning
2.3.99 Knowledge Patterns NOS

2.4 *Learning*

2.4.1   Potential for Alteration
2.4.2   Altered Learning Processes
2.4.99 Learning Patterns NOS

2.5 *Memory*

2.5.1   Potential for Alteration
2.5.2   Altered Memory
    2.5.2.1 Amnesia
    2.5.2.2 Distorted Memory
    2.5.2.3 Long-Term Memory Loss
    2.5.2.4 Memory Deficit
    2.5.2.5 Short-Term Memory Loss
2.5.99 Memory Patterns NOS

2.6 *Thought Processes*

2.6.1   Potential for Alteration
*2.6.2   Altered Thought Processes
    2.6.2.1 Altered Abstract Thinking
    2.6.2.2 Altered Concentration
    2.6.2.3 Altered Problem Solving
    2.6.2.4 Confusion/Disorientation
    2.6.2.5 Delirium
    2.6.2.6 Delusions
    2.6.2.7 Ideas of Reference
    2.6.2.8 Magical Thinking
    2.6.2.9 Obsessions
    2.6.2.10 Suspiciousness
    2.6.2.11 Thought Insertion
2.6.99 Thought Processes NOS

3. HUMAN RESPONSE PATTERNS IN ECOLOGICAL PROCESSES

3.1 *Community Maintenance*

3.1.1   Potential for Alteration
3.1.2   Altered Community Maintenance
    3.1.2.1 Community Safety Hazards
    3.1.2.2 Community Sanitation Hazards
3.1.99 Community Maintenance Patterns NOS

3.2 *Environmental Integrity*

3.2.1   Potential for Alteration
3.2.2   Altered Environmental Integrity
3.2.99 Environmental Integrity Patterns NOS

3.3 *Home Maintenance*

3.3.1   Potential for Alteration
*3.3.2   Altered Home Maintenance
    3.3.2.1 Home Safety Hazards
    3.3.2.2 Home Sanitation Hazards
3.3.99 Home Maintenance Patterns NOS

4. HUMAN RESPONSE PATTERNS IN EMOTIONAL PROCESSES

4.1 *Feeling States*

4.1.1   Potential for Alteration
    4.1.1.1 Anticipatory Grieving
4.1.2   Altered Feeling State
    4.1.2.1 Anger
    *4.1.2.2 Anxiety
    4.1.2.3 Elation
    4.1.2.4 Envy
    *4.1.2.5 Fear
    *4.1.2.6 Grief
    4.1.2.7 Guilt
    4.1.2.8 Sadness
    4.1.2.9 Shame
4.1.3   Affect Incongruous in Situation
4.1.4   Flat Affect
4.1.99 Feeling States NOS

4.2 *Feeling Processes*

4.2.1   Potential for Alteration
4.2.2   Altered Feeling Processes
    4.2.2.1 Lability
    4.2.2.2 Mood Swings
4.2.99 Feeling Processes NOS

5. **HUMAN RESPONSE PATTERNS IN INTERPERSONAL PROCESSES**

5.1   Abuse Response Patterns

    5.1.1   Potential for Alteration
    5.1.2   Altered Abuse Response
        *5.1.2.1   Post-trauma Response
        *5.1.2.2   Rape Trauma Syndrome
        *5.1.2.3   Compound Reaction
        *5.1.2.4   Silent Reaction
    5.1.99   Abuse Response Patterns NOS

5.2   Communication Processes

    5.2.1   Potential for Alteration
   *5.2.2   Altered Communication Processes
        5.2.2.1   Altered Nonverbal Communication
      *5.2.2.2   Altered Verbal Communication
           5.2.2.2.1   Aphasia
           5.2.2.2.2   Bizarre Content
           5.2.2.2.3   Confabulation
           5.2.2.2.4   Echolalia
           5.2.2.2.5   Incoherent
           5.2.2.2.6   Mute
           5.2.2.2.7   Neologisms
           5.2.2.2.8   Nonsense/Word Salad
           5.2.2.2.9   Stuttering
    5.2.99   Communication Processes NOS

5.3   Conduct/Impulse Processes

    5.3.1   Potential for Alteration
      *5.3.1.1   Potential for Violence
      5.3.1.2   Suicidal Ideation
    5.3.2   Altered Conduct/Impulse Processes
        5.3.2.1   Accident Prone
        5.3.2.2   Aggressive/Violent Behavior Toward Environment
        5.3.2.3   Delinquency
        5.3.2.4   Lying
        5.3.2.5   Physical Aggression Toward Others
        5.3.2.6   Physical Aggression Toward Self
           5.3.2.6.1   Suicide Attempt(s)
        5.3.2.7   Promiscuity
        5.3.2.8   Running Away
        5.3.2.9   Substance Abuse
        5.3.2.10   Truancy
        5.3.2.11   Vandalism
        5.3.2.12   Verbal Aggression Toward Others
    5.3.99   Conduct/Impulse Processes NOS

5.4   Family Processes

    5.4.1   Potential for Alteration
      *5.4.1.1   Potential for Altered Parenting
      *5.4.1.2   Potential for Family Growth
   *5.4.2   Altered Family Processes
      5.4.2.1   Ineffective Family Coping
        *5.4.2.1.1   Compromised
        *5.4.2.1.2   Disabled
    5.4.99   Family Processes NOS

5.5   Role Performance

    5.5.1   Potential for Alteration
   *5.5.2   Altered Role Performance
      5.5.2.1   Altered Family Role
        5.5.2.1.1   Parental Role Conflict
        5.5.2.1.2   Parental Role Deficit
      5.5.2.2   Altered Play Role
      5.5.2.3   Altered Student Pole
      5.5.2.4   Altered Work Role
   *5.5.3   Ineffective Individual Coping
      *5.5.3.1   Defensive Coping
      *5.5.3.2   Ineffective Denial
    5.5.99   Role Performance Patterns NOS

5.6   Sexuality

    5.6.1   Potential for Alteration
    5.6.2   Altered Sexual Behavior Leading to Intercourse
    5.6.3   Altered Sexual Conception Actions
    5.6.4   Altered Sexual Development
    5.6.5   Altered Sexual Intercourse
    5.6.6   Altered Sexual Relationships
   *5.6.7   Altered Sexuality Patterns
    5.6.8   Altered Variation of Sexual Expression
   *5.6.9   Sexual Dysfunction
    5.6.99   Sexuality Processes NOS

5.7   Social Interaction

    5.7.1   Potential for Alteration
   *5.7.2   Altered Social Interaction
      5.7.2.1   Bizarre Behaviors
      5.7.2.2   Compulsive Behaviors
      5.7.2.3   Disorganized Social Behaviors
      5.7.2.4   Social Intrusiveness
      *5.7.2.5   Social Isolation/Withdrawal
      5.7.2.6   Unpredictable Behaviors
    5.7.99   Social Interaction Patterns NOS

6. HUMAN RESPONSE PATTERNS IN PERCEPTION PROCESSES

6.1 *Attention*

   6.1.1   Potential for Alteration
   6.1.2   Altered Attention
       6.1.2.1 Hyperalertness
       6.1.2.2 Inattention
       6.1.2.3 Selective Attention
   6.1.99 Attention Patterns NOS

6.2 *Comfort*

   6.2.1   Potential for Alteration
 *6.2.2   Altered Comfort Patterns
       6.2.2.1 Discomfort
       6.2.2.2 Distress
     *6.2.2.3 Pain
          6.2.2.3.1 Acute Pain
        *6.2.2.3.2 Chronic Pain
   6.2.99 Comfort Patterns NOS

6.3 *Self Concept*

   6.3.1   Potential for Alteration
   6.3.2   Altered Self Concept
    *6.3.2.1 Altered Body Image
    *6.3.2.2 Altered Personal Identity
    *6.3.2.3 Altered Self Esteem
      *6.3.2.3.1 Chronic Low Self Esteem
      *6.3.2.3.2 Situational Low Self Esteem
     6.3.2.4 Altered Sexual Identity
       6.3.2.4.1 Altered Gender Identity
   6.3.3   Undeveloped Self Concept
   6.3.99 Self Concept Patterns NOS

6.4 *Sensory Perception*

   6.4.1   Potential for Alteration
 *6.4.2   Altered Sensory Perception
       6.4.2.1 Hallucinations
        *6.4.2.1.1 Auditory
        *6.4.2.1.2 Gustatory
        *6.4.2.1.3 Kinesthetic
        *6.4.2.1.4 Olfactory
        *6.4.2.1.5 Tactile
        *6.4.2.1.6 Visual
       6.4.2.2 Illusions
   6.4.99 Sensory Perception Processes NOS

7. HUMAN RESPONSE PATTERNS IN PHYSIOLOGICAL PROCESSES

7.1 *Circulation*

   7.1.1   Potential for Alteration
       7.1.1.1 Fluid Volume Deficit
   7.1.2   Altered Circulation
       7.1.2.1 Altered Cardiac Circulation
        *7.1.2.1.1 Decreased Cardiac Output
       7.1.2.2 Altered Vascular Circulation
        *7.1.2.2.1 Altered Fluid Volume
        *7.1.2.2.2 Fluid Volume Excess
        *7.1.2.2.3 Tissue Perfusion
          *7.1.2.2.3.1 Peripheral
          *7.1.2.2.3.2 Renal
   7.1.99 Altered Circulation Processes NOS

7.2 *Elimination*

   7.2.1   Potential for Alteration
   7.2.2   Altered Elimination Processes
    *7.2.2.1 Altered Bowel Elimination
      *7.2.2.1.1 Constipation
      *7.2.2.1.2 Diarrhea
      7.2.2.1.3 Encopresis
      *7.2.2.1.4 Incontinence
    *7.2.2.2 Altered Urinary Elimination
      7.2.2.2.1 Enuresis
      *7.2.2.2.2 Incontinence
        *7.2.2.2.2.1 Functional
        *7.2.2.2.2.2 Reflex
        *7.2.2.2.2.3 Stress
        *7.2.2.2.2.4 Total
        *7.2.2.2.2.5 Urge
      *7.2.2.2.3 Retention
     7.2.2.3 Altered Skin Elimination
   7.2.99 Elimination Processes NOS

7.3 *Endocrine/Metabolic Processes*

   7.3.1   Potential for Alteration
   7.3.2   Altered Endocrine/Metabolic Processes
    *7.3.2.1 Altered Growth and Development
     7.3.2.2 Altered Hormone Regulation
       7.3.2.2.1 Premenstrual Stress Syndrome
   7.3.99 Endocrine/Metabolic Processes NOS

7.4 *Gastrointestinal Processes*

   7.4.1   Potential for Alteration
   7.4.2   Altered Gastrointestinal Processes

7.4.2.1   Altered Absorption
7.4.2.2   Altered Digestion
*7.4.2.3   Tissue Perfusion
7.4.99   Gastrointestinal Processes NOS

7.5   *Musculoskeletal Processes*

7.5.1   Potential for Alteration
   *7.5.1.1   Potential for Disuse Syndrome
   *7.5.1.2   Potential for Injury
7.5.2   Altered Musculoskeletal Processes
   7.5.2.1   Altered Coordination
   7.5.2.2   Altered Equilibrium
   7.5.2.3   Altered Mobility
   7.5.2.4   Altered Motor Planning
   7.5.2.5   Altered Muscle Strength
   7.5.2.6   Altered Muscle Tone
   7.5.2.7   Altered Posture
   7.5.2.8   Altered Range of Motion
   7.5.2.9   Altered Reflex Patterns
   7.5.2.10 Altered Physical Mobility
   7.5.2.11 Muscle Twitching
7.5.99   Musculoskeletal Processes NOS

7.6   *Neuro/Sensory Processes*

7.6.1   Potential for Alteration
7.6.2   Altered Neuro/Sensory Processes
   7.6.2.1   Altered Level of Consciousness
   7.6.2.2   Altered Sensory Acuity
      7.6.2.2.1   Auditory
      *7.6.2.2.2   Dysreflexia
      7.6.2.2.3   Gustatory
      7.6.2.2.4   Olfactory
      7.6.2.2.5   Tactile
      7.6.2.2.6   Visual
   7.6.2.3   Altered Sensory Integration
   7.6.2.4   Altered Sensory Processing
      7.6.2.4.1   Auditory
      7.6.2.4.2   Gustatory
      7.6.2.4.3   Olfactory
      7.6.2.4.4   Tactile
      7.6.2.4.5   Visual
   *7.6.2.5   Cerebral Tissue Perfusion
   *7.6.2.6   Unilateral Neglect
   7.6.2.7   Seizures
7.6.99   Neuro/Sensory Processes NOS

7.7   *Nutrition*

7.7.1   Potential for Alteration
   *7.7.1.1   Potential for More Than Body Requirements
   *7.7.1.2   Potential for Poisoning

7.7.2   Altered Nutrition Processes
   7.7.2.1   Altered Cellular Processes
   7.7.2.2   Altered Eating Processes
      7.7.2.2.1   Anorexia
      *7.7.2.2.2   Altered Oral Mucous Membrane
   7.7.2.3   Altered Systemic Processes
      *7.7.2.3.1   Less Than Body Requirements
      *7.7.2.3.2   More Than Body Requirements
   7.7.2.4   Impaired Swallowing
7.7.99   Nutrition Processes NOS

7.8   *Oxygenation*

7.8.1   Potential of Alteration
   *7.8.1.1   Potential for Aspiration
   *7.8.1.2   Potential for Suffocating
7.8.2   Altered Oxygenation Processes
   7.8.2.1   Altered Respiration
      *7.8.2.1.1   Altered Gas Exchange
      *7.8.2.1.2   Ineffective Airway Clearance
      *7.8.2.1.3   Ineffective Breathing Pattern
   *7.8.2.2   Tissue Perfusion
7.8.99   Oxygenation Processes NOS

7.9   *Physical Integrity*

7.9.1   Potential for Alteration
   *7.9.1.1   Potential for Altered Skin Integrity
   *7.9.1.2   Potential for Trauma
7.9.2   Altered Oral Mucous Membrane
   *7.9.2.1   Altered Skin Integrity
   *7.9.2.2   Altered Tissue Integrity
7.9.99   Physical Integrity Processes NOS

7.10   *Physical Regulation Processes*

7.10.1   Potential for Alteration
   *7.10.1.1   Potential for Altered Body Temperature
   *7.10.1.2   Potential for Infection
7.10.2   Altered Physical Regulation Processes
   7.10.2.1   Altered Immune Response
      7.10.2.1.1   Infection
   7.10.2.2   Altered Body Temperature
      *7.10.2.2.1   Hyperthermia
      *7.10.2.2.2   Hypothermia
      *7.10.2.2.3   Ineffective Thermoregulation
7.10.99   Physical Regulation Processes NOS

8. **HUMAN RESPONSE PATTERNS IN VALUATION PROCESSES**

8.1 Meaningfulness

    8.1.1   Potential for Alteration
   *8.1.2   Altered Meaningfulness
        8.1.2.1   Helplessness
      *8.1.2.2   Hopelessness
        8.1.2.3   Loneliness
      *8.1.2.4   Powerlessness
    8.1.99 Meaningfulness Patterns NOS

8.2 Spirituality

    8.2.1   Potential for Alteration

    8.2.2   Altered Spirituality
        8.2.2.1   Spiritual Despair
      *8.2.2.2   Spiritual Distress
    8.2.99 Spirituality Patterns NOS

8.3 Values

    8.3.1   Potential for Alteration
    8.3.2   Altered Values
        8.3.2.1   Conflict with Social Order
        8.3.2.2   Inability to Internalize Values
        8.3.2.3   Unclear Values
    8.3.99 Value Patterns NOS

Glossary

abandonment A legal concept that applies when practitioners refuse to give care or make arrangements for such care to their patients, who are in immediate need of treatment.

abreaction The conscious memory and emotional reliving of a past painful experience.

accountability Liability for one's behavior.

accreditation The method by which a group or agency recognizes a program of study or an institution as meeting predetermined standards or criteria.

acting in The expression of unconscious wishes, needs, conflicts, and feelings in actions rather than words, within a therapy session.

acting out The expression of unconscious wishes, needs, conflicts, and feelings in actions rather than words.

activities of daily living Self-care activities—such as eating, personal hygiene, recreational activities, and socialization—that are performed daily by healthy individuals as part of independent living. During periods of illness, individuals may not be able to perform some or all of these self-care activities.

addiction Physical and emotional dependence on an object or activity, such as drugs, alcohol, or work.

adjustment The manner by which one fits with one's peer group, family, and society, and copes with life.

adolescence Period of growth and development beginning at puberty (usually 12 or 13 years) and ending at adulthood (usually 20 or 21 years).

aerophagia Excessive pathologic air swallowing.

affect One's internal and external emotional tone.

affective psychosis Psychosis characterized by changes in the emotional state, usually elation or depression.

aggression Forceful physical or verbal behavior.

agitation Severe restlessness and anxiety.

agnosia Inability to recognize and grasp the meaning of sensory stimuli owing to organic brain disorder.

agoraphobia Fear of going outside or of open spaces.

agranulocytosis Pronounced reduction in polymorphonuclear leukocytes, a side effect of some psychotropic medications.

akathisia Continuous restlessness and uncontrolled movements.

akinesia Lethargy, subjective sense of fatigue, muscle weakness often mistaken for withdrawal and apathy, but actually a side effect of some antipsychotic medications.

alcoholism Habituation, dependence, or addiction to alcohol, leading to poor physical or mental health, disturbed interpersonal relations, and decreased personal effectiveness.

alienation A feeling of detachment.

allied ancillary personnel Non-nurse health-care workers, such as nursing assistants and licensed practical nurses (LPNs).

alternative family A group of people living communally to achieve common goals.

Alzheimer's disease A fatal disease characterized by brain deterioration leading to loss of memory, judgment, and interest.

ambivalence Simultaneous strong feelings that are the opposite of one another, for example, love and hate.

amnesia Loss of short-term or long-term memory owing to organic or functional causes.

amphetamines Antidepressant drugs that produce temporary elation through cortical stimulation.

anaclitic Characterized by strong dependence.

anaclitic depression Depression associated with loss of strong dependence like that experienced in infancy.

anal character The psychoanalytic term for one who is excessively orderly, restricted, controlled, stubborn, or miserly owing to events occurring in the anal stage.

anal erotism Erotic feelings arising from anal functions or activity.

analgesia Absence or reduction of pain.

analogic communication Communication without words.

anal stage The period of growth and development between 1½ and 3 years, when toilet training occurs.

analysand A person in psychoanalytic therapy.

anger A feeling of power and aggression resulting from frustration, anxiety, and helplessness.

anhedonia A state characterized by a lack of pleasure.

anilingus Oral stimulation of the anus.

anima A Jungian term for the inner, feminine self of a man.

animus A Jungian term for the inner, masculine self of a woman.

anniversary reaction An emotional state that occurs on the anniversary of a traumatic event in one's past, for example, death of a parent.

anorexia Lack of appetite.

anorexia nervosa A disease characterized by severe loss of appetite and weight, along with other symptoms.

anticholinergic Antagonistic to the action of parasympathetic or other cholinergic nerve fibers, a category of neurological side effects of psychotropic medications.

anticipatory guidance A method of counseling whereby the person is helped to plan for possible future events before they occur.

anxiety An unpleasant feeling of tension resulting from a physical or emotional threat to self.

apathy Absence of emotions, interest, and activity.

aphasia Inability to pronounce words, name common objects, or arrange words in sequence owing to organic brain disease.

aphonia Inability to produce normal speech owing to physical or organic causes.

"as if" behavior Unconsciously derived false behavior designed to cover up or compensate for unconscious thoughts, feelings, need, or conflicts.

assaultive Physically or verbally attacking.

assertive behavior Behavior designed to achieve one's goals without disturbing another's self-respect.

assertiveness training A form of therapy that aims to help individuals to ask for what they want without violating the rights of others, and to refuse requests without feeling guilty.

assessment The systematic process of collecting relevant client data for the purpose of determining actual or potential health problems and functional status. Methods used to obtain data include interviews, observations, physical examinations, review of records, and collaboration with colleagues.

assignment (of benefits) Legal authorization by the insured for an insurance company to directly reimburse the provider.

attachment Interpersonal, emotional connectedness, as between a mother and infant.

attachment phase The stage of infancy when the mother and infant become emotionally connected.

attention-deficit/hyperactivity disorder A disorder usually occurring in children, characterized by inattention, hyperactivity-impulsivity, and impairment in social, academic, or occupational functioning.

attitude therapy A form of milieu therapy in which staff members all assume consistent, prescribed attitudes designed to be therapeutic toward clients.

atypical developmental psychosis An early childhood disorder characterized by autistic behavior.

aura A physical experience that signals the onset of another experience, such as hallucinations before a grand mal seizure or visual changes before a migraine headache.

autism, autistic thinking Thinking that is self-gratifying without regard for reality.

autistic Private, within the self without regard for reality.

autoaggression Aggression directed toward oneself.

autoerotism Sexuality directed toward oneself.

autonomy Self-direction, independence.

aversion therapy Therapy that provides unpleasant stimuli or punishment for undesirable behavior.

bad trip An acute anxiety reaction following the use of psychedelic drugs.

basic human needs therapy Abraham Maslow's theory based on a hierarchy of physical and emotional needs.

behavior modification Therapy based on Pavlovian conditioning and designed to change behavior in a desired direction.

beneficiary The person (not necessarily the patient) eligible for benefits under an insurance contract, usually synonymous with the "insured."

benefit period Usually a 12-month period, often based on the calendar year or contract year. After this time new deductibles must accumulate before benefits will be paid, and yearly benefit limits that were exceeded are not applicable.

bestiality Sexual relations between humans and animals; also called zoophilia.

bipolar disorder A condition characterized by manic and depressive phases.

birth defect An abnormality found in an infant at birth owing to genetic or nongenetic causes.

birth trauma Otto Rank's term referring to the shock of the birth process, which leads to anxiety and neurosis.

bisexual One who engages in sex with both males and females.

blended family A family composed of members who originated from two separate nuclear families, as occurs when divorced people marry, each bringing children into the new family.

blind spot A repressed area in one's life.

blocking Involuntary stopping of a thought process owing to unconscious emotional factors.

blotting paper syndrome The acting out by staff of a feeling held by a client who is unable to express it, for example, anger.

blunting of affect A state characterized by an absence of emotional tone.

body image The conscious and unconscious picture one holds of one's own body.

bonding The process of developing emotional connectedness, as between a mother and infant.

borderline personality disorder A personality disorder characterized by wide fluctuations of mood, behavior, and self-image. These clients are often angry, self-destructive, and manipulative and frequently abuse drugs and alcohol.

brief therapy Treatment that focuses on the resolution of a specific problem or behavior in a limited number of sessions.

bulimia A state of increased hunger and morbid eating.

burnout A state of apathy resulting from stress; in mental care settings, characterized by detached, automatic, dehumanized care of clients.

capitation Payment to a provider, or group of providers, as a set fee for each enrollee, rather than for services rendered.

carrier Insurance company or other organization responsible for administration of third-party claims; sometimes refers only to true insurers and at other times to all third-party reimbursers.

carve-out benefits Alternative to traditional coordination of benefits in which the secondary carrier reimburses the insured only for the difference between the coverage provided by the primary carrier and the coverage of the secondary insurer.

case management An intervention in which health care is integrated, coordinated, and advocated for individuals, families, and groups who require services. The aim of case management is to decrease fragmentation and ensure access to appropriate, individualized, and cost-effective care. As a case manager, the nurse has the authority and accountability required to negotiate with multiple providers and obtain diverse services.

castration Surgical removal of the ovaries in females and the testes in males.

castration anxiety Literally, a fear of loss or injury of the genitals; figuratively, tension resulting when one fears the loss of any vital object or state.

catalysts Group members who stimulate others to move forward.

catatonia A state characterized by immobility, muscular inflexibility, and sometimes excitability.

catchment area Geographic area of 75,000 to 200,000 persons served by a community mental health center.

catharsis Verbalization of thoughts and feelings, usually in therapy sessions.

cathexis Conscious or unconscious investment in an object or idea.

cephalalgia Head pain or headache.

cerea flexibilitas Condition in which the client's arm or leg remains in the position in which it was placed by another person; also called waxy flexibility.

certification The formal process by which clinical competence is validated in a specialty area of practice.

certified specialist in psychiatric–mental health nursing (RN, CS) A psychiatric–mental health clinical nurse specialist who is nationally certified and qualified for autonomous advanced practice.

change agent One who acts for another deliberately to improve a situation.

child ego state In transactional analysis theory, the aspect of the adult that is left over from childhood.

childhood psychosis A state characterized by disordered thinking, affect, mobility, perception, reality testing, speech, and object relations.

circumstantiality Disturbed thinking process whereby a person includes many unnecessary details in verbal communications before reaching the central idea.

Civilian Health and Medical Program of the Uniformed Service (CHAMPUS) Health care benefit program for families of active and retired military personnel.

claim A request for payment, sent by patient or practitioner, to a third-party reimburser.

client The term used instead of "patient" by mental health professionals desiring a less medical, more humanistic view of mental health care.

client system The individual, family, group, or community for whom the nurse is providing formally specified services.

clinical psychologist A doctorally prepared psychologist who provides psychotherapy, behavior modification techniques, and psychological testing.

clinical social worker (CSW) A social worker with at least master's-level preparation who provides psychotherapy and case management.

COBRA (Consolidated Omnibus Budget Reconciliation Act) Provides options for continued group insurance coverage for a limited period of time to employees who have lost group insurance benefits because of job termination or reduced work hours.

cognitive Referring to thought, comprehension, judgment, memory, and reasoning as opposed to emotional processes.

cognitive therapy Therapy that concentrates on the empirical investigation of a client's cognitions and attitudes.

cohesiveness The result of all the forces that act on individuals to remain in a group and to feel they belong.

collateral visit A session with a relative, friend, or employer of a patient, which is part of the treatment of the patient.

collective unconscious A Jungian term referring to the aspect of the unconscious common to all people; also called racial unconscious.

commitment The process of hospitalizing clients for psychiatric care by legal means.

communal family A group of persons living and working together to accomplish shared goals.

community mental health center A community-based facility for the prevention and treatment of mental illness. Services may include inpatient, outpatient, day hospital, emergency, consultation, and educational services.

community psychiatry Psychiatry that concentrates on the environmental factors in mental illness and seeks to prevent and treat clients close to home.

community rating As opposed to "experience rating," an insurance company or managed care organization charges the same premium for all subscribers, rather than adjusting the rates based on the claims experience of the employer, union, or group.

compensation The attempt to cover up unconscious feelings, needs, or conflicts by acting in a way opposite to them.

complementarity A term referring to the two-sidedness of relationships and all communication.

complementary message A nonverbal message that augments a verbal message.

compromise A solution to a conflict whereby both sides give up something, and both feel relatively satisfied with the outcome.

compulsion A consistent urge to perform an act repetitively, in response to unacceptable unconscious wishes, needs, or feelings.

compulsive ritual A series of acts carried out compulsively, in response to unacceptable unconscious wishes, needs, or feelings.

concreteness Primitive thinking that employs literal meanings for ideas, as opposed to abstract meanings; also called concrete thinking.

condensation The boiling down of several concepts into a single idea or symbol, as occurs in dreams.

conditioning Associating specific stimuli with specific responses.

conduct disorder A repetitive and persistent pattern of behavior in which the basic rights of others or major age-appropriate societal norms or rules are violated.

confabulation The filling in of memory gaps with data that have no basis in fact, but that the teller believes to be true.

confirmation Validation by one person of the other person's thoughts or ideas.

conflict A clash between two equal opposing forces within oneself or between people or groups.

confrontation Communication designed to alert a person to thoughts, ideas, and concepts previously unconsidered and often threatening.

connotative meaning Meaning that comes from personal experience rather than objective sources.

conscious Readily accessible to an individual through thoughts and feelings.

consensual validation The process of checking with another person to determine that one's thoughts and feelings are realistic.

consumer A client or patient receiving mental health services.

contract A mutually agreed-upon plan of action between client and mental health worker. The contract emphasizes client behavior and worker accountability.

contradicting message A nonverbal message that communicates the opposite meaning of the concurrent verbal message.

conversion The expression of an unconscious wish by somatic means, for example, blindness that has no physical basis.

coordination of benefits A procedure, defined by various laws and contract language, which provides for payment by the *primary* and *secondary carrier* and prevents patients from being reimbursed for more than the actual cost of care.

copayment A fixed amount of percentage, per service, that is the responsibility of the patient, rather than of the third party.

coping mechanisms Unconscious methods by which an individual defends against anxiety.

coping skill A conscious method developed by a person to overcome a problem.

coprolalia Obscene language or speech.

coprophagia Eating feces.

coprophilia The desire to defecate on a partner or to be defecated on by a partner.

corrective emotional experience The reliving in a positive, therapeutic situation of a past traumatic event, such that the person grows and benefits emotionally.

counseling A specific, time-limited interaction of a nurse with a client, family, or group experiencing immediate or ongoing difficulties related to their health or well-being. The difficulty is investigated using a problem-solving approach for the purpose of understanding the experience and integrating it with other life experiences.

counterphobic Inclining toward an object or situation that a person unconsciously fears.

countertransference An irrational, unrealistic response to a client by a mental health worker, based on the worker's unconscious needs, wishes, conflicts, or feelings, or on the client's projections that are introjected by the worker.

covered services Services defined by the insurance contract as eligible for reimbursement.

covert Hidden or disguised.

creative arts therapist A therapist who uses dance, movement, art, and poetry to help clients express feelings, interact with others, and improve self-esteem.

crime victim program Usually a state-funded program to pay medical and other expenses caused by the crimes of others.

crisis A state of psychological disequilibrium brought on by an event that causes extreme anxiety not assuaged by the person's usual coping mechanisms.

crisis counseling Brief emergency individual, group, or family therapy designed to help persons cope with a specific issue.

crisis intervention Intervention designed to help an individual cope with a sudden problem and emerge at a level of functioning equal to or higher than the precrisis state.

critical incident stress debriefing (CISD) Intervention following a disaster designed to help victims ventilate, share experiences, and work through their feelings.

critical path A standard written plan and timetable for care that identifies routine treatments, activities, medications, expected length of stay, and discharge planning.

cultural completeness A multidimensional concept involving knowledge, attitude, and skills related to cultures other than one's own.

cultural sensitivity Awareness of and respect for cultures other than one's own.

culture The organized set of ideas, values, and beliefs held commonly by a group.

cunnilingus Oral stimulation of the female genitalia.

current procedure terminology (CPT-4) code Five-digit codes that are used to identify the service being provided (e.g., 90844—individual psychotherapy—45 to 50 minutes).

customary charge The typical fee charged for a service by providers in a community. Both "typical" and "community" may be defined by the insurer.

cyclothymic behavior Alternating elation and sadness.

day hospital A psychotherapeutic program for clients who attend during the day and return home at night.

death instinct A Freudian term for the unconscious drive toward death.

decompensation The breakdown of a stable emotional adjustment or defensive system.

deductible A specific amount the insured must pay, usually at the beginning of each benefit year, before insurance reimbursement may begin. The deductible may apply to all medical or just mental health benefits. There may be both individual deductibles (e.g., $250) and a family deductible (e.g., $500), so that if either is met, benefits will begin.

defense mechanism The unconscious operations used by an individual to defend against anxiety; also called mental mechanisms, coping mechanisms, security operations.

déjà vu The feeling that a current experience happened before.

delirium A state of confusion and disorientation caused by an acute organic reaction.

delusion A false, fixed belief inconsistent with reality and arising from unconscious needs.

dementia Loss of mental functioning with organic causes.

dementia praecox An obsolete term for schizophrenia.

denial An unconscious mechanism whereby disturbing thoughts, feelings, and events are kept out of conscious awareness.

denotative meaning A meaning that is commonly understood by most people in a culture, as opposed to connotative meaning, which is personal to an individual.

dependency Infantile reliance on others for mothering, love, assurance, affection, shelter, protection, security, warmth, and food.

depersonalization A feeling of strangeness or unreality about the self, the environment, or both.

depression A feeling of profound sadness, low self-esteem, and hopelessness about one's life.

desensitization The gradual exposure of a client to an object or situation that was previously feared, until the client is no longer afraid.

detachment Emotional unrelatedness characterized by aloofness, denial, intellectualization, and superficiality.

devaluation Consistent, exaggerated criticism used as a defense against feelings of inadequacy; seen in borderline personality disorder.

developmental crisis A crisis that is linked to the developmental stage of the client.

developmental lag Emotional or physical development that is lower than expected considering chronological age.

developmental stages The phases of growth and development from infancy to late adulthood.

deviance Behavior that is markedly different from the usual behavior in a group.

diagnosis-related groups (DRGs) Categories of illnesses for which Medicare pays a hospital a set amount, regardless of the actual days and services provided. Seen as a model for other carriers and also as one which may be extended to individual practitioners.

Diagnostic and Statistic Manual of Mental Disorders (DSM-IV) An American Psychiatric Association manual that, along with ICD-9-CM, lists terminology and diagnosis codes.

differentiation Healthy separateness and independence from others.

digital communication Communication that is verbal and can be validated.

direct recognition statutes Also known as *Freedom of Choice Laws,* laws requiring insurance companies that reimburse for services of psychiatrists to reimburse for the same services if provided by other specific providers (usually psychologists, sometimes social workers, and psychiatric clinical nurse specialists).

disconfirmation Communication that invalidates another's sense of self-worth.

discrimination The ability to note differences between similar objects or circumstances.

disengaged families Families in which members are emotionally disconnected.

disorientation The inability to identify time, place, or person.

displacement The transfer of feelings about one person to another, less threatening person.

disqualification Communication that invalidates other communication.

dissociation The removal from conscious awareness of thoughts, feelings, and actions that would cause anxiety, were they acknowledged openly.

dissociative disorders Response to stress by massive dissociation, for example, amnesia, fugue, depersonalization disorder, and dissociative identity disorder.

dissociative identity disorder The presence of two or more distinct identities or personality states, each with its own relatively enduring pattern of perceiving, relating to, and thinking about the environment and self.

distance In family therapy, the emotional and physical space between members.

double-bind communication Communication that gives two conflicting messages simultaneously, so that the receiver cannot respond adequately.

Down's syndrome A congenital developmental disability characterized by mental deficiency, defective brain development, and other deformities; also called mongolism.

dream analysis Used in psychoanalytic therapy to observe and understand unconscious behavior by careful exploration of the client's dreams.

drive Basic motivation, urge, or instinct.

drug addiction Overpowering, chronic dependency on drugs.

drug dependence Drug addiction leading to the client's inability to function, need for ever-increasing doses, physical withdrawal symptoms if the drug is stopped, and psychological dependence.

dynamics Emotional forces that work to produce behavior patterns or symptoms.

dysarthria Inability to speak normally, owing to organic disease.

dysattention Failure to pay attention to the environment.

dysmenesia Inability to recall and retain information.

dyspareunia Pelvic pain, emotional in origin, experienced by women during intercourse.

dysphagia Painful or difficult swallowing.

dysthymic disorder Depression lasting over 2 years with symptoms of poor appetite, overeating, insomnia, hypersomnia, low energy, fatigue, low self-esteem, poor concentration, difficulty making decisions, or feelings of hopelessness.

dystonia Severe, often rapidly developing contractions of muscles of tongue, jaw, neck, and extraocular muscles seen as a side effect with some antipsychotic medications.

echolalia Continuous repetition of words said in the client's presence; usually seen in schizophrenia.

echopraxia Imitation of motions made in the client's presence; usually seen in schizophrenia.

ECT Treatment used most often in depression, whereby an electrical current is passed to the brain, resulting in unconsciousness and a convulsion; also called electroconvulsive therapy.

EEG A method of recording the electrical activity of the brain; also called electroencephalogram.

ego The aspect of personality that includes intellectual, perceptual, governing, and defensive operations.

egocentric Self-involved to the point of a lack of interest in others.

ego-dystonic Incongruent with one's conscious wishes or values, for example, homosexuality in a client who wants to be heterosexual.

ego functions Those conscious functions that help regulate one's life, such as judgment, problem solving, reality testing, and impulse control.

ego ideal Standards set for oneself that eventually become a part of the superego.

ego psychology Personality theory that is concerned with adaptation to reality, object relations, and interpersonal relations.

ego strength Ability to maintain reality and manage the forces of the id and superego.

ego-syntonic Congruent with one's conscious wishes and values.

Electra complex Erotic attachment of a daughter for her father.

elopement Client's departure from a psychiatric inpatient unit without permission.

emotional shock waves In family therapy, symptoms that appear after a crisis has passed.

empathy Emotional understanding of another's experience; differs from sympathy, which is subjective and contains elements of pity, agreement, and condolence.

employee assistance plan (EAP) Employer-sponsored plan to provide limited counseling services to employees and their families.

encounter group A method of group interaction popular in the 1960s and early 1970s, which emphasized confrontation, the "here-and-now," and the expression of feelings; still used in drug treatment centers.

enmeshed families Families characterized by power struggles, overcontrolling mothers, and a lack of open affection among members.

enuresis Bed-wetting.

epigenetic principle Erickson's concept that both physical and psychosocial growth are in the genetic makeup of each individual and are triggered by social expectations.

epilepsy A disorder characterized by periodic motor or sensory seizures, sometimes with loss of consciousness; may be without known organic causes (idiopathic) or caused by organic lesions (symptomatic).

ERISA (Employee Retirement Insurance Security Act) A federal law that not only protects pension benefits, but also allows companies to skirt state insurance mandates when they set up self-insurance trusts.

ethics Standards of morality regulating rules of conduct.

etiology Cause.

euphoria An exaggerated feeling of well-being that is not congruent with objective facts. The cause may be functional or organic.

exclusions Specific illnesses, treatments, or circumstances that are not subject to reimbursement under an insurance contract.

exhibitionism The practice of exposing the genitals in public for sexual self-stimulation; also used to describe behavior whereby the individual enjoys public attention.

existential psychotherapy Therapy that focuses on the client's development of a thorough exploration of past and present experiences, and designed to change the client's "mode of being in the world."

expert power Power attained through expert skill and knowledge.

extended family The nuclear family and relatives from descent, adoption, or marriage.

extinction The removal of a behavior through lack of reinforcement.

extrapyramidal syndrome A disorder characterized by muscular rigidity, tremors, and other involuntary movements, and caused by improper use of psychotropic drugs.

extraterritoriality An exception to *Freedom of Choice Laws* in some states that allows companies with plans written out of state to not comply with provisions of the law.

eye movement desensitization and reprocessing (EMDR) A cognitive behavioral therapy technique that employs rapid eye movement and recall of negative events to relieve anxiety and other symptoms.

facilitative communication Communication designed to initiate, carry on, and maintain satisfying relationships with others.

factitious disorders Simulations of physical or mental disorders to obtain treatment and attention.

false memories "Memories" of past trauma usually stimulated by therapy or reading by suggestible clients. False memories are "recollections" of uncorroborated events.

family and marital therapy Approaches used to enhance the family's or couple's relationship and patterns of communication. Diagnoses, interventions, and outcomes emphasize the observable, interrelated behaviors that characterize the family or couple system.

family boundaries Informal rules about who participates in the family system and how.

family ego mass The aspect of a family characterized by a lack of personal boundaries, retarding the individual's progress toward individuation.

family life chronology The psychosocial history of a family.

family lifestyle Automatic method in a family for living out their self-images.

family myths A set of unrealistic beliefs held by family members about each other and family roles.

family themes A family's ideas about its origins and history.

fantasy A daydream.

fear A physical and emotional reaction to real or imagined danger.

federal employees health benefit programs (FEHB) A series of group health plans covering federal employees.

feedback Negative or positive reinforcement conveyed through communication.

fee for service Traditional form of insurance in which the provider is paid for each service performed; contrasted with *capitation*.

feminism Ideology aimed at social, political, and economic rights for women.

feminist therapy Therapy aimed at addressing problems resulting from gender inequality.

fetish An inanimate object such as an article of clothing that produces excitement and sexual pleasure.

fixation The arrest or concentration of psychic energy at a developmental stage where emotional needs have been either overgratified or undergratified.

flagellantism Masochistic or sadistic acts in which one or both partners derive sexual satisfaction from whipping or being whipped.

flashbacks Reliving of painful past experiences.

flatness of affect A lack of emotional tone and instead an apathetic, unrelated feeling tone.

flight of ideas A rapid shift from one idea to another with only vague associations between the ideas; seen in mania and schizophrenia.

flowchart A method of diagramming events and their interrelationships in a system.

folie à deux A condition in which two closely related persons share the same delusions or pathologic ideas; also called shared paranoid disorder.

forensic psychiatry The branch of psychiatry concerned with legal aspects of psychiatric disorders.

foreplay Sexual stimulation preceding intercourse.

forgiveness Accepting the insurance reimbursement as payment and waiving all or part of the copayment.

formication The tactile hallucination that insects are crawling on the body, seen in clients suffering delirium tremens.

fornication Voluntary sexual intercourse between unmarried people.

fourth party Utilization review company hired by a third party.

free association Uncensored verbalization by the client of whatever comes to mind.

free-floating anxiety Intense, severe, persistent anxiety.

freezing A family therapy technique whereby the client pantomimes a problem situation and then remains motionless at an important point.

frigidity The female's inability to participate in or enjoy sexual intercourse.

frustration The feeling resulting from inability to meet one's goals.

fugue state A condition in which clients suffer amnesia without knowing this and wander from their homes to unconsciously avoid a current anxiety-provoking situation.

functional Having a psychological rather than an organic cause.

functional status Level of the client's ability to independently perform activities related to self-care, social relations, occupational functioning, and use of leisure time.

fusion Enmeshment of individuals into a state of oneness.

gatekeeper Individuals such as primary care physicians or EAP counselors who control access of patients to specialists in a managed care organization.

gender identity The child's experience of being a male or female.

gender role The behaviors expected by society according to whether one is male or female.

General Adaptation Syndrome (GAS) Measurable body changes produced by stress and occurring in the stages of alarm, resistance, and exhaustion.

generalization The process of transferring learning from one situation to other similar situations.

genogram A family chart showing births, deaths, marriages, and so forth, over three generations.

genuineness Spontaneous and authentic communication.

Gestalt therapy Therapy that focuses on here-and-now experiences and attempts to treat the "whole person" and the interrelations of its component parts.

Global Assessment of Functioning (GAF) Scale Scale used as a part of multiaxial assessment in the *DSM-IV* to measure psychological, social, and occupational functioning.

globus hystericus A feeling of a lump in the throat with difficult swallowing, caused by anxiety.

grandiosity An exaggerated, unrealistic perception of one's wealth, power, fame, or ability.

grand mal epilepsy A disorder characterized by seizures and loss of consciousness, and often preceded by an aura.

grief A self-limited reaction to loss of a person, object, place, or idea.

grief work The process of consciously separating from a person, object, place, or idea and reinvesting in a new person, object, and so forth.

group Two or more persons interacting in such a way that they influence one another.

group therapy Psychotherapy based on the examination of group interaction with a view toward understanding and eventually changing the ways clients interact with others.

groupthink "Party line" thinking engaged in by members of a highly cohesive in-group in which agreement and uniformity are crucial and critical thinking is unacceptable.

guilt Self-reproach.

habituation Psychological dependence on drugs or alcohol.

hallucination A sensory perception based on internal stimuli and lacking external reality.

hallucinogen A drug producing distorted perceptions and delirium.

HCFA-1500 An insurance claim form developed by the Health Care Financing Administration, required for Medicare and accepted by most insurance companies.

Health Care Financing Administration (HCFA) A government agency that sets regulations for Medicare and other federal programs.

health maintenance organization (HMO) A prepaid managed health plan that rewards practitioners for providing as few services as necessary, usually through *capitation*. In principle, HMOs should cut costs by encouraging disease prevention and avoiding unnecessary and expensive procedures. HMOs now take many forms and often are hybrids of *preferred provider organizations* and HMOs. They may use professionals who are their employees or who are in independent practice. Patients must see HMO providers to receive any reimbursement.

hedonism Consistent pursuit of pleasure and avoidance of pain.

helplessness A real or imagined state in which one is at the mercy of fate or others, unable to change.

here-and-now approach In therapy, a tendency to focus on what is happening in the present, as opposed to the past.

hidden agenda A goal held by one or more people that is hidden from the others in a group.

hirsutism Presence of excessive bodily and facial hair, especially in women.

holistic Concerned with the whole person rather than discrete systems or parts.

holistic treatment Provision of comprehensive care that identifies physical, emotional, social, economic, and spiritual needs as they relate to the individual's response to illness and to the ability to perform activities of daily living.

homosexual One who engages in sex with members of the same sex.

hopelessness A feeling of extreme pessimism about the future.

hostility Anger that is destructive in nature and purpose.

hot line A crisis telephone answering service employing counselors, usually on a 24-hour basis.

hyperactivity Increased activity, usually accompanied by emotional lability and flight of ideas.

hyperkinesis Increased activity seen in some neurologic conditions, especially in children.

hyperpyrexia Extremely high fever; can be an adverse effect with antiparkinsonian medications.

hypnogogic state The state just before sleep when mental images occur involuntarily.

hypnosis An altered state of consciousness during which one may be receptive to suggestion and direction.

hypochondriasis Excessive preoccupation with one's physical health, without organic pathology.

hypomania A mild state of manic behavior.

hysterical personality disorder A disorder characterized by dramatic, emotionally intense, unstable behavior; also called histrionic personality disorder.

iatrogenic Disorders or problems induced by treatment.

id A psychoanalytic term for the unconscious aspect of personality containing primitive urges and desires, and ruled by the pleasure principle.

idealization Imbuing persons or principles with exaggeratedly positive attributes.

ideas of reference The false perception that events relate directly to oneself.

identification The unconscious mechanism whereby one takes on characteristics of another.

identity The sense of one's self based on experience, memories, perceptions, and emotions.

illness trajectory The course of the illness or chronic condition, which depends on the individual, the interventions, and unpredictable events that occur during the course of the illness.

illusion Misperception or misinterpretation of a real experience.

immediacy A communication technique in which the nurse responds to interaction between the nurse and client in the here-and-now.

impotence Inability of the male to achieve or to maintain an erection.

impulsive behavior Unpredictable, unexpected behavior motivated by immediate needs rather than long-range goals.

inadequate personality disorder. A disorder in which one reacts with ineptness and social instability.

inappropriate affect Emotional tone not in keeping with one's thoughts, actions, or genuine feelings.

incest Sexual relations between persons who are biologically related or between parents and their stepchildren.

"incident to" services Medicare services provided by a supervisee that are reimbursable.

incorporation The symbolic, unconscious taking of a person or the person's attributes inside of oneself.

independent practice association (IPA) A health maintenance organization model using practitioners who are not employees of the HMO.

individual provider profile An insurance company's record or the *usual* fees charged by a provider over a period of time for each service.

individuation The process of becoming a separate, distinct, autonomous person.

infantile autism Psychosis in a young child.

informational power Power attributed to a person based on information the person is believed to have.

insanity A legal term used for mental illness or psychosis.

insight Understanding the connection between one's unconscious wishes and one's behavior. Intellectual insight is a cognitive connection only, whereas emotional insight is believed to produce lasting change in behavior.

insurance A system of protection against loss in which a number of individuals agree to pay premiums periodically for a guarantee that they will be compensated under certain conditions for certain losses.

insured See *beneficiary*.

insurer The company actually taking the financial risk, by promising to pay claims for specified treatments. Insurance companies may serve as insurers or administrators.

integrated health plan A single benefit plan that combines elements of choice with managed care, often giving subscribers some choice, at extra cost, either through higher annual premiums or through *point of service* options.

intellectualization The use of thinking and talking to avoid emotions and closeness.

intelligence The ability to learn, remember, apply learning to new situations, think logically, and reason abstractly.

intermediary A company that handles paperwork and transfer of funds for an insurer (e.g., a self-insured trust) or government program.

intermittent explosive disorder A disorder leading to loss of control of aggression, serious assault, and destruction of property.

International Classification of Diseases, 9th ed. (ICD-9-CM) Mental health portion of international diagnostic listings compiled by the World Health Organization. Most insurance companies accept ICD-9-CM listings, which closely parallel those of *DSM-IV.*

interpersonal theory of psychiatry Harry Stack Sullivan's theory that mental illness is the result of anxiety generated in early interpersonal interaction, and that therapy consists of corrective interpersonal interaction between the therapist and client.

interpretation The process by which the therapist offers an explanation of the client's behavior to the client, based on the therapist's objective observations and theory.

intimacy Emotional closeness.

intoxication Excessive use of a drug or alcohol, leading to maladaptive behavior.

intrapsychic Within the self.

introjection The unconscious taking in of either loved or hated aspects of a person, usually a parent or significant other.

introjective identification The taking in of another's projections, so that one feels what the other is feeling.

introjects Those aspects of a person that have been taken in as a result of interaction with a significant other.

intuition Emotional knowing without thinking or talking.

involuntary commitment Confinement in a psychiatric setting without personal consent.

isolation The dissociation of feelings from a past thought, memory, or experience.

jealousy A painful feeling brought on by the notion that a person with whom one has a close, intimate relationship has an even closer relationship with a third person.

judgment The capacity for appropriate, realistic behavior based on an awareness of the consequences of one's behavior.

kinesics The study of body movement.

kinesthesia Awareness of the movements and positions of the body.

kin network A collection of related families who exchange goods and services.

kleptomania The failure to resist impulses to steal objects that are then given away, returned secretly, kept, or hidden.

Korsakoff's disease A disorder characterized by thiamine deficiency owing to prolonged, heavy use of alcohol.

labeling A method of describing and categorizing deviant behavior.

la belle indifference An inappropriate lack of concern, seen in clients with conversion hysteria.

language disorders Disorders involving problems learning or using language.

lanugo Fine, soft hair appearing on the forehead, ears, and flanks.

latency The stage of growth and development between age 6 years and puberty.

latent Hidden, covert.

learned helplessness Presumed powerlessness brought about by the lack of reward for assertive behavior and the extinction of assertiveness.

legitimate power Power brought about by the belief in a group that this person has the right to influence others.

lesbian A female homosexual.

lethality assessment A study of the seriousness of a client's intent to commit suicide.

libido Sexual drive or motivation.

lithium therapy The use of lithium salts to treat mental disorders.

local adaptation syndrome (LAS) The signs of stress in a discrete part of the body.

looseness of association The free flow of thoughts or ideas that appear to have little or no connection to one another.

loyalty commitments Unconscious bonds between family members.

loyalty conflict A pull toward loyalty to one person that leads to disloyalty to another.

LSD (lysergic acid diethylamide) A drug that can induce a psychotic-like state.

magical thinking The belief that thinking something can make it happen, seen in children and psychotic clients.

major medical An adjunct to basic hospitalization and medical services policies that usually adds hospital days, amounts for medical services, and additional services. Outpatient mental health is often covered under major medical provisions.

male erectile disorder Persistent or recurrent inability to attain or maintain an adequate erection until completion of the sexual activity.

male orgasmic disorder Persistent or recurrent delay in or absence of orgasm following a normal sexual excitement phase during sexual activity that the clinician, taking into account the person's age, judges to be adequate in focus, intensity, and duration.

malingering The presentation of false or exaggerated physical or psychological symptoms to accomplish conscious goals, such as avoiding military service, obtaining drugs, or obtaining financial compensation.

managed care Attempting to control costs of health care through controls in advance, or during the course of health care.

mania A condition of extreme excitement and euphoria, with loss of reality testing.

manic depressive illness A severe condition characterized by extreme mania or deep depression; also called bipolar disorder.

manifest content The remembered content of a fantasy or dream as opposed to the latent content that is disguised.

manipulation The influencing of another for self-gratification.

MAO inhibitor (monoamine oxidase inhibitor) A type of antidepressant that acts by inhibiting the enzyme monoamine oxidase, which oxidizes norepinephrine and serotonin.

masochism Unconscious or conscious pleasure when experiencing mental or physical pain.

masturbation Sexual stimulation of oneself or another manually, orally, or mechanically.

maternal deprivation The absence of adequate physical and emotional care in infancy or childhood.

maturational crises Crises triggered by expected developmental life changes, as opposed to situational crises, which are triggered by unexpected events.

maximums Limits on the amount of insurance reimbursement per session, per year, or per lifetime.

Medicaid Also known as medical assistance. A combined federal and state program to provide health services for low-income individuals.

medical assistance See *Medicaid*.

medically necessary A provision in most health insurance policies that allows the insurer to reimburse only for those treatments that the company deems to be required.

Medicare A federal program to provide health services to individuals 65 and older and those with severe disability. Part A covers hospital expenses and Part B covers practitioner fees.

Medigap Medicare supplement policies that reimburse the patient for copayments and deductibles on treatments accepted by Medicare.

mental health State of well-being in which individuals function well in society and are generally satisfied with their lives.

mental retardation A developmental disorder characterized by subnormal intellectual functioning, learning, social adjustment, and maturation.

mental status exam An assessment of the client's cognitive impairment used when the client appears disoriented or confused.

metacommunication Communication about communication.

metarules Rules about rules.

migraine A disorder characterized by intense, recurrent, usually one-sided headaches accompanied by nausea and vomiting and thought to be caused by a combination of emotional factors, hormonal levels, and dietary intake.

milieu therapy Therapy focused on positive manipulation of the client's environment.

minimal brain dysfunction (MBD) A disorder characterized by impaired perception, conceptualization, language comprehension, control of attention, motor function, and impulse control.

modeling Behaving in a way designed to set an example for another.

multigenerational transmission In family theory, the passing on of ideas, values, and behavior patterns from generation to generation.

multi-infarct dementia A disorder caused by vascular disease and characterized by progressive neurologic deterioration, with some intellectual functions left intact. There is disturbance in memory, abstract thinking, judgment, impulse control, and personality.

multiple personality A dissociative disorder in which different distinct "personalities" reappear from time to time in the client, now called dissociative identity disorder.

mutism Refusal to speak for conscious or unconscious reasons.

narcissism Self-love or self-involvement seen as normal in childhood but pathologic when extended to the same degree into adulthood.

narcissistic personality disorder. A personality disorder characterized by a grandiose sense of importance and an exhibitionistic need for attention and admiration.

narcolepsy A disorder characterized by involuntary, brief, uncontrollable episodes of sleep.

narcosynthesis Interventions used by the therapist in narcotherapy.

narcotherapy The use of drugs to interview a client, facilitating the client's expression of feelings.

necrophilia Sexual relations with a dead body.

neologism A word invented by the client, having no public, consensual meaning.

neuroleptics A group of antipsychotic drugs that produce CNS side effects that mimic extrapyramidal disease such as Parkinson's disease.

neurosis A group of disorders characterized by anxiety and nonpsychotic symptoms.

neurotransmitters Neurochemicals released during the transmission of nerve impulses.

nihilism The delusion that the self or part of the self does not exist.

nondeferrable care Treatment that cannot be postponed.

nonverbal communication Communication without words, such as body language, gestures, and facial expressions.

norms Rules established by a group for the ways members should behave.

nuclear family Parents and their children, including two generations only.

nurse practice act State statutes that define the legal limits of practice for registered nurses.

nursing care plan A plan for nursing care including the client's needs, goals for care, and suggested interventions.

nursing diagnosis classification A name, taxonomy label, or summarizing group of words that conveys a nursing assessment conclusion regarding actual or potential health problems of the client. Identifying a nursing diagnosis involves a clinical judgment that the problem being addressed is one that nurses have the legal authority to treat.

nursing practice standards Authoritative statements that describe a level of care or performance, common to the profession of nursing, by which the quality of nursing practice can be judged. They include activities related to assessment, diagnosis, outcome identification, planning, implementation, evaluation, quality of care, performance appraisal, education, collegiality, ethics, collaboration, research, and resource utilization.

nursing process A systematic and interactive problem-solving approach that includes individualized patient/client assessment, planning, implementation/intervention, and evaluation.

object relations Emotional attachments with others.

obsession A recurring thought, idea, or impulse that the person is unable to stop or control.

obsessive-compulsive disorder A disorder characterized by recurrent obsessions or compulsions, rigidity, perfectionism, overconformity, and self-doubt.

occupational therapy A type of therapy designed to help clients to express thoughts and feelings through creative activities and to learn new skills for creative expression.

Oedipus complex Sexual feelings toward the parent of the opposite sex and jealousy toward the parent of the same sex, occurring in childhood, between 3 and 6 years of age, and often appearing in unconscious ways in adulthood.

omega sign Furrowing between the eyebrows, occurring with depression (Ω).

omnipotence Fantasies of greatness or exaggerated importance.

one-to-one relationship A client–therapist relationship formed in the process of crisis intervention or individual therapy.

operational mourning A technique in family therapy whereby family members grieve the loss of family members who may have died some years ago without the emotional "working through" of the survivors.

orality The persistence of oral pleasure in adulthood seen in eating, smoking, drinking, and excessive dependency.

oral phase The first phase of psychosexual development in which psychic energy is invested in the mouth, sucking, and eating.

organic brain syndrome (OBS) Psychotic or nonpsychotic behavior caused by organic brain damage.

organicity Brain damage demonstrated by errors in judgment and memory and loss of coordination.

orientation Awareness of time, place, and person.

orthomolecular medicine The treatment of schizophrenia with large doses of niacin (B_3); also called megavitamin therapy, niacin therapy.

outcome The client's goal, or the result of interventions, that includes the degree of wellness and the continued need for care, medication, support, counseling, and education.

overcompensation A coping mechanism whereby the person experiences an "unacceptable" thought or feeling and acts exaggeratedly opposite to the thought or feeling.

overt Open to observation, not hidden.

panic The experience of high anxiety.

panic attacks Periods of sudden apprehension or terror, characterized by palpitations, chest pain, choking or smothering sensations, and fear of losing control or going crazy.

paradoxical injunction Therapeutic technique in which clients are instructed by the therapist to do consciously what they are doing unconsciously.

paralanguage Verbal communication other than words, such as sobs, laughs, moans, and voice quality; also called paralinguistics.

paranoid disorder A psychotic disorder characterized by delusions of reference and persecution, and grandiosity.

paranoid personality disorder A disorder characterized by suspiciousness, pathological jealousy, hypersensitivity, hypervigilance, and secretiveness.

paranoid schizophrenia A type of schizophrenia in which the client has a concrete and pervasive delusional system that is usually persecutory.

parataxic mode Sullivan's concept describing the experience of events or objects connected on the basis of one or two similarities, yet treated as though they were the same.

parentification The process by which children are forced to take on the role of "parent" to their own parents or to younger siblings.

participating provider A practitioner who agrees to see patients enrolled in a program, usually agreeing to accept the insurance company's set reimbursement and usually receiving payment directly from the insurance company.

passive-aggressive behavior Behavior that is seemingly passive but is motivated by unconscious anger and calls out anger and frustration in others, such as lateness, obtuseness, forgetting, and "mistakes."

pastoral counseling Counseling by a clergy member usually geared to helping clients with situational or maturational crises.

pathologic gambling A condition in which the person has a chronic, progressive compulsion to gamble.

pavor nocturnus Night terror brought on by an anxiety dream or nightmare.

pederasty Sodomy between a man and boy.

pedophilia Sexual activity between an adult and child.

penis envy A Freudian term that originally referred to little girls' envy of little boys' penises but later came to mean the female desire for attributes traditionally held by men.

perception The process of sensation, interpretation, and comprehension of stimuli in a personal, individual way.

perseveration A symptom of organic brain disease whereby the client persists in a single response or idea continually.

persona A Jungian term for the external mask or facade that people present to the world.

personality The deeply ingrained traits and thoughts characteristic of each individual.

personality disorder A mental disorder that originates in the personality and in which there is minimal anxiety or distress, such as compulsive personality or passive-aggressive personality.

personal space The area around an individual that the person prefers to have empty or free of intrusion by another.

petit mal epilepsy A disorder characterized by sudden, brief lapses of consciousness, twitches, and loss of muscle tone.

phallic stage The stage of growth and development between age 3 and 6 years.

phallic symbols Objects that represent the penis, such as guns, knives, cigars, bananas.

phenomena of concern Actual or potential mental problems that are of concern to psychiatric–mental health nurses.

phenothiazine derivative A substance derived from phenothiazide and used as an antipsychotic drug.

phobia A persistent, irrational fear leading to a compelling desire to avoid the feared object, activity, or situation.

pica Persistent eating of a nonnutritive substance, such as plaster, dirt, paint, string, hair, or cloth.

placebo A pharmacologically inert substance, such as a sugar or flour pill, used for research or because of its potential psychological effect.

plasticity Malleability, the ability to be formed or molded.

pleasure principle The tendency to seek pleasure and avoid pain.

point of service A managed care concept in which patients can choose from a network of providers, at extra cost to the patient, on a one-time or ongoing basis, at the time the service is needed.

postpartum psychosis Psychosis following childbirth and associated with organic or interpersonal influences.

posttraumatic stress disorder A disorder arising after a traumatic event that is generally outside the range of common experience, for example, military combat, rape, earthquake, or flood. Symptoms of anxiety and depression are common.

poverty of content of speech Speech that is abundant but conveys little information.

poverty of speech Speech that is brief and unelaborated.

power The ability to influence others.

precocity Unusually early appearance of intellectual or physical characteristics.

preconscious Thoughts and feelings on the fringe of awareness that can be brought into awareness with concentration.

preexisting condition An illness that existed before a patient first enlisted in an insurance program. Companies frequently will not pay for preexisting conditions for at least 1 year.

preferred provider organization (PPO) A managed care structure, with some resemblance to health maintenance organizations, in which participating providers agree to see patients at a lower cost. Patients receive a financial incentive (lower copayments) for seeing participating providers.

pregenital The oral and anal stages of development in children.

premature ejaculation Male ejaculation early in intercourse before the female partner reaches orgasm.

premature grieving Survivor grief felt during the time a person is dying, characterized by emotional withdrawal from the dying person.

premorbid Before the disease.

prescription of the symptom A therapeutic strategy whereby the client is encouraged to increase the symptom with the hope that this will ultimately decrease it.

prescriptive authority The statutory/regulatory authority to prescribe drugs and devices as a component of a profession's scope of practice.

pressure of speech Speech that is abundant, rapid, and difficult to interrupt.

prevailing charge Another term for *customary charge*.

primal scene Sexual intercourse viewed or fantasized by a child.

primary carrier The insurance carrier with first responsibility for payment, if the patient is covered by two different policies.

primary gain The main function or use of a symptom for a client, for example, hysterical blindness that prevents the client from reading unpleasant news.

primary impotence Abiding inability to obtain or maintain an erection in a man who has never done so.

primary mental health care A mode of service delivery that is initiated at the first point of contact with the mental health care system. It involves the continuous and comprehensive mental health services necessary for promotion of optimal mental health, prevention of mental illness, and intervention, health maintenance, and rehabilitation.

primary orgasmic dysfunction Abiding inability of a female who has never done so to reach orgasm.

primary prevention Attempts to obviate illnesses before they occur by removing possible causes.

primary process thinking Primitive thinking such as that of early development, dreams, and psychosis, in which syntaxic logic is absent.

primitive idealization An archaic form of intense idealization to protect one from recognizing strong, aggressive, angry tendencies; seen in borderline personality disorders.

problem-oriented records Psychiatric records that include a database, problem list, initial plans, and progress notes.

process The nonverbal aspect of interaction between two or more people, such as tone of voice, sequence of topics, and body language.

prodromal Early signs or symptoms of a disorder.

professional code Statement of ethical guidelines for nursing behavior that serves as a framework for decision making.

projection The attribution to others of one's own "unacceptable" thoughts and feelings.

projective identification The infusion of unwanted feelings into another, who introjects these feelings.

projective tests Personality tests in which relatively unstructured and ambiguous material is presented to the client, who is asked to describe it, thereby allowing the client to project certain aspects of the personality onto the material and thus reveal unconscious thoughts, feelings, wishes, and conflicts. Examples are the Rorschach (inkblot) test and the thematic apperception test (TAT).

prostitution The provision of sex for money.

prototaxic mode Sullivan's term for the most primitive mode of thought, in which each moment is isolated from the moment before or after it.

provider The individual or corporation providing the health service.

pseudomutuality Behavior between two or more persons who appear superficially to be close and happy, but do not have a close emotional connection.

pseudoparkinsonian syndrome Extrapyramidal side effects mimicking Parkinson's disease, including masklike face, shuffling gait, rigidity with flexion of arms, and outward rotating tremor of hands, seen as a side effect of some antipsychotic medications.

psychedelic Drugs that affect the mind dramatically, for example, LSD.

psychiatric aide A paraprofessional trained to work with psychiatric clients.

psychiatric audit An evaluation of psychiatric care, usually done by comparing patient records to predetermined standards of care.

psychiatric clinical nurse specialist A nurse who has graduated from a master's program providing clinical theory and practice in psychiatric nursing, including individual, group, and family therapy.

psychiatric–mental health nursing A specialized area of nursing practice that employs theories of human behavior as its science and the purposeful use of "self" as its art; the diagnosis and treatment of human responses to actual or potential mental disorders and their long-term effects. Interventions include the continuous and comprehensive primary mental health care services necessary for the promotion of optimal mental health, the prevention of mental illness, psychotherapy, rehabilitation from mental disorders, and health maintenance.

psychiatric–mental health registered nurse A baccalaureate-prepared registered nurse who demonstrates clinical skills exceeding those of a beginning registered nurse or novice in the specialty and who is employed in the specialized practice of psychiatric–mental health nursing (see *psychiatric–mental health nursing*). This designation is for those who are nationally certified within the specialty. In this basic practice level, the nurse can function in clinical, administrative, consultative, educative, research, and advocacy roles.

psychiatric social worker A graduate of a 2-year master's program in social work, with specialization in psychiatry.

psychiatrist A medical doctor who has specialized in psychiatry.

psychic determinism The idea that behavior is not random or accidental, but rather is set in motion by earlier events.

psychoanalysis A treatment modality, first described by Freud, that uses an examination of the client's unconscious processes through dream analysis, fantasies, free association, and examination of the client's transference.

psychoanalyst A mental health professional who has undergone psychoanalytic training and provides psychoanalysis to clients.

psychodrama A type of therapy in which clients' emotional and interactional problems are simulated or acted out dramatically under the direction of a therapist.

psychodynamic theory The idea that current behavior is understandable in light of past behavior.

psychogenic Caused by psychological factors, in the absence of organic pathology.

psychological pillow A position in which the person's head and neck are elevated as though resting on a pillow.

psychological tests Personality tests or intelligence tests usually administered and interpreted by clinical psychologists.

psychomotor agitation Nonproductive and repetitious motor activity that is excessive and accompanied by anxiety.

psychomotor retardation Excessively slow movement and speech often seen in depressed persons.

psychophysiologic disorder A physical condition brought on by psychological factors. Examples are obesity, tension headaches, neurodermatitis, asthma, ulcer, and ulcerative colitis.

psychosexual development Emotional and sexual growth from birth to adulthood.

psychosexual disorder Disorders of sexual functioning caused by psychological factors. Examples include transsexualism, gender identity disorder, paraphilia, fetishism, transvestism, zoophilia, pedophilia, exhibitionism, voyeurism, sexual masochism, and sexual sadism.

psychosexual dysfunctions Disorders of psychophysiologic or appetite changes during the sexual response cycle. These include frigidity, impotence, and ego-dystonic homosexuality.

psychosis A condition of grossly impaired reality testing usually accompanied by delusions and hallucinations.

psychosurgery Surgical removal or interruption of specific areas or pathways in the brain, especially the prefrontal lobes.

psychotherapy A method of treatment based on the development of an intimate relationship between client and therapist for the purpose of exploring and modifying the client's behavior in a satisfying direction.

psychotropic Affecting the brain.

pyromania A condition in which there is an obsession with setting fires and watching them burn.

rage Overpowering angry feelings, usually related to frustration and originating in infantile frustration.

rape Carnal knowledge forcibly and against one's will, including sexual penetration of the victim's vagina, rectum, or mouth.

rapport A conscious feeling of mutual respect, harmony, and affection between two people.

rationalization An unconscious mechanism whereby a person creates a logical, socially acceptable explanation for a thought, feeling, or action considered unacceptable.

reaction formation An unconscious mechanism whereby a person acts the opposite of the actual unconscious feeling experienced, to avoid the true feeling.

reading disorder Significant impairment in reading development not accounted for by chronologic age, mental age, or inadequate schooling; also called dyslexia.

reality principle A learned ego function in which people learn to delay gratification or tension release.

reality testing The ability to differentiate one's subjective thoughts and feelings from the objective thoughts and feelings of others.

reasonable charge The amount deemed "reasonable" by the insurance company for a particular service. This may be the lower of *actual* and *customary* or an arbitrary figure. To avoid challenges, insurance companies may further limit reimbursement by such statements as "payment will be made for reasonable charges, not to exceed $40 per visit."

recall Recent memory; the process of retrieving recent memories.

reciprocal inhibition The pairing of an anxiety-provoking stimulus with another stimulus of the opposite quality, but strong enough to reduce the anxiety.

recreational therapist A mental health worker who provides activities designed to help clients socialize and express thoughts and feelings in a socially acceptable way.

referent power Power accorded to a person because others identify with, or want to be like, the person.

registered nurse (RN) An individual educationally prepared in nursing and licensed by the state board of nursing to practice nursing in that state. Registered nurses may qualify for specialty practice at two levels: basic and advanced. These levels are differentiated by educational preparation, professional experience, type of practice, and certification.

regression A return to earlier behavior, usually prompted by anxiety.

reinforcement Reward for a behavioral response.

relative value scales Listings of health care procedures that evaluate their worth compared to each other.

remission Abatement of illness.

REM sleep The part of the sleep cycle in which rapid eye movement and dreaming occurs. REM sleep is necessary to restore one mentally and emotionally, and occurs for longer periods after a stressful day.

repressed memory Recall at a later time of an actual traumatic event that has been forgotten as a psychic defense.

repression The unconscious defense of keeping "unacceptable" thoughts and feelings out of awareness.

rescue fantasy The unrealistic narcissistic need to relieve a client of symptoms or problems.

residual The stage of an illness that follows the remission of florid symptoms or the full syndrome.

resistance A process whereby powerful unconscious forces prevent clients from giving up defenses and distortions.

retardation of thought Excessive slowness in expressing thoughts.

reversal The process by which a person acts, thinks, or feels the opposite of an instinctual wish experienced unconsciously.

reward power Power attributed to a person in a position to reward others or remove negative aspects of their lives.

ritual A behavior repeated for religious, cultural, or pathological reasons.

role Behavior expected of one person by others.

role model One who behaves in a way designed for others to copy.

role-playing A technique in group or family therapy whereby members act out the behavior of others in the group or family.

role reversal Exchange of usual behavior between two persons.

Rorschach test (inkblot test) A projective personality test in which the person is asked to say what comes to mind when viewing each of 10 inkblot cards.

rum fits Major motor seizures during withdrawal from alcoholism.

rumination Continual thinking and discussions about a specific subject.

rumination disorder of infancy A disorder characterized by repeated regurgitation of food, with weight loss or failure to gain expected weight, developing after a period of normal functioning.

sadism Sexual pleasure and erotic gratification obtained from inflicting physical or emotional pain.

satyriasis Exaggerated sexual drive in the male.

scapegoat The member of a group or family who becomes the target of the group's anger, and is perceived as bad or sick by the others.

schismatic family A family that has constant controversy and conflict, particularly between the parents.

schizoaffective disorder An uninterrupted period of illness during which, at some time, there is either major depression, a manic episode, or a mixed episode concurrent with schizophrenia.

schizoid personality disorder A personality disorder in which there is a defect in the capacity to form social relationships; the absence of warm, tender feelings for others; and indifference to praise, criticism, and the feelings of others.

schizophrenic disorders A group of psychotic disorders characterized by regression, thought disturbances, including delusions and hallucinations, bizarre dress and behavior, poverty of speech, abnormal motor behavior, ritualistic behavior, and withdrawal.

schizophreniform disorder A schizophrenic state lasting less than 6 months.

schizotypal personality disorder A personality disorder in which there are various oddities of thought, perception, speech, and behavior without the extremes found in schizophrenia.

school phobia A disorder characterized by a fear of leaving major attachment figures or home; also called separation anxiety disorder.

scope of practice A range of nursing functions differentiated according to level of practice, role of the nurse, and work setting. The parameters are determined by each state's nursing practice act, professional code of ethics, and nursing practice standards, as well as each individual's personal competency to perform particular activities or functions.

screen memory A consciously acceptable memory that serves as a cover for a deeper memory that is more painful.

sculpting A family therapy technique whereby one member creates a living tableau of the family members, placing them in actual positions vis-à-vis each other, representing their relationships and interactions with one another.

secondary carrier The insurance company responsible for only that portion left after the *primary carrier* has fulfilled its obligation. This payment may be through *coordination of benefits* or *carve-out benefits.*

secondary gains The advantages clients derive from their illnesses, for example, sympathy, attention, and financial support.

secondary impotence A current inability to achieve or maintain an erection in a man who has done so successfully in the past.

secondary prevention The early discovery and treatment of disease.

security operation Sullivan's term for defense mechanisms used to lessen or avoid anxiety.

selective inattention The process of filtering out aspects of an experience under conditions of moderate or severe anxiety.

self-actualization Becoming all one is capable of becoming by using all of one's potential.

self-awareness Sensitivity to one's own motives, thoughts, feelings, wishes, and so forth.

self-concept A person's image of the self.

self-esteem A person's degree of confidence, worth, and competence.

self-fulfilling prophesy A self-destructive process by which a person holds a certain distorted belief and then unconsciously goes about making that belief a reality.

self-insured company A company that underwrites its own insurance and pays benefits (through an insurance trust) for its employees. These corporations may use insurance companies to administer the plan and may even have insurance for their own catastrophic losses. These plans are usually not subject to state insurance laws but are governed through the federal *ERISA.*

self-mutilation Self-disfigurement of one's own body, frequently seen in clients with borderline personality disorders.

self-system Sullivan's concept of the self developed during childhood as a result of reflected appraisals of significant others.

senile dementia Progressive memory impairment, apathy, and withdrawal in clients over 65 years of age.

sensorium Consciousness.

sensory deprivation Diminution of sensory stimuli, leading to personality changes and inner perceptual distortions.

sensory overload Increased sensory stimuli leading to signs of stress.

separation anxiety Tension experienced in relation to moving away from a significant person.

separation anxiety disorder A disorder of childhood and adolescence characterized by stomachaches, headaches, nausea, and vomiting when there is the threat of separation from the home or parents; also called school phobia.

sex therapy Treatment of sexual dysfunction by a qualified therapist.

shaping A technique designed to change a client's behavior.

shared psychotic disorder A disorder developing as a result of a close relationship with another person who has persecutory delusions, such that the delusions are partially shared; also called folie à deux.

sibling position A person's position vis-à-vis brothers and sisters in terms of birth order.

sibling rivalry Competition among brothers and sisters.

sick role A position of "patient" adopted by a person to satisfy dependency needs.

sign An objective manifestation of pathology, observable by others.

significant other Sullivan's term for those who played an important role in development of a child's self-system; today, used to designate those who are important to a client.

single-parent family A family consisting of a mother or father and offspring.

situational crisis A crisis brought on by a traumatic external event.

situational orgasmic dysfunction A disorder whereby a woman is able to achieve orgasm only under certain situations.

skewed families Families in which one parent has a serious personality problem that is covered over through tacit agreement so that the family appears to function without conflict.

sleep terror disorder A disorder characterized by continual episodes of abrupt awakening from sleep, screaming, intense anxiety, and agitation; also called pavor nocturnus.

sleepwalking disorder A disorder characterized by continual episodes of awakening from sleep and walking, followed by amnesia for the event.

SOAP A method of record keeping used in problem-oriented records. The acronym is formed as follows: S for *subjective* (client's view of the problem), O for *objec-tive* (clinical findings), A for *assessment* (analyses and syntheses of subjective and objective data), P for *plan* (proposed method of handling the client's problems).

social network One's system of social relationships that can be used as a support system in a crisis.

social network therapy Therapy designed to mobilize those around the client to be helpful, or clients to help one another.

social phobia A disorder in which the client has a persistent fear of situations where there may be scrutiny by others, for example, public speaking or performance, using public toilets, or eating in public.

sociopathic personality The client who engages in chronic antisocial behavior, is unable to sustain jobs, and often abuses drugs; also called antisocial personality disorder.

sociotherapy Therapy that focuses on the environment rather than intrapsychic factors.

sodomy Any sex act other than face-to-face coitus between a man and woman. The legal meaning varies from state to state.

somatic delusion A false belief that the body is changing in an unusual way, for example, rotting inside.

somatic language Messages that are translated into physical symptoms.

somatic therapy Treatment of mental illness by physical means, for example, drug therapy or electroconvulsive therapy.

somatization disorders Disorders characterized by recurrent and multiple somatic complaints of several years' duration for which medical attention has been sought but which are apparently not caused by physical disorders.

somatoform disorders A category of disorders, including somatization disorder and conversion disorder, in which physical symptoms occur without demonstrable organic findings.

somnambulism Sleepwalking; a dissociative state in which the person walks about while sleeping.

split personality See *dissociative identity disorder.*

splitting Active separation of affects of opposite quality so that one does not contaminate the other. The client sees people or events as all good or all bad.

SRO (single-room occupancy) A hotel or boardinghouse where deinstitutionalized clients may live.

Stanford-Binet Scale An intelligence test for children.

status A collection of rights and duties accorded to a group member by other members.

stereotyped behavior Repeated speech or motor behavior, often seen in schizophrenia. Examples include echolalia and echopraxia.

stereotyped movement disorder A group of disorders involving an abnormality of gross motor movements. Examples include all tics and Tourette's disorder.

stop-loss limit A protection for the insured; a monetary limit at which a plan that was paying a proportion of costs (often 80%) will reimburse subsequent expenses at 100%. Mental health benefits are often not afforded stop-loss limits.

stress Tension.

stress adaptation therapy A framework for understanding the effect of stress on individuals.

stressor A person or experience that produces tension.

sublimation The conscious or unconscious channeling of "unacceptable" drives into acceptable activities.

substance use disorder A group of disorders characterized by the abuse of addictive substances such as alcohol, drugs, and tobacco.

substitution The unconscious replacement of an "unacceptable" wish, goal, or emotion with an acceptable one.

suicidal thoughts Thoughts of self-annihilation. Active suicidal thoughts involve a fantasy or plan of killing oneself. Passive suicidal thoughts involve a wish to die without taking action, for example, "I wish I were dead."

suicide Self-inflicted death.

superbill A detailed receipt that can also serve as an insurance claim.

superego The aspect of personality, known as the conscience, that includes one's ego ideals.

superficiality Lightness of interpersonal contact used to protect one from intimacy or emotional closeness.

supportive psychotherapy Therapy aimed at reinforcing the client's strengths and resources.

support system Aspects of the environment that provide comfort or security, including people or material objects (home, place, money, job).

suppression The process by which disturbing or "unacceptable" thoughts and feelings are consciously forced out of awareness.

symbiosis The close bond between infant and mother in which both appear fused. When occurring between adults, this seeming lack of boundaries is considered pathological.

symbolization The abstract process whereby one object or idea represents another, for example, a big car may represent power and prestige.

symmetrical relationships Relationships in which equality is a priority.

symptom An objective or subjective manifestation of pathology.

symptom substitution The replacement of one symptom with another when the first is removed. Adversaries of behavior modification believe that when one symptom is removed or extinguished, another may take its place, since the underlying problem may not be solved.

syndrome A group of symptoms that occur together and that constitute a recognizable condition.

synesthesia Seeing colors when a loud sound is heard.

syntaxic mode Sullivan's term for the mode of experience in which past, present, and future are recognized and events are perceived in logical sequence.

system A group of people in interaction or interrelationship, where there is a boundary around them, the whole is more than the sum of its parts, and any change in one part affects the whole group.

tangentiality The tendency to deviate from the central idea in a communication and to move the conversation off in another direction.

tardive dyskinesia A condition occurring after years of antipsychotic drug treatment. The client has involuntary movements of the face, jaw, and tongue, lip smacking, drooling, and protrusion of the tongue.

task-oriented groups Groups brought together to accomplish a task, for example, "activities of daily living" groups.

TAT (thematic apperception test) A projective test in which subjects are shown a series of drawings suggesting life situations, and are asked to tell a story about each drawing.

territoriality The tendency to perceive a space or function as "belonging" to oneself or one's group.

tertiary prevention The elimination or reduction of the aftermath of illness; rehabilitation.

therapeutic That which is thought to heal.

therapeutic alliance A relationship between a client and a helping person with the goal of helping the client.

therapeutic community A method of therapy whereby clients are helped to understand their interpersonal problems through continual examination of their interactions with one another and with staff. Elements are democratization, permissiveness, communalism, and reality confrontation.

therapeutic community meetings Regularly held meetings with all clients and staff in a therapeutic community.

third party Insurance company, employer, parent, or friend who pays part or all of one's health care fees.

third-party administrators (TPAs) Administrators of self-insured or ASO contracts.

thought disorder A condition seen often in schizophrenia in which the client shows loose, bizarre, illogical, confused, or abrupt thinking.

tic An involuntary, rapid movement of a related group of muscles or the involuntary production of noises or words.

tobacco dependence The continual use of tobacco for at least 1 month with either (1) unsuccessful attempts to stop or reduce the amount of tobacco use permanently, (2) the development of tobacco withdrawal, or (3) the presence of a serious physical disorder, for example, respiratory or cardiovascular disease, that the individual knows is exacerbated by tobacco use.

tolerance The condition in drug or alcohol addiction when increasing amounts are needed to produce the desired effects.

Tourette's disorder A disorder characterized by recurrent, involuntary, repetitive, rapid movements (tics), including multiple verbal tics resembling clicks, grunts, yelps, barks, sniffs, coughs, or words.

trance A state of diminished activity and consciousness resembling sleep and seen in hypnosis, hysteria, and ecstatic religious states.

tranquilizer A drug that depresses central nervous system function, calming the person without impairing the client's ability to function.

transcendental meditation (TM) A learned meditation technique in which the individual sits quietly with closed eyes, concentrating on a mantra with the goal of relieving tension and improving body sensations and interpersonal relations.

transference The attribution to the therapist of thoughts, feelings, wishes, and needs originally felt toward the parent or significant other.

transient situational disturbance A group of disorders that invite maladaptive reactions to an identifiable psychosocial stressor, occurring within 3 months after the onset of the stressor; also called adjustment disorder.

transsexual An individual who longs to belong to the opposite gender.

transvestite An individual who dresses in clothing of the opposite gender.

trauma An event producing intense anxiety.

triangle An interpersonal configuration or event involving three persons.

triangulation Dysfunctional communication and behavior in an interpersonal triangle, usually involving the alliance of two people against the third.

tricyclics A category of antidepressant drugs.

unconscious Mental processes that are dissociated or out of conscious awareness.

undoing A compulsive act whereby the person reverses a previous act that caused anxiety.

urolangia Sexual pleasure from urinating on another or being urinated on.

usual charge The most common charge made by a particular practitioner for a particular service over a period of time.

usual, customary, and reasonable (UCR) A system in which the insurance company pays the lower of the *usual, customary* (or prevailing), or *reasonable* charge.

utilization review A procedure in managed care that usually involves preauthorizing services, either before treatment begins or after a set number of sessions.

vaginismus Involuntary contraction of the vagina, making intercourse painful or impossible.

values Internal priorities about the worth of various aspects of life.

values clarification A process by which clients become aware of their values and behave accordingly.

Varaguth's sign A sign of depression in which there is angulation of the inner end of the fold of skin in the upper eyelid.

vertigo Dizziness associated with faintness.

vocational rehabilitation Usually a state-funded program designed to help people who are unable to work productively.

voluntary commitment The process whereby a client or guardian agrees in writing to enter a mental hospital.

voyeur One who receives sexual pleasure from looking at others.

waxy flexibility A condition seen in catatonic schizophrenia in which the client remains in a position in which he or she is placed; also called cerea flexibilitas.

Wernicke-Korsakoff disease A disorder caused by thiamine deficiency associated with prolonged alcohol use. Symptoms are amnesia, confusion, and disorientation.

withdrawal Movement away from reality or from interpersonal conflict.

withdrawal symptoms Physical and psychological manifestations occurring when a person stops using an addictive substance.

word salad The use of words and phrases without logical connection.

workers' compensation A program required by all states but administered privately, to reimburse employees for illnesses and conditions caused through their employment.

zoophilia Sexual relations with animals.

Index